IADVL

Handbook of Geriatric Dermatology

IADVL

Handbook of Geriatric Dermatology

Chief Editor

Vibhu Mendiratta MD, FIMSA
Director-Professor and Head
Department of Dermatology and Venereology
Lady Hardinge Medical College
Sucheta Kriplani Hospital and
Kalawati Saran Children Hospital
New Delhi

Associate Editor

Leelavathy Budamakuntla
MD, FRGUHS (Aesthetic Dermatology)
Professor and Head
Department of Dermatology
Bowring and Lady Curzon Hospital
Bowring Medical College
and Research Institute
Bengaluru

Assistant Editors

Aarti Sarda MS, MRCP (SCE)
Consultant Dermatologist
Wizderm, Kolkata

Samipa S Mukherjee
MBBS, DDV, DDVL, FRGUHS (Pediatric Dermatology)
Consultant, Pediatric Dermatology at Cloud Nine
An alumnus of Christian Medical College, Vellore
Fellowship in Pediatric Dermatology at
Bangalore Medical College and Research Institute
Bengaluru

CBS

CBS Publishers & Distributors Pvt Ltd

New Delhi • Bengaluru • Chennai • Kochi • Kolkata • Mumbai
Hyderabad • Jharkhand • Nagpur • Patna • Pune • Uttarakhand

IADVL
Handbook of
Geriatric Dermatology

ISBN: 978-81-947082-0-9

First Edition: 2021

Published by Satish Kumar Jain and produced by Varun Jain for

CBS Publishers & Distributors Pvt Ltd
4819/XI Prahlad Street, 24 Ansari Road, Daryaganj, New Delhi 110 002
Ph: 23289259, 23266861, 23266867 Fax: 011-23243014 Website: www.cbspd.com
e-mail: delhi@cbspd.com; cbspubs@airtelmail.in

Corporate Office: 204 FIE, Industrial Area, Patparganj, Delhi 110 092
Ph: 4934 4934 Fax: 4934 4935 e-mail: publishing@cbspd.com; publicity@cbspd.com

Branches

- **Bengaluru:** Seema House 2975, 17th Cross, K.R. Road, Banasankari 2nd Stage, Bengaluru 560 070, Karnataka
  Ph: +91-80-26771678/79 Fax: +91-80-26771680 e-mail: bangalore@cbspd.com
- **Chennai:** 7, Subbaraya Street, Shenoy Nagar, Chennai 600 030, Tamil Nadu
  Ph: +91-44-26260666, 26208620 Fax: +91-44-42032115 e-mail: chennai@cbspd.com
- **Kochi:** 42/1325, 1326, Power House Road, Opp KSEB Power House, Ernakulam 682 018, Kochi, Kerala
  Ph: +91-484-4059061-65 Fax: +91-484-4059065 e-mail: kochi@cbspd.com
- **Kolkata:** No. 6/B, Ground Floor, Rameswar Shaw Road, Kolkata-700014 (West Bengal), India
  Ph: +91-33-2289-1126, 2289-1127, 2289-1128 e-mail: kolkata@cbspd.com
- **Mumbai:** PWD Shed, Gala No. 25/26, Ramchandra Bhatt Marg, Next to JJ Hospital Gate No. 2, OPP. Union Bank of India, Noorbaug, Mumbai-400009, Maharashtra
  Ph: +91-22-66661880/9 Mob: 0-8424005858 e-mail: mumbai@cbspd.com

Representatives

• **Hyderabad**	0-9885175004	• **Jharkhand**	0-9811541605	• **Nagpur**	0-9421945513
• **Patna**	0-9334159340	• **Pune**	0-9623451994	• **Uttarakhand**	0-9716462459

Printed at Magic International Pvt. Ltd., Greater Noida, UP, India

Foreword

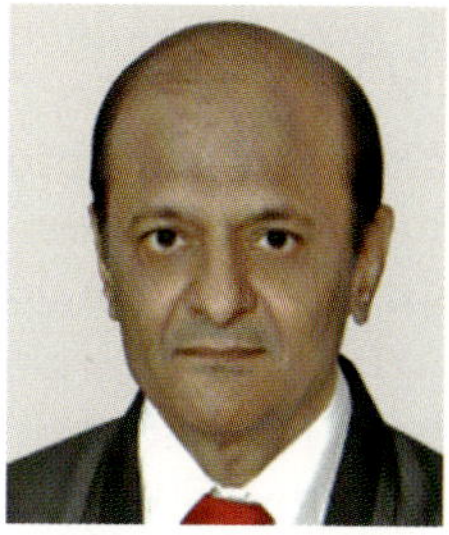

I am immensely pleased to know that *IADVL Handbook of Geriatric Dermatology* is now ready and will shortly go to press. My sincere appreciation to one and all involved in this laborious task.

Globally, the population aged 65 years and over is growing faster than all other groups and by the year 2050, one in six people in the world will be over the age 65 years (16% of global population). It is very timely that IADVL is coming out with a handbook on geriatric dermatology, a vast and fast growing branch of dermatology.

There are 30 chapters in this handbook covering basic aspects, complete range of common skin conditions, psychocutaneous and environmental dermatoses, and aesthetic concerns. Inclusion of topical and systemic therapies, drug interactions, dermatosurgical and cosmetic procedures makes it a complete document. A chapter on dermoscopy adds a value to it. I am sure that this comprehensive handbook will be very much useful to postgraduate students, those in academics and in clinical practice.

Overall, the project was well conceived and well delivered. This project has seen light of the day because of constant efforts and a lot of persuasion by Dr Deepika Pandhi, Chairperson, IADVL Academy, and Dr Vibhu Mendiratta, the Chief Editor of the book.

I realised that many of our colleagues have agreed to write chapters at short notice and as a substitute, even some of them have written two chapters facilitating timely completion of this project. I am indebted to them all.

As a parting note, I would like to say that geriatric dermatology is an important subject. Let us try to strengthen our efforts towards promoting it through IADVL. Let us create brilliance together.

Yours in academic endeavour.

Yogesh Marfatia

Past National President of IADVL, 2017

Foreword

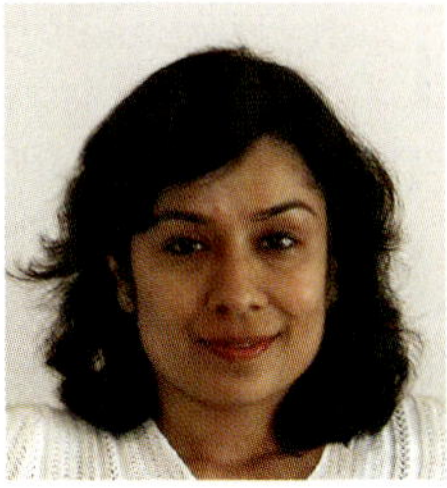

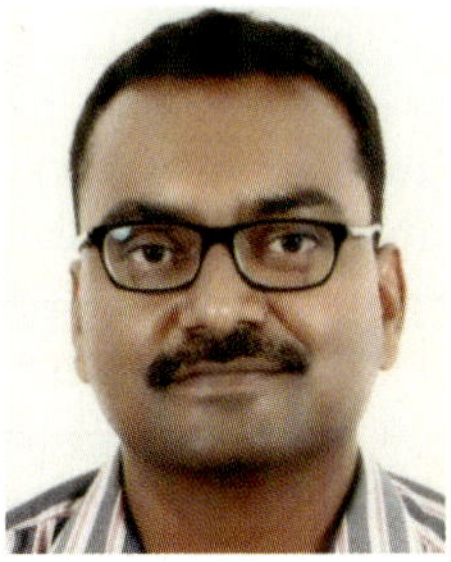

We are immensely happy to write the Foreword for the *IADVL Handbook of Geriatric Dermatology*. With increasing life expectancy and increasing proportion of elderly patients, it was a felt need that Indian Association of Dermatologists, Venereologists and Leprologists came out with a dedicated textbook of geriatric dermatology.

Practicing geriatric dermatology and caring for elderly patients may be a lot different from caring for adult patients, because of the heterogeneity of their clinical presentation, comorbidities, polypharmacy and special needs based on how much they can care for themselves. They need much more time than an average adult patient to express their problems and also to understand remedies prescribed thereof.

The editorial team of this handbook with Dr Vibhu Mendiratta as Chief Editor and eminent authors come out with a masterpiece encompassing 30 chapters that discuss very important and relevant topics from physiology of ageing skin to drug interactions due to polypharmacy in an easy-to-understand write-up. We are sure that this work is going to fill the gap in our understanding of the skin and its diseases in the elderly, that is different from the skin of adults in many ways and will be a help for dermatologists in managing dermatological diseases in this age group.

On behalf of the IADVL Academy we convey our appreciation to the editorial team and all the authors for this superlative effort and wish this book on a much-needed topic great success.

Deepika Pandhi
Chairperson, IADVL Academy

Dipankar De
Convener, IADVL Academy

Foreword

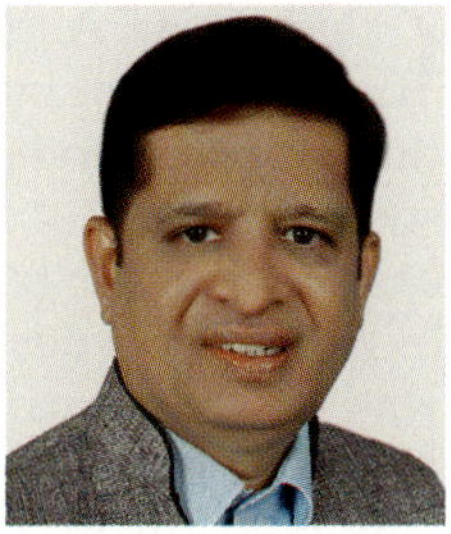

Globally, the population is ageing and the World Health Organisation predicts that, by 2050, the population aged 60 years or more will double and those aged 80 years will exceed 400 million persons. Therefore, it is obvious that dermatologists are likely to see more geriatric patients in their clinical practice and it is now imperative to be cognizant about the variations in presentation and frequency of dermatoses in this population as well as the unique impact of polypharmacy and the complications and higher risk profile of pharmacotherapy in this age group. Further, inappropriate prescribing is frequent for these patients, with instances of both over-treatment and under-treatment leading to adverse outcomes. The need for an updated detailed text on this topic is therefore obvious. IADVL is happy to present a synopsis in the form of this *IADVL Handbook of Geriatric Dermatology* that can serve as a ready reckoner for the practical aspects of managing dermatological diseases in this age group. The core editorial team belongs to the special interest group of geriatrics of the Indian Association of Dermatologists, Venereologists and Leprologists. There are detailed descriptions of the clinical manifestations of important dermatoses with practical tips for their management in this age group. These are well illustrated with several high quality images. It is noteworthy that the editors have included chapters on aesthetic concerns, principles of topical and systemic therapy in elderly, polypharmacy, psychocutaneous disorders and nursing care.

I am confident that the book will serve the needs of our students and physicians who would like to keep updated about management of dermatoses in the geriatric age group. I appreciate the editorial team headed by Prof Vibhu Mendiratta as the Chief Editor, for this commendable and painstaking effort.

Prof Kiran Godse MD
President, IADVL 2020

Foreword

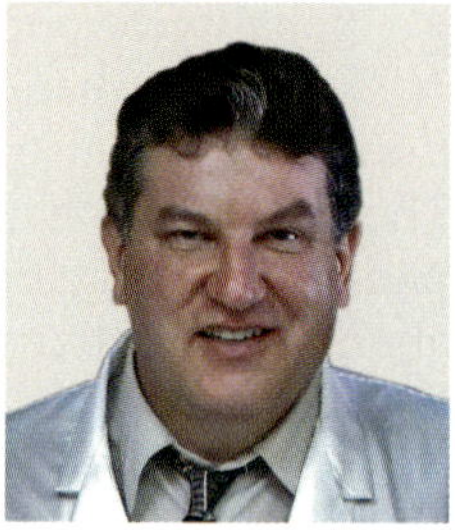

Old is new. Although there have always been some people who have lived well into their eighties or even beyond, the magnitude of this longevity today is a very recent development among the human species. It was not until the 20th century that human longevity began to commonly climb to its current extent of 75-plus years for most people in technologically developed societies. In 1900 AD, the average age of death was 49 years, primarily due to problems of high infant mortality. However, by the mid-century mark, the rapid ascent of human longevity was well on its way and has not yet stopped climbing. Today, dermatology is practiced in the face of an unprecedented demographic event marked by common and extreme longevity.

The elderly population has a rapidly increasing need for comprehensive skin care. The demographics of global aging allow a profound insight into this need. A record-breaking rate of 800,000 new members enter the 65+ cohort per month. The geographic distribution of this growth is surprisingly uneven. More than three-quarters of this burgeoning global growth is still in developing countries. Italy has the highest national percentage of 65+ citizens. However, for the oldest cohort (80+ population), more than 33% live in three nations: China, the United States and India.

The world population of older adults is increasing significantly. According to World Population Prospects 2019 (United Nations, 2019), by 2050, 1 in 6 people in the world will be over the age of 65, up from 1 in 11 in 2019. There were 703 million persons aged 65 years or over in the world in 2019. Globally, a person aged 65 years in 2015–2020 could expect to live, on average, an additional 17 years. The number of older persons is projected to double to 1.5 billion in 2050. The age group 85 and older is the fastest growing segment of the population. The vast majority of people older than 70 years of age have at least one bothersome skin condition, and approximately 10% have 3–4 dermatological problems.

India is riding the crest of the wave of the silver tsunami of aging. The increase in average life expectancy has shifted the Indian demography and the providers for the elderly must be prepared for the important tasks ahead.

For almost four decades I have been working with the elderly and examining what can be done to improve their care. We have cared for over 800,000 elderly in nursing homes and in our office practice and I have been fortunate to be able to contribute to the improvement of skin and general health in this needy population. I have outlined my ideas and insights in the 25 + textbooks that I have written and edited and the many lectures I have provided. I hope that they will contribute to the care of our elderly.

The recent COVID-19 pandemic has turned our focus on the socio-economic factors that contribute to the care of our seniors and the devastating effect on health that goes along with putting tens of thousands of our elderly in close quarters in nursing facilities. Just when we thought we could continue to focus on chronic disease as our major nemesis, the horrible virus erupted and has produced more fatalities in the elderly population than in any other portion of society. The high geriatric incidence of those at high-risk for severe illness from COVID-19 highlights the fact that geriatric health will be among the top healthcare system challenges in all of our futures.

Thank you for the privilege to write the Foreword for the upcoming handbook on geriatric dermatology under the aegis of the Indian Association of Dermatology. The invitation by Dr Vibhu Mendiratta has allowed me to appreciate this concise text on various geriatric dermatoses. We are all primarily the same in our description of geriatric skin diseases, although I found that certain cultural expressions and diseases were both enlightening and important, including *bindi* dermatitis, Buddha ears, and certainly more cases of myiasis or facies leprosa were noted than a dermatologist in the USA would likely encounter.

The excellent chapters included have been contributed by various Indian dermatologists, including those on infestations, infections, chronic venous insufficiency and adverse drug reactions. The book will create an enhanced awareness of geriatric skin care for all readers at every level of their career.

As Dr Sarda and Dr Vaidyanathan quote at the beginning of their excellent chapter, "Youth is a gift of nature but age is a work of art." As physicians, we share the task in creating the best in each of our patient's health and appearance. I urge all of us throughout the world to improve the care of our elderly and carry on this important mission.

Thank you.

Robert Norman
Drrobertnorman@gmail.com

Preface

There is a perceptible change in the demography of the Indian population. The elderly constitute a sizeable part of our population and suffer from unique dermatoses requiring a specialised approach.

During course of several meetings and discussions with IADVL fraternity, colleagues and trainee dermatologists, several knowledge and practice gaps related to geriatric skin diseases emerged. The need to have a consolidated guide for addressing this neglected segment was strongly felt. The *IADVL Handbook of Geriatric Dermatology* is a collective effort by dermatologists involved in the care of elderly from several parts of India. The text has been written with the objective to highlight special characteristics of geriatric dermatoses.

The book incorporates chapters on common and relevant topics are of practical interest including pruritus in elderly psoriasis, autoimmune diseases, hair and nail disorders, eczemas, pigmentary issues, aesthetic concerns, skin tumours and sexually transmitted infections to name a few.

Management of skin diseases in elderly is delicate, tedious and fraught with challenges. This work is fruit of a joint vision of the editorial team and seniors with the goal of providing improved care of skin diseases in elderly. We hope that this compendium shall serve its purpose of enlightening the readers about the nuances of geriatric skin care.

Vibhu Mendiratta

Acknowledgements

Life is a great teacher.

My personal involvement in the care of my octogenarian parents made me realise the inadequacies in both the existing literature and knowledge domain in this area. An undiagnosed skin rash in geriatric patients evokes set of differential diagnoses from the simplest to the most sinister.

I dedicate this book to my parents I am indebted to all my patients who bore with my repeated interrogations.

I thank my family for allowing me shots of time from their depleted bank, enabling me to end this race to the finish.

Vibhu Mendiratta

List of Contributors

A Selvam MD
Senior Consultant Dermatologist
AKJN Skin and Advanced Laser Centre
8/13, MG Road Adyar
Chennai
Website: www.akjnskinandlaserchennai.com
Email: dr.a.selvam@gmail.com

Aarti Sarda MD
Consultant Dermatologist
Wizderm Speciality Skin and Hair Clinic
Kolkata, West Bengal
Email: draartisarda@yahoo.co.in

Amit Sureshchandra Gulati DVD
Consultant Dermatologist
AKIRA Skin and Hair Clinic
Mumbai, Maharashtra, India.
Email: dr.gulatiamit@gmail.com

Amritha A Hongal
Assistant Professor
Department of Dermatology
Bangalore Medical College and Research Institute
Bengaluru
Email: amritahongalleo@gmail.com

Angoori Gyaneswari
Professor and Head
Department of Dermatology
SVS Medical College
Mahbubnagar,Telangana
Email: dr_a_g_rao@yahoo.co.in

Asit Mittal MD (DVL)
Senior Professor
Department of Dermatology
RNT Medical College
Udaipur, Rajasthan, India
Email: asitmittal62@gmail.com

Bela Shah
Professor and Head
Department of Dermatology, STI and Leprosy
BJ Medical College and Civil Hospital
Ahmedabad, Gujarat
Email: shah.drbela@gmail.com

Chander Grover MD, DNB, MNAMS
Professor
Department of Dermatology and STD
University College of Medical Sciences and
GTB Hospital, Delhi, India
Email: chandergroverkubba@rediffmail.com

Faiz Riyaz Arakkal MD, DDVL, FIMSA
Consultant Dermatologist
IQRAA Community Hospital
Vazhakkad, Malappuram, Kerala, India
Email: faizderm@gmail.com

Indrashis Podder MD, DNB
Assistant Professor
Department of Dermatology, Venereology and
Leprosy
College of Medicine and Sagore Dutta Hospital
Kolkata, West Bengal
Email: ipodder88@gmail.com

Kapil Vyas MD (DVL)
Assistant Professor
Department of Dermatology
Geetanjali Medical College and Hospital
Udaipur, Rajasthan, India
Email: kapilvyas23@gmail.com

Kinjal Deepak Rambhia
MD, DNB, Fellowship in Diagnostic Dermatology
Assistant Professor
Department of Dermatology
HBT Medical College and Dr RN Cooper Hospital
Mumbai, Maharashtra, India
Email: kinjal_rambhia@hotmail.com

Krishna Bhalala MBBS
Resident
Department of Dermatology
KJ Somaiya Medical College
Mumbai

Lalit Gupta
Senior Professor
Department of Dermatology
Venereology and Leprology
RNT Medical College
Udaipur, Rajasthan
Email: lalitanj@yahoo.com

Leelavathy Budamakuntla
MD, FRGUHS (Aesthetic Dermatology)
Professor and Head
Department of Dermatology
Bowring and Lady Curzon Hospital
Bowring Medical College and Research Institute
Bengaluru
Email: drleelaskincare@gmail.com

Manjeet Ramteke MD
Assistant Professor
Department of Dermatology and Venereology
Grant Medical College
Mumbai
Email: manjeetramteke@gmail.com

Manoj Pawar
Assistant Professor
Department of Dermatology
Dr Vasantrao Pawar Medical College
Nashik, Maharashtra, India

Megha Valjibhai Kakani
Junior Resident
Department of Dermatology
Venereology and Leprosy
Grant Government Medical College
Sir JJ Group of Hospitals
Mumbai, Maharashtra, India
Email: meghakakani.8@gmail.com

Meghana Madhukar Phiske MD, DNB, DVD, DDV
Associative Professor
MGM Medical College and Hospital
Kamothe, Navi Mumbai
Consultant Dermatologist
Dr Meghana's Skin Clinic
Sector 17, Vashi, Navi Mumbai
Ex Associate Professor
Department of Dermatology, TNMC and BYL
Nair Ch. Hospital, Mumbai, India
Ex Assistant Professor and Associate Professor
LTMMC and LTMGH, Sion, Mumbai, India
Email: phiskemeghana@gmail.com

N Asokan MD, DVD, Dip NB
Professor and Head
Department of Dermatology and Venereology
Government Medical College
Thrissur, Kerala, India
Email: asokann65@gmail.com

Najeeba Riyaz
MD, DVD, DNB, MRCP (UK), SCE Derm, FRCP (Glasg), FIMSA, FIAD
Professor and Head
Department of Dermatology
KMCT Medical College
Calicut, Kerala, India
Email: najeebaderm@gmail.com

Nirmala Devi Palanivel MBBS, MD
Professor and Head
Department of Dermatology, Venereology and Leprosy
Tirunelveli Medical College
Tirunelveli, Tamil Nadu, India
Email: nirmaladevipalanivel@gmail.com

Pratik Gahalaut MBBS, MD
Professor and Head
Department of Dermatology, Venereology and Leprosy
Shri Ram Murti Smarak Institute of Medical Sciences, Bareilly, Uttar Pradesh, India
Email: drpratikg@rediffmail.com

Priyadarshini Sahu MD, DNB, MNAMS
Assistant Professor
Department of Dermatology, Venereology and Leprology
Pt. BD Sharma University Health Sciences
Rohtak, Haryana, India
Email: priyadarshini.sahu.9@gmail.com

Rajesh Kumar MD, FAAD (USA)
Associate Professor
Department of Dermatology and Venereology
Grant Medical College
Mumbai
Email: rkderm@gmail.com

Rashmi Modak MBBS, DDVL, FIADVL (Dermatosurgery)
Clinical Dermatology, Dermatosurgery
Consultant Dermatologist
Ra'Derm Clinic
Mulund, Mumbai, India
Email: dr.rashmi.dermat@gmail.com

Reema R Baxi
Postgraduate Student
Department of Skin and VD
Medical College Baroda and SSG Hospital
Vadodara, Gujarat, India
Email: reema_baxi@yahoo.in

Richa Chaudhary MD
Ex Assistant Professor, NDMC, Delhi
Consultant Dermatologist
Jaipur Golden Hospital, Delhi
and Skin Castle, Rohini, Delhi
Email: richapgims99@gmail.com

Roshin Anish MBBS, DDVL
Consultant Dermatologist
Moulana Hospital
Perinthalmanna, Malappuram, Kerala, India

Samipa S Mukherjee
MBBS, DDV, DDVL, FRGUHS (Pediatric Dermatology)
Consultant Pediatric Dermatologist and Dermatologist, Cloudnine Hospitals
Bengaluru
Email: drsamipamukherjee@gmail.com

Sheilly Kapoor
Senior Visiting Consultant
Medanta-The Medicity Hospital, Sector 39
Gurugram, and Director
Rejuva Skin Clinic
Gurugram, Haryana, India
Email: rajneeshsheilly@yahoo.com

Shital Poojary MD, DNB, FCPS
Professor and Head
Department of Dermatology
KJ Somaiya Medical College
Mumbai, Maharashtra, India
Email: spoojary2004@gmail.com

Subrata Malakar MBBS, DCH, MD (DVL)
GD 225 Salt Lake Sector 3
Kolkata
Landmark: Tank No 12
Email: subr3575@gmail.com

Sudip Das MD
Professor and Head
Department of Dermatology
Calcutta National Medical College
Kolkata, West Bengal

Sulochana Paul MD (DVL)
Postgraduate Student
Department of Dermatology
Venerology and Lepropsy
Tirunelveli Medical College
Tirunelveli, Tamil Nadu, India
Email: drsulopaul@gmail.com

Sunil Kumar Gupta MD
Associate Professor
Department of Dermatology
Venerology and Leprosy
All India Institute of Medical Sciences
Gorakhpur, UP, India
Email: dr.sunil_30@yahoo.co.in

Surabhi Dayal MD
Senior Professor and Head
Department of Dermatology
Venereology and Leprology
Pt. BD Sharma University Health Sciences
Rohtak, Haryana, India
Email: mini_md44@rediffmail.com
surabhidayal7@gmail.com

Sweta Hasmukh Rambhia MBBS, DVD
Consultant Dermatologist
Just Care Skin Clinic
Malad West, Mumbai
Maharashtra, India
Email: drswetarambhia@gmail.com

Usha Naraindas Khemani MD (Skin and VD), DDV, FAAD
Associate Professor and Head of Unit
Gokuldas Tejpal Hospital (GTH)
Department of Dermatology
Venereology and Leprosy (DVL)
Grant Government Medical College
Sir JJ Group of Hospitals
Mumbai, Maharashtra, India
Email: ushakhemani@gmail.com

Varsha Vaidyanathan MD, DNB
Senior Resident
Department of Dermatology
North DMC Medical College and Hindurao Hospital, Delhi
Email: drvarshavaidyanathan@gmail.com

Vibhu Mendiratta MD, FIMSA
Director-Professor and Head
Department of Dermatology and STD
Lady Hardinge Medical College and associated Sucheta Kriplani Hospital and Kalawati Saran Children Hospital
Saheed Bhagat Singh Marg
New Delhi, India
Email: vibhumendiratta@rediffmail.com

Vijay Zawar
Professor
Department of Dermatology
Dr Vasantrao Pawar Medical College
Nashik, Maharashtra, India
Email: drvijayzawar@rediffmail.com

Vivekananda Ittigi MBBS, DDVL, FRGUHS
Senior Resident
Dermatologist
Hassan Institute of Medical Sciences
Hassan, Karnataka, India
Email: v.ittigi@yahoo.com

Yogesh S Marfatia MD (Skin and VD)
Professor
Department of Skin and VD
Medical College Baroda and SSG Hospital
Vadodara, Gujarat, India
Email: ym11256@gmail.com

Contents

CHAPTER 1

An Overview of Geriatric Dermatoses

• *Leelavathy Budamakuntla* • *Amritha Hongal*

Geriatrics is a speciality that focuses on health care of elderly people. It aims to promote health by preventing and treating diseases and disabilities in older adults. The term Geriatrics is derived from Greek word *geron* meaning "old man", and *iatros* meaning "healer". With the increase in lifespan of humans, chronic diseases are becoming more prevalent that includes the skin diseases *per se* and the diseases of other organ systems having skin manifestations as well. Thus, geriatric dermatology is a vast and fast growing branch of dermatology.

With ageing, due to chronology (intrinsic) and environmental insults (extrinsic), several qualitative and quantitative changes occur in the skin. These changes include epidermal barrier changes, immunosenescence and altered wound healing capacity. The epidermal barrier changes include slow epidermal cell turnover and retention, loss of acidification of skin mantle and decreased production of sebum and sweat, which leads to xerosis and pruritus, and predisposes to contact dermatitis and secondary infections. Delayed wound healing process in addition to impaired vascular response, reduced nerve endings in skin and reduced support from fat and bone underneath due to atrophies predispose to development of pressure ulcers in elders. Delayed wound healing is characterised by delay in the re-epithelisation, increased time in fibroblast proliferation, abnormal matrix degradation.[1]

Photoageing refers to ultraviolet radiation induced damage of an ageing skin (Fig. 1.1A). In few individuals who get exposed to sunlight chronically may develop skin lesions in the form of senile comedones, epidermal cysts on an actinically damaged skin. This is known as Favre-Racouchot syndrome (Fig. 1.1B).

Common dermatoses seen in elderly are pruritus, xerosis and eczemas. Pruritus in elderly being a chronic problem, significantly affects quality of life. However, it is difficult to determine the cause. Even after determining the cause, choosing the correct treatment is not easy due to the presence of co-morbidities and polypharmacy due to multiple medications[2] (Fig. 1.2).

With advancing age and impaired mobility, the geriatric population is at a higher risk of developing chronic venous insufficiency which further worsens the mobility due to oedema, pain, ulcers and secondary infections. This necessitates help in day-to-day activities. Considering the chronicity and recurrence of eczemas, it is important to educate the patient regarding the triggering factors like xerosis, immobility (leading to stasis), medications and others[3] (Fig. 1.3).

With immunosenescence, the cell-mediated immune response is impaired in elderly, thus making them more susceptible to infections. Thus, dermatophytoses, candidiasis, herpes zoster and post-herpetic neuralgia are common in elderly[4] (Fig. 1.4A and B). Leprosy

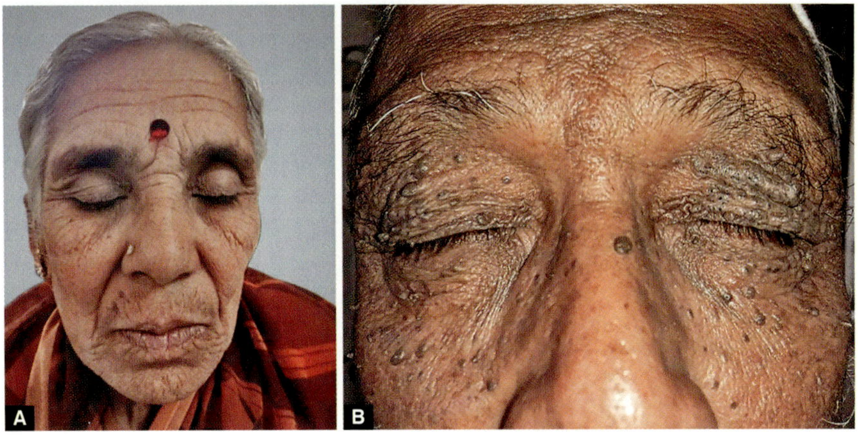

Fig. 1.1A and B: Photoageing and Favre-Racouchot syndrome

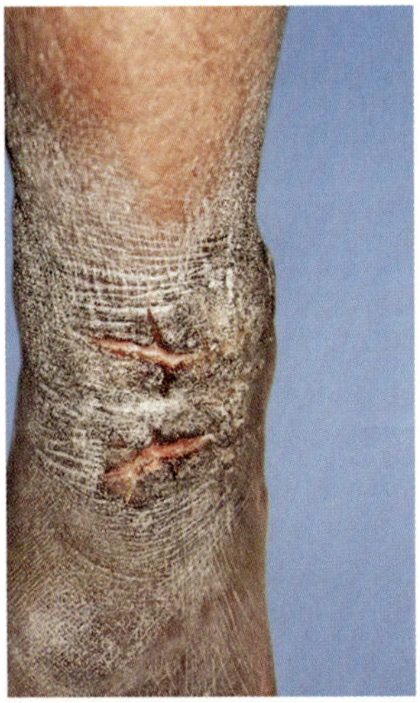

Fig. 1.2: Lichen simplex chronicus with fissures

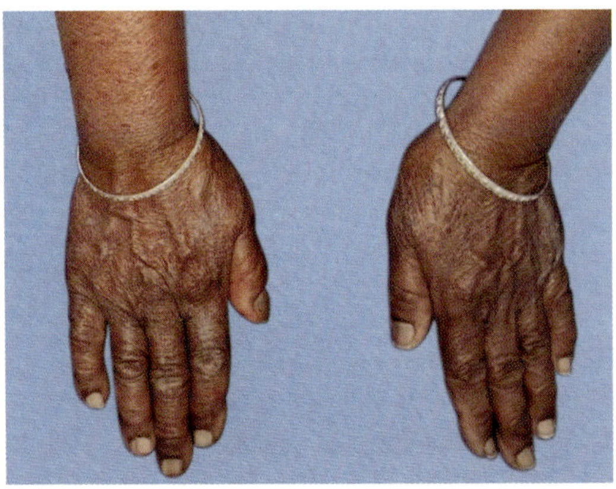

Fig. 1.3: Senile xerosis

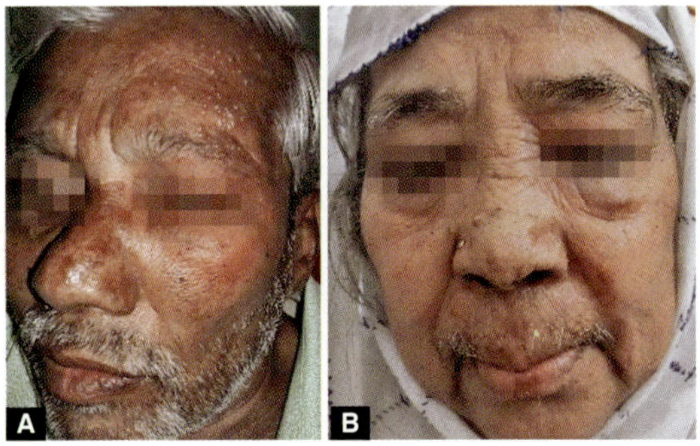

Fig. 1.4A and B: Herpes zoster involving left ophthalmic nerve and tinea faciei

can affect any age but in the elderly, lepromatous leprosy, trophic ulcer and the deformities are more commonly encountered (Fig. 1.5A to C).

Elderly individuals are sexually active thus accounting for STIs like syphilis, Chlamydia and HIV occurrence. Increased time to attain erection, decreased vaginal lubrication, psychosocial factors like loss of spouse and infrequent or no use of condoms are the predisposing factors for STIs in elderly.[5]

Papulosquamous disorders, also a class of inflammatory dermatoses, are less common in elderly due to decline in immune response with age. Plaque psoriasis, nail psoriasis and sebopsoriasis are the common variants of psoriasis. Due to the presence of comorbidities

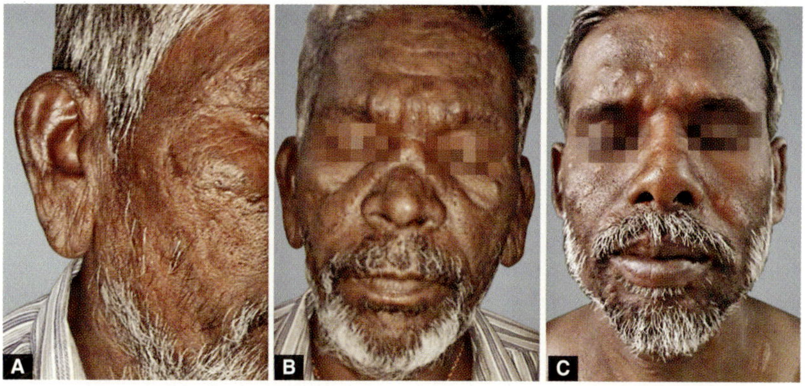

Fig. 1.5A to C: Buddha ear, facies leprosa and lepromatous leprosy

in elderly the aim of treatment of psoriasis is to substantially improve the condition to a level that does not interfere with daily life activities[6] (Fig. 1.6A to C).

Connective tissue disorders are immune complex mediated autoimmune disorders. With immunosenescence, the susceptibility of the elderly to these autoimmune disorders declines, however, some variants like giant cell arteritis and polymyalgia rheumatica selectively emerge in old age. Also, the association of malignancy with polymyositis/dermatomyositis increases with advanced age[7] (Fig. 1.7A and B).

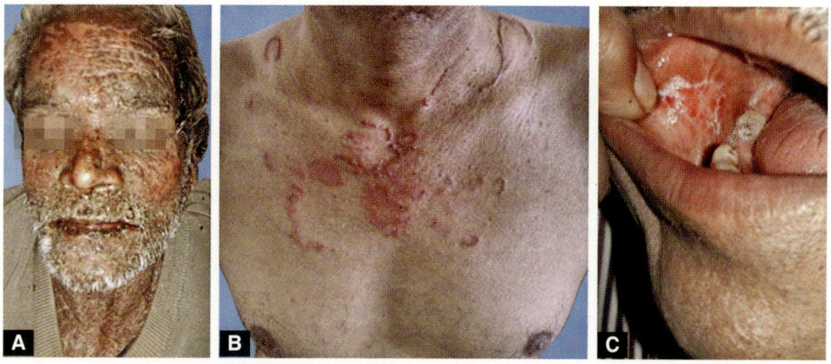

Fig. 1.6A to C: Erythrodermic psoriasis, granuloma annulare and oral erosive lichen planus

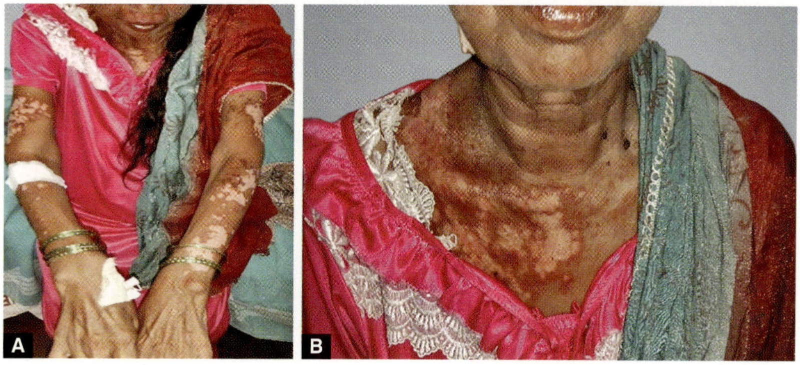

Fig. 1.7A and B: Subacute cutaneous lupus erythematosus

However, a few inflammatory dermatoses like the vesiculobullous disorders, namely bullous pemphigoid and Grover's disease are common in older patients over the age of 60. Bullous pemphigoid is a chronic, subepidermal blistering disorder that presents with tense blisters commonly over the legs and arms, with spontaneous remissions and exacerbations. The duration of appearance of blisters can vary from weeks, months or years, but most experience spontaneous remission in 1 to 5 years (Fig. 1.8). Grover's disease, also called transient acantholytic dermatosis, presents with erythematous to brown non-follicular papules over the trunk that can become pustular, vesicular or rarely bullous. Steroids (topical/oral, chosen based on severity) are the 1st line of treatment. Since these diseases are rarely fatal, avoid use of strong immunosuppressants in elderly.[8]

In addition to patterned hair loss with ageing, diffuse hair loss is common in elderly due to nutritional deficiency (iron/protein), hypothyroidism, medications taken for their comorbidities. We need to investigate for the underlying pathology if the hair loss is not typically patterned or if there is associated scarring which is relatively rare in elderly. Unwanted hair growth is common in women after menopause due to altered estrogen–androgen balance. With increasing age, nails show changes in thickness, colour, shape and growth rate and become more dry and brittle. Subungual hyperkeratosis and longitudinal ridging are commonly seen in elderly. Subungual hyperkeratosis can be idiopathic (onychogryphosis) (Fig. 1.9) or a result of fungal infection or papulosquamous disorders. Terry nails caused by hypoalbuminemia and half nails caused by renal insufficiency are common in elderly.[9]

Skin tumours in elderly can be epidermal, melanocytic or mesodermal in origin. Benign skin tumours that commonly occur are seborrheic keratosis (Fig. 1.10A), lentigo, sebaceous hyperplasia, epidermal cyst and keratoacanthoma; Premalignant tumours are actinic keratosis, oral leukokeratosis (Fig. 1.10B) and Bowen's disease; and the malignant tumours are basal cell carcinoma (Fig. 1.10C), squamous cell carcinoma, melanoma and cutaneous lymphomas (Fig. 1.10D).[10]

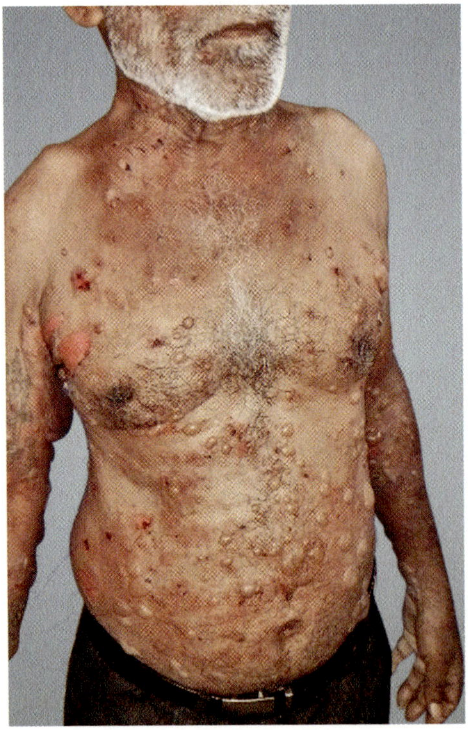

Fig. 1.8: Bullous pemphigoid

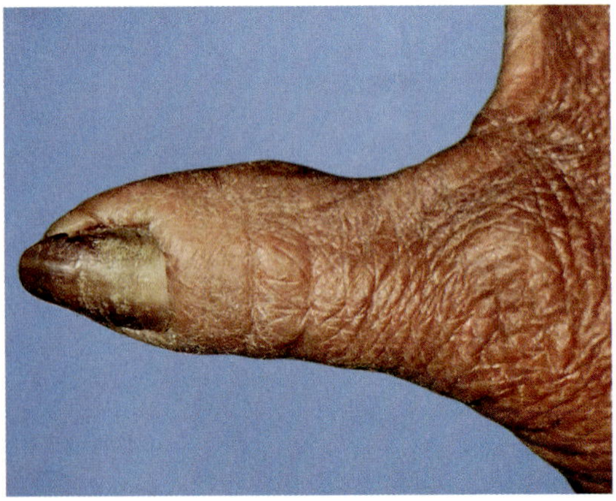

Fig. 1.9: Onychogryphosis

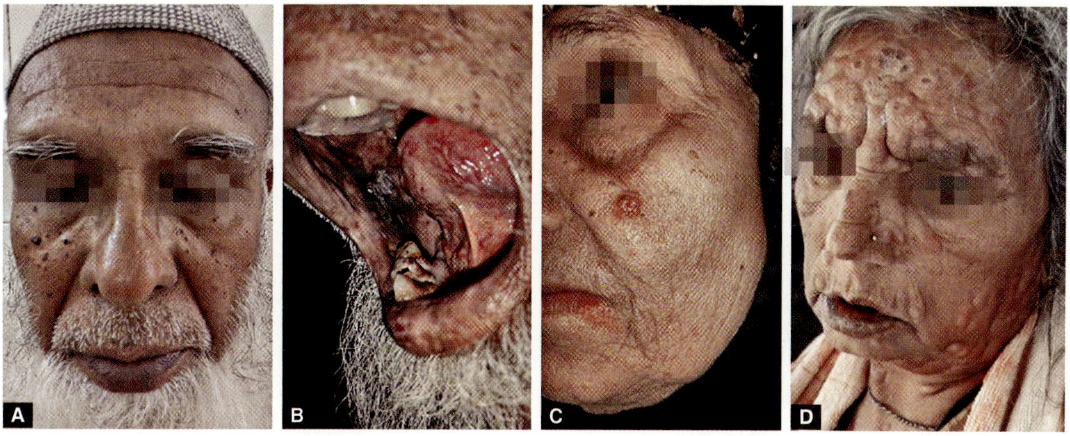

Fig. 1.10A to D: Seborrhoeic keratosis and dermatosis papulosa nigra, oral leukokeratosis in a tobacco chewer, basal cell carcinoma and cutaneous T cell lymphoma

The important risk factor for skin cancers in elderly is the cumulative ultraviolet radiation exposure with the age and others include fair skin type and family history of skin cancer.[11] Skin acts a window into the various internal malignancies. Cutaneous manifestations that are highly associated with internal malignancy are tripe palms, Bazex syndrome, paraneoplastic pemphigus, erythema gyratum reopens, necrolytic migratory erythema and hypertrichosis lanuginosa acquisita, and weakly associated are acanthosis nigricans, acquired ichthyosis and multiple seborrhoeic keratoses. A detailed history, thorough cutaneous and systemic examination and relevant investigations aid in the early diagnosis of internal malignancy.

Skin is a mirror of underlying systemic metabolic disorders as well. Xanthelasma is a marker of hypertriglyceridemia which needs prompt management in order to prevent atherosclerosis and other cerebrovascular events (Fig. 1.11).

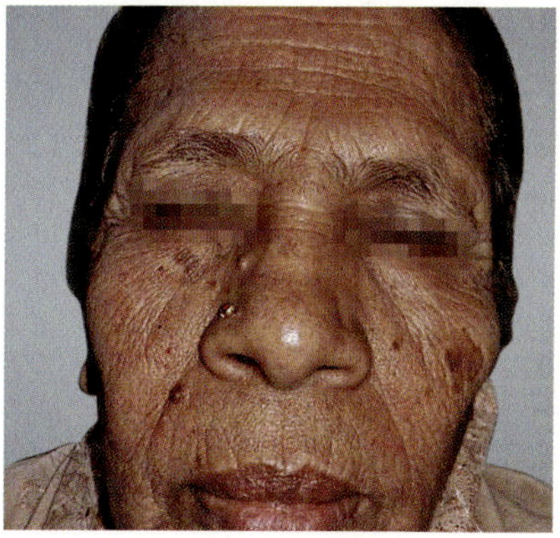

Fig. 1.11: Xanthelasma

Skin is a common site for adverse effects of drugs. With ageing, the hepatic and renal clearance of drugs is altered resulting in their altered metabolism and hence the increased incidence of adverse effects. Elderly patients have multiple comorbidities and are on multiple medications. Such instances of polypharmacy should be avoided as they are associated with poor health outcomes. Polypharmacy is defined as unintentional prescription of many drugs, taking medications with duplicate mechanism of action or inadvertent addition of drug that has interactions with other drug.[12] All physicians should judiciously prescribe medications to avoid polypharmacy. Considering the physiological changes with ageing (delayed wound healing and immunosenescence increasing the risk of wound dehiscence and infection respectively), presence of multiple comorbidities and polypharmacy, it is a challenge to opt for dermatosurgical management in elderly.[13]

The geriatric population is a growing presence in psychodermatology. It is important to understand the unique challenges that they present with, a decreased cognitive impairment with age and physical disability which would require them to become dependent on caregivers. The most common psychocutaneous disorders in elderly would be delusional parasitosis and neurotic excoriation The first line treatment would depend on the underlying psychiatric diagnosis, anxiety or depression. It is essential not to overlook these conditions as simply an old man or woman with an itch.[14]

Lastly dermatologists should be aware of cutaneous signs of elderly abuse and neglect as they are easily visible and must be differentiated from pathological causes.[15]

References

1. Chang A, Wong J, Endo J, Norman R. Geriatric Dermatology Review: Major Changes in Skin Function in Older Patients and Their Contribution to Common Clinical Challenges. Journal of the American Medical Directors Association. 2013; 14(10):724–730.
2. Cohen KR, Frank J, Salbu RL, Israel I. Pruritus in the Elderly: Clinical Approaches to the Improvement of Quality of Life. Pharmacy and Therapeutics. 2012; 37(4):227–239.
3. Weyer K, Stücker M, Pientka L, Reich-Schupke S. Chronic venous insufficiency in a geriatric collective. Phlebologie. 2015; 44(5):239–246.
4. Elgart M. Skin Infections and Infestations in Geriatric Patients. Clinics in Geriatric Medicine. 2002; 18(1):89–101.
5. Johnson B. Sexually Transmitted Infections and Older Adults. Journal of Gerontological Nursing. 2013; 39(11):53–60.
6. van Voorhees A, Vittorio C, Werth V. Papulosquamous disorders of the elderly. Clinics in Geriatric Medicine. 2001; 17(4):739–768.
7. Nagaratnam N, Nagaratnam K, Cheuk G. Connective Tissue Disorders and Vasculitis in the Elderly. Diseases in the Elderly. 2016; 379–388.
8. Scheinfeld N. Skin disorders in older adults. Papulosquamous and bullous diseases, Part 1. Consultant 360. 2011; 51 (3):25–29/37.
9. Scheinfeld N. Skin disorders in older adults: age-related changes to hair and nails. Consultant 360. 2012; 52(1).
10. Common skin tumors in the elderly. Am Fam Physician. 1992; 46(1):163–8.
11. Malaguarnera G, Giordano M, Cappellani A, Berretta M, Malaguarnera M, Perrotta R. Skin Cancers in Elderly Patients. Anti-cancer Agents in Medicinal Chemistry. 2013; 13(9):1406–1411.
12. Endo J, Wong J, Norman R, Chang A. Geriatric dermatology. Journal of the American Academy of Dermatology. 2013; 68(4):521.e1–521.e10.
13. Meissner M, Kaufmann R. Dermatosurgery in the elderly. Der Hautarzt. 2016; 67(2):153–159.
14. Nguyen TV, Wong JW, Koo JYM. Clinical cases in psychocutaneous disease. London: Springer; 2014.
15. Chang A, Wong J, Endo J, Norman R. Geriatric dermatology. Journal of the American Academy of Dermatology. 2013; 68(4):533.e1–533.e10.

CHAPTER 2

Physiology of the Ageing Skin

• Samipa S Mukherjee

Introduction

The skin is the largest organ of the body contributing approximately about 7% of the body weight. It forms the interface between the external and the internal environment. The principal functions of the skin include protection, excretion, secretion, absorption, thermoregulation, pigmentogenesis, accumulation, sensory perception and regulation of immunological processes. These functions are all affected by the structural changes in the skin with ageing and, after middle age, most functions are reduced, some by as much as 50–60%. Skin changes associated with chronologic ageing or photoageing, such as wrinkling, laxity, and changes in pigmentation, prompt patients to seek cosmetic procedures to improve the appearance of their skin.

Theories for ageing skin

1. **Oxidative stress:** The free radical or oxidative stress theory of ageing suggests that accumulation of oxidative cellular damage is a major factor in the ageing process and a prime determinant of longevity.

   The damage is the result of production of reactive oxygen species (ROS) produced as a by-product of the cellular metabolism. Ageing is associated with changes in the molecular structure of DNA, proteins, the lipids, and prostaglandins. These changes may at times be the result not only due to damage as a result of increased oxidative stress but also due to spontaneous errors and mutations. During the alteration of the oxidative stress balance in the body the internal antioxidant mechanism is impaired leading to DNA damage. Damaged DNA due to high levels of ROS can then result in genomic instability at large. Accelerated senescence is a protective response by the body to eliminate damaged DNA and encounter increased oxidative stress in the cells.

2. **Role of mitochondria:** An error in the coding process due to exposure to oxidative stress may form the basis of the mitochondrial theory for ageing. In the pathogenesis of ageing, accumulation of mutations in mitochondrial DNA, decreased oxidative phosphorylation occurs and imbalance in the ratio of antioxidant enzymes and free radicals perpetuate the increased production and accumulation of ROS. Mitochondrial dysfunction and ROS production leads to a vicious cycle which is the basis of mitochondrial free radical theory of ageing.

3. **Cellular senescence and telomeres:** Skin cells undergo huge turnovers during the life cycle of a human being. The telomeres act as a watchdog to prevent the proliferation of cancerous cells. With each cell division the length of the telomere is reduced. A consequence of this protective effect and telomere shortening results in cellular senescence and cell ageing.

4. **Role of ultraviolet radiations:** Recent evidence demonstrates that parts of chronologically aged skin or irradiated with UV has major changes in molecular characteristics, including the transduction signaling pathways that promote expression matrix metalloproteinase, a decrease in procollagen synthesis and tissue damage. Earlier although photoageing and chronological ageing were considered different entities there have been studies to prove significant overlaps in the pathways. UV radiation has now shown to accelerate many important steps in the chronological ageing pathway. Recent studies have also show that intrinsic ageing and photoageing share a common pathway involving telomere-generated signaling that is responsible for most clinical manifestations of skin ageing.
5. **Effects of smoking:** Matrix metalloproteinases, which degrade collagen, are induced dose-dependently by tobacco smoke extract. Smoking induces dryness of the skin, altered blood circulation, depletion of nutrients and oxygen supply to the skin thereby leading to cutaneous manifestations of early wrinkling, lusterless dry skin.
6. **Role of pollution:** The skin serves as a barrier to the entry of chemicals and particles from the external environment into the intérieur milieu. Percutaneous penetration of pollutants, pesticides, chemicals and cosmetics have a damageing effect on the skin. The exposure to environmental pro-oxidant agents leads to the formation of ROS and the generation of bioactive molecules that can damage skin cells.
7. **Vascular theory:** Intrinsically aged skin shows decrease in vessel size and density, whereas UV irradiation results in generation of immature blood vessels due to upregulation of VEGF and downregulation of angiogenesis inhibitor thrombospondin-1.

EFFECTS OF AGEING ON SKIN ARCHITECTURE

The Epidermis

The thickness of the epidermis reduces with flattening of the rete ridges at the dermo-epidermal junction. The loss of surface area of the dermo-epidermal interface contributes to increased skin fragility and reduced nutrient transfer between dermis and epidermis making them prone for bullous disorders like bullous pemphigoid and acquired epidermolysis bullosa. Epidermal cell turnover decreases, which may account for slower wound healing and less effective desquamation. With age, there is a prominent loss of melanocytes and Langerhans cells. A reduction in surface contact between the epidermis and dermis, results in a reduced exchange of nutrients and metabolites between the two layers.

The Dermis

The dermis becomes atrophic with reduced numbers of fibroblasts (reducing the skin regenerating and wound healing capacity) and there is a decrease in subdermal adipose tissue leading to loss of turgor of skin and loss of elasticity. The number and diameter of collagen fiber bundles decreases with age and the ratio of type III collagen to type I collagen increases, thereby leading to more wound gaping and reduced shearing stress of the skin.

Vasculature

The vessels become fragile and lifted on the skin thereby becoming more prone to injury and easy bruisability. Recent studies suggest that damaged collagen also contributes to the plethora of new blood vessels that are often seen in damaged skin, particularly in aged individuals with a light complexion. Ageing leads to drastic reduction in dermal blood vessels, and a shortening of capillary loops in the dermal papillae due to the changes in the dermoepidermal junction and the rete ridges. This results in the pallor, decreased temperature and impaired thermoregulation often found in the skin of older people making them more prone to injuries due to vasoconstriction and cold temperatures.

Subcutaneous tissue: The loss of subcutaneous tissue leads to volume loss resulting in loss of turgor, compromised insulation and padding. This makes them susceptible to injuries especially over bony prominences and decreased adaptation to colder weather.

EFFECTS OF SKIN AGEING

Clinical signs of photoageing include dryness, rhytides, irregular pigmentation, loss of elasticity, telangiectasias, and areas of purpura. The contributors to wrinkles and skin sagging include persistent gravitational force, persistent traction by the musculature of skin tension lines and loss of subcutaneous fat. This leads to deepening of forehead lines, lines at the angles of mouth and eyes and sagging and prominence of the nasolabial fold. As the fat undergoes resorption the malar prominence diminishes and the jowls become prominent due to gravitational pull exerted on the fat compartments.

CONCLUSION

Ageing is an inevitable process resulting due to the consequence of genetic programming and cumulative 'wear and tear' damage. With progressive ageing there is a change in the structure, function and response adaptability of the skin to the external stimulus. Although ageing of skin is an inevitable consequence the psychological impact upon an individual may be reduced owing to the advancement in dermatoaesthetics.

Key Message

Chronological skin ageing is the result of increased oxidative stress and imbalance in the antioxidant mechanism of the body. External factors like pollution, diet, lifestyle and smoking have an important implication in the chronological ageing. The skin undergoes structural modifications with chronological ageing which predisposes it to the development of disorders of the elderly.

Further Reading

1. Barja, G. Updating the Mitochondrial Free Radical Theory of Ageing: An Integrated View, Key Aspects and Confounding Concepts. Antioxidants Redox Signaling. 2013; 19:1420–1445.
2. Du, C, Anderson, A, Lortie, M, Parsons, R, Bodnar, A. Oxidative Damage and Cellular Defense Mechanisms in Sea Urchin Models of Ageing. Free Radical Biology Medicine. 2013; 63:254–263.
3. Fisard, M, Ravussin, E. Energy Metabolism and Oxidative Stress: Impact on the Metabolic Syndrome and the Ageing Process. Endocrine. 2006; 29:27–32.
4. Ott, M, Gogvadze, V, Orrenius, S, Zhivotovsky, B. Mitochondria, Oxidative Stress and Cell Death. Apoptosis. 2007; 12:913–922.
5. Rastogi, RP, Richa, KA, Tyagi, MB, et al. Molecular Mechanisms of Ultraviolet Radiation-induced DNA, 280 Damage and Repair. Journal of Nucleic Acids, 2010, Article ID: 592980.
6. Viña, J, Borras, C, Abdelaziz, KM, Garcia-Valles, R. and Gomez-Cabrera, MC. The Free Radical Theory of Ageing Revisited: The Cell Signaling Disruption Theory of Ageing. Antioxidants Redox Signaling. 2013; 19:779–787.

CHAPTER 3

Cutaneous Manifestation of Skin Ageing

• *Rashmi Modak*

Key Points

- Ageing is a complex and a multifactorial phenomenon which includes intrinsic and extrinsic ageing.
- Xerosis and pruritus are the most common dermatologic afflictions in the aged, amounting for as many 80% of dermatologic complaints among the elderly population.
- Inflammatory dermatoses including eczema and psoriasis are also very common.
- An understanding of the skin helps to identify technologies most likely to be effective in improving pigment, lines, volume loss and skin laxity.

Introduction

There is an increased focus on geriatric dermatology due to the growing trend of ageing populations in many countries worldwide. Ageing is an inevitable and continuous process occurring in all organ systems including skin. In skin, however, this process is influenced by the various cumulative environmental insults of physical, chemical, and mechanical injuries. Advancement in molecular sciences had helped to corroborate the role of genetic and immunologic factors in skin ageing. Ageing skin not only has medical and cosmetic implications but also social ramifications. This chapter will mainly focus on the cutaneous manifestations of ageing skin.

EPIDEMIOLOGY

The geriatric population consists of persons over 65 years of age and as it is increasing in numbers, the incidence of geriatric skin diseases is becoming more widely acknowledged. In a study conducted in Turkey in three senior homes on 300 elderly patients, fungal infection (49.7%) and xerosis (45.3%) were found to be the most common dermatoses.[1] In Taiwan, eczematous dermatitis was most common, followed by fungal infection, xerosis, benign tumors, and viral infections, whereas in Tunisia fungal infections were most common, followed by benign tumors, eczematous dermatitis, bacterial and viral infections, and then xerosis.[2,3] Differences exist between male and female skin and the same is reflected in ageing skin of both. Females are known to have more of sagging and wrinkling but a smoother texture as compared to their male counterparts. However, males are more prone to infections with increased susceptibility to photoageing and skin cancers with delayed wound healing. According to Fitzpatrick classification, a majority of Indians have 3 and 4 skin type.[4,5] Fair-skinned people are more prone to pre-malignant and malignant lesions as compared to dark-skinned individuals. India has a huge ethnic variation and hence extrapolation of Asian skin to Indian population would be inapt. General ethnic variations exist—Asians tend to have more pigmentary problems but less severe wrinkling compared to Caucasians and African-Americans.[6,7]

PATHOPHYSIOLOGY/ETIOPATHOGENESIS[8,9]

Intrinsic ageing includes genetically determined skin changes occurring due to gradual physiological decline while extrinsic ageing is due to external factors that can be controlled.

In general, the balance between DNA damage and repair, controls the rate of ageing in both types of ageing. The diverse cellular, molecular and immunologic mechanism/ theories pertaining to skin ageing have been discussed below.

Cell senescence (telomere) theory: Ageing is due to cell senescence activation occurring due to shortening of telomeres as a result of continuous cell replication. Telomeres are small DNA sequences present at the ends of chromosomes that extend the life of the cells when intact. In addition, various oxidative stress including UV radiation and environmental exposures can also cause telomere damage and shortening.

Genetic theory: The polymorphism in MCR1 (melanocortin 1 receptor) gene that maps to chromosome 16q24.3 and is located on the surface of melanocytes is a known risk factor for photoageing.

Theory of ROS (reactive oxygen species): Increase in free radicals or ROS during aerobic metabolism coupled with decrease in antioxidative mechanism with age cause cumulative damage to various biomolecules including cellular and mitochondrial damage resulting in cellular senescence and thus apoptosis. UV radiation primarily can induce ROS formation. ROS activates cell surface receptors which then leads to intracellular signaling, inducing the transcription of nuclear factors—activator protein 1 (AP-1) and nuclear factor kappa light chain enhancer of activated B cells (NFκB). AP-1 decreases gene expression of collagen I and III leading to reduced collagen synthesis and stimulates synthesis of matrix metalloproteinases (MMP) that degrade mature collagen. NFκB triggers the transcription of inflammatory cytokines and is involved in collagen degradation.

Protein oxidation theory: Cellular proteosomes are required for degradation of proteins. Ageing cells show a decline in proteosomal activities and accumulation of oxidized proteins leading to accelerated tissue dysfunction and ageing. UV-induced protein oxidation and accumulation progressively inhibits proteosomal activities resulting in ageing.

ECM (extracellular matrix) theory: Transforming growth factor β is a cytokine responsible for inducing synthesis of ECM proteins and growth inhibitor of epidermis. UV radiation impairs TGF-β pathway by downregulating TGF-β type II receptors and upregulating Smad 7, a negative regulator of TGF resulting in reduction of type I procollagen transcription and thus collagen production. Ageing fibroblasts lead to reduction in collagen production and UV-induced upregulation of fibroblast elastase damage elastic fibres, facilitating wrinkle formation. Thus, there is decrease in collagen synthesis, abnormal accumulation of elastic fibres and proteoglycans.

Vascular theory: Intrinsically aged skin shows decrease in vessel size and density, whereas UV irradiation results in generation of immature blood vessels due to upregulation of VEGF and downregulation of angiogenesis inhibitor thrombospondin-1.

Immune system theory: Immune system of skin contributes to skin ageing by chronic and persistent inflammation. UV radiation increases IL-1, IL-6 and TGF-α which increases keratinocyte proliferation. Decreased epidermal growth factor receptors and amphiregulin expression in aged skin leads to decreased migration and proliferation of fibroblast leading to impaired wound healing. Decreased toll-like receptor (TLR) expression and function in ageing skin lead to poor adaptive immunity and increased susceptibility to pathogens.

CLINICAL FEATURES

Cutaneous manifestation of intrinsic, extrinsic ageing and various age-related dermatoses have been described.

Cutaneous Manifestation of Intrinsic Ageing

Intrinsic ageing or chronological ageing is the natural ageing occurring in all skin types continuously and gradually in a person's lifetime. It occurs due to endogenous factors such as genetic predisposition, cellular metabolic pathways, and hormonal alterations.[10] Typically seen in the ages of 40–60 years, and in women earlier than men. The prominent cutaneous manifestations include fine wrinkling, dryness and atrophy. There is slight decrease in the elasticity of the skin leading to fine wrinkling while the skin surface markings are maintained. The skin is smooth, homogenous with only slight alteration in the pigmentation leading to pallor. There is a slight decrease in the skin thickness resulting in mild atrophy and dryness.[6] It is observed in its purest form in UV protected skin including inner aspect of arms (Fig. 3.1) and on hips and buttocks.[9]

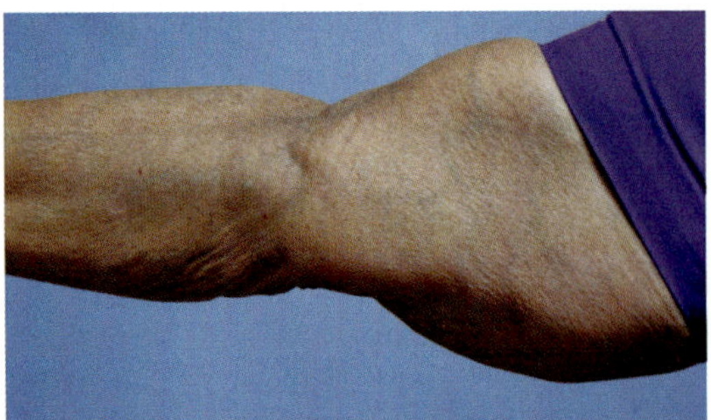

Fig. 3.1: Features of intrinsic ageing including fine wrinkles and homogenous colour seen over inner aspect of arm and forearm

Ethnicity: Wrinkling in Asians is known to occur later and with less severity than in Caucasians.[6] Pigmentary problems are more common in Asians as compared to African-Americans.[7] In fair skinned individuals, the aged skin is more atrophic with multiple telangiectasias and more prone for pre-malignant and malignant lesions including basal cell carcinoma and squamous cell carcinoma. Dark skinned individuals develop deep furrows and severe elastosis.[7,11]

Gender differences: Men have rough texture due to thicker stratum corneum and more prone to develop enlarged pores due to higher amount of sebum secretion. They have dull skin due to increased trans-epidermal water loss (TEWL) and darker and red complexion due to increased melanin, haemoglobin and carotene (Fig. 3.2A). Males are more susceptible to extrinsic ageing and to develop bacterial and viral infections. Females have lighter skin tone and vascularity and less TEWL due to presence of ceramides in the stratum corneum but more of wrinkles and sagging (Fig. 3.2B).

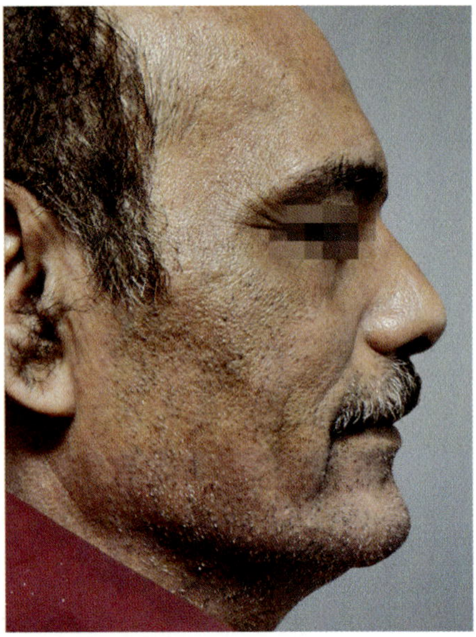

Fig. 3.2A: Rough texture and darker complexion in an aged male

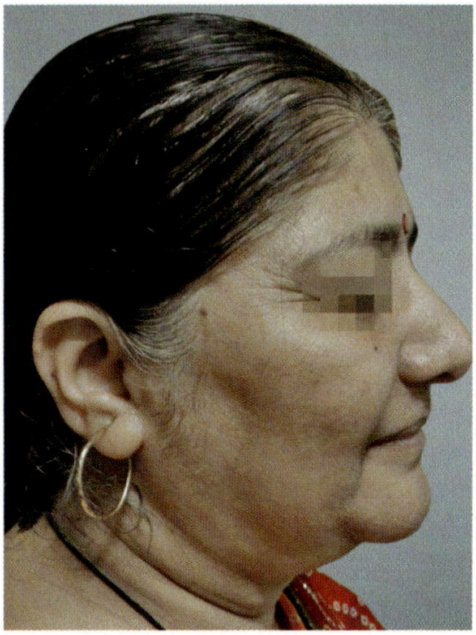

Fig. 3.2B: Lighter skin tone but more sagging in an aged female

Due to decreased estrogen in *menopausal* women, there is increased skin dryness and decreased elasticity and dermal thickness.[9] Vaginal epithelium atrophies, cervico-vaginal secretions become sparse, vaginal pH rises, leading to atrophic vaginitis and increased susceptibility to infection. Labia majora loses subcutaneous fat as also labia minora, vestibule atrophies. Pubic hair grays and becomes sparse.[6,9]

Genetics: Chronological ageing is a pre-ordained process determined genetically and supported by telomere cell senescence theory showing classical features of intrinsic ageing.[9] Skin changes in gene mutations accompanying progeroid syndromes (Hutchinson-Gilford progeria and Werner's syndrome) include skin atrophy and sclerosis, telangiectasias, poikiloderma, alopecias, thinning and graying of hair and several malignancies.

Dermatoporosis: It is a chronic cutaneous syndrome in which there is age associated functional impairment in skin in which the integrity of skin is severely compromised.[9] It occurs due to decreased hyaluronic acid in skin, primarily resulting from chronological ageing and long-term and unprotected sun exposure or secondarily due to long-term use of topical or systemic corticosteroids.[12] Following four stages of dermatoporosis have been described:

Stage I: Characterised by the presence of extreme skin atrophy, senile purpura and pseudoscars.

Stage II: In addition to the lesions found in stage I, there are some localized skin lacerations.

Stage III: Skin lacerations are larger (>3 cm) and extensive and may involve entire extremity.

Stage IV: Advanced lesions result in dissecting hematomas and skin necrosis.

Cutaneous Manifestation of Extrinsic Ageing

Extrinsic ageing or photoageing (dermatoheliosis) is due to the effects of or superimposition of chronic UV radiation on an intrinsically aged skin. It occurs as a result of exogenous factors, primarily UV light exposure and secondary to exposure of pollutants, temperature and humidity, smoking, alcohol, drugs and lifestyle influences including nutrition.[10] It may be seen as early as late teens. The salient cutaneous manifestations are coarse wrinkles, dyspigmentation and telangiectasias.[9] There is marked decrease in the elasticity of the skin leading to deep wrinkles and furrows with markedly altered skin surface markings. The skin is leathery, blotchy with irregular pigmentation. The skin thickness is increased resulting in nodular and rough texture.[6] It is usually observed on sites that are exposed to UV radiation including face, neck, upper chest, extensor aspect of forearms and dorsum of hands (Fig. 3.3A and B).

Photoageing variants: Atrophic and hypertrophic photoageing are the two variants of extrinsic photoageing described by Gilchrest and others.[13] Atrophic ageing is characterised by epidermal atrophy, telangiectasias,

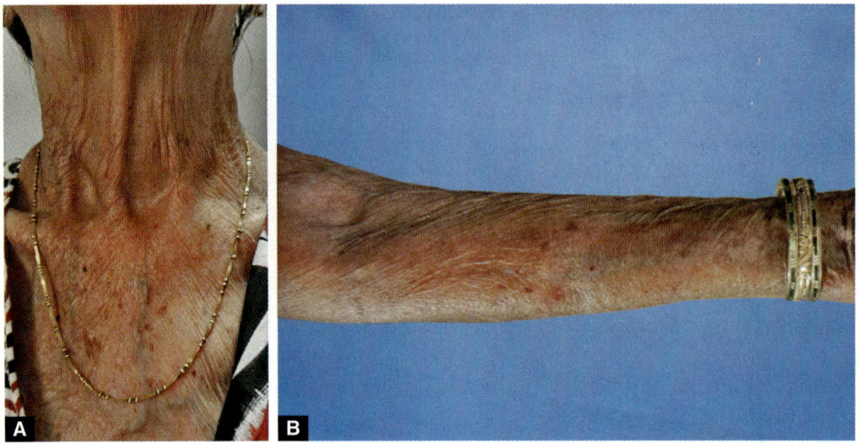

Fig. 3.3: (A) Features of extrinsic ageing including coarse wrinkles and dyspigmentation seen over neck and (B) upper chest

dyspigmentation seen usually in Fitzpatrick skin types I and II. This variant is predisposed to pre-cancerous and cancerous skin lesions. Hypertrophic ageing, the less common variant, is characterised by epidermal hypertrophy, coarse wrinkling, tanning, lentigines and less tendency for neoplasms. It is usually seen in Fitzpatrick skin types III and IV. Even though the collagen damage is equal in both variants, hypertrophic variants show more of solar elastosis.

Infrared and visible light: Infrared light (700 nm–1 mm) and visible light (400–700 nm) are implicated in producing features similar to photoageing. While infrared light induces heat damage and alters mitochondrial integrity of skin cells, visible light causes oxidative damage to skin cells.[14]

Smoking: Smoker's face is characterised by a greyish skin hue with static linear lines or wrinkles radiating perpendicular from eyes and lips (smoker's lines) are seen in individuals with long-standing exposure to tobacco smoke.[6,9] Smoking is considered an independent risk factor having a clear dose–response relationship with wrinkling.[6,15,16]

Alcohol: Signs of skin ageing in an alcoholic include a necklace of telangiectasia, spider nevi, goose flesh and palmar erythema, again showing a dose–response relationship with alcohol intake.[17]

Pollution: Airborne particulate matter exposure may cause prominent skin ageing signs including pigment spots and wrinkles by generation of free oxygen radicals or ROS.[11]

Environmental temperature and humidity: Skin ageing can also be influenced by environmental temperature and humidity as structural proteins and lipids of the skin are critically dependent on temperature for appropriate conformation. Low temperature decreases the evaporative water loss and stiffens the skin.[6,18]

Medications: Some medications, contribute to ageing, particularly hypocholesterolemic drugs, such as statins by inducing abnormal increased desquamation and dryness of skin.[6,19]

Nutrition: Consumption of foods containing advanced glycation end products (AGEs) can stiffen collagen, elastin, vitronectin and laminin in skin and blood vessels leading to skin ulcers and slow wound healing.[20] Foods containing high AGEs include browning/ brown crust of toasted bread, donuts, grill marks on grilled meat, barbecued meats, brown colour of malted barley, dark coloured soft drinks, etc.[21]

Psychological stress: Chronic psychological stress alters the homeostatic mechanisms of the body leading to increased production of ROS, chronic immune dysfunction and DNA damage in skin cells contributing to features of ageing.[22]

Cutaneous Manifestation of Age-related Dermatoses[23–25]

As ageing skin undergoes progressive degenerative structural and physiologic changes that occur as a natural consequence of intrinsic ageing combined with the effects of cumulative extrinsic damage, elderly patients are more susceptible to dermatological disorders. As skin ages, the vasculature, supporting dermis, the immune function of skin progressively deteriorates. Due to these changes, the elderly are more prone to vascular disorders like stasis dermatitis, skin injuries such as pressure sores and ulcers as also various infections and autoimmune diseases. Also due to polypharmacy there is increased risk of drug reactions. A list of age-related dermatoses has been enumerated in Box 3.1. The pathophysiology, clinical features and complications are described in Table 3.1.

Box 3.1: List of age-related dermatoses

Common skin lesions:
- Telangiectasia, senile purpura, poikilodermic changes
- Freckling, lentigines, solar comedones, colloid milia
- Guttate hypomelanosis (Fig. 3.4), cutis rhomboidalis nuchae, stellate pseudoscars, lichen sclerosus et atrophicus

Inflammatory dermatoses:
- Pruritus
- Xerosis and asteatotic eczema
- Nummular dermatitis
- Seborrheic dermatitis
- Contact dermatitis
- Drug eruptions

Vascular disorders:
- Chronic venous insufficiency (stasis dermatitis) and ulceration
- Pressure ulcers

Infectious diseases:

Bacterial
- Impetigo/folliculitis
- Cellulitis

Viral
- Herpes zoster
- Molluscum contagiosum

Fungal
- Onychomycosis
- Tinea pedis
- Tinea cruris
- Intertrigo

Infestation
- Pediculosis
- Scabies

Neoplasms:

Benign tumors
- Seborrheic keratosis
- Skin tags
- Cherry angiomas

Premalignant tumours
- Actinic keratosis
- Actinic cheilitis /leukoplakia
- Morbus Bowen
- Lentigo maligna

Malignant tumours
- Malignant melanoma
- Basal cell carcinoma
- Squamous cell carcinoma

Psychodermatoses:
- Lichen simplex chronicus
- Prurigo nodularis
- Neurotic excoriations
- Delusion of parasitosis
- Dermatitis artefacta

Autoimmune dermatoses:
- Lupus erythematosus
- Psoriasis
- Vitiligo

Vesiculobullous dermatoses:
- Bullous pemphigoid
- Para-neoplastic pemphigus
- Epidermolysis bullosa acquisita

Orogenital:
- Glossodynia, xerostomia
- Vulvodynia, other vulvar problems
- Balanitis

TABLE 3.1: Pathophysiology, clinical features and complications of age-related dermatoses

Age-related dermatoses	Pathophysiology/ etiopathogenesis	Clinical features	Complications
Common skin lesions	Loss of dermal collagen and fat coupled with vascular fragility may predispose the elderly to purpuric lesions	*Bateman purpura (senile purpura)*—ecchymotic patches on photodamaged extensor surfaces of the arms and dorsal hands that appear with or without antecedent trauma.[9] *Favre-Racouchot syndrome (nodular elastosis)*—comedones, follicular cysts, and large folds of furrowed and yellowish skin around the eyes and extends onto the cheeks in the elderly, especially in men.[26] *Cutis rhomboidalis nuchae*—the skin over the back of the neck is thickened, rough, and leathery, skin markings become exaggerated.[23]	
Inflammatory dermatoses			
Pruritus	Age-related changes in the nerves leading to increased touch and pain thresholds, possibly due to subclinical neuropathy, have been suggested.[27] Associated with a release of histamine, which can induce a perpetuating cycle.[28] In up to 30% of patients, pruritus remains idiopathic and occurs more severely and frequently with increasing age.[29,30] Dermatological causes include xerosis (most common), inflammatory eczematous disorders, lichen simplex chronicus, urticaria, and others.[31] Underlying systemic diseases or conditions, including iron deficiency anaemia, thyroid disease, diabetes mellitus, cholestatic liver disease, renal dysfunction, drug reaction, and malignancy.	Most common dermatological complaint. It can be intense, may be accompanied by sensations of tingling or even burning and increases in severity at night.[33] Clinically skin is dry, and an abnormality of keratinization is implicated.[30] Generalised pruritus may indicate psychological stress or internal disease or intake of systemic drugs.[29] Chronic pruritus (>6-week duration) is a distressing symptom. Chronically scratched skin can become thickened and hyperpigmented (lichenification).[34]	Chronic scratching may lead to secondary infections, non-healing wounds

(contd.)

TABLE 3.1: Pathophysiology, clinical features and complications of age-related dermatoses (*contd.*)

Age-related dermatoses	Pathophysiology/ etiopathogenesis	Clinical features	Complications
	Emotional or psychological stresses.[29,32] Medications causing pruritus include antibacterials, diuretics, NSAIDs, and calcium channel antagonists.[29]		
Xerosis and asteatotic eczema	Increased transepidermal water loss, reduced sebum and sweat production, and decreased natural moisturizing factors, in ageing skin lead to dryness.[35] Irregular alignment of corneocytes because of abnormal maturation and adhesion of keratinocytes results in rough and scaly skin.[36] Extrinsic aggravating factors include low ambient humidity, excessive bathing (using harsh soaps or detergents), irritating clothing, use of products containing alcohol or acetone, drugs including diuretic drugs and cholesterol-lowering agents.[37] Asteatotic eczema (eczema craquele) is seen secondary to epidermal lipid and free fatty acid depletion.[38]	Xerosis, or dryness of the skin, is the most common skin disorder in the elderly, the chief complaint of which is pruritus.[39] Usually seen on anterior shin (Fig. 3.5), dorsum of hands, forearm.[23] Often accompanied by excoriation, or inflammatory changes including varying degrees of erythema, cracking, fissuring, or present with a "crazy paving" appearance.[25]	In cases of extensive or generalized eczema craquele internal malignancy, such as malignant lymphoma must be ruled out.[40] More prone for secondary infections and ulcers.
Nummular dermatitis	Discoid eczema is often associated with low humidity, xerosis, or emotional stress.[25]	Pruritic oval- or coin-shaped plaques, which may weep or become crusted, scaly, or infected. Commonly found on lower legs and forearms.[25]	Predisposed to secondary infection
Seborrhoeic dermatitis	*Malassezia yeast* is implicated in its pathogenesis.[41] Commonly seen in those with neurological disorders, such as Parkinson's disease, Alzheimer's disease, or emotional stress.[42]	Erythema and greasy red-brown papules covered with scaly yellow flakes and plaques in areas rich in sebaceous glands, including scalp, eyebrows, glabella, paranasal fold, postauricular area, and intertriginous areas.[43]	

(*contd.*)

TABLE 3.1: Pathophysiology, clinical features and complications of age-related dermatoses (*contd.*)

Age-related dermatoses	Pathophysiology/ etiopathogenesis	Clinical features	Complications
Contact dermatitis	Contact with antimicrobials (i.e. neomycin, nitrofurazone in topical medications); Lanolin; parabens (in topical medications, cosmetics, or moisturizers); dyes; plants; balsams; rubber; and nickel.[44,45] Alkaline soaps, detergents, or cleaners.[46]	In 11% of the elderly population, includes allergy and irritant-type reactions.[47] Less vesiculation or inflammation and early appearance of scaling, hyperpigmentation, and lichenification is seen secondary to a decreased ability to mount a delayed-type hypersensitivity reaction.[48]	Predisposed to secondary infection. Less responsive to treatment, tends to run a more chronic course.
Drug eruptions	Physiologically, the respiratory, excretory, and metabolic functions are generally deteriorated, and multiple drugs are apt to accumulate in the body, leading to a high incidence. Polypharmacy leads to higher risk.	Incidence: 10–30%, most common being exanthematic eruptions.[48,49] Other presentation: *Exanthematic eruption*—maculopapular, morbilliform, or erythematous lesions. *Drug-induced vasculitis*—purpuric maculopapular eruption on limbs, accompanied by fever, aching, and fatigue. *Fixed drug eruption*—rounded single erythematous or bullous lesions, which typically recur at the same spot upon re-challenging with the same medication. common sites are hands, feet, genitals, and around mouth or eyes. *Erythema multiforme*—minor or major forms, a hypersensitivity reaction characterised by target-like lesions on the extremities and trunk accompanied by systemic symptoms. Other presentations include urticaria, contact dermatitis, purpura, and photodermatitis.[50]	May present as more serious life-threatening Stevens-Johnson syndrome or toxic epidermal necrolysis.[49]

(*contd.*)

TABLE 3.1: Pathophysiology, clinical features and complications of age-related dermatoses (*contd.*)

Age-related dermatoses	Pathophysiology/ etiopathogenesis	Clinical features	Complications
Vascular disorders			
Chronic venous insufficiency (stasis dermatitis) and ulceration	It is due to venous insufficiency and venous hypertension related to valvular incompetence. Decreased endothelial cell permeability, leukocyte adhesion contribute to compromised immune reaction.[8]	Stasis dermatitis (hypostatic eczema) presents as ill-defined dark erythema, dermatitis, variable scaling, varicose veins, and edema of feet and ankles. Chronic stage shows lichenification, hyperpigmentation, or lipodermato- sclerosis. Excoriation or trauma to the fragile skin results in painful, well marginated ulcers.	Secondary bacterial infection may lead to cellulitis and lymphangitis.
Pressure ulcers	Pressure on tissue over an extended period of time causes ischemia and results in tissue damage. Ageing skin is rendered more susceptible to injury, less capable of undergoing modification or repair as well as impaired inflammatory responses.[51] High risk individuals—critical care patients, quadriplegics, terminal cancer patients, diabetics, patients with end-stage renal disease, and incontinent, immobile, immunosuppressed, and malnourished.	Decubitus ulcer/ bed sores are seen usually over bony prominences and as tissue damage starts from deep in the muscle bone interface, an apparently small ulcer may turn out to be a much deeper /extensive ulcer after debridement. It is divided into stages depending on the severity.[52,53]	Marjolin ulcer—a cancer arising in chronic wounds and burn scars.[54]
Infectious diseases			
Bacterial infections	Various physical factors, malnourishment, nutritional deficiencies may cause alteration in skin architecture and loss of barrier function.[52] Causative organisms include *Staphylococcus aureus* or Group A beta-hemolytic streptococci.	Both superficial and infection of subcutaneous tissue including bullous and non-bullous forms of impetigo, cellulitis, erysipelas are seen.[55]	Abscess, or necrosis or lymphangitis.

(*contd.*)

TABLE 3.1: Pathophysiology, clinical features and complications of age-related dermatoses (*contd.*)

Age-related dermatoses	Pathophysiology/ etiopathogenesis	Clinical features	Complications
Viral infections	Impaired immune function. Causative organisms include herpes simplex and varicella zoster virus, pox virus.	Herpes zoster/shingles associated with prodromal pain and with classical vesicles seen in higher numbers in adults older than 60 years (Fig. 3.6).[56] Others include herpes simplex and molluscum contagiosum (MC).[57] HSV-I is shown to be a major factor for Alzheimer's disease in elderly.[58]	Postherpetic neuralgia (PHN), the duration and severity of PHN are related to age.[59]
Fungal infections	Predisposing factors—diabetes mellitus, obesity, systemic/topical glucocorticoids, broad-spectrum antibiotics, immunosuppressive drugs, and chronic debilitation. Causative organisms—dermatophytes, most commonly *Trichophyton rubrum*, *Trichophyton mentagrophytes*, *Epidermophyton floccosum*, and *Candida species*.	Onychomycosis, tinea pedis, tinea cruris, and candidiasis (intertrigo, angular cheilitis, genital candidiasis, oral thrush, balanitis, vulvitis chronic paronychia) occur commonly in the aged population.	
Infestation	*Mite Sarcoptes scabiei*, head louse (*Pediculus humanus capitis*) and pubic lice (*Pthirus pubis*).	Scabies—clinical presentation in the elderly can vary markedly due to pre-existing dermatoses. Pediculosis capitis (pruritus and nits cemented to the hair shaft) or *Pthirus pubis* (pruritic papular eruption).	Secondary infection and eczematisation is common in elderly.
Neoplasms Benign tumours		Seborrhoeic keratosis—well-circumscribed tan to brownish papules or plaques with a greasy feel, often occurs on face (Fig. 3.7), trunk, and upper extremities. Skin tag (acrochordons or soft fibroma)—soft, skin-coloured to brownish, round or pedunculated, fibro-epithelial polyp seen over neck, intertriginous areas. Cherry angiomas (senile angiomas)—bright red, dome-shaped papules, distributed on the trunk (Fig. 3.8).	

(*contd.*)

TABLE 3.1: Pathophysiology, clinical features and complications of age-related dermatoses (*contd.*)

Age-related dermatoses	Pathophysiology/ etiopathogenesis	Clinical features	Complications
Pre-malignant tumours		*Actinic keratosis*—scaly hyperpigmented or erythematous plaques over hands, forehead, and the ears that may ulcerate.[61] *Lentigo maligna*—a brown-black irregularly pigmented freckle, usually occurring on the face (malignant cells confined to epidermis). *Actinic cheilitis*—dryness, scaling, atrophy, telangiectasia, fissures leukoplakia over lower lip. *Leukoplakia*—white patches on mucosal surfaces,which cannot be rubbed off, associated with alcohol and/or tobacco.	
Malignant tumours	Lowered immunity and the harmful effects of ultraviolet light on the skin.	*Melanomas*—brownish or black plaques, with irregular borders and irregular pigmentation.[62] *Basal cell carcinoma (BCC)*—pearly papules, rolled edges, and telangiectasia. *Squamous cell carcinomas (SCC)*—irregular growths with an indurated base. *Keratoacanthoma*—erythematous dome-shaped, 1–10 cm nodule with a keratin plug in the centre, mostly on the sun-exposed areas, considered to be subtype of SCC.	BCC—deep invasion and extensive destruction of muscle and bone.
Psychodermatoses			
Lichen simplex chronicus (LSC), prurigo nodularis	Skin disorders with psychological impact and psychiatric disorders with skin manifestations.[63,64] Secondary to habitual scratching and picking. Suggested damage to the peripheral nervous system, such as radiculopathy and neuropathy.[65]	*Lichen simplex chronicus*—lichenified red scaly plaque. *Prurigo nodularis*—erythematous or hyperpigmented, scattered, and discrete keratotic nodules on the extremities.	Severe cases may ulcerate.

(*contd.*)

TABLE 3.1: Pathophysiology, clinical features and complications of age-related dermatoses (*contd.*)

Age-related dermatoses	Pathophysiology/ etiopathogenesis	Clinical features	Complications
Neurotic excoriations, Delusion of parasitosis	Delusional parasitosis—patients firmly believe that their bodies are infested by some type of organisms despite lack of supporting evidence.[66]	*Neurotic excoriations* (pathological skin picking)—a type of impulse control disorder, variety of excoriated papules at different stages of healing in the background of post-inflammatory scars.[67,68] *Delusion of parasitosis*—small bits of excoriated skin, debris, and unrelated insects or insect parts—the match box sign.	
Autoimmune dermatoses			
Systemic lupus erythematosus (SLE)	Senescence of the skin immunological system with reduction in immune response but increase in autoantibodies and inflammatory response.[69]	Atypical features, insidious presentation are more common.[70] Lung involvement and Sjogren's syndrome observed more frequently.[71]	
Vesiculobullous dermatoses[72]			
Bulluous pemphigoid	Autoantibodies to hemidesmosomal proteins present in the basement membrane of stratified squamous epithelia.	Tense blisters in flexural areas of the skin, eye and the oral cavity.	Lesions frequently result in scar formation, which may cause blindness.
Paraneoplastic pemphigus	Autoantibodies to multiple antigens within the desmosomes.	Severe stomatitis and polymorphous skin eruption.	Associated with neoplasms, leukaemia and lymphoma.
Epidermolysis bullosa acquisita	Autoantibodies to type VII collagen in the anchoring fibrils of the basement membrane.	Lesions may either arise on an inflammatory base or be non-inflammatory and result primarily from trauma.	
Orogenital			
Glossodynia, xerostomia	Saliva undergoes chemical changes with ageing and along with polypharmacy in elderly, leads to xerostomia and finally glossodynia.[73]	Dryness, cracking and fissuring of the oral mucosa, pain and halitosis.	Dental caries
Vulvodynia and other vulvar problems	Vulva is affected by cessation of estrogen after menopause.[74] Vulvodynia is a diagnosis of exclusion.	Pain, burning, stinging, irritation, tenderness on pressure, varying degrees of erythema.	Increased risk of SCC
Balanitis	Inflammation of the glans, or the head, of the penis, due to infection or another cause.[75]	Reddish, shiny, pruritic plaque over glans.	

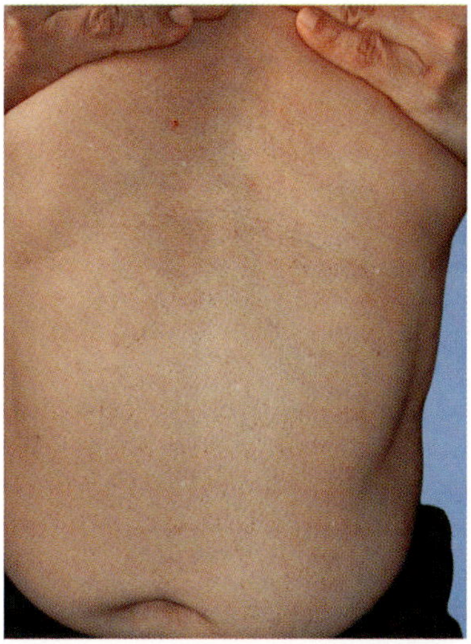

Fig. 3.4: Multiple guttate hypomelanotic lesions over the trunk of an elderly male

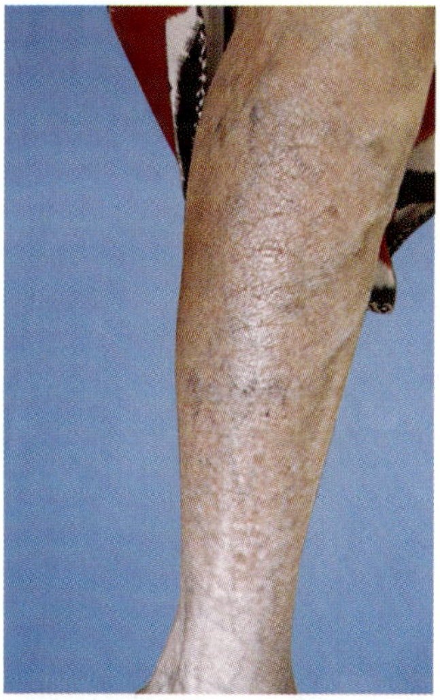

Fig. 3.5: Dryness of the skin seen commonly on anterior shin of the legs with varicose veins

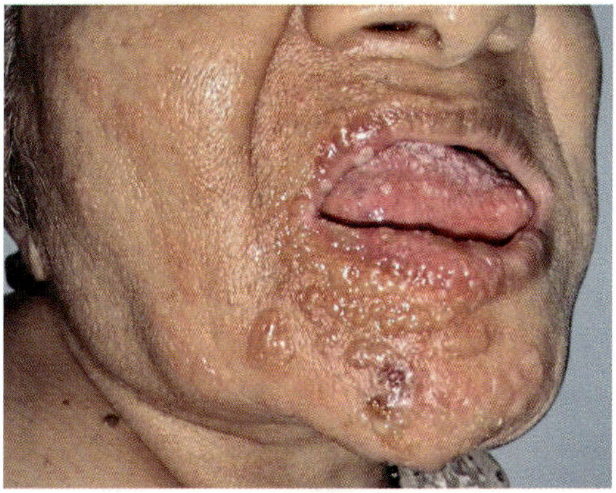

Fig. 3.6: Lesions of herpes zoster distributed along maxillary and mandibular division of trigeminal nerve in an elderly female

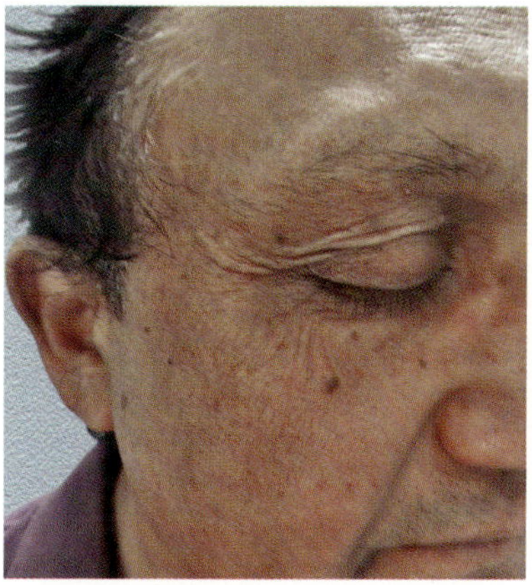

Fig. 3.7: Multiple seborrhoeic keratoses over face including upper eyelid in an elderly male

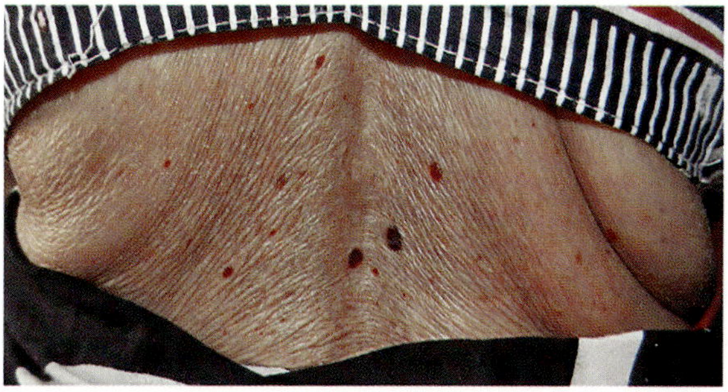

Fig. 3.8: Multiple cherry angiomas seen over trunk in an elderly female

MANAGEMENT

Skin ageing, especially photoageing, can be quantified on histology and yield important clinical information on the risk of actinic keratosis and skin cancer development. As histological quantification is not practical in a clinical setup, various non-invasive tools have been developed for both intrinsic and extrinsic ageing are listed in Box 3.2. Treatment of intrinsic ageing includes use of anti-ageing products and procedures, while for extrinsic ageing avoidance of implicated exogenous factors, modification of lifestyle and habits and appropriate use of sunscreens and skin care products. Various products and procedure help in improving texture and colour and have been given in Table 3.2. Management of various age-related dermatoses have been mentioned in Table 3.3.

Box 3.2: Various non-invasive tools to measure skin ageing[9]

- Reflectance confocal microscopy (RCM)
- Spectrophotometry
- Skin surface topography
- Fluorescence lifetime imaging microscopy (FLIM)
- SCINEXA score

TABLE 3.2: Various products and procedures to treat skin ageing[76,77]

Cosmeceutical products		Procedures
Topical	Systemic	
Sunscreen	Hormone replacement therapy (estrogen/progesterone/dihydro-epiandrosterone sulphate) especially in peri- and post-menopausal women	Chemical peeling
Antioxidants including vitamins, coenzymes, botanicals, etc. which help in reducing collagen degradation caused by free radicals.	Antioxidants	Microdermabrasion
Cell regulators including retinoids, peptides, growth factors, stem cells, etc. which influence dermal metabolism and cause synthesis of collagen.		Lasers and lights
		Radiofrequency/electrocautery
		Injectables (fillers, botulinum toxin, PRP) for soft tissue augmentation and contouring

TABLE 3.3: Management of age-related dermatoses

Age-related dermatoses	Investigations	Treatment
Common skin lesions		
Senile purpura		Resolves slowly, no effective treatment
Favre-Racouchot syndrome		Comedone extraction, EC/RF

(contd.)

TABLE 3.3: Management of age-related dermatoses (*contd.*)

Age-related dermatoses	Investigations	Treatment
Inflammatory dermatoses		
Pruritus	Careful diagnostic evaluation including CBC, S. ferritin, urine analysis, LFT, RFT, chest X-ray, thyroid function test to rule out any underlying diseases.	Correcting existing xerosis or any underlying systemic cause. Topical steroids, antihistamines, soothing agents, and emollient creams. Systemic antihistamines and corticosteroids. Psychogenic cause of pruritus responds best to local or systemic doxepin.[63]
Xerosis and asteatotic eczema	Investigations for malignant lymphoma in case of extensive eczema craquele.[40]	Avoidance of aggravating factors and hydration of skin. Advised to bathe less frequently using a moderate—temperature bath, mild soaps, or soap substitutes, application of bath oil, etc. Moisturizers containing occlusive and humectant properties need to be applied immediately after bath.[47] Topical steroids, topical pimecrolimus indicated for asteatotic eczema.[78–80]
Nummular dermatitis	Potassium hydroxide (KOH) preparation and microscopic examination—helpful for differential diagnosis from tinea corporis.	Topical corticosteroids, topical calcineurin inhibitors, and emollients.
Seborrhoeic dermatitis	KOH preparation and microscopic examination.	Scalp is usually treated with shampoos containing cytostatic agents (zinc pyrithione, selenium sulfide); keratolytics (salicylic acid); ketoconazole; or tar preparations. Glabrous skin is treated with mild topical corticosteroids, calcineurin-inhibitors and antifungal creams.[25]
Contact dermatitis	Patch testing—useful in identifying the allergens.	Irritant dermatitis—emollients and mild corticosteroids Allergic contact dermatitis—potent topical corticosteroids, oral antihistamines, or corticosteroids.[81–84]
Drug eruptions	Careful investigation of medication history, including over-the-counter or herbal drugs.	Withdrawal of the inducing drug, supportive management.

(*contd.*)

TABLE 3.3: Management of age-related dermatoses (*contd.*)

Age-related dermatoses	Investigations	Treatment
Vascular disorders		
Chronic venous insufficiency (stasis dermatitis) and ulceration	Venous Doppler to locate the valvular incompetency.	*Treatment of stasis dermatitis*—application of mild topical corticosteroid preparations, controlling edema, leg elevation, and compression dressings or stockings.[85,86] *Venous ulceration*—astringent soaks (e.g. aluminum acetate solution or potassium permanganate solution soaks); debridement; or systemic antibiotics in the case of secondary infection.[87] Surgical treatment for varicose veins may be required. Calcium dobesilate is indicated as an adjuvant therapy in patients with venous ulcers and leg ulcerations.[88]
Pressure ulcers	Investigations for associated medical condition. Cultures for Gram stain prior to antibiotic therapy.	*Prevention*—treatment of associated medical condition, proper nourishment, increasing mobility, using device repositioning schedules, reducing shearing forces, careful skincare, reducing skin to skin contact, daily skin examinations.[89] *Relief of pressure or friction*—position/mobilization techniques, pressure-reducing devices, frequent repositioning. *Wound care*—debridement, dressings, and control of bacterial infection.
Infectious diseases		
Bacterial infections	Skin swabs (open lesions) or aspiration (bullae) to be sent for detection of causative organism and tested for antibacterial sensitivity.[25]	*Penicillinase*—resistant penicillin, such as flucloxacillin or dicloxacillin for 10 days or macrolide antibiotics MRSA—vancomycin, teicoplanin, linezolid, and quinupristin-dalfopristin.[55,90]
Viral infection	Tzanck smear	*Oral antivirals*—acyclovir, valacyclovir, famciclovir Steroids and NSAIDs added according to severity *Topical*—topical lidocaine, dressings with Burow's solution, calamine lotion.[59] *Preventive*—zoster vaccine (Zostavax) helps by decreasing incidence and severity.[91] PHN—tricyclic antidepressants (amitriptyline, desipramine); gabapentin. MC—cryotherapy and electrodesiccation and curettage.

(*contd.*)

TABLE 3.3: Management of age-related dermatoses (*contd.*)

Age-related dermatoses	Investigations	Treatment
Fungal infections	KOH preparation and microscopic examination, fungal cultures.	*General measures*—affected areas need to be kept dry, control of predisposing factors. *Topical*—imidazoles (clotrimazole, sulconazole), allylamines (terbinafine, butenafine), keratolytic agents (salicylic acid, lactic acid). *Oral*—fluconazole, itraconazole, terbinafine, griseofulvin.
Infestation	Mite orova faeces identified in scrapings.	*Topical*—permethrin, crotamiton, benzoyl benzoate, GBH, sulphur. *Oral*—ivermectin
Neoplasms		
Benign tumours		Electrodesiccation, and cryotherapy.
Pre-malignant tumours	Punch biopsy	Sunlight avoidance and use of sunscreens, topical emollients and corticosteroids (actinic keratosis). Oral corticosteroids and azathioprine in chronic cases.[92] Avoidance of alcohol and tobacco (leucokeratosis). 5-fluorouracil—actinic cheilitis/leucokeratosis. Electrodesiccation and cryotherapy.
Malignant tumours		Excision of the tumour
Psychodermatoses		
LSC, prurigo nodularis		*Psychotherapy*—behaviour modification, habit reversal therapy. *Topical*—steroid ointments, doxepin cream. *Oral*—gabapentin.
Neurotic excoriations, delusion of parasitosis		*Psychotherapy*—cognitive behavioural therapy *Oral*—atypical antipsychotics, antidepressants, lamotrigine, gabapentin, naltrexone, and topiramate.[66,93]
Autoimmune dermatoses[94]		
SLE, Sjögren's syndrome	Higher prevalence of autoantibodies such as rheumatoid factor, anti-Ro and anti-cardiolipin antibodies, anti-double-stranded DNA antibodies.	Sun protection, oral and topical corticosteroids, other immunosuppressants.

(*contd.*)

TABLE 3.3: Management of age-related dermatoses (*contd.*)

Age-related dermatoses	Investigations	Treatment
Vesiculo-bullous dermatoses		
Bullous pemphigoid	Skin biopsy, immunofluorescence.	Oral corticosteroids or immunosuppressive agents such as azathioprine.
Para-neoplastic pemphigus		Treatment of the underlying neoplasm or may require immunosuppressive therapy.
Epidermolysis bullosa acquisita		Corticosteroids, dapsone, cyclosporine, plasmapheresis and immunoglobulin G.
Oro-genital		
Glossodynia and xerostomia		Hydration, artificial saliva substitutes, selective serotonin reuptake inhibitors (sertraline).[95]
Vulvodynia		*Vulvar care measures* *Topical anesthetics* (e.g 5% lidocaine ointment) *Tricyclic antidepressants* (e.g. amitriptyline) or anticonvulsants (e.g. gabapentin) (orally or compounded into a vulvar cream) *Biofeedback* and physical therapy *Surgery* (vestibulectomy with vaginal advancement) usually a last resort
Balanitis	Biopsy to r/o malignancy/other dermatoses in persistent cases	Treatment of the underlying cause. Circumcision, Topical steroids, Topical and systemic antibiotics.

CONCLUSION

Ageing is a complex and a multifactorial phenomenon wherein progressive intrinsic changes in the skin combine with cumulative environment factors to produce both structural and functional disturbances. Xerosis and pruritus are the most common dermatologic afflictions in the aged, amounting for as many as 80% of dermatologic complaints among the elderly population. Inflammatory dermatoses including eczema and psoriasis are also very common. The cumulative effects of environment insults, especially solar radiation, also contribute to the marked increase in neoplastic diseases in old age. Even though skin problems sometimes may not seem significant compared to the other systemic diseases which are commonly seen in this age group, proper diagnosis and management of age-related dermatoses help reduce the morbidity and improve quality of life in these patients.

References

1. Kilic A, Gul U, Aslan E, Soylu S. Dermatologic findings in the senior population of nursing homes in Turkey. Arch Gerontol Geriatr 2008; 47:93–8.
2. Liao YH, Chen KH, Tseng MP, Sun CC. Pattern of skin diseases in a geriatric population in Taiwan: a 7-year survey from the outpatient clinic of a university medical center. Dermatology 2001; 203:308–13.
3. Souissi A, Zeglaoul F, El Fekih N, et al. Skin diseases in the elderly: a multicentre Tunisian study. Ann Dermatol Venereol. 2006;133:231–4.
4. Verma SB. Redefining colour of Indian skin. J Eur Acad Dermatol Venereol. 2008;22:1263–4.
5. Hourblin V, Nouveau S, Roy N, de Lacharrière O. Skin complexion and pigmentary disorders in facial skin of 1204 women in 4 Indian cities. Indian J Dermatol Venereol Leprol. 2014;80(5):395–401.
6. Farage MA, Miller KW, Elsner P, Maibach HI. Intrinsic and extrinsic factors in skin ageing: a review. Int J Cosmet Sci. 2008 Apr;30(2):87–95.
7. Singh G.Can we prevent skin aging? Indian J Dermatol Venereol Leprol. 2009;75(5):447–51.
8. Mina Y, Barbara AG. Aging of skin. In: Goldsmith Al, Katz I S, Gilrchrest AB et al, editors. Fitzpatrick's dermatology in general medicine. 8th ed. United States, McGraw-Hill,2012; p 1213–20.
9. Sachs D, Fisher G, Voorhees J. Skin Aeging. In: Griffiths CEM, Barker J, Bleiker T, Chalmers R, Creamer D, editors. Rook's Textbook of Dermatology. 9th Ed. UK: Wiley Blackwell; 2016. p 155.1–155.9.
10. Nikolakis G, Makrantonaki E, Zouboulis CC. Skin mirrors human aging. Horm Mol Biol Clin Investig. 2013;16(1):13–28.
11. Vierkötter A and Krutmann J. Environmental influences on skin aging and ethnic-specific manifestations. Dermatoendocrinol. 2012;4(3): 227–31.
12. G. Kaya, JH. Saurat. Dermatoporosis: A new concept in skin aging. European Geriatric Medicine. 2010;1:216–19.
13. Yaar M, Gilchrest BA. Photoageing: mechanism, prevention and therapy. *Br J Dermatol* 2007;157 (5):874–87.
14. Dupont E, Gomez J, Bilodeau D. Beyond UV radiation: a skin under challenge. Int J Cosmet Sci. 2013; 35(3):224–32.
15. Leow, YH and Maibach, HI. Cigarette smoking, cutaneous vasculature, and tissue oxygen. Clin. Dermatol. 1998;16:579–84.
16. Kennedy C, Bastiaens, MT, Bajdik, CD, et al. Leiden. Skin Cancer Study. Effect of smoking and sun on the aging skin. J. Invest. Dermatol. 2003;120:548–54.
17. Bashir KR. A necklace of telangiectases: an early clinical sign of alcohol abuse. Can Fam Physician. 1984 Oct;30:2067–74.
18. McCallion, R. and Li Wan Po, A. Dry and photo-aged skin: manifestations and management. J. Clin. Pharm. Ther. 1993;18:15–32.
19. Jackson, SM, Williams, ML, Feingold, KR and Elias, PM. Pathobiology of the stratum corneum. West. J. Med. 1993;158:279–85.
20. Draelos ZD. Aging skin: the role of diet: facts and controversies. Clin Dermatol. 2013;31(6):701–6.
21. O'Brien J, Morrissey PA. Nutritional and toxicological aspects of the Maillard browning reaction in foods. Crit Rev Food Sci Nutr. 1989;28(3):211–48.
22. Dunn JH, Koo J. Psychological stress and skin aging: a review of possible mechanisms and potential therapies. Dermatol Online J. 2013;19(6):18561.
23. Jafferany M, Huynh TV, Silverman MA, Zaidi Z. Geriatric dermatoses: a clinical review of skin diseases in an aging population. Int J Dermatol. 2012;51(5):509–22.
24. Zouboulis CC, Makrantonaki E. Clinical aspects and molecular diagnostics of skin aging. Clin Dermatol. 2011;29(1):3–14.
25. Wey SJ, Chen D. Common cutaneous disorders in the elderly. Journal of Clinical Gerontology and Geriatrics. 2010;1(2):36–41.
26. Sawicki J, Barankin B. Dermacase: Favre-Racouchot syndrome. Can Fam Physician. 2010; 56:247–8.
27. Nusbaun NJ. Aging and sensory senescence. South Med J 1999;92:267–75.
28. DeWitt S. Nursing assessment of the skin and dermatologic lesions. Nurs Clin North Am 1990; 25:235–45.
29. Fleischer AB. Pruritus in the elderly: management by senior dermatologists. Adv Dermatol 1993; 28:603–9.
30. Long CC, Marks R. Stratum corneum changes in patients with senile pruritus. J Am Acad Dermatol 1992;27:560–4.
31. Thaipisuttikul Y. Pruritic skin diseases in the elderly. J Dermatol 1998;25:153–7.

32. Stander S, Weisshaar E, Mettang T, Szepietowski JC, Carstens E, Ikoma A, et al. Clinical classification of itch: a position paper of the International Forum for the Study of Itch. Acta Derm Venereol. 2007; 87:291–4.
33. Yosipovitch G. Assessment of itch: more to be learned and improvements to be made. J Invest Dermatol. 2003;121:1301–5.
34. Braun M, Lowitt MH. Pruritus. Adv Dermatol. 2001;17:1–27.
35. Norman RA. Xerosis and pruritus in elderly patients, part 1. Ostomy Wound Manage. 2006; 52:12–4.
36. Richey ML, Richey HK, Fenske NA. Aging-related skin changes: development and clinical meaning. Geriatrics. 1988;43:49–64.
37. Smoker A. Skin care in old age. Nurse Stand. 1999; 13:47–53.
38. Akimoto K, Yoshikawa N, Higaki Y, et al. Quantitative analysis of stratum corneum lipids in xerosis and asteatotic eczema. J Dermatol. 1993; 20:1–6.
39. Beauregard S, Gilchrest BA. A survey of skin problems and skin care regimens in the elderly. Arch Dermatol. 1987;123:1638–43.
40. Sparsa A, Liozon E, Boulinguez S, et al. Generalized eczema craquale as a presenting feature of systemic lymphoma: a report of seven cases. Acta Derm Venereol. 2005; 85:333–6.
41. Falk MHS, Linder MT, Johansson C, Bartosik J, Bäck O, Särnhult T, et al. The prevalence of *Malassezia yeast* in patients with atopic dermatitis, seborrhoeic dermatitis and healthy controls. Acta Derm Venereol. 2005;85:17–23.
42. Mastrolonardo M, Diaferio A, Logroscino G. Seborrheic dermatitis, increased sebum excretion, and Parkinson's disease: a survey of (im)possible links. Med Hypotheses 2003;60:907–11.
43. Moschella S. Skin diseases of the elderly. In: Norman R, editor. Geriatric dermatology. New York: Parthenon, 2001:17–34.
44. Beacham BE. Common dermatoses in the elderly. Am Fam Physician. 1993;47:1445–50.
45. Kleinsmith DM, Perricone NV. Common skin problems in the elderly. Dermatol Clin. 1986;4:214–7.
46. Gilchrest BA. Geriatric skin problems. Hosp Pract (Off Ed). 1986;21:59–65.
47. Fitzpatrick JE. Common inflammatory skin diseases of the elderly. Geriatrics. 1989;44:40–6.
48. Naldi L, Conforti A, Venegoni M, et al. Cutaneous reaction to drugs: an analysis of spontaneous reports infour Italian regions. Br J Clin Pharmacol. 1999; 48:839–46.
49. Sullivan JR, Shear NH. Drug eruptions and other adverse drug effects in aged skin. Clin Geriatr Med. 2002;18:21–42.
50. Nedorost ST, Stevens SR. Diagnosis and treatment of allergic skin disorders in the elderly. Drugs Aging 2001;18:827–35.
51. Martini F. Fundamentals of anatomy and physiology. San Francisco, CA: Benjamin-Cummings; 2004.
52. Norman RA. Geriatric dermatology. Dermatol Ther. 2003; 16:260–8.
53. Norman R. Dermatologic problems and treatment in long term/nursing home care. In: Norman R, ed. Geriatric Dermatology. New York: Parthenon, 2001: 5–16.
54. Esther RJ, Lamps L, Schwartz HS. Marjolin ulcers: secondary carcinomas in chronic wounds. J South Orthop Assoc 1999;8:181–7.
55. Laube S, Farrell AM. Bacterial skin infections in the elderly. Drug Aging 2002;19:331–42.
56. Rimland D, Moanna A. Increasing incidence of herpes zoster among veterans. Clin Infect Dis. 2010; 50: 1000–5.
57. Elgart ML. Skin infections and infestations. Clin Geriatr Med. 2002; 18:89–101.
58. Itzhaki RF, Wozniak MA. Herpes simplex type I in Alzheimer's disease: the enemy within. J Alzheimers Dis. 2008;13:393–405.
59. Beutner KR. Clinical management of herpes zoster in the elderly patient. Compr Ther. 1996;22:183–6.
60. Nanda A, Mamon HJ, Fuchs CS. Sign of Leser-Trélat in newly diagnosed advanced gastric adenocarcinoma. J Clin Oncol. 2008;26:4992–3.
61. Schwartz RA. The actinic keratosis: a perspective and update. Dermatol Surg. 1997;23:1009–19.
62. Testori A, Soteldo J, Sances D, et al. Cutaneous melanoma in the elderly. Melanoma Res. 2009; 19:25–34.
63. Jafferany M. Psychodermatology: a guide to understanding common psychocutaneous disorders. Prim Care Companion J Clin Psychiatry. 2007;9:203–13.
64. Jafferany M, Vander Stoep A, Dumitrescu A, Hornung RL. The knowledge, awareness and practice patterns of dermatologists towards psychodermatology: results of a survey study. Int J Dermatol. 2010;49:784–9.

65. Solak O, Kulac M, Yaman M, et al. Lichen simplex chronicus as a symptom of neuropathy. Clin Exp Dermatol. 2009;34:476–80.
66. Lepping P, Freudenmann RW. Delusional parasitosis: a new pathway for diagnosis and treatment. Clin Exp Dermatol. 2008; 33:113–7.
67. Odlaug BL, Grant JE. Pathological skin picking. Am J Drug Alcohol Abuse 2010;36:296–303.
68. Odlaug BL, Grant JE. Clinical characteristics and medical complications of pathological skin picking. Gen Hosp Psychiatry 2008;30:61–6.
69. Watad A, Bragazzi NL, Adawi M, Amital H. Autoimmunity in the Elderly: Insights from Basic Science and Clinics—A Mini-Review. Gerontology 2017; 63:515–23.
70. Ramos-Casals M, Brito-Zerón P, López-So A. Autoimmune diseases in the elderly: systemic lupus erythematosus and Sjögren's syndrome. Aging health 2004; 4:4.
71. Vadasz Z, Haj T, Kessel A, Toubi. Age-related autoimmunity. *BMC Medicine* 2013;11:94.
72. Mutasim DF. Autoimmune bullous dermatoses in the elderly: diagnosis and management. Drugs Aging. 2003;20(9):663–81.
73. Astor FC, Hanft KL , Ciocon JO. Xerostomia: a prevalent condition in the elderly.Ear, Nose, and Throat Journal 1999:78(7):476–79.
74. Barhan S, EzenaguL. Vulvar problems in elderly women. Original Article Postgraduate medicine, 2015; 121–32.
75. Singh S , Bunker C. Male genital dermatoses in old age. *Age and Ageing* 2008;37(5):500–4.
76. Ganceviciene R, Liakou A, Theodoridis A, et al**.** Skin anti-aging strategies**.** Dermatoendocrinol. 2012; 4(3):308–19.
77. Ramos-e-Silva M, Celem LR, Ramos-e-Silva S, Fucci-da-Costa AP. Anti-aging cosmetics: facts and controversies. Clin Dermatol. 2013;31(6):750–8.
78. Davies A. Management of dry skin conditions in older people. Br J Community Nurs 2008;13(6):250, 252, 254–7.
79. Day I, Lin AN. Use of pimecrolimus cream in disorders other than atopic dermatitis. J Cutan Med Surg 2008; 12:17–26.
80. Schulz P, Bunselmeyer B, Brautigam M, Luger TA. Pimecrolimus cream 1% is effective in asteatotic dermatitis: a result of randomized double blind vehicle controlled study in 40 patients. J Eur Acad Dermatol Venereol. 2007;21:90–4.
81. Chew AL, Maibach HI, editors. Irritant dermatitis. Berlin/Heidelberg, Germany: Springer 2005; p 187–207.
82. Levin C, Zhai H, Bashir S, Chew AL, Anigbogu A, Stern R, et al. Efficacy of corticosteroids in acute experimental irritant contact dermatitis? Skin Res Technol 2001;7:214–8.
83. Levin C, Zhai H, Maibach H. Corticosteroids of clinical value in lipid-soluble chemical-induced irritation in man? Exog Dermatol 2002;1:97–101.
84. Nedorost ST, Stevens SR. Diagnosis and treatment of allergic skin disorders in the elderly. Drugs Aging 2001;18:827–35.
85. Gupta AK, Koven JD, Lester R, et al. Open label study to evaluate the healing rate and safety of the profore extra four-layer bandage system in patients with leg ulceration. J Cutan Med Surg. 2000;4:8–11.
86. Johnson S. Compression hosiery in the prevention and treatment of venous leg ulcers. J Tissue Viability 2002;12:72–4.
87. Brem H, Tomic-Canic M, Tarnovskaya A, Ehrlich HP, Baskin-Bey E, Gill K, et al. Healing of elderly patients with diabetic foot ulcers, venous stasis ulcers and pressure ulcers. Surg Technol Int. 2003:11:161–7.
88. Kaur C, Sarkar R, Kanwar AJ, et al. An open trial of calcium dobesilate in patients with venous ulcers and stasis dermatitis. Int J Dermatol. 2003;42: 147–152.
89. Jaul E. Assessment and management of pressure ulcers in the elderly: current strategies. Drugs Aging 2010;27:311–325.
90. Weinberg JM, Scheinfeld NS. Cutaneous infections in the elderly: diagnosis and management. Dermatol Ther. 2003;16:195–205.
91. Sanford M, Keating GM. Zoster vaccine (zostavax): a review of its use in preventing herpes zoster and postherpetic neuralgia in older adults. Drugs Aging 2010;27:159–76.
92. Forsyth EL, Millard TP. Diagnosis and pharmacological treatment of chronic actinic dermatitis in the elderly: an update. Drugs Aging 2010;27:451–56.
93. Grant JE, Odlaug BL. Update on pathological skin picking. Curr Psychiatry Rep 2009; 11:283–8.
94. Loo WJ, Burrows NP. Management of autoimmune skin disorders in the elderly. Drugs Aging 2004; 21(12):767–77.
95. Akira Toyofuku, Miho Takenoshita, Haruhiko Miyako. Two cases of recovery from glossodynia in elderly patients with the use of sertraline. Japanese journal of psychosomatic dentistry. 2007; 22(2):84–7.

CHAPTER 4

Pruritus in Geriatrics

• *Bela Shah*

Key Points

- Pruritus is a very common complaint in geriatric age group.
- Many a times, these patients require detailed work-up.
- Many dermatological as well as systemic diseases are associated with pruritus.
- Pruritus may be paraneoplastic in nature especially in this age group.
- Pros and cons of first and second generation antihistamines are mandatory to learn.
- Systemic and topical steroids are to be used sparingly and with a caution.
- Therapies like opiates, agonists and antagonists are other therapeutic options available to us to address refractory cases.

Introduction

Pruritus is the most common complaint in people over the age of 60 years. 60% of the elderly individuals are affected by pruritus in more or less manner.[1] Pruritus in elderly imparts a diagnostic and therapeutic challenge to the treating physician. Aging skin is susceptible to pruritic disorders because of the cumulative effects that the environment has on the skin and because of changes to the skin structure that occur as we age. Chronic itch in elderly can be due to several causes, commonest due to dry skin (Fig. 4.1), immunosenescense and neural degeneration, many dermatological disorders and systemic conditions, such as end-stage renal disease and diabetes. Chronic itch impairs quality of life and results into sleep disturbances.

CHANGES OCCURRING IN SKIN IN OLD AGE

- Impaired skin barrier
- Impaired immune system response
- Reduction in subcutaneous fat
- Decreased skin turnover
- Decreased vascularity of skin
- Decreased sweat and sebaceous gland secretion.

Ageing primarily affects 3 systems of body, which leads to inflammation of skin and itching

1. Epidermal barrier function
2. Immune system
3. Skeletal and neural system

1. Epidermal Barrier Defect due to Ageing

The surface pH of the epidermis becomes alkaline with ageing. Alkaline pH affects enzymatic activity leading to decreased production of ceramides, decreased level of natural moisturizing factors and decreased lamellar body secretion. Initially they develop irritation after exposure to mild allergens. Increase in pH also increases activity of serine proteases which activate protease-activated receptor 2 (PAR2) receptors, which induce itch. Aquaporin-3, a glycerol and water membrane channel which maintains skin

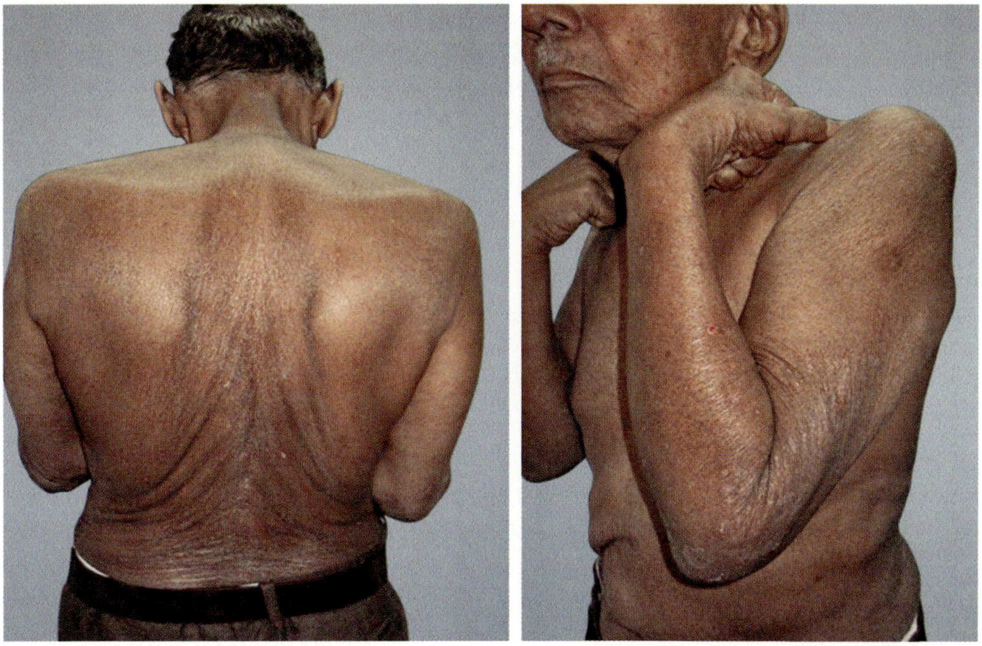

Fig. 4.1: Xerosis of skin

hydration is also reduced in age group. All these changes lead to defect in epidermal barrier, which make them prone to develop contact dermatitis.

2. Changes in Immune System due to Ageing (Immunosenescence)

Immunosenescence affects both innate and adaptive immunity, and has been associated with increased levels of autoreactivity. Bullous pemphigoid (BP), which is more common in the elderly, may manifest with itch and a nonspecific urticarial rash accompanied by circulating autoantibodies.

With age:

- The immune system becomes proinflammatory.
- There is aberration of T and B cell function which make them "allergic" phenotype, or there occurs an apparent Th2 dominance.
- There is loss of naive T cells, which reduce the T cell repertoire. It reduces the ability of patient to react effectively to infectious agents to which he/she has not been previously exposed.

3. Degenerative Musculoskeletal and Neural Changes with Age

Age-related changes in the nerves lead to increased touch and pain thresholds, possibly due to subclinical neuropathy.

Idiopathic itch in elderly patients in some cases may be a result of this subclinical neuropathy.

Most common sensory ganglionitis known to cause pruritus is shingles (herpes zoster) which can activate itch neurons.

Elderly patients frequently are afflicted with degenerative diseases of the spine. It leads to nerve impingement occurring during old age can lead to localised pruritus. *For example,* brachioradial pruritus and notalgia paresthetica.

Diabetes mellitus induced small fibre polyneuropathy also manifests as itch usually involving scalp and trunk.

CUTANEOUS CONDITIONS LEADING TO PRURITUS

Nummular eczema: It is an extremely pruritic skin condition, characterised by coin-shaped plaques. It can be considered as a late-onset form of atopic dermatitis.

There is decreased epidermal nerve fibres in patients with NE compared with healthy controls.[4] It is due to increased sensitivity to environmental aeroallergens compared with age-matched controls. This impaired cutaneous barrier may lead to increased susceptibility to allergic contact dermatitis to materials such as metals, soaps, and chemicals.

Seborrhoeic dermatitis (Fig. 4.2): It is characterised by erythematous patches and plaques with overlying adherent, greasy scales. Oily areas of the body, such as the scalp, eyebrows, eyelids, periauricular area, nasolabial folds, cheeks, sternal area and interscapular areas are mainly affected. The SD reported prevalence in the elderly population is 31%[2] and is also associated with localized itch. SD is a particularly common skin manifestation in elderly patients with Parkinson's disease, depression or anxiety.

Drugs like levodopa and carbidopa can cause itching as side effects.

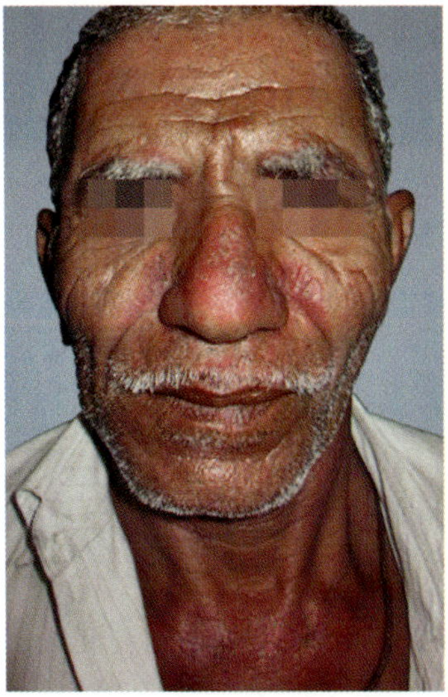

Fig. 4.2: Seborrhoeic dermatitis

Contact dermatitis: It results from direct skin exposure to chemical substance.

Studies have determined that the prevalence of allergic contact dermatitis in the elderly is between 33 and 64% in European countries.[3]

Contact dermatitis is divided into allergic and irritant forms. Allergic contact dermatitis consists of a reaction to an external stimulus that is mediated by the adaptive immune system, whereas irritant contact dermatitis consists of a non-specific reaction that is mediated by the innate immune system.

Skin barrier defects and immunosenescence are the risk factors for the development of contact dermatitis in the elderly. In addition to this, topical medications may cause contact dermatitis and hence prescribed with caution in this age group.

Chronic venous insufficiency (CVI), as a result of valvular incompetence, results in retrograde flow of blood in the lower extremities. CVI results in several skin manifestations, such as telangiectasias, reticular veins, varicose veins, oedema, pigmentation and lipodermatosclerosis. These skin changes increase the risk of chronic pruritus especially in elderly patients.

Psoriasis is chronic inflammatory disease, which is not uncommon in elderly. Associations have been made between psoriasis and metabolic syndrome, cardiovascular diseases, malignancy and psoriatic arthritis. Itch is the most common symptom in elderly psoriatic patients. Genital area evaluation is necessary in patients with psoriasis because of the high prevalence of genital itch in this population.

Chronic idiopathic urticaria (CIU) is a pruritic condition, characterised by the presence of wheals on a near daily basis for greater than 6 weeks. CIU is common in the elderly. It is usually described as "stinging, tickling, or burning sensation". The itch is often worse at night and may be triggered by ambient heat and sweating.

Bullous diseases: Bullous pemphigoid may be associated with pruritus. Intense and generalised pruritus precedes the development of skin lesions by periods greater than 3 months. Scratching can be so intense that in many cases blisters are uncommonly observed compared to secondary excoriations and crusting. Pruritus in dermatitis herpetiformis has burning, stinging or "firey" character, especially on the scalp.

Transient acantholytic dermatosis, or Grover's disease (GD) is characterised by very pruritic papules and papulovesicles affecting the trunk and proximal limbs. This disease most commonly affects elderly Caucasian men. Several factors have been related to Grover's disease, such as exposure to sunlight, hot temperatures and sweat. Malignancies and cutaneous infections are also associated with Grover's disease. Tumour necrosis factor-α and other inflammatory mediators are possible causes of itch in this disease.

Scabies is a parasitic infestation caused by the mite *Sarcoptes scabiei* (var. *hominis*). In elderly people, the scabies mite no longer respects the "preferential areas" of involvement. The finger webs may be completely spared. The face may have lesions. In the patient with "invisible" scabies, the number of lesions may be very limited, and a careful search of the finger webs, genitalia, navel, breasts of women, axillary lines, and soles of the feet is paramount. The soles are a particularly "rich" area to look for burrows in elderly people. They are at risk of developing crusted scabies (Norwegian scabies) due to immunosuppression and neuropathy.

In elderly patients, misdiagnosis can lead to unnecessary use of topical steroids, with a delay in proper diagnosis and treatment.

Basal cell carcinoma (BCC) is the most common skin cancer in the elderly. 32% of patients with BCC had itch, intensity correlates with the degree of inflammation and the type of inflammatory infiltrate.[4]

Advanced stages of **cutaneous T cell lymphoma (CTCL)** (Fig. 4.3) such as tumoral mycosis fungoides or erythroderma, present with intense itch. Folliculotropic MF is one of the variants, is associated with severe itching. In patients with CTCL associated with itch, increased interleukin 31 (IL-31) expression has been seen.[5]

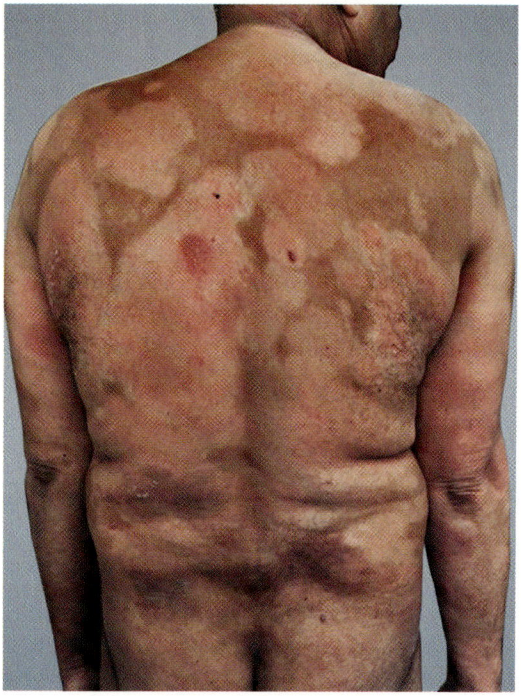

Fig. 4.3: Plaque stage of cutaneous T cell lymphoma

SYSTEMIC CAUSES OF PRURITUS

Various systemic conditions including renal diseases and liver diseases, various neoplasms, neural conditions and infectious conditions have been related to chronic itch. Systemic disorders manifest as pruritus with or without rash.

There is an increased risk of developing malignancies in elderly population and the itch related to cancer is known as **paraneoplastic itch**. New onset itch without a rash in elderly, we have to have a high index of suspicion for malignancy.

Various cancers such as low-grade lymphoma and other haematological malignancies, including chronic lymphocytic leukaemia (CLL) and multiple myeloma, are common in old age and are associated with chronic itch.

Hepatobiliary diseases also lead to chronic pruritus. It is known as cholestatic pruritus. Autotaxin (ATX) and lysophosphatidic acid (LPA) are the potential mediators of cholestatic pruritus. In cholestatic pruritus, liver transplantation may be the only treatment.

Itch associated with chronic kidney disease (CKD) may be referred to as **uremic pruritus** or CKD itch. The prevalence of CKD itch in geriatric patients has not been assessed. The glomerular filtration rate decreases with age. It is of interest to determine if there is any correlation between chronic itch and a decrease in the glomerular filtration rate.

Elderly people are affected by stroke more commonly. Itch has been anecdotally reported as a post-stroke complication. In patients of cerebrovascular accidents, pruritus develops in contralateral side.[5]

Trigeminal trophic syndrome (TTS) is a specific presentation of itch due to the infarction of the lateral medulla. This is characterised by intense pruritus in addition to facial ulceration in the area distributed by the trigeminal nerve.

In **HIV** patients, chronic itch is one of the most common dermatological complaints reported which affect the quality of life.

DRUGS CAUSING CHRONIC PRURITUS

Polypharmacy in elderly can cause drug interactions and the development of drug related itch. Drug-related itch use may be acute (lasting less than 6 weeks) or chronic and may present with or without a rash. It may present hours, weeks, months or years after drug ingestion. It may appear following the first dose of medication or at any other time during a treatment regimen.

When a medication is suspected to be the cause of itch, it should be discontinued. However, itch may persist for months following cessation of medication use.

List of drugs causing pruritus:

- Aspirin and other NSAIDs
- Penicillins
- Cephalosporins
- Fluoroquinolones
- Methoxsalen
- Vancomycin
- Antimalarials—chloroquine
- Hydroxyethyl starch
- Quinidine
- Amiodarone
- Iodinated contrast medium
- EGFR inhibitors
- Calcium channel blockers
- Angiotensin receptor blockers
- Thiazides
- Tamoxifen
- Bleomycin
- Opioid agonists
- Lithium
- Phenothiazines
- Nicotinic acid derivatives anticonvulsants
- Statins
- Benzodiazepines

PSYCHOGENIC CONDITIONS

Multiple psychiatric disorders have been related to itch: Depression, obsessive compulsive disorder, anxiety, somatoform disorders, mania, psychosis, substance abuse and delusion of parasitosis. Depression and anxiety disorders are especially common in elderly patients.

Chronic itch in certain dermatological conditions, such as psoriasis, LSC, nummular eczema and itch localized to the scalp and genital area is common in the elderly and can be exacerbated by anxiety or stress.

MANAGEMENT

History Taking

History taking is a important part to reach accurate diagnosis during examination. First, it is important to determine whether the patient has acute (<6 week) or chronic itch (>6 week). Various points to be covered are:

- Onset and total duration of itch
- Intensity
- Localization
- Course and variation during day
- Triggering factors
- Relieving/exacerbating factors
- Behavioural response to itch
- Association to bath
- Impairment in quality of life, burden, sleep disturbance
- Medications, including topical agents: Prescribed, over-the-counter: Duration of use and relationship to onset of pruritus
- Past medical history: Thyroid, liver or renal dysfunction, other systemic diseases
- Family history of atopy, skin disease or similar pruritic condition
- Personal history

Physical Examination

- Look for presence of primary lesions over entire skin including mucous membranes, scalp, hair, nails, and anogenital region.
- Lichenification is a secondary change that requires as much as 90 h of scratching, or as many as 140,000 scratches.
- Butterfly area of the back is a useful site for examination in neurotic itch.
- Examination of the genitalia for nodular scabies, LSC.
- Inspection of hair and nail to r/o systemic disease.
- Palpation of abdomen for organomegaly, major lymphatic groups, and the thyroid.

INVESTIGATIONS

Baseline evaluation:

- CBC with differential, ESR
- Thyroid function (TSH, T3, T4 levels)
- BUN, creatinine
- Alkaline phosphatase, bilirubin
- Fasting and post-prandial glucose levels
- Parathyroid function (calcium and phosphorus levels)
- Serum iron, ferritin
- Chest X-ray
- Stool for ova, parasites and occult blood
- Urinalysis
- Age-appropriate cancer screening
- Biopsy from primary skin lesion

General Measures

- Patient education is an important component of successful treatment of pruritus
- Frequent liberal application of emollients, especially after bathing
- Avoid hot and prolonged showers
- Avoid irritating soaps, and all soaps except to apocrine-gland bearing areas
- Avoid friction
- Keeping finger nails short
- Wearing soft and loose cotton clothing
- Avoiding cleansers with a high pH or those containing alcohol.

Topical Treatment

Emollients

It is considered as first-line therapy for localized itch, itch associated with CKD, and xerosis. They optimize skin barrier function and prevent excessive transepidermal water loss. Acidic topical treatments (pH 4.5–6) help maintain a low pH within the skin surface and reduce the activity of itch-inducing serine proteases.

The level of urea, a natural moisturizing factor, has been shown to be decreased within the SC of elderly patients. Use of urea may be beneficial in a variety of pruritic conditions, including xerosis, CKD itch, neuropathic itch, atopic dermatitis, contact dermatitis and psoriasis.

Menthol activates the transient receptor potential melastatin 8 (TRPM-8) receptor on A-delta afferents to elicit a cooling sensation. It is used as antipruritic agent at 1–5% concentration. It is short acting. Its effect lasts up to 30 minutes. Chronic use of menthol can lead to hypersensitivity and transient burning sensations.

Capsaicin (8-methyl-*N*-vanillyl-6-nonenamide) is an active component of chili peppers has been used in the treatment of postherpetic neuralgia, notalgia parasthetica and brachiradial pruritus. It causes local desensitization of peripheral nerves, perhaps through activation of transient receptor potential vanilloid 1 (TRPV-1) receptors. Burning sensation during the initial usage may limit its compliance. Pre-treatment with EMLA (lidocaine/prilocaine), has been shown to reduce this burning sensation.

Topical corticosteroids in chronic itch may be used in dermatological conditions such as psoriasis, LSC or NE, in which inflammation is the underlying aetiology. Long-term use should be avoided whenever possible as it leads to atrophy of skin.

Topical immunomodulators such as tacrolimus and pimecrolimus have promising results in pruritus of atopic dermatitis, seborrhoeic dermatitis, contact dermatitis.

Side effects include burning and stinging sensations.

Pramoxine, a local anaesthetic, has been shown to reduce itch in patients with CKD. Side effects include skin irritation and dryness at the site of application.

Topical 5% doxepin cream, a potent H1 and H2 antagonist, has been shown in a randomized, controlled trial to reduce pruritus in patients with atopic eczema. Side effects may include localized stinging or burning sensations, and drowsiness.

Systemic Agents

Antihistamines: First-generation antihistamines (hydroxyzine, diphenhydramine) and second-generation antihistamines (cetirizine, fexofenadine, loratadine) are useful in chronic pruritus.

Second-generation antihistamines are useful in the treatment of histamine-mediated pruritic conditions, such as chronic urticaria. First-generation antihistamines may also be useful in helping patients who experience nocturnal pruritus to sleep at night, because of their soporific effects.

Comparison between first and second generation antihistamines is given in Table 4.1.

TABLE 4.1: Antihistamine agents

First generation	Second generation
• Sedative	Less or no sedation
• Anticholinergic effects: Slurred speech, urinary retention, dry mouth, constipation	No anticholinergic effect
• Motor incoordination	No motor incoordination
• Impairment of psychomotor performance	No impairment of psychomotor function
• α-adrenergic blocking action → hypertension	Loratidine has cardiotoxic properties
• Genitourinary system—erectile dysfunction, dysuria	Less antipruritic effects

- Relatively safe drugs in liver dysfunction:
  - Chlorpheniramine
  - Mizolastine
  - Levocetrizine
  - Fexofenadine
  - Loratadine (low dose)
- Relatively safe in kidney dysfunction:
  - Chlorpheniramine
  - Hydroxyzine
  - Doxepin
  - Mizolastine
  - Loratadine (low dose)

- *Selective norepinephrine reuptake inhibitors:* Mirtazapine is an effective treatment for pruritus in patients with chronic leukaemia, systemic lymphoma, CTCL, CKD or cholestasis.

  Dose: 15–45 mg/day

  It may be useful in treating chronic pruritus in patients with comorbid anxiety and/or depression. Drowsiness, dry mouth, increase in appetite and weight gain can occur as side effects.
- *Selective serotonin reuptake inhibitors:* Paroxetine and fluvoxamine have been reported to have an antipruritic effect in patients with atopic dermatitis, systemic lymphoma or solid carcinomas. **Sertraline** reduces pruritus associated with chronic liver disease. Insomnia, dry mouth and sexual dysfunction are the side effects of paroxetine.

  Dose: Paroxetine: 10–40 mg PO qd

  Fluvoxamine: 25–150 mg PO qd

  Sertraline: 75–100 mg PO qd
- *Tricyclic antidepressants:* Amitriptyline can be useful in treating neuropathic itch. The anticholinergic side effects of this agent, such as urinary retention, constipation, dizziness, dry mouth, cardiac conduction abnormalities and blurred vision are more commonly seen in elderly patients as they are more susceptible.

  Doxepin, which acts as both a tricyclic antidepressant (TCA) and an H1 antagonist, may be used to treat psychogenic itch and NI.
- *μ-opioid receptor antagonists:* Naltrexone, a μ-opioid receptor antagonists is shown to be effective in cholestatic pruritus and atopic dermatitis. Side effects include nausea, loss of appetite, diarrhoea, hepatotoxicity and reversal of analgesia. These agents should be used with caution in the elderly population.

  Dose: 25–50 mg PO qd
- *Kappa-opioid agonists and μ-opioid antagonists:* Butorphanol, administered intranasally, has been shown to be an efficacious treatment for chronic, severe and intractable pruritus. Side effects include somnolence, dizziness, nausea and vomiting.

  Dose: Butorphanol: 1–4 mg intranasally qd

  Nalfurafine: 2.5–5 μg PO qd
- *Kappa-opioid agonists:* Nalfurafine is a kappa opioid agonist. This reduces itch in patients with uraemic pruritus who are undergoing haemodialysis. Side effects include insomnia and headache.
- *Analogues of gamma-aminobutyric acid:* Gabapentin and pregabalin are effective antipruritic agents, which act by inhibiting neuronal transmission. They are useful for itch due to CKD and treating neuropathic itch from conditions such as prurigo-nodularis, postherpetic itch and BRP.

  In the elderly, doses should be started low and titrated.

  Side effects include drowsiness, weight gain, ataxia, leg swelling, blurred vision and constipation. Withdrawal symptoms are common so cessation should be tapered.

  Dose: Gabapentine: 100–3600 mg PO qd

  Pregabalin: 150–300 mg PO qd
- *Thalidomide:* It is an immunomodulatory agent, has been used in the treatment of refractory pruritus due to CKD. It has also been mentioned as a potential treatment for paraneoplastic itch.
- *Selective neurokinin-1 receptor antagonists:* Aprepitant has been used in the treatment of chronic pruritus associated with seizary syndrome. It acts by preventing substance P from binding to its NK_1 receptor. Substance P, a tachykinin neuropeptide, mediates nausea pathways in the brainstem and itch pathways from the skin to spinal cord. Aprepitant can be used at a dose of 80 mg daily or for three consecutive days every two weeks at dosages of 125 mg on day 1 and 80 mg on days 2–3.

- *UVB phototherapy* is effective in treating uraemic pruritus, cholestatic pruritus and HIV-associated pruritus. In uremic pruritus, UVB phototherapy acts by induction of apoptosis of cutaneous mast cells and thus relieves itch. It also inhibits T-helper 1 (Th1)-mediated immune responses and promotes decreased IL-2 production.

  In elderly, the advantages of phototherapy include avoidance of drug interactions and compliance issues.

CONCLUSION

- In many cases of geriatric pruritus, 'pruritus' can not be dismissed as a vague complaint, as it may give a clue to underlying sinister systemic diseases like CKD or even internal malignancies.
- Disease quality of life may be severely impaired in few patients and it may result into sleep disturbances.
- In patients with impaired sleep, sedative antihistamines have a definitive role.
- Anticholinergic side effects of first generation antihistamines result in retention of urine and precipitation of glaucoma, hence needs to be avoided.

References

1. Beauregard S, Gilchrest BA. A survey of skin problems and skin care regimens in the elderly. Arch Dermatol 1987; 123:1638–43.
2. Fitzpatrick JE. Common inflammatory skin diseases of the elderly. Geriatrics. 1989; 44(7):40–6.
3. Balato A, Balato N, Di Costanzo L, Ayala F. Contact sensitization in the elderly. Clin Dermatol. 2011; 29(1):24–30.
4. Yosipovitch G, Mills KC, Nattkemper LA, Feneran A, Liang TH, et al. Association of pain and itch with depth of invasion and inflammatory cell constitution in skin cancer: results of a large clinicopathologic study. JAMA Dermatol. 2014; 150(11):1160–6.
5. Singer EM, Shin DB, Nattkemper LA, Benoit BM, Klein RS, et al. IL-31 is produced by the malignant T-cell population in cutaneous T cell lymphoma and correlates with CTCL pruritus. J Invest Dermatol. 2013; 133(12):2783–5.

CHAPTER 5

Eczema in Elderly

• *Asit Mittal* • *Kapil Vyas*

Key Message

- Proportion of geriatric population is continuously growing and so is the prevalence of elderly eczema.
- Age-related barrier dysfunction, immunosenescence and neural degeneration make integument susceptible to eczema.
- Different clinico-morphologically patterns of eczema seen in older population are influenced by environment, cultural practices, comorbidities, and lifestyle.
- The eczematous process secondary to drugs and systemic diseases, needs special attention due to their different course and prognosis.
- Key to successful management is holistic approach addressing multiple factors that aggravate eczema and optimum use of the available therapy in cost effective manner.

Introduction

The integument is the dynamic tissue that changes across the ages. The characteristic structural and physiochemical changes associated with the ageing process make elderly skin prone to myriad dematoses and eczema are no exceptions.[1,2] Eczema is the common concern in the elderly subjects and is the leading cause of localized and generalized pruritus.

Aging-specific changes; that is, the immunosenescence, hormonal changes, barrier dysfunctions, appendageal hypoactivity, and neural degeneration underlie the higher prevalence of eczema in elderly.[3] Moreover, presence of comorbidities, exposure to various medications, psychogenic factors may further dictate the course and prognosis of various eczema in elderly.[4–6] Most of complications secondarily to eczema in the elderly are preventable or treatable, so proper skin care and treatment should be emphasized in general health care for the elderly. In this section we will discuss various eczemas seen in the geriatric population.

EPIDEMIOLOGY

Eczema is one of the commonest dermatoses of elderly with prevalence varying from country to country. The geriatric population is continuously growing and so is the prevalence of geriatric eczema.[7] Studies from different geographical areas reveal differing statistical data on various epidemiological determinants of eczema in elderly subjects.[8–12] In India, there is scarcity of studies on various eczematous conditions in the elderly people though several studies have been carried out in the west. Age, gender, ethinicity, climatic conditions, cultural practices can all contribute to varying patterns of eczematous dermatoses.[13,14] A study from Turkey conducted on 4099 geriatric patients found eczematous dermatitis to be the most common disorder in the population studied.[1] Similarly, studies from Singapore,[14] Taiwan[15] and UK[16] revealed eczematous dermatitis as the leading cause of skin problem in elderly subjects.

Various Indian studies, revealed that, approximately one-third of the geriatric population had eczema of different clinico-morphological type.[17,18]

Broadly, eczema in elderly, can be divided into endogenous and exogenous types but in clinical scenario, considerable overlap is seen between the two types. Asteotic eczema is the most common endogenous eczema in elderly followed by nummular, stasis, atopic and seborrheic eczema.[19] Infectious dermatitis has been reported to be the most common cause of exogenous eczema followed by contact dermatitis (allergic or irritant).[20,21] It is hypothesized that allergic contact dermatitis, would be less prevalent in elderly owing to shift of balance to Th2 response. The pattern and distribution of different eczema may also be influenced by humidity, temperature, seasonal changes, and cultural practices. Several triggering factors specific to elderly population such as poor dietary and fluid intake, multiple medications, physical limitations, urinary or faecal incontinence, mental state, personal hygiene and chronic illness may induce or exacerbate the eczematous dermatitis in elderly subjects.[22]

Pathophysiology of Eczema in Elderly

To understand, the pathophysiology of eczematous disorders in elderly patients, it is important to consider changes in the integument across ageing. Physiological changes that occur with ageing and that may play an important role in causation of eczema are: (a) **Epidermal barrier dysregulation**, (b) **Immunosenescence**; (c) **Neurodegeneration.** Physical inactivity, hormonal influences, appendageal hypoactivity, and comorbidities associated with ageing may further contribute to eczematous process.

Epidermal Barrier Dysregulation

The cutaneous permeability barrier resides in the outer layer of the epidermis, the stratum corneum (SC) which is both metabolically active and interactive with the underlying nucleated cell layers of the epidermis.[23,24] With ageing, rate of production of lipids and aquaporin-3 gene expression is reduced resulting in defects in epidermal barrier function and hydration.[25,26] In addition to this metabolic perturbation, abnormalities in amphiregulin and interleukin 1α signalling of barrier homeostasis in aged epidermis, results in altered threshold to proinflammatory and immunological stimuli and resultant eczematous dermatitis.[27,28] In addition to these intrinsic tissue specific alteration, the role of extrinsic factors cannot be neglected. Use of soaps, contact with hot and hard water and vigorous rubbing of skin for cleaning are such extrinsic factors that may contribute to barrier disruption and delayed repair. Barrier defects further facilitate the entry of irritants, pathogens and allergens, and promote the expression of pro-inflammatory cytokines responsible for systemic sensitization.

Immunosenescence

Immunosenescence involves thymic involution and subsequent age-related declines in T cell functions. Naïve T cells are reduced with ageing, but memory T cells are concomitantly increased.[29,30] The pool of allergen-specific T_{reg} cells which have a role in peripheral immune tolerance is maintained by the expansion of existing naïve and memory-like T_{reg} cells, and possible conversion of non-regulatory T cells (e.g. Th17 cells) into T_{reg} cells. However, such renewal may lead to alterations in phenotypes. and functions of T_{reg} cells, resulting in collapsed immune tolerance and activation of hypersensitivity reactions to environmental allergens/antigens in elderly patients.[31] Also tendency for the systemic Th1/Th2 balance to shift towards Th2 cytokine responses with aging might also be associated with the etiology of elderly eczema.[32] It has been observed that sex hormones influence the immune system in humans. Decline in androgen and estrogen level with ageing may alter cytokine milieu (IL-4 vs INF-γ) and production capacity of T cells.[33]

Degenerative Skeletal and Neural Disease

Elderly patients frequently are affected with degenerative diseases of bone and nervous system which may produce itching.[34] This along with age specific triggers, may lead to chronic itch scratch cycle that further disrupt barrier function by inflicting repeated trauma.[35,36]

CLINICAL FEATURES

The chief complaint of elderly is often a pruritic rash heralding an eczematous disease. Clinically, eczematous dermatoses are characterised by variable degree of itching, redness, excoriation, exudation, papulation and vesiculation in early course and fissuring, hyperkeratosis, lichenification, and scaling with chronicity. The different clinico-morphologically patterns of eczema in older population, that are seen commonly in clinical practice are asteotic eczema, stasis eczema, seborrheic eczema, nummular eczema , atopic eczema, hand eczema and contact dermatitis. The eczematous process secondary to drugs and systemic diseases, also needs attention due to their different course and prognosis.

Asteatotic eczema, also known as ''eczema craquele''occur mainly in dry environment with low relative humidity and is seen in patients who have dry skin. In addition to ageing, xerotic skin may be seen in atopic eczema, chronic renal or liver failure, AIDS, myxedema, malabsorption states and diuretic therapy.[37] Asteatotic eczema occurs most often on the anterolateral portion of the lower legs with cracked porcelain or ''crazy paving'' appearance (Fig. 5.1).

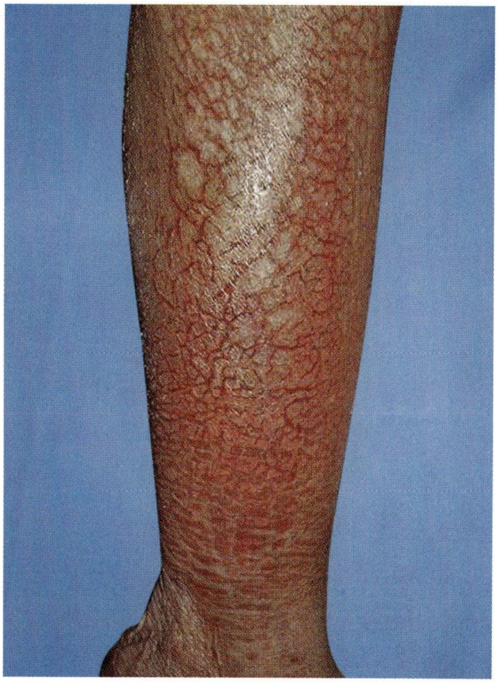

Fig. 5.1: Crazy pavement appearance seen in asteatotic eczema

Stasis dermatitis, also known as venous eczema, affects around 6–7% of elderly subjects.[38] Venous skin changes usually develop in swollen legs in the presence of established chronic venous hypertension, which in turn is due to defective or damaged bileaflet valves in the legs. Pitting oedema and pigmentatry changes due to haemosiderin deposition are often present. These pigment changes are commonly known as staining and are important indicator of venous disease. The affected skin is itchy, erythematous and scaly, and may ooze, crust and crack. Venous eczema often coexists with lipodermatosclerosis that can be misdiagnosed as cellulitis. An acute exacerbation of stasis dermatitis can result in "id" reaction or autosensitization dermatitis, producing a secondary, acute, papulovesicular, often symmetrical distribution on the extremities. In setting of stasis dermatitis, allergic contact dermatitis is not uncommon due to frequent use of potential sensitizers (Fig. 5.2).

Seborrhoeic dermatitis is a chronic relapsing inflammatory skin disorder clinically characterized poorly defined erythematous patches and greasy scales. It usually affects seborrhoeic

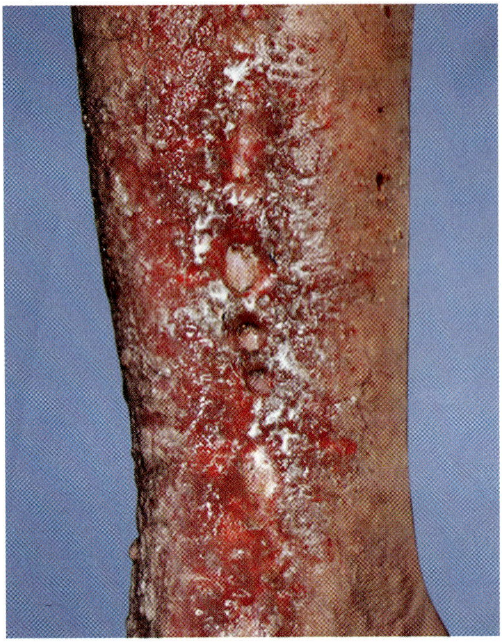

Fig. 5.2: Allergic contact dermatitis superimposed on venous stasis eczema

areas such as scalp, face, chest, back, and flexures. The prevalence of adult seborrheic dermatitis is estimated at 5%. Although the exact cause of seborrheic dermatitis has yet to be understood, *Malassezia yeasts*, hormones (androgens), sebum levels and immune response are known to play important roles in its development. Additional factors including drugs, winter temperatures and stress may exacerbate seborrhoeic dermatitis. The incidence is much higher in those with HIV infection and Parkinson's disease.[39]

Nummular eczema is morphological type of eczema characterised by multiple coin-shaped eczematous lesions, most commonly affecting the extremities and trunk.[40] It may be associated with atopy, infections, alcohol, drugs and the contact allergens.[41,42] Positive patch test to the allergen *Dermatophagoides farinae* and the house dust allergen were reported in elderly patients with nummular eczema.[43] Clinical relevance of positive patch tests is yet not known in this entity.

Contact dermatitis: Contact dermatitis can be classified into irritant contact dermatitis and allergic contact dermatitis. Delayed repair of the aged epidermal barrier after skin irritation is of high relevance in the development of irritant contact dermatitis. In the elderly, ICD as well as ACD are often found on the hands and in the perineal region in older incontinent patients.[44] Asteatotic and perineal irritant dermatitis are the most important subtypes of irritant contact dermatitis in the elderly.[45]

Patients coming from rural background use detergent soap for cleansing skin. This may severely compromise their skin barrier and increased chances of ICD. Similarly, use of medicated soaps (chlorxylenol) can produce dryness and itch, consistent with asteatotic ICD.

Other important chemical and physical irritants include solvents oil, acids and alkalis, heat, sweat, ultraviolet (UV) irradiation, and occlusion.[46]

Perineal or incontinence dermatitis is typical for older individuals and is mostly related to urinary or fecal incontinence, or both.[47] There is risk of superinfection with *Staphylococcus aureus*, and candidiasis.[48] In severe cases, ulcers may develop. Depending on the type of incontinence, the disease begins in the perianal (fecal incontinence) or vulvar region (urine incontinence).[49]

Theoretically, risk of allergic contact dermatitis should be low in elderly subjects as previously discussed, however, in clinical practice this may not be true. If any eczema is not responding to the usual measures or is getting worse after some topical application, possibility of ACD should be considered. Some of the contact allergen seems important in the Indian context are related to various cultural practices, viz. para-tertiary butyl phenol in bindi dermatitis as seen in married woman of India.[50] PPD as in hair dye dermatitis in elderly subjects. Another unusual cause in India is parthenium dermatitis, a phytophotodermatitis due to the plant parthenium hysterophorus, which grows wild and causes an intractable allergic contact dermatitis.[51] Patch test with different allergens are usually required to confirm such cases.

Atopic eczema, is a chronic, relapsing, severely pruritic eczematous dermatitis, characterized by allergic inflammation and skin barrier defects. Previously, considered as a pediatric disease. It is now, frequently reported in elderly subjects.[52] New subgroup of elderly AE has been added to the classification of AE.[53] Clinical and histopathological features of elderly AE have been characterised as both IgE-mediated allergic and non-IgE-mediated allergic forms. Most frequent environmental allergens involved in the IgE-mediated allergic form are house dust mites (e.g. *Dermatophagoides* species), followed by pollens and foods.[54] Skin manifestations of elderly patients with atopic eczema (AE) include atopic red face with Hertoghe's sign, diffuse eczematous erythema; atopic hand eczema, nummular eczema, prurigo nodularis, lichenified eczema of the flexures with scarcely involving folds (reverse sign).

Psychogenic eczema includes disorders such as lichen simplex chronicus, prurigo nodularis, neurotic excoriations, and delusions of parasitosis. These disorders have either their onset primarily as dermatological disease, viz. atopy or having psychiatric element right from outset.[55]

Neurogenic eczema (autonomic denervation eczema), SKINTED, an acronym for "surgery of the knee, injury to infrapatellar branch of saphenous nerve and traumatic eczematous dermatitis" has been recently described in Indian patients. It is thought to be due to nerve injury following knee replacement surgery, thereby, disturbing the sensory functions of the skin leading to xerosis and inflammation.[56]

Eczematous conditions associated with systemic causes and drugs

Eczema are associated with comorbidities of ageing such as hypertension, diabetes, thyroid diseases, epilepsy, asthma, and malignancies. Comorbidity of ageing also predispose subjects to polypharmacy which may be responsible for eczematous drug eruptions. CCBs and ACE inhibitors have been reported with eczema, drugs such as statins causes eczemas by disrupting barrier.[57]

DIAGNOSIS AND MANAGEMENT

Eczema in elderly is essentially a clinical diagnosis, however, skin biopsy may be needed occasionally where eczema mimics as psoriasis or mycosis fungoides. Patch test may aid in detection of different allergens in situation of allergic contact dermatitis. Serum IgE may help to detect underlying atopic state. Battery of routine hematological, biochemical, endocrinal and microbiological laboratory studies are justified in detecting ageing specific causes responsible for eczematous eruptions of senescence (Table 5.1). Usually, eczema in elderly is chronic relapsing condition and successful management includes searching for underlying etiology and removing triggers responsible for recurrent flares[58] (Table 5.2).

TABLE 5.1: Differential diagnosis of eczematous eruptions in elderly

- Atopic dermatitis
- Contact dermatitis (both allergic and irritant)
- Cutaneous T cell lymphoma (mycosis fungoides, Sézary syndrome)
- Atypical psoriasis
- Eczema-like cutaneous drug eruption (especially in polymedicated elderly patients)
- Seborrhoeic dermatitis
- Factitious dermatitis
- Dermatophytosis
- Scabies
- Dermatitis herpetiformis
- Ichthyosis
- Actinic prurigo
- Erythroderma due to other causes

Adapted: Silvestre Salvador JF, et al. J Investig Allergol Clin Immunol, 2017.

TABLE 5.2: Usual triggers for eczema

- Xerotic skin
- Woolen clothings
- Skin infections
- Irritants and allergens (detergents, dust mites, pollen)
- Low humidity heat, sweating
- Physical inactivity and emotional stress

Adapted: Silvestre Salvador JF, et al. J Investig Allergol Clin Immunol, 2017.

Principles in management of elderly eczema are:

a. Restoration of the Skin Barrier

Most patients with eczema have sensitive skin that is prone to xerosis and irritation. Using hypoallergenic skin care products, liberal use of emollients and optimizing the bathing method may promote the integrity of the skin's barrier function. Limiting bathing to ten minutes per day, replacing high pH based soap with syndet soap, using warm (rather than hot) water, will help to minimize barrier disruption.

b. Reducing Inflammatory Drive

Depending upon the severity of eczema and the body surface area involved by it, either topical, systemic or physical mode of therapies may be required for controlling inflammation. An overview of treatment options is provided in Table 5.3. Mild to moderate eczema, can be controlled with topical therapy while more severe disease usually require phototherapy or systemic therapy.

TABLE 5.3: Overview of treatment options in eczema

Topical therapy		Simple moisturizers (petroleum jelly) are the most useful option. Liberal use to be practiced Barrier enhancing creams Topical corticosteroids (consider pitfalls of its use in the frail skin) Topical calcineurin inhibitors
Phototherapy		Narrowband UVB (311 nm), broadband UVB (280–315 nm) (available at equipped centres) UVA (315–400 nm), UVA 1 (340–400 nm) (not available widely in India)
Systemic therapies	Anti-inflammatory and immunomodulators	Corticosteroids Cyclosporine, azathioprine, methotrexate, mycophenolate mofetil
	Antipruritic	Sedating and non-sedating antihistaminics (chlorpheniramine, cetrizine, loratadine, ebastine) Neuromodulators of itch (SSRIs, opiates, antipsychotics, anticonvulsants)
	Anti-infectives	Penicillins, cephalosporins, FQ, vancomycin, linezolide, rifampicin, amikacin, etc.
Newer therapies		Interferon-γ Omalizumab Mepalizumab Intravenous immunoglobulin Tumor necrosis factor-alpha inhibitors Rituximab
Lifestyle interventions		Healthy diets, exercise, proper bathing technique, avoidance of irritants, humidification, stress management

For mild disease, topical steroids with liberal use of emollients are the first choice. Judicious use of topical steroid is warranted considering thin skin of elderly subjects and issue of systemic absorption. Topical corticosteroids work by activation of nuclear glucocorticoid receptors to alter expression of cytokines involved in the inflammatory response.[59] Topical calcineurin inhibitors are second line agents for episodic flare and inhibit the immune response in a more targeted fashion. The most effective therapeutic approach is combining and sequencing the therapy to gain maximum benefit yet avoiding side effect of individual agents. Prescription barrier creams containing hyaluronic acid, telmesteine, *Vitis vinifera* and glycyrrhetinic acid, which have moisturizing, anti-inflammatory, and antioxidant properties are another useful agents with multitude action. For moderate to severe eczema, physical therapy and systemic agents are required. Physical therapy in form of NBUVB may be a good alternate in the elderly subjects due to its less interaction with drugs and favourable adverse effect profile.[60] It also overcomes some of the physical and cognitive concern that are the reason for noncompliance with other treatment modalities. The disadvantage with this modality is its availability at the higher centres only and the need for frequent visits. This is why it has failed to gain the wide acceptance. Systemic therapy consists of medication that can reduce inflammation and target the itch scratch cycle. Systemic agents include antihistaminics, corticosteroids, and steroid sparing agents such as cyclosporine, methotrexate, azathioprine, mycophenolate mofetil, and most recently leflunamide.[61] Systemic steroids although useful cannot be used for long periods in elderly subjects for obvious reasons, however short-term use of low dose prednisolone is well justified to achieve control over the stubborn eczema. Low dose methotrexate in dose of 5–7.5 mg per week is an another cost effective alternate in elderly subjects but interactions with drugs should be cautiously evaluated. To effectively target the itch scratch cycle, antihistaminics should be considered along with immune modulation. The nonsedating antihistaminics are safer but are nonefficacious. Sedative antihistaminics have greater efficacy but there is concern about impaired cognition so one has to strike a right balance by starting with low dose and gradually escalating the dose. Today, a range of anti-pruritic medications are available and among them neuromodulating agents are gaining popularity.[62] Use of neuromodulating agents such as SSRIs, antiepileptics, antipsychotics are increasing and physician can choose them depending on their expertise.

c. Addressing Complications

It seems prudent to prevent or treat the complications at an early stage. Infections are the most often seen complication and should be managed with timely administration of antibiotics. Erythroderma is fortunately rare complication but a medical emergency that should be dealt in ICU settings. The management of erythroderma is beyond the scope of this chapter.

d. Proper Counselling and Lifestyle Modification

One cannot underestimate the role of counselling and lifestyle modification in the management of eczema. Dietary modification, exercise, skin hydration, stress reduction, and proper compliance along with trigger avoidance is needed to avoid acute flare and maintaining remissions. Therapeutic patient education and a psychodermatological approach are also useful approach for modifying habitual scratching.[63]

Finally, the treatment should be tailored according to the individual needs. The most effective therapy will involve short-term treatment of flares with long-term maintenance approach to skin care designed to prevent or minimize flares. In recent years, new groups of therapeutics as immunotherapy and biologics are on the horizon, but only time will tell, how useful and safe they will be in elderly eczema.

CONCLUSION

Eczema in elderly subjects is a common and chronic relapsing condition which is often frustrating for both patients and treating physician. This need to be addressed in a systematic way with formulation of standard protocol for diagnosis and management and optimizing the benefits of therapy by curtailing down the adverse effect in a cost effective manner.

References

1. Norman RA. Geriatric dermatology. Dermatol Ther. 2003; 16:260–8.
2. Farage MA, Miller KW, Elsner P, Maibach HI. Characteristics of the Aging Skin. Adv Wound Care (New Rochelle). 2013; 2:5–10.
3. Tanei R, Hasegawa Y. Atopic dermatitis in older adults: A viewpoint from geriatric dermatology. Geriatr Gerontol Int. 2016; 16 (Suppl. 1):75–86
4. Nair PA, Vora RJ. Association of systemic diseases with cutaneous dermatosis in elderly population: preliminary observation at a rural tertiary care centre. Family Med Prim Care. 2015; 4:74–78.
5. Joly P, Benoit-Corven C, Baricault S, et al. Chronic eczematous eruptions of the elderly are associated with chronic exposure to calcium channel blockers: results from a case-control study. J Invest Dermatol 2007; 127:2766–71.
6. Klockk M, Gotestamet KG, Mykletun A. Factor accounting for association between anxiety and depression and eczema, BMC Dermatol. 2010; 10:3.
7. Rajan SI, Sarma PS, Mishra US. Demography of Indian aging, 2001–2051. J Aging Soc Policy. 2003; 15:11–30.
8. Polat M, Ýlhan MN, Dermatological complaint of elderly attending a dermatology outpatient clinic in Turkey, Acta Dermatovenerol Croat. 2015; 23:277–81.
9. Jindal R, Jain A , Roy S, Rawat SDS, Bhardwaj N. Skin Disorders Among Geriatric Population at a Tertiary Center in Uttarakhand. J Clin Diagn Res. 2016; 10:WC06–WC08.
10. Yalcin B, Tamer E, Toy GG, Oztas P, Hayran M, Alli N. The prevalence of skin diseases in the elderly: analysis of 4099 geriatric patients. Int J Dermatol. 2006;45:672–76.
11. Bilgili G, Karadag AS, Ozkol HU, Calka O, Akdeniz N. The prevalence of skin diseases among the geriatric patients in Eastern Turkey. J Pak Med Assoc. 2012; 62:535–39.
12. Smith DR, Kubo H, Tang S, Yamagata Z. Skin disease among staff in a Japanese nursing home. J Occup Health. 2003; 45:60–2.
13. Patange VS, Fernandez RJ. A study of geriatric dermatoses. Ind J Dermatol Venerol Leprol. 1995; 61:206–8.
14. Yap BK, Siew GM, Goh LC. Pattern of skin diseases in the elderly at the National Skin Centre (Singapore) 1990. Singapore Med J 1994; 35:147–150.
15. Liao YH, Chen KH, Tseng MP, Sun CC. Pattern of skin diseases in a geriatric population in Taiwan: a 7-year survey from the outpatient clinic of a university medical center. Dermatology 2001; 203: 308–313.
16. Deo MS, Kerse N, Vandai AC, Jarrett P. Dermatological disease in the older age group: a cross-sectional study in aged care facilities. BMJ Open 2015; 5:e009941.
17. Sayal SK, Rajbhandari S, Malkit AK, Gupta CM. A study of dermatological disorders in geriatric age group. Indian Journal of Dermatol Venereal Leprol. 1998; 64:270–2.
18. Goyal A, Balai M, Mittal A, Khare AK, Gupta LK. Pattern of geriatric dermatoses at a Tertiary Care Teaching Hospital of South Rajasthan, India. Our Dermatol Online. 2017; 8:237–41.
19. Ingram J. Eczematous disorders. In: Griffiths C, Barker J, Blekier T, Chalmers R, Creamer D (eds) Rook's Textbook of Dermatology 2016; 39:1–31.
20. Suter-Widmer J, Elsner P. Age and irritation. In: van der Valk PGM, Maibach H, editors. The irritant contact dermatitis syndrome. Boca Raton: CRC Press; 1996. p. 257–61.
21. Farage MA, Miller KW, Berardesca E, Maibach HI. Incontinence in the aged: contact dermatitis and other cutaneous consequences. Contact Dermatitis 2007; 57:211–7.

22. Kim BJ, Lee SY, Kim HB, Lee E, Hong SJ. Environmental changes, microbiota, and allergic diseases. Allergy Asthma Immunol Res. 2014; 6: 389–400.

23. Schurer NY, Elias PM. The biochemistry and function of stratum corneum lipids. Adv Lipid Res. 1991; 24:27–56.

24. Elias PM, Wood LC, Feingold KR. Epidermal pathogenesis of inflammatory dermatoses. Am J Contact Dermat. 1999; 10:119–26.

25. Jensen JM, Förl M, Winoto-Morbach S, et al. Acid and neutral sphingomyelinase, ceramide synthase, and acid ceramidase activities in cutaneous aging. Exp Dermatol. 2005; 14:609–18.

26. Li J, Tang H, Hu X, et al. Aquaporin-3 gene and protein expression in sun-protected human skin decreases with skin ageing. Australas J Dermatol. 2010; 51:106–12.

27. Gilchrest B, Stoff J, Soter N. Chronologic aging alters the response to ultraviolet induced inflammation in human skin. J Invest Dermatol. 1982; 79:47–53.

28. Thivolet J, Nicolas JF. Skin aging and immune competence. Br J Dermatol. 1990; 122:77–81.

29. Hirokawa K. Immunity and aging. In: Pathy J, ed. Principles and Practice of Geriatric Medicine. New York: John Wiley and Sons, 1998; 35–47.

30. Czesnikiewicz-Guzik M, Lee WW, Cui D, et al. T cell subset-specific susceptibility to aging. Clin Immunol 2008; 127:107–18.

31. Fessler J, Ficjan A, Duftner C, Dejaco C. The impact of aging on regulatory T cells. Front Immunol. 2013; 4:231.

32. Sandmand M, Bruunsgaard H, Kemp K, et al. Is ageing associated with a shift in the balance between type 1 and type 2 cytokines in humans Clin Exp Immunol. 2002; 127:107–14.

33. Pietschmann P, Gollob E, Brosch S, et al. The effect of age and gender on cytokine production by human peripheral blood mononuclear cells and markers of bone metabolism. Exp Gerontol. 2003; 38:1119–27.

34. Veien NK, Laurberg G. Brachioradial pruritus: A follow-up of 76 patients. Acta Derm Venereol. 2011; 91:183–85.

35. Canavero S, Bonicalzi V, Massa-Micon B. Central neurogenic pruritus: A literature review. Acta Neurol Belg. 1997; 97:244–47.

36. Yamaoka H, Sasaki H, Yamasaki H, et al. Truncal pruritus of unknown origin may be a symptom of diabetic polyneuropathy. Diabetes Care. 2010; 33:150–55.

37. EllisC, et al. Cost of atopic dermatitis and eczema in the United States. J Am Acad Dermatol. 2002; 46:361–70.

38. Sundaresan S, Migden MR, Silapunt S. Stasis Dermatitis: Pathophysiology, Evaluation, and Management. Am J Clin Dermatol. 2017; 18: 383–90.

39. Bukviæ Mokos Z, Kralj M, Basta-Juzbašiæ A, Lakoš Jukiæ I. Seborrheic dermatitis: an update. Acta Dermatovenerol Croat. 2012; 20(2):98–104.

40. Rollins TG. From xerosis to nummular dermatitis. The dehydration dermatosis. JAMA. 1968; 206:637.

41. Fleming C, Parry E, Forsyth A, Kemmett D. Patch testing in discoid eczema. Contact Dermatitis. 1997; 36:261–64.

42. Adachi A, Horikawa T, Takashima T, Ichihashi M. Mercury-induced nummular dermatitis. J Am Acad Dermatol. 2000; 43:383–85.

43. Aoyama H, Tanaka M, Hara M, Tabata N, Tagami H. Nummular eczema: An addition of senile xerosis and unique cutaneous reactivities to environmental aeroallergens. Dermatology. 1999; 199:135–39.

44. Frosch PJ. Cutaneous irritation. In: Rycroft RCG, Menne T, Frosch PJ, Benezra C, editors. Textbook of Contact Dermatitis. Berlin: Springer; 1992. p. 28–61.

45. Seyfarth F. et al. Dry skin, barrier function, and irritant contact dermatitis in the elderly Clin Dermatol. 2011; 29:31–36.

46. Farage MA, Miller KW, Berardesca E, Maibach HI. Incontinence in the aged: contact dermatitis and other cutaneous consequences. Contact Dermatitis 2007; 57:211–17.

47. Roberts RO, Jacobsen SJ, Reilly WT, et al. Prevalence of combined fecal and urinary incontinence: a community-based study. J Am Geriatr Soc 1999; 47:837–41.

48. Gray M. Preventing and managing perineal dermatitis: a shared goal for wound and continence care. J Wound Ostomy Continence Nurs 2004; 31:S2–9.

49. Elsner P, Maibach HI. The effect of prolonged drying on transepidermal water loss, capacitance and pH of human vulvar and forearm skin. Acta Derm Venereol. 1990; 70:105–9.
50. Ghosh S, Mukhopadhyay S. Chemical leucoderma: a clinicoaetiological study of 864 cases in the perspective of a developing country. Br J Dermatol. 2009; 160:40–47.
51. Lakshmi C, Srinivas CR. Parthenium: a wide angle view. Indian J Dermatol Venereol Leprol. 2007; 73:296–306.
52. Tanei, R. Atopic dermatitis in the elderly. Inflamm. Allergy Drug Targets 2009; 8:394–404.
53. Bieber, T, Bussmann, C. Atopic dermatitis. In Dermatology, 3rd ed.; Bolognia, JL, Jorizzo, JL, Schaffer, JV, Eds.; Elsevier: Amsterdam, The Netherlands, 2012; 1:203–17.
54. Tanei, R, Katsuoka, K. Clinical analyses of atopic dermatitis in the aged. J. Dermatol. 2008; 35: 562–69.
55. Fried RG. Evaluation and treatment of "psychogenic" pruritus and self excoriation. J Am Acad Dermatol 1994; 30:993–99.
56. Madke B, Mhatre M, Kumar P, Singh AL, Patki A. Autonomic denervation dermatitis: A new type of eczematous dermatitis. Clin Dermatol Rev. 2017; 1:61–64.
57. Summers EM, Bingham CS, Dahle KW, Sweeney C, Ying J, Sontheimer RD. Chronic eczematous eruptions in the aging: further support for an association with exposure to calcium channel blockers. JAMA Dermatol. 2013; 149:814–18.
58. Eichenfield LF, et al. Guidelines of care for the management of atopic dermatitis: Section 1. Diagnosis and assessment of atopic dermatitis. J Am Acad Dermatol. 2014; 70:338–51.
59. Hanifin JM, Cooper KD, Ho VC, et al. Guidelines of care for atopic dermatitis, developed in accordance with the American Academy of Dermatology (AAD)/American Academy of Dermatology Association" Administrative Regulations for Evidence-based Clinical Practice Guidelines". J Am Acad Dermatol. 2004; 50:391–404.
60. Reynolds NJ, Franklin V, Gray JC, Diffey BL, Farr PM. Narrowband ultraviolet B and broad-band ultraviolet A phototherapy in adult atopic eczema: a randomised controlled trial. Lancet. 2001; 357:2012–16.
61. Spergel JM. Immunology and treatment of atopic dermatitis. Am J Clin Dermatol. 2008; 9:233–44.
62. Szepietowski JC, Weisshaar E (eds). Itch—Management in Clinical Practice. Curr Probl Dermatol. Basel, Karger, 2016; 50:192–201.
63. Tanei R. Clinical Characteristics, Treatments, and Prognosis of Atopic Eczema in the Elderly J. Clin. Med. 2015; 4:979–97.

CHAPTER 6

Chronic Venous Insufficiency in Elderly

• *Sudip Das* • *Indrashis Podder* • *Aarti Sarda*

Introduction

Chronic venous insufficiency (CVI) is a relatively under reported condition which often results in significant morbidity, adversely affecting the quality of life. This condition may present with a plethora of varied manifestations, thus obscuring the diagnosis at the early stages. CVI refers to a cluster of conditions occurring due to disturbed venous circulation of the lower extremities, characterised by persistent ambulatory venous hypertension leading to various pathologies, including pain, oedema, skin changes, and ulcerations. If untreated, more advanced forms of venous pathologies may occur like hyperpigmentation, venous eczema, lipodermatosclerosis, atrophied blanche, and healed or active ulcers.[1] Varicose veins are the commonest manifestations of CVI, usually associated with reflux of the great saphenous vein (GSV).[2]

The incidence of this condition varies greatly by geographic location. It is primarily a disease of the Western hemisphere, affecting almost 25% of their adult population.[2] This condition shows a female preponderance [female:male 3:1]; although recent reports indicate a higher male prevalence.[3–4] The prevalence increases with advancing age, most cases being reported >50 years age.[2]

Etiopathogenesis

Normal Venous Anatomy and Function

It is of foremost importance to first understand the normal venous anatomy and function to imbibe a clear idea regarding the etiopathogenesis of CVI. The peripheral venous system is a reservoir to pool blood and subsequently returns it to the heart acting as a conduit.

The veins of the lower extremity are further divided into superficial, deep, and perforator veins depending on their position relative to the muscle fascia.[4] The superficial venous system (located above the muscular fascial layer) comprises an interconnecting vascular network, including the great saphenous vein (GSV), small saphenous vein and several smaller accessory veins, which may develop pathology resulting in CVI. The deep venous system (located underneath the muscle fascia) serves as a collection chamber for the entire outflow from the extremity. These deeper veins can be categorized into axial veins, which follow the course of the major arteries, and intramuscular veins, including venous sinusoids and plexi. The perforating veins traverse the anatomic fascial layer to connect the superficial to the deep venous system.

All these veins have a lining of unidirectional bicuspid valves on their intramural surface. These valves ensure the flow of blood against gravity, to the heart but prevent their return to the feet, especially in the upright posture.[4] The density of these valves increases proximo-distally to counter-elevated venous pressure distally because of gravitational effects. Additionally, valves in the perforating veins only allow blood flow from the superficial to the deep veins. These valves function in unison with the venous muscle pumps (most notably calf muscle pump) to maintain the flow of blood against gravity to the heart.[1]

Proper functioning of the peripheral venous system depends on the patency of these vessels, their valves and the surrounding muscular pumps. Pathology pertaining to any component may result in dysfunction of the venous system, leading to CVI.

There are several factors which play an important role in the development of this condition and the associated pathologic skin changes as discussed below:

Venous stasis: This is the most important etiopathologic factor leading to the different skin manifestations of CVI. Long-standing accumulation of blood in tortuous, non-functioning and dilated skin veins results in subsequent tissue anoxia and cell death leading to the characteristic skin changes and ulceration. Development of physiologic arteriovenous fistulae in the varicose limbs have been reported to counter-tissue hypoxia.[5]

Venous hypertension: Venous stasis coupled with dysfunctional muscular pump function leads to increased venous hydrostatic pressure in the varicose limbs. Initially the deeper veins are affected, the superficial veins remaining free. However, incompetent venous valves lead to transmission of this pressure to the weaker superficial veins, leading to the typical skin changes and ulceration.[6]

Fibrin cuff: Formation of pericapillary fibrin cuff further impedes the diffusion of oxygen from the vessels to tissue acting as a barrier, thus aggravating tissue hypoxia and cell damage. Recently, fibrin cuff has been recognized as the marker of endothelial cell damage and leucocyte trapping.[7]

Water Hammer effect: This theory was propounded by Raju and Frederick,[8] which states that increased venous pressure is transmitted to the superficial veins by the dysfunctional perforators.

Leukocyte trapping: Venous stasis and increased intravascular hydrostatic pressure damages the vessel walls, which in turn leads to peripheral margination of the white cells.[9] As a result, capillary plugs are formed which further impede blood flow, thus aggravating tissue hypoxia and cellular damage. These white cells also secrete free radicals and cytokines (interleukin-1, tumor necrosis factor) which promote tissue damage and apoptosis. Lately, Mustoe[10] has proposed a unifying hypothesis encompassing leukocyte trapping and venous hypertension as the most important pathologic factor.

Predisposing Factors

There are several predisposing factors which enhances the chance of developing CVI. Some of the important factors are briefly discussed below:

Age and gender: Multiple studies have shown that CVI predominantly affects the elderly age group. The overall prevalence of varicose veins has been reported to be 22%, 35%, and 41% at ages 40, 50, and 60 years respectively.[11] This condition shows a female preponderance [F:M 3:1], as the former usually follow a sedentary lifestyle.[2]

Pregnancy: Pregnancy is an important predisposing factor for the development of CVI and varicose veins, and the risk increases with successive pregnancies. The gravid uterus exerts pressure on the pelvic vasculature, subsequently resulting in lower extremity venous hypertension, venous distention, and valve rupture. The altered hormonal milieu during pregnancy may also be a causative factor, as oestrogen and progesterone receptors have been found on the saphenous veins.[12]

Genetic predisposition: CVI develops more frequently in genetically predisposed individuals, as positive family history is an important risk factor. Mutations of the desmuslin gene, thrombomodulin gene and other structural genes regulating the extracellular matrix and vascular smooth muscle have been implicated.

Several syndromes have been associated with varicose veins like Klippel-Trénaunay syndrome, lymphedema distichiasis syndrome and other syndromes associated with delayed wound healing. Rarer syndromes include cerebral autosomal dominant arteriopathy with subcortical infarcts and leukoencephalopathy (CADASIL) and Chuvash polycythemia.[13]

Lifestyle: Sedentary work and prolonged standing at work (traffic constables, security guards and bus conductors) are independent risk factors for the development of CVI.

Increased body mass index (BMI) (>30 kg/m^2) is also a notable risk factor, as subcutaneous deposition of adipose tissue further narrows the blood vessels thus interfering with normal blood flow.[2]

Clinical Features

CVI is an umbrella term which can present with a plethora of clinical manifestations. Telangiectasias or reticular veins comprise the early presentation, while advanced stages may present with leg pain, leg oedema, varicose veins, skin fibrosis, venous ulceration and other cutaneous changes.

Leg oedema starts in the lower part gradually ascending upwards, often associated with a dull/aching pain and heaviness of the legs. Both oedema and pain are relieved by elevation of the leg.

Varicose veins are the most common and classical presentation characterised by dilated and tortuous superficial veins, visible from above the skin. Superficial thrombophlebitis commonly occurs in these patients.

Excessive dilatation of the varicose veins may result in tenderness along the veins.

In advanced stages, the deep venous system may be obstructed leading to venous claudication, or intense leg cramping with ambulation.

Cutaneous changes: · Skin hyperpigmentation due to deposition of hemosiderin in the perivascular tissue and dermis.

- Eczematous changes due to pooling of blood (stasis dermatitis)—stasis dermatitis (hypostatic eczema) occurs on the lower legs because of underlying insufficient venous drainage. Varicose veins are often present, and chronic pruritic dermatitis develops with periods of exacerbations. The dermatitis may be weepy or dry, scaly or lichenified.
- Venous ulcers: Ulcers are the most common complication of hypostatic eczema. Usually a solitary lesion is present with clear floor and sloping margins, around the medial malleolus (gaiter region).
- Thickening of skin due to proliferation of fibrous tissue in the dermis and subcutis, called lipodermatosclerosis.
- There is an increased risk of developing cellulitis, leg ulceration and delayed wound healing.

Assessment of the severity of CV:[12, 14, 15] Several tools have been proposed for objective assessment of the severity of CVI. Amongst them the CEAP (clinical, etiology, anatomic, pathophysiology) classification (Table 6.1) is most widely accepted. A venous severity score has also been developed to complement the CEAP classification for a more detailed assessment and to evaluate response to treatment. The venous clinical severity score consists of 10 attributes (pain, varicose veins, venous oedema, skin pigmentation, inflammation, induration, number of ulcers, duration of ulcers, size of ulcers, and compressive therapy) with 4 grades (absent, mild, moderate, severe). The venous disability score measures the ability to perform normal activities of daily living with or without compressive stockings. The venous anatomic segmental score assigns a numerical value to segments of the venous system in the lower extremity to identify the site of reflux and/or obstruction. The anatomical score may be used in conjunction with CEAP, called the advanced CEAP classification.

TABLE 6.1: CEAP classification for chronic venous disease

Clinical classification		Anatomic classification	
C0	No visible or palpable signs of venous disease	As	Superficial veins
C1	Telangiectasias or reticular mass	Ap	Perforator veins
C2	Varicose veins	Ad	Deep veins
C3	Edema	An	No venous location identified
C4	Pigmentation or eczema		
C5	Healed venous ulcer		
C6	Active venous ulcer		
S	Symptomatic: Ache, pain, tightens, skin irritation, heaviness, muscle cramps		
Etiologic classification		**Pathophysiologic classification**	
Ec	Congenital	Pr	Reflux
Ep	Primary	Po	Obstruction
Es	Secondary (post-thrombotic)	Pr, o	Reflux, obstruction
En	No venous cause identified	Pn	No venous pathophysiology identifiable

Diagnosis

Chronic venous insufficiency is essentially a clinical diagnosis, which is sufficient in most cases. Besides, several imaging tests are present to confirm the diagnosis.

Physical examination: A thorough clinical examination is of paramount importance when CVI is suspected. It involves inspection of the skin for signs of CVI like hyperpigmentation, stasis dermatitis, atrophic blanche (white scarring at the site of previous ulcerations with a paucity of capillaries) and lipodermatosclerosis. Presence of thickened, engorged and tortuous superficial veins suggest varicose veins. Usually, pitting oedema is the finding, however, long standing cases may result in non-pitting oedema due to fibrosis. Peripheral pulsations should be checked to rule out any arterial pathology.

A bed-side test called the Trendelenburg test or tourniquet test may be performed to assess the location of venous pathology (superficial/deep reflux). The test is performed with the patient lying down to empty the lower extremity veins. The upright posture is then resumed after applying a tourniquet or using manual compression at various levels. In the presence of superficial disease the varicose veins remain collapsed if compression is distal to the point of reflux. With deep (or combined) venous insufficiency, the varicose veins appear despite the use of the tourniquet or manual compression.

Doppler duplex imaging: Doppler duplex imaging study of the limb vasculature remains the gold standard to confirm the diagnosis of CVI. The goal of duplex imaging is to rule out any obstruction or reflux in the deep veins or detection of deep vein thrombosis and assess the patency of superficial veins (great saphenous vein and small saphenous vein) and other perforator or branch veins. Low-frequency transducers (2–3 MHz) are usually used to evaluate the iliac veins and inferior vena cava while high-frequency transducers (5–10 MHz) are used to evaluate the distal veins. In almost 65% of all cases of CVI, reflux has been noted at the confluence of GSV and common femoral vein.[16] However, duplex imaging alone has limited role, it provides valuable information when used in conjunction with clinical examination.

Plethysmography: Plethysmography (PPG) is a diagnostic investigation in which we assess the changes in the volume of blood present in dermis by measuring the back scatter of light emitted from a diode with a photosensor. The venous refill time is the time required for the PPG tracing to return to 90% of the baseline after cessation of calf contraction. A venous refill time less 20 seconds is suggestive of CVI.

Air plethysmography (APG) is a modified version employed to evaluate the venous outflow during rapid cuff deflation on an elevated limb that has a proximal venous occlusion cuff applied. The parameter assessed is called venous filling index (venous outflow at 1 second expressed as a percentage of the total venous volume). Venous filling index (>4–7 ml/s) suggests CVI, and is directly proportional to its severity.

Computed tomography and magnetic resonance venography: These are advanced imaging techniques used to diagnose rarer causes of CVI like May-Thurner syndrome, nutcracker syndrome, pelvic congestion syndrome, venous malformations and atriovenous malformations.[2] Computed tomography helps us to rule out thromboembolism in the proximal veins, while magnetic resonance venography evaluates the age of thrombus.

Treatment

The treatment of CVI may be classified under the following heads:

- General/conservative measures
- Specific measures
  - Non-invasive modalities
  - Invasive modalities

General/Conservative Measures

Some of the important general measures which may be adopted to prevent the worsening of CVI are briefly discussed below. All these measures provide best results when used as adjuncts to specific therapy.

- *Behavioural modifications*: Avoidance of prolonged standing and elevating the legs should be advised to prevent the peripheral pooling of blood and venous hypertension.
- *Compression therapy:* The use of compressive stockings forms the backbone of conservative management. The Bisgaard regimen helps in the healing of venous ulcers. This regimen consists of 4 components—patient education, foot elevation, elastic compression garments and evaluation using the CEAP classification. Non-elastic ambulatory below knee compression is also effective.

  Compression helps to reduce the blood vessel diameter and pressure, thus preventing the backflow of blood. Recent reports also suggest several additional effects like decreased release of inflammatory cytokines, reduced capillary leak and delayed clotting by inactivation of thrombin and promoting plasmin formation.[2]

  Both elastic and non-elastic compressive bandages, stockings or specially designed boots may be used for this purpose. Patients should be encouraged to apply maximum compression within his/her comfort limits. Graded elastic compressive stockings (20–50 mm Hg pressure) are most widely used for this purpose. May Berry et al[17] have demonstrated optimum results with compressive pressure of 30–40 mm Hg.
- *Muscular exercise:* Graded exercise programs to strengthen the calf and foot muscle pumps have been found to be beneficial as they help in maintaining normal blood flow thus preventing its peripheral pooling.[2]

Specific Measures

The specific measures may be categorized under two heads—non-invasive and invasive, as discussed below.

Non-invasive treatment modalities: The non-invasive treatment modalities are used in milder forms of CVI with predominant involvement of the superficial veins, patients unfit for surgery and those not consenting for surgical procedures.

- **Endovenous laser ablation (EVLA):** The basic principle of this modality is laser-induced thermal ablation and shrinkage of the damaged superficial veins. Laser beam having wavelength 1320 nm has been found to be most effective. Water in the vein wall is the main chromophore, presence/absence of blood in the vein does not play any role. Recently, laser ablation using lower wavelengths has been used (810, 940 and 980 nm).

We should be cautious to avoid overheating as it may lead to severe damage of the veins and surrounding tissues resulting in perforation, haematoma and postoperative pain.[18] The target veins should be freed of blood prior to therapy, as haemoglobin has a chance of getting overheated increasing the chance of damage.

- **Radiofrequency ablation (RFA):** Thermal ablation of the damaged veins may also be achieved by using radiofrequency waves. Several studies have highlighted the superiority of RFA to EVLA in terms of pain, bruising and postoperative recovery, with comparable rates of GSV occlusion.[2] Almeida et al[19] have demonstrated similar efficacy of RFA and surgical ligation with stripping of GSV in their patients after 2 years.

Invasive treatment modalities

- **Venous sclerotherapy:** Venous sclerotherapy is a minimally invasive technique in which a sclerosing agent is injected within the affected vein to cause its occlusion after draining its blood. Polidocanol sulphate is the commonest sclerosant used, often injected under ultrasound guidance.[2]

  Sclerotherapy is indicated for several conditions like spider veins, telangiectasias, venous lakes, varicose veins up to 4 mm diameter, bleeding varices and small vascular malformations.

  Some uncommon complications of this procedure include pigmentation, capillary dilatation (telangiectatic matting) and post-procedure pain.

- **Surgical therapies:** Two surgical therapies are commonly practiced: (1) Surgical ligation and stripping of the great saphenous vein (GSV) and (2) valvuloplasty or valve reconstruction surgery.

  Indications of surgery

  Some of the important indications for surgery in CVI are given below:

  i. Presence of venous ulcer not responding to conventional and minimally invasive therapy.
  ii. Recurrent episodes of varicose vein.
  iii. Disabling symptoms and persistent discomfort not amenable to other therapies.
  iv. As a complement to conservative and minimally invasive modalities to obtain best results.

- **Surgical ligation and stripping of the great saphenous vein (GSV):** Surgical ligation of great saphenous vein (GSV) at the saphenofemoral junction along with its stripping (phlebectomy) is the gold standard treatment for advanced varicose veins (CEAP class 2 to 6). Recently transilluminated powered phlebectomy has been introduced, which is an advanced technique comprising of tumescent dissection, transillumination and powered phlebectomy.

  Some of the complications of this procedure include pain, bruising, occasional nerve injury and postoperative morbidity. Powered phlebectomy improves the postoperative recovery time, however, the risk of other complications remain unchanged.

- **Valve reconstruction surgery/valvuloplasty:** Valve reconstruction surgery/valvuloplasty is indicated in advanced cases of CVI presenting with recurrent ulcerations and disabling symptoms, as venous valve dysfunction/incompetence is one of the primary causative factors of this disorder. Initially open valve replacement was performed, however, recently transcommisural valvuloplasty is being performed for valve repair. Valve replacement is being performed using axillary vein valve, profunda femoris valve or cryopreserved valve allografts.

- **Subfascial endoscopic perforator surgery (SEPS):** This surgical procedure is performed in cases of incompetence of the perforator veins. The incompetent perforator vein is accessed from a remote site (away from lipodermatosclerosis or ulcers) and ligated. Bianchi et al[20] have reported better healing rates when SEPS is performed along with ligation and stripping of GSV.

References

1. Eberhardt RT, Raffetto JD. Chronic venous insufficiency. Circulation 2014; 130:333–46.
2. Youn YJ, Lee J. Chronic venous insulticiency and varicose veins of the lower extremities. Kor J Intern Med. 2019 Mar;34(2):269–83.
3. Labropoulos N, Kang SS, Mansour MA, Giannoukas AD, Buckman J, Baker WH. Primary superficial vein reflux with competent saphenous trunk. Eur J Vasc Endovasc Surg. 1999;18:201–06.
4. Gloviczki P, Yao JS, Mózes G, Carmichael SW, Gloviczki P. Development and anatomy of the venous system. In: Gloviczki P, Yao JS, eds. *Handbook of Venous Disorders*, 2nd Edition. New York, NY: Arnold Publisher; 2001:11–24.
5. Gourdin FW, Smith JG Jr. Etiology of venous ulceration. South Med J. 1993; 86:1142–46.
6. Recek C. Calf pump activity influencing venous hemodynamics in the lower extremity. Int J Angiol. 2013; 22:23–30.
7. Scheur M, Falanga V. Pericapillary fibrin cuffs in venous disease. Dermatologic Surgery 1997; 23:955–60.
8. Raju S, Frederick R. Evaluation of methods for detecting venous reflux: perspectives in venous insufficiency. Archives of Surgery 1990; 125: 1463–67.
9. Hahn TL, Unthank JL, Lalka SG. Increased hindlimb leukocyte concentration in a chronic rodent model of venous hypertension. Journal of Surgical Research 1999; 81:38–41.
10. Mustoe T. Understanding chronic wounds: a unifying hypothesis on their pathogenesis and implications for therapy. The American Journal of Surgery 2004; 187:S65–70.
11. Laurikka JO, Sisto T, Tarkka MR, Auvinen O, Hakama M. Risk indicators for varicose veins in forty-to sixty-year-old in the tampere varicose vein study. World journal of surgery 2002; 26:648–51.
12. Ciardullo, AV, Panico, S, Bellati, C, Rubba, P, Rinaldi, S, Iannuzzi, A, Cioffi, V, Iannuzzo, G and Berrino, F. High endogenous estradiol is associated with increased venous distensibility and clinical evidence of varicose veins in menopausal women. Journal of Vascular Surgery 2000; 32:544–49.
13. Anwar MA, Georgiadis KA, Shalhoub J, Lim CS, Gohel MS, Davies AH. A review of familial, genetic, and congenital aspects of primary varicose vein disease. Circulation: Cardiovascular Genetics 2012; 5:460–66.
14. Eklöf B, Rutherford RB, Bergan JJ, Carpentier PH, Gloviczki P, Kistner RL, Meissner MH, Moneta GL, Myers K, Padberg FT, Perrin M. Revision of the CEAP classification for chronic venous disorders: consensus statement. Journal of Vascular Surgery 2004; 40:1248–52.
15. Vasquez MA, Rabe E, McLafferty RB, Shortell CK, Marston WA, Gillespie D, Meissner MH, Rutherford RB. Revision of the venous clinical severity score: venous outcomes consensus statement: special communication of the American Venous Forum Ad Hoc Outcomes Working Group. Journal of Vascular Surgery 2010; 52:1387–96.
16. García-Gimeno M, Rodríguez-Camarero S, Tagarro-Villalba S, Ramalle-Gomara E, González-González E, Arranz MA, García DL, Puerta CV. Duplex mapping of 2036 primary varicose veins. Journal of Vascular Surgery 2009; 49:681–9.
17. Mayberry JC, Moneta GL, Taylor LM, Porter JM. Fifteen-year results of ambulatory compression therapy for chronic venous ulcers. Surgery 1991; 109:575–81.
18. Proebstle TM, Sandhofer M, Kargl A, Gül D, Rother W, Knop J, Lehr HA. Thermal damage of the inner vein wall during endovenous laser treatment: key role of energy absorption by intravascular blood. Dermatologic Surgery 2002; 28:596–600.
19. Heller J. Treatment of Chronic Venous Insufficiency. Endovascular Today 2011; 12–5.
20. Bianchi C, Ballard JL, Abou-Zamzam AM, Teruya TH. Subfascial endoscopic perforator vein surgery combined with saphenous vein ablation: results and critical analysis. Journal of Vascular Surgery 2003; 38:67–71.

CHAPTER 7

Infestations in Elderly

• Kinjal Deepak Rambhia • Sweta Hasmukh Rambhia • Amit Sureshchandra Gulati

Introduction

Infestations of the skin may be caused by mite, louse, flea or flies. Overcrowding, low standards of hygiene, neglect, delayed diagnosis, inadequate treatment and insufficient control measures lead to frequent epidemics and endemics of such infestations. In geriatric population, these infestations are commonly encountered owing to other associated comorbidities, neglect of medical issues, improper self-care and grooming practices which are prevalent amongst the elderly population. This chapter will discuss these infestations in detail.

SCABIES

Key Points

- Scabies is caused by a mite *Sarcoptes scabiei* of the order acarina
- Close contact for 15–20 minutes with an infected person is sufficient for disease transmission
- Nocturnal itching is the most common symptom and burrows are the characteristic lesions of scabies
- Treatment with oral ivermectin and topical permethrin are the mainstay of treatment
- Prophylactic treatment of close contacts is indicated to prevent recurrences.

- Mites (Acari)
- Suborder Astigmata
- Family Sarcoptidae

Introduction

Scabies is a disease affecting humans and other animals like cats and dogs. It is caused by a mite *Sarcoptes scabiei* of the order Acarina. This disease entity has been well described in ancient Indian medicine textbooks dating back to 800 BC.[1] The etiological role of the itch mite in scabies was established by Bonomo and Cestoni.[2]

Epidemiology

Scabies is mainly known to occur in children. It has the highest prevalence among children below the age of 5 years and the prevalence of scabies infection decreases with an increasing age.[3] It occurs in all parts of the world and affects all races and social classes with no sexual predilection.

Climatic factors favouring survival of the mite are high humidity and low temperature. Environmental factors affect transmission of this disease with an increased affection noted in overcrowded areas. It was believed that prolonged, intimate personal contact is a significant factor in the transmission of scabies. However, close contact for 15–20 minutes with an infected person is sufficient for disease transmission.[4]

Etiopathogenesis

Transfer of fertilized female mites to a new host is essential for establishing infection in a new host. Indirect spread via fomites like bedding or clothing is relatively uncommon.[5] *Sarcoptes scabiei* var. *hominis* are ovoid whitish mites, dorsoventrally flattened and approximately 0.4 × 0.3 millimetres in dimensions. The body has transverse corrugations, spines and bristles. They have four pairs of legs—the front two pairs end in suckers and the 2 pairs at the posterior side end in long trailing bristles in females. The male mites are smaller in size as compared to the females and their 4th pair of legs also ends in suckers.

Copulation occurs in a burrow which is excavated into the skin by the female mite. Later, the fertilized female enlarges the burrow downwards and begins laying the eggs while the male dies. In a lifespan of 4–6 weeks, the female mite lays 40–50 eggs. Six-legged larvae emerge from the eggs after 3–4 days; escape the burrow by breaking its roof and dig short burrows (moulting pockets) where they undergo moults to become mature nymphs. After further moults they transform into adult males and females (Fig. 7.1).

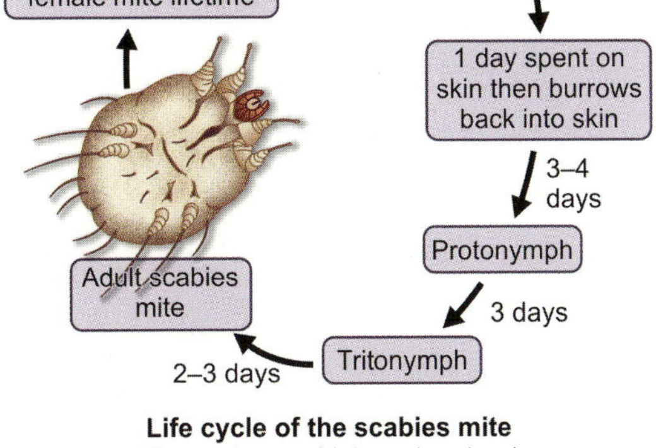

Fig. 7.1: Life cycle of scabies mite [*From:* Dermatology Bolognia JL, Jorizzo JL, Rapini RP (editors), 2nd edition, Meinking TL, Burkhart CN, Burkhart CG, Elgart G. Infestations, Elsevier (2008), page 1295]

Habitat: The mites prefer certain sites, whereas they avoid areas with high density of pilosebaceous glands. On an average, a scabies affected individual harbours approximately 12 adult mites.[6,7]

However, there are numerous mites in the crusted form of scabies (Norwegian scabies) pruritus and lesions other than burrow occur due to allergic sensitivity to the mite and its products. However, the exact immunological events are not known. There is speculation regarding the role of both immediate and delayed type of hypersensitivity.

Clinical Features

Itching is the most common symptom and usually worse at night. The onset of symptoms is 3–4 weeks after the infection. Burrows (raised brownish, serpentine, tortuous lesions with a slight scaly appearance at the entry and a tiny vesicle at the distal end) are the characteristic lesions of scabies. These burrows are commonly found on the web spaces of the fingers, flexor aspects of the wrists, elbows, anterior axillary folds, umbilicus, periumbilical areas, thighs, knees, ankles, nipples, areola and genitals (Fig. 7.2A to D). In uncomplicated adult cases, the scalp, face, palms and soles are characteristically spared. On the other hand, these areas are commonly involved in infants and children. This pattern of distribution of mites is probably due to their preference for non-hairy and low sebum areas.

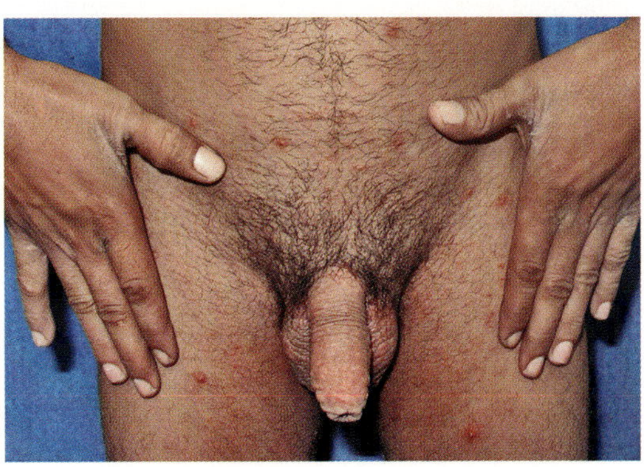

Fig. 7.2A: Scabies affecting web spaces and genitals

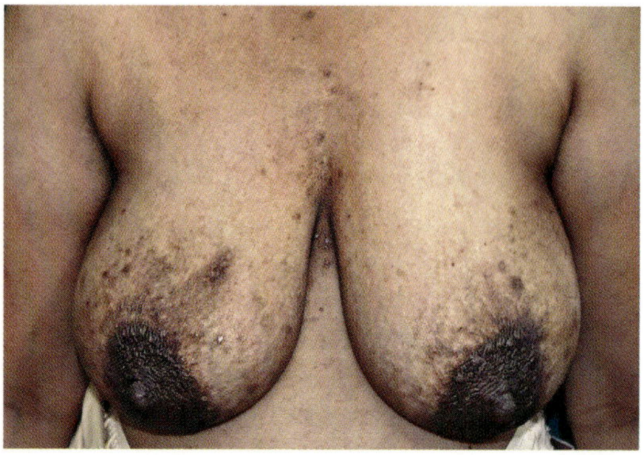

Fig. 7.2B: Involvement of areola in a case of scabies

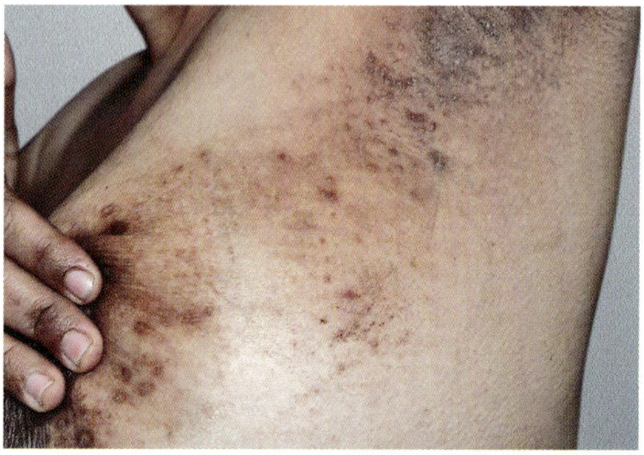

Fig. 7.2C: Excoriated papules over the axilla and areola

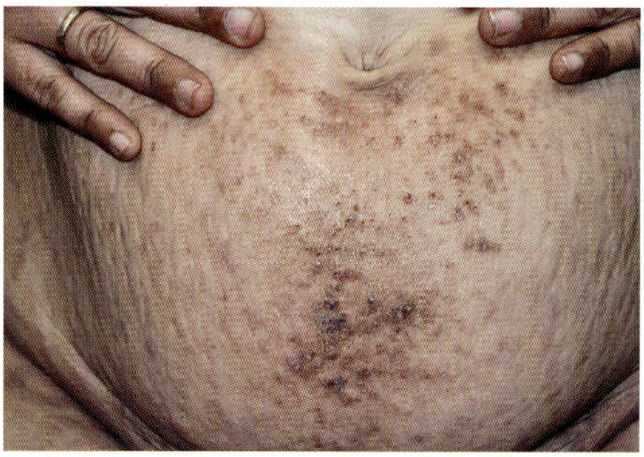

Fig. 7.2D: Periumbilical area involvement in a case of scabies

Cutaneous examination reveals erythematous papules and papulovesicles, excoriation marks, eczematisation and signs of secondary infection. Secondary infection in the form of impetigo or folliculitis may be seen.

Histopathological examination reveals epidermal spongiosis, intraepidermal neutrophilic and eosinophilic abscesses, a moderately dense perivascular infiltrate of lymphocytes, eosinophils and histiocytes.

Scabies in Babies

In infants affected with scabies, there is extensive distribution of burrows. There are vesicular and vesiculopustular lesions on the hands and the feet. There may be extensive eczematisation and secondary infection.

Scabies in the Elderly

In elderly individuals with scabies, there are numerous burrows on the characteristic sites. In addition, the lesions on the trunk are surmounted with burrows and extensive eczematisation is frequently encountered.

Nodular Scabies

Persistent nodules occur on the elbow, axilla, genitalia and the gluteal areas (Fig. 7.3A to C). These nodules persist for weeks, months or even years and represent foreign body reaction to retained products of the mites.

Scabies in Clean

In hygienic individuals mild-moderate itching with few papular lesions at the sites of predisposition occur.

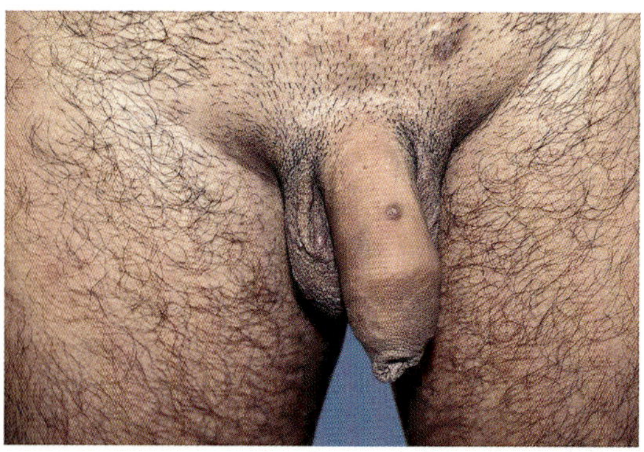

Fig. 7.3A: Nodular scabies involving the penile shaft

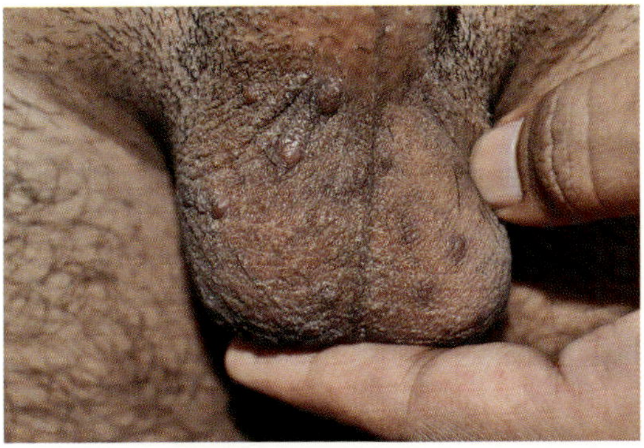

Fig. 7.3B: Nodular scabies involving the scrotum

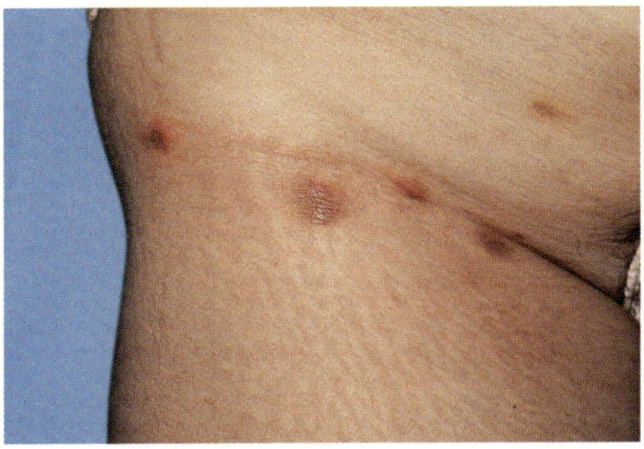

Fig. 7.3C: Nodular scabies involving the groin and thigh

Occasionally, scabies may present as chronic urticaria with lesions localised to the buttocks and axillae.

Crusted Scabies (Norwegian Scabies)

Crusted scabies was first described by Danielssen and Boeck in Norway as a type of scabies with numerous mites.[8] In this entity the mite population may reach up to millions; and such cases may cause an outbreak of common scabies.

In common scabies the scratching caused by intense pruritus destroys the burrows and controls the mite population. In cases with immunosuppression, the host response to the mites is modified and their multiplication continues. Other settings where crusted scabies may be encountered include poor cutaneous sensation (do not perceive itch; do not scratch), poor personal hygiene, defective cell-mediated or humoral immunity.

Clinically, crusted scabies is characterised by hyperkeratotic, scaly crusted lesions with numerous mites. In addition to the typical sites the scalp, face, palms, soles, neck and lumbosacral area are commonly involved (Fig. 7.4A to C). It may present as erythroderma. Nail involvement in the form of subungual hyperkeratosis, dystrophy and discolouration may occur.

Scabies Incognito

Scabies treated with topical or systemic corticosteroids may have unusual clinical

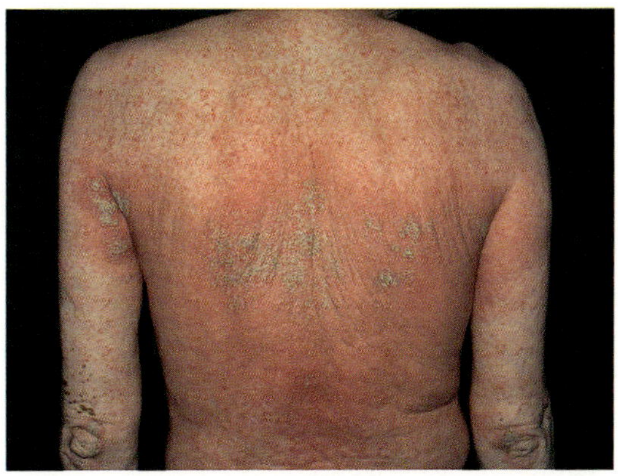

Fig. 7.4A: Norwegian scabies in a patient on chemotherapy. Note the hyperkeratotic, crusted lesions on the back

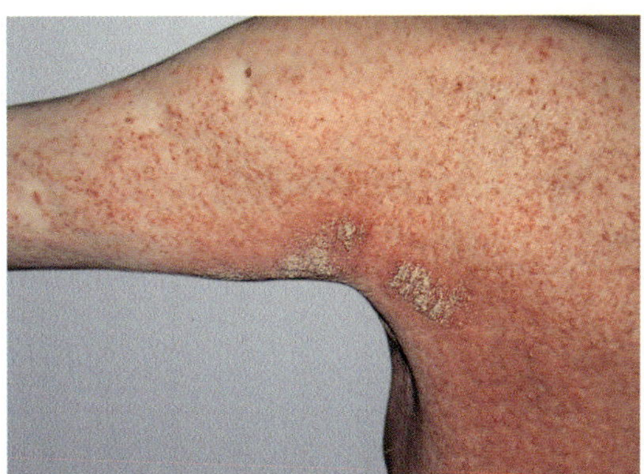

Fig. 7.4B: Hyperkeratotic crusted lesions in a case of Norwegian scabies

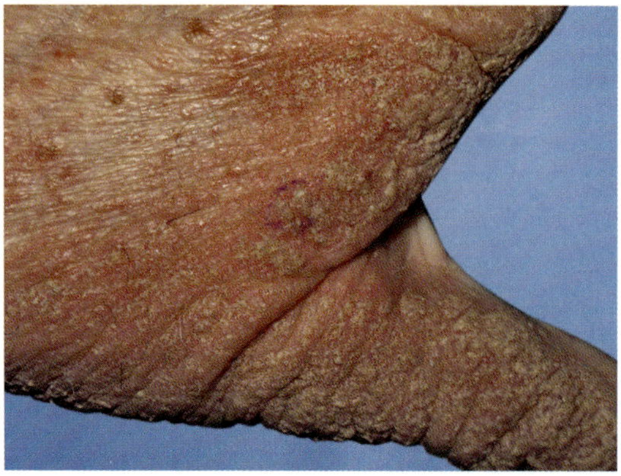

Fig. 7.4C: Crusted scabies with characteristic site involved

features, affection of atypical sites and simulate various other dermatological disorders. Such cases have reduced pruritus due to the effect of corticosteroids and an increase mite population.

Animal Transmitted Scabies (Pseudoscabies)

Dogs are the most common cause of animal transmitted scabies. Canine scabies affects forearm, lower chest, abdomen, thighs, and areas in contact with the person carrying the pet. Interdigital web spaces and genitals are characteristically spared.

Other Rare Variants

1. Bullous pemphigoid like eruption.[9]
2. Cutaneous vasculitis.[10]

Complications

The various cutaneous and systemic complications of scabies are listed in Table 7.1.

TABLE 7.1: Complications of scabies infestation

Cutaneous	Systemic
Secondary pyodermas	Acute glomerulonephritis
Impetigo	
Ecthyma	
Cellulitis	
Furunculosis	
Lymphangitis	

Diagnosis

Table 7.2 provides the clues to diagnosis of scabies.

TABLE 7.2: Diagnosis of scabies

1. Typical history
   - Nocturnal itching
   - Family history
2. Clinical examination
   - Distribution of lesions
   - Presence of burrows
   - Genital lesions
3. Dermoscopy
   - Mite in its burrow—'jet with contrail sign'
4. Microscopy
   - Scraping of burrow and 10% KOH mount—visualisation of mites, eggs or fragments of egg shells.
5. Histopathology (Fig. 7.5A and B)
   - Mites or mite products in the stratum corneum· spongiotic dermatitis with neutrophilic and eosinophilic exocytosis
   - Moderate to dense superficial perivascular infiltrate of lymphocytes, eosinophils and histiocytes

Treatment

The treatment of scabies includes general measures and correct use of scabicidal drugs. Detailed instructions regarding the proper application of these agents should be given to affected individuals.

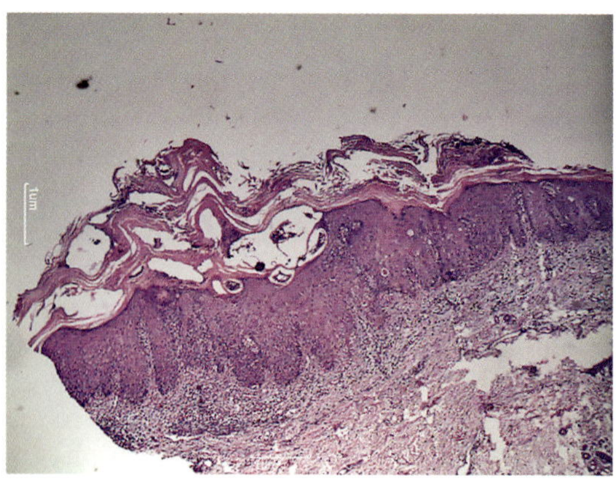

Fig. 7.5A: Psoriasiform hyperkeratosis with spongiotic dermatitis. Note the thickened, parakeratotic stratum corneum in a case of crusted scabies

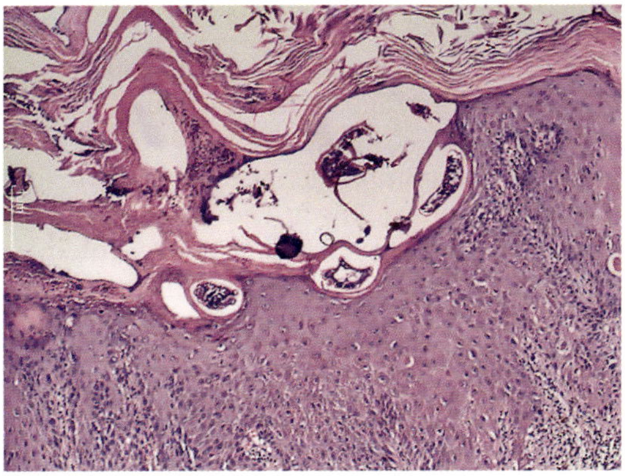

Fig. 7.5B: Burrow, mite and its products in the stratum corneum

General Measures

All topical antiscabetics should be applied all over the body except the head and scalp. Special attention should be given to the classic sites of scabies. Generally, 30 gram of cream is sufficient for a single application in a single adult patient. A thorough bath should be taken after the completion of the desired contact period of the antiscabetic drug. A second application 1–2 weeks later may be advised to eliminate the eggs which have hatched later and were unaffected by the previous scabicidal agent. In geriatric patients, the topical treatment modalities may fail due to incorrect application resulting from impaired mobility of the patient; oral ivermectin may be added.

Therapeutic Agents

The various therapeutic agents used for the treatment of scabies include permethrin 5%, lindane 1%, crotamiton 10%, sulfur 2–10% and ivermectin tablets (Table 7.3).

TABLE 7.3: Treatment of scabies

S. No.	Drug	Formulations	Mechanism of action	Contact period	Side effects	Pregnancy category
1.	Permethrin 5%	Lotion, cream	Disruption of the sodium channel current of the nerve cells of parasite causing delayed repolarisation, paralysis and death	8–12 hours	Allergic contact dermatitis	B
2.	Gamma benzene hexachloride (lindane) 1%	Lotion, cream, shampoo	Inhibition of gamma aminobutyric acid gated chloride channels	8–12 hours, overnight	Neurotoxicity (convulsions, dizziness, headache) especially in elderly, crusted scabies	C
3.	Benzyl benzoate 25%	Lotion, ointment	Scabicidal	Three consecutive overnight application	Skin irritation, dermatitis, convulsions	Contra-indicated in pregnancy
4.	Crotamiton 15%	Ointment, lotion, cream		Overnight for 3–5 days	Irritant contact dermatitis	C
5.	Sulphur 5–10%	Ointment		Overnight for 3 consecutive nights	Irritant contact dermatitis especially denuded areas	Not established but considered safe
6.	Ivermectin 200 μg/kg	Tablets	Inhibition of GABA gated chloride channels	Once. May be repeated after 10–14 days		C

Permethrin is a synthetic pyrethroid with high insecticidal activity and less side-effects. Permethrin cream or lotion in a concentration of 5% applied for a single overnight application is highly efficacious with less toxicity. The action of permethrin is due to disruption of the sodium channel current of the nerve cells of parasite causing delayed repolarisation, paralysis and death. Less than 2% of the applied dose is absorbed by the human skin; the absorbed amount being rapidly metabolised by the tissue esterases. The inactive by-products of tissue metabolism are then excreted through the kidneys. It has a cure rate of 89–100% as described in several studies and is considered superior to other antiscabetic drugs.[11]

Gamma-benzene hexachloride or lindane 1% is a scabicidal agent which is applied topically for 8–12 hours or overnight and repeated after one week to eliminate any newly hatched larvae. Adverse reactions like irritability, insomnia, ataxia, tremors, seizures, headache, dizziness may be seen in individuals who inadvertently apply the medication daily. To avoid percutaneous absorption, GBH should be washed off well with soap and water after 12 hours.[12]

Benzyl benzoate lotion 25% is as an economical scabicidal agent. It is applied overnight for three consecutive nights. It may cause skin irritation due to incorrect use.

Crotamiton 10% lotion or cream may be used for the treatment of scabies. In addition to its scabicidal effect, it also has an antipruritic effect. It is applied daily for 5 consecutive days.

Ivermectin is a macrocyclic lactone derivative and shares some structural similarities to antibiotic macrolides and antifungal polyenes. It acts by inhibition of GABA gated chloride channels. A single dose of 200 µg/kg is effective. A repeat dose after 10–14 days may increase the cure rate up to 95%.

Topical ivermectin 0.8%/weight/volume in a dose of 25 ml single overnight topical application is found to be effective. A second application after one week is recommended.[13]

CONCLUSION

Scabies is a common infestation which poses a significant public health problem. Geriatric patients with scabies present with atypical features and involvement of uncommon sites which cause a delay in the diagnosis. Oral ivermectin 200 µg/kg and topical permethrin 5% lotion may be used with excellent results.

PEDICULOSIS

Key Points

- Pediculosis capitis is a common infestation seen in all socio-economic groups.
- Body louse infestation is seen in individuals with poor hygiene and low socio-economic groups.
- Pubic louse infestation is predominantly transmitted through sexual or close contact.
- Though uncommon louse may be responsible of the transmission of certain systemic illnesses.
- Treatment includes permethrin, malathion, lindane and ivermectin.

Order: Phthiraptera

Suborder: Anoplura (blood sucking ectoparasites of mammals)

Family: Pediculidae

Genus: Pediculus

Introduction

Pediculosis is caused by lice. *Pediculus humanus* (head and body louse) (Table 7.4) and *Phthirus pubis* (pubic louse) are host-specific, obligate ectoparasites of man, suck the blood of the host and spend their entire life on humans.

Epidemiology

The incidence of pediculosis has been increasing worldwide.[14] The prevalence of head lice is more in girls than in boys due to the longer length of hair especially in the rural population.[15] The most common mode of transmission is direct head to head contact, fomites like comb, hair brush and towels. The

TABLE 7.4: Differentiation of head and body louse	
Head louse	**Body louse**
1. *Pediculus humanus capitis*	*Pediculus humanus corporis*
2. Smaller 2.4–3.3 mm	Larger 3.8–4.0 mm
3. Darker in colour	Lighter compared to head louse
4. Segments of the antennae are smaller	Segments of antennae are larger
5. Lives for 30 days	Lives for 60 days
6. Female lays 100 eggs	Lays 300 eggs
7. Habitat—hair	Clothing of host; visits skin to feed
8. Nits—close to the scalp to favour incubation of the eggs	Nits—seams of the clothes

incidence of pediculosis capitis is higher in overcrowded places, populations with low standards of hygiene and lower socio-economic strata of society.

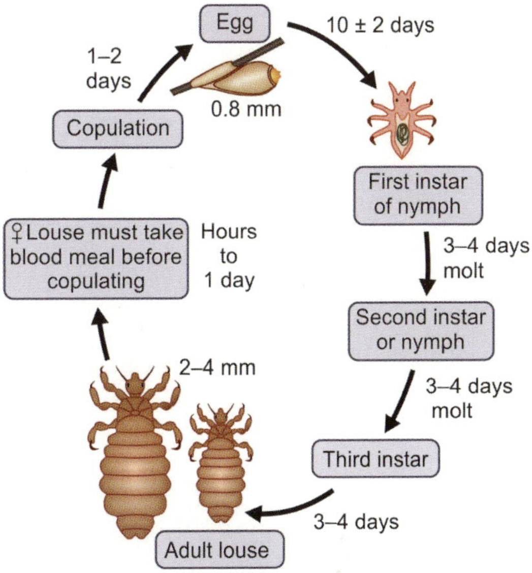

Life cycle of a louse (*Pediculus capitis*)

Fig. 7.6: Life cycle of pediculosis [Dermatology, Bolognia JL, Jorizzo JL, Rapini RP (editors), 2nd edition, Meinking TL, Burkhart CN, Burkhart CG, Elgart G. Infestations, Elsevier (2008), page 1295]

Etiopathogenesis

Lice are wingless, dorsoventrally flattened insects. They have a head which has 5 segmented antennae and mouth parts modified for sucking blood. The thorax which is a small area has 3 short pairs of legs which end with conspicuous claws. The claws at the distal end of the legs help the lice to hold on to the hair and fibres of the clothing of the host. The third part is the abdomen which is larger than the head and thorax. It comprises nine segments of which only seven are apparent.

Unless mechanically removed, lice spend their entire life on the host. Their life cycle is depicted in Fig. 7.6. Each louse takes 2–3 blood meals per day from the host. They can survive without a blood meal for approximately 10 days. In case of severe infestation, the host loses 10–20 ml of blood per day due to lice. A female head louse lives for 30 days; while the body louse lives for 60 days.

The nits are cemented to the individual hair with proteinaceous matrix that closely resembles the amino acid constituents of the human hair.[16] Mode of transmission is direct contact with infected individual or fomites, combs, brushes, hair accessories, helmets.

Clinical Features

The most important site of involvement in pediculosis capitis is the suboccipital depression; also termed the louse pit.[17] Other commonly involved sites on the scalp include posterior auricular and temporal regions of the scalp. Besides the scalp, lice infestation can also occur on the other hairy areas of the body including the beard and the pubic area. The eggs of the lice also called nits are more easily visualised and are an important sign of the infestation.[18] Nits are oval, whitish, glistening, translucent capsule like structures with an overlying lidor operculum (Fig. 7.7A and B). They are firmly attached to the hair by a sticky secretion from the accessory glands of the adult lice. An important sign of differentiation of the nit from scales of dandruff is that nits cannot be flicked off from the hair.

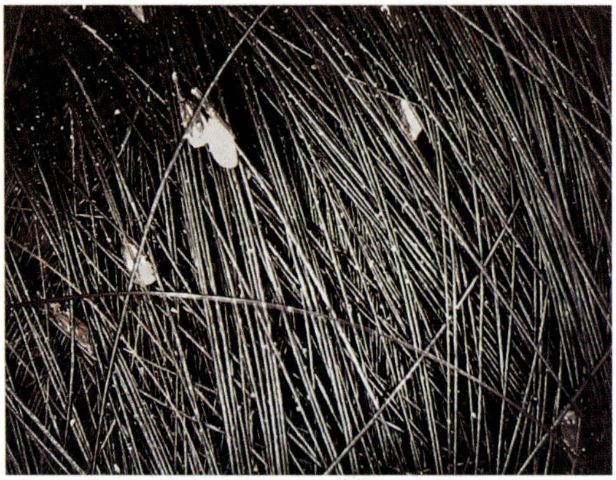

Fig. 7.7A: Nits attached to the hair shafts

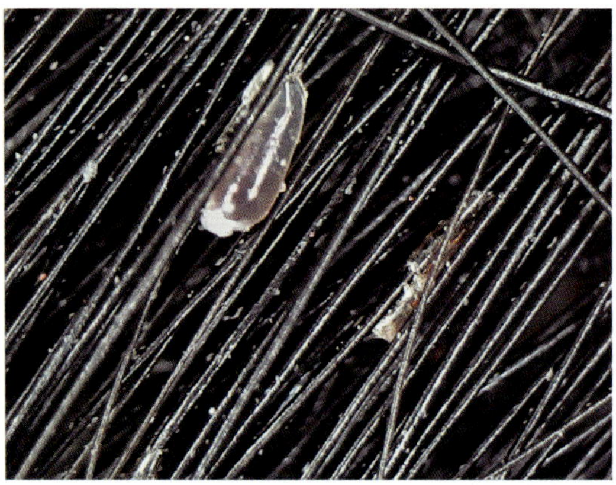

Fig. 7.7B: Dermoscopic visualisation of nits attached to the hair shafts

Occasionally, nits may mimic white piedra. Nits are usually found attached close to the skin (<1 cm) as it provides a temperature which is suitable for their incubation. However, as the hair shaft grows, they are carried away from the scalp. Thus, the distance of the nits from the scalp gives an approximate duration of the infestation.

The most common symptom of lice infestation is itching which may vary from mild to severe or intolerable. The itching is probably caused by a sensitization reaction to the saliva or excreta of the louse. Excessive scratching leads to secondary pyoderma. Cutaneous examination may reveal oozing, crusting, papular eruptions on the nape of the neck, eczematisation of the neck or scalp with cervical lymphadenopathy.

Severe infestation which is neglected and left untreated leads to plica polonica; where the scalp hair gets matted together. Head lice can carry *Staphylococcus aureus* and *Streptococcus pyogenes* on their surface due to the pus and exudation.[19]

Pediculid is the occurrence of generalised erythematous macules, maculopapular rash involving the trunk as a result of sensitization reaction to the head louse.[20]

Diagnosis

The following Table 7.5 enlists the points to be noted for diagnosis of pediculosis.

TABLE 7.5: Diagnosis of pediculosis

1. History
   - Itching over the scalp
   - Characteristic location: Occipital area
2. Clinical examination
   - Nits
   - Louse
   - Excoriation
   - Erythema
   - Scaling over scalp
   - Pyoderma
   - Lymphadenopathy
3. Microscopy
   - Identification of nits, adult lice on the hair (Fig. 7.8)

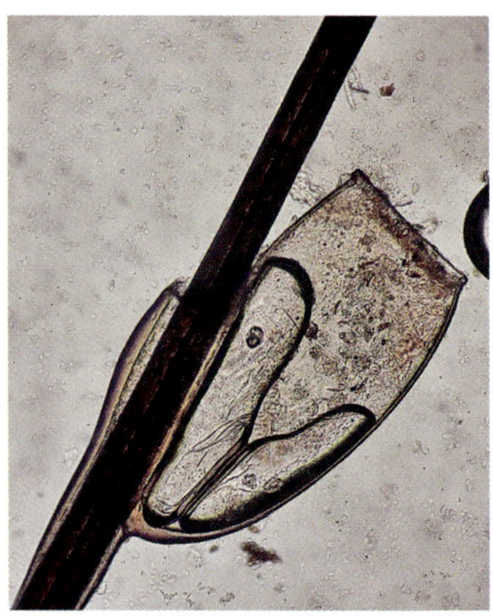

Fig. 7.8: Nit cemented to the hair shaft

Differential Diagnosis

The differential diagnosis of pediculosis capitis is enlisted in Table 7.6.

TABLE 7.6: Differential diagnosis of pediculosis capitis

1. Seborrhoeic dermatitis
2. Psoriasis
3. White piedra
4. Dried hair products (pseudocasts)

Complications

1. Secondary pyoderma
2. Infections
3. Plica polonica

Treatment

The choice of treatment of pediculosis capitis depends on convenience of applications, resistance patterns to various pediculicides, adverse effects and cost of therapy. The management of pediculosis includes treatment with pediculicide, general measures (Table 7.7) and local therapies along with systemic therapy.

TABLE 7.7: General measures

1. Maintenance of hygiene of self, clothes and surroundings
2. Evaluation and treatment of all the family members even if they are asymptomatic
3. Instructions for parents and school teachers
4. Wet hair combing with a fine light coloured nit comb to facilitate removal of lice and nits
5. Avoid sharing of combs, hair brushes, towels and hair clips

Topical Treatment of Pediculosis Capitis (Table 7.8)

Head lice may be treated with topical malathion 0.5% which is left over the scalp for 12 hours and washed off later; this kills the larvae and adult lice. A second application of malathion after 10–14 days is generally recommended to kill the larvae which have hatched later.[21] Gamma-benzene hexachloride (lindane) 1% lotion is an effective topical pediculicide to be applied as a short contact therapy for 5 minutes.[22] However, it is contraindicated in infants, pregnancy and lactation.

TABLE 7.8: Topical treatment of pediculosis capitis

Topical agent	Larvicidal pediculosis capitis/corporis	Ovicidal	Application	Adverse effects	Pregnancy category/ lactation/children
Permethrin 1%	Yes	Yes	Short contact of 10 minutes to dry hair	Allergic contact dermatitis to formaldehyde in predisposed individuals	Pregnancy category B/ approved in infants above 2 months
Malathion 0.5%	Yes	Yes	Application for 12 hours to dry hair	Irritation	Pregnancy category B/ Children above 6 years
GBH 1% shampoo	Yes	No	Local application to dry hair for 4–5 minutes	Central nervous system toxicity	Category C/not approved in children
Ivermectin 1%			Topical application to dry hair for 10 mintues		
Spinosad 0.9% cream	Yes	Yes	Topical application to dry hair for 10 mintues	None	Category B/children above 4 years

Crotamiton 10% is safe but less effective and has to be applied and kept for at least 24 hours. Permethrin 1% (synthetic pyrethroid) is a safe and effective pediculicide. It is applied for 10 minutes to dry hair and later rinsed. It can be safely used in pregnancy. Ivermectin 1% lotion has also been used for the topical treatment of pediculosis capitis. The common causes of treatment failure are described in Table 7.9.

Oral Pediculicides

Oral medications may be used as second-line therapy in pediculosis. The oral agents used for the treatment of pediculosis include ivermectin, albendazole, levamisole and cotrimoxazole. Cotrimoxazole is especially helpful in cases of pediculosis with secondary infection where it controls the secondary infection as well as acts as a pediculicide. The drugs used for oral treatment are included in Table 7.10.

TABLE 7.9: Causes of treatment failure with common topical pediculicides

1. Noncompliance of treatment
2. Reinfestation from the source
3. • Incorrect application of the topical agent
   • Insufficient quantity of agent used
   • Overexposure to the drug due to repeated use
   • Dilution of the drug due to simultaneous use of oil, hair gels
   • Applying of the drug on wet hair
4. Use of the medication as a prophylactic agent
5. Resistance—mutation in sodium channel subunit gene (knockdown resistance type mutation, T929I and L932F)—permethrin resistance[15]

PEDICULOSIS CORPORIS (*PEDICULUS HUMANUS* VAR. *CORPORIS*)

The body louse or clothing louse is called pediculus corporis. It is commonly seen in low socio-economic populations and people with poor hygiene living in overcrowded conditions.

Epidemiology

Pediculosis corporis is a disease of poverty affecting individuals of low socio-economic strata of society, families or populations living in overcrowded areas with low standards of hygiene. It is rare in developed countries. There is no predilection for any age, sex or race.

Etiopathogenesis

The body louse is larger, longer, grey coloured and has longer segments in its antennae (Fig. 7.10). The development and life cycle of the body louse is similar to the head louse. It attaches to the clothing with the hind legs and reaches the skin.

TABLE 7.10: Oral treatment for pediculosis capitis

Drug	Dose	Mechanism of action	Pregnancy category
Ivermectin	200 µg/kg. Repeat after 7–10 days	Flaccid paralysis of the lice due to interference with the chloride channels in the nerve and muscle of the organism	Not approved in pregnancy and lactation
Albendazole	400 ml single dose. Repeat after 7–10 days	Mitochondrial disruption, ATP depletion and cell death	Not approved in pregnancy and lactation
Cotrimoxazole		Interfere with the folate metabolism in louse gut by destruction of the bacteria Not approved as a pediculicide	Not approved
Levamisole	3.5 ml/kg for 10 days	Acetylcholine receptor agonist leads to tonic paralysis of the lice	Not approved

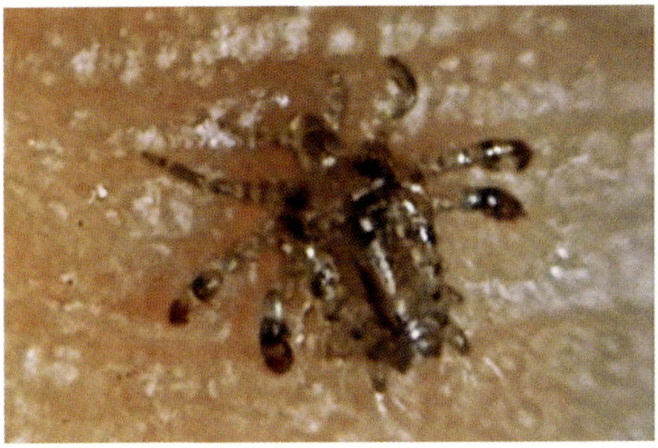

Fig. 7.9: Dermoscopic visualisation of body louse on the hand of a patient

Pediculus corporis is the prime vector for (Table 7.11):

1. Rickettsia
2. Borrelia
3. Bartonella infections

Clinical Features

The main symptom is severe pruritus; which most commonly involves the back, neck, shoulder, trunk. Pruritus is believed to be an immunological response to sensitization to the salivary antigens of the lice. Cutaneous examination of the infested host reveals pin-point red macules, erythematous papules, excoriations, crust. The seams of the clothing that are in contact with the neck, axilla and waistline reveal nits and adult lice. Stains of blood and fecal pellets of adult lice may be found on the clothing and bedding. Chronic long-standing lice infestation results in lichenification, post-inflammatory hyper-pigmentation and severe excoriation marks which is called Vagabond's disease.

TABLE 7.11: Medical importance of pediculus corporis

Vector	Causative agent	Diseases
Pediculus corporis	*Rickettsia prowazekii* *Borrelia recurrentis* *Bartonella quintana*	Epidemic typhus Relapsing fever Trench fever Bacillary angio-matosis Endocarditis

Differential Diagnosis (Table 7.12)

TABLE 7.12: Differential diagnosis of pediculosis corporis

1. Scabies
2. Other infestations
3. Pruritus secondary to liver or renal disease
4. Atopic dermatitis
5. Contact dermatitis
6. Drug reaction
7. Viral exanthema

Diagnosis

Diagnosis is confirmed by visualisation of lice or nits in the seams of the clothing or in the bedding of the affected individual.

Complications

1. Secondary infection
2. Vagabond's disease

Treatment

General Measures

Laundering of clothing including the under-clothes and bedding at high temperature (hot water >50°C is effective in controlling the lice infestation. Hot ironing of the seams of the clothing help to destroy the lice and the nits. The patient is advised to maintain good personal hygiene and have a scrub bath. Frequent changing and washing of the clothes is recommended.

Topical pediculicides are applied over the body with regimens similar to scabies treat-ment. Dusting powders containing DDT, malathion, dieldrin, lindane, permethrin may be used for mass treatment in large populations.

Prevention

Treatment of clothing with permethrin based repellent may help to prevent infestations.

PHTHIRIASIS PUBIS (CRAB LOUSE)

Phthiriasis pubis is the infestation of a host with pubic louse. The pubic louse is broad, short, grey with long legs with morphological resemblance to a crab. Males are smaller than females. The first pair of legs is slender than the other two and has serrated edges. It is a mobile insect and travels 10 cm in a day.

Habitat: Pubic hair is the most common site. But they can also be found on the thighs, trunk, perianal area, beard and moustache. Children residing with infected parents may harbour lice over the eyelids.

Lice lay 20–30 eggs per day in their lifespan of 2 weeks. An adult crab louse can survive for up to 36 hours away from the host.

Epidemiology

Pubic lice infestation is known to occur all over the world. The incidence of this infection is higher in men due to coarse body hair. There is a direct correlation between the incidence of the disease with the sexual promiscuity and to poor hygienic conditions.[23] Pediculosis pubis is often found to occur in association with syphilis and gonorrhoea; in the same age group as that of other venereal diseases which indicates sexual mode of transmission.[24]

Clinical Features

Pruritus is the predominant symptom. The patient may notice moving insects on the skin. Secondary infection and eczematisation secondary to louse infestation may occur. 'Maculae caerulae' are seen on the thighs and trunk in individuals with chronic lice infestation. They are slate-grey to bluish, irregularly shaped macules 0.5–1 cm in diameter. Maculae caerulae are believed to be caused due to the breakdown of bilirubin to biliverdin by enzymes in louse saliva.

Diagnosis

The diagnosis of pubic lice is included in Table 7.13 and differential diagnosis of pediculosis is included in Table 7.14.

TABLE 7.13: Diagnosis of pubic lice infestation

1. **History:** Itching crawling of insects
2. **Clinical examination:** Maculae caerulae visualisation of lice
3. **Microscopic visualisation of lice** (Fig. 7.10)

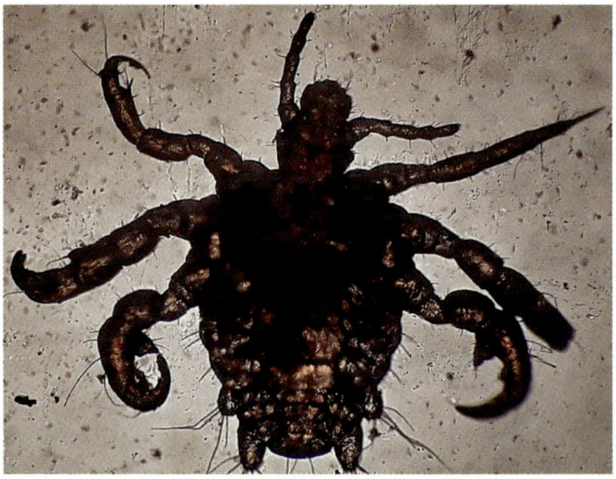

Fig. 7.10: Microscopic examination of the pubic louse

TABLE 7.14: Differential diagnosis of pediculosis

Pediculosis capitis	Pediculosis corporis	*Phthirus pubis*
Seborrhoeic dermatitis	Scabies	Scabies
Cosmetics, e.g. hair spray, gels	Atopic dermatitis	White piedra
Hair casts	Allergic contact dermatitis	Allergic contact dermatitis
White piedra	Irritant contact dermatitis	Irritant contact dermatitis
Black piedra	Drug reaction	Trichomycosis pubis
Trichorrhexis nodosa	Viral exanthema	Hair casts
Psoriasis	Pruritus secondary to liver or renal impairment	
	Autosensitization dermatitis	

Treatment

Treatment of pubic louse infestations is presented in Table 7.15.

TABLE 7.15: Treatment of pubic louse infestation

Drug	Route	Day 1	Repeat application day 8	Adverse effects	Efficacy	Pregnancy category
Permethrin 1% cream	Topical application; contact time 10 minutes to dry hair	Yes	Yes	Not commonly seen allergic contact dermatitis	Fair	B
Permethrin 5% cream	Topical application for 8–12 hours	Yes	Yes	ACD in individuals with sensitivity to formaldehyde	Good	B
Lindane 1% shampoo	Topical application for 4–5 minutes to dry hair, then add water to lather and rinse	Yes	Yes	Potential CNS toxicity; risk of seizures not recommended for, infants, children, pregnant or lactating women, elderly	Poor	C
Ivermectin	200 µg/kg oral dose	Yes	Yes	Potential CNS toxicity not recommended for children <15 kg, pregnancy and lactation	Fair	C

TABLE 7.16: Treatment options for phthiriasis palpebrarum

1. Occlusive agent: White soft paraffin, petrolatum (Vaseline)
   Interferes with the respiratory function of the louse by blocking its spiracles
   Twice daily for 2–3 weeks
   Treatment of choice
2. Fluorescein 10–20%
3. Cryotherapy
4. Mechanical removal of nits with forceps
5. Epilation of eyelashes
6. Physostigmine ointment
7. Oral ivermectin

CONCLUSION

Lice infestations can cause significant distress to the patients. In addition, body louse may be responsible for causing various systemic disorders. In geriatric population the condition may occur because of reduced self-care and neglect by the other family members. It is important to differentiate it from other conditions which commonly cause pruritus in the elderly. Careful examination of clothes may be of value in the diagnosis body louse infestation. The treatment options include permethrin, malathion, lindane and ivermectin. Treatment options for phthiriasis palpebrarum are given in Table 7.16.

DEMODICIDOSIS (FOLLICLE MITES)

Key Points

- Demodicidosis or demodicosis is caused by an obligate human ectoparasite demodex mite.
- *Demodex folliculorum* is most commonly found on the face; while *Demodex brevis* is commonly found over the neck and chest.
- Demodicosis is classified into primary and secondary forms based on the clinical manifestations and diagnostic criteria.
- Diagnosis can be done by biopsy or skin surface biopsy technique (KOH preparation) for visualisation of demodex mites (count >5 per square centimetre).
- Treatment includes antibiotics and anti-inflammatory agents like azelaic acid and metronidazole.

Introduction

Demodicidosis or demodicosis is caused by obligate human ectoparasite Demodex mites who belong to the family Demodicidae and the suborder prostigmata. The Demodex mite is found in or near the pilosebaceous units. Infestation with Demodex mites is usually asymptomatic. There are two species of Demodex. Their details are given in Table 7.17.

Cutaneous diseases caused or associated with Demodex mites are termed demodicosis or demodicidosis. A classification of demodicidosis into primary and secondary forms has also been described.[25]

Epidemiology

Demodex mite is most commonly found on the human facial skin. The prevalence of human Demodex mites varies between 23% and 100%; is highest in 20–30 age group when sebum secretion is highest and is low in infants and children. It is most commonly seen in the middle age group and elderly population where it affects the healthy facial skin; though their density remains low.[26] Histologically, density of Demodex mites greater than 5 mites per follicle is considered significant.[27] Infestation of both the species is more common in males than in females; males having higher colonisation rates and harbouring more *Demodex brevis* than females.

TABLE 7.17: Differences between *Demodex folliculorum* and *Demodex brevis*

Demodex folliculorum	*Demodex brevis*
1. Elongated (0.2–0.4 mm)	Smaller (0.1–0.2 mm)
2. Inhabits the hair follicles; upper part of pilosebaceous unit	Lives in the sebaceous and Meibomian glands; burrows deeper into the duct and sebaceous glands
3. More common	Less common
4. Localised to face	Commonly found on neck and chest
Striated body, 4 pairs of short legs, elongated abdomen, worm-like appearance	

Sites of Involvement

Demodex folliculorum is most commonly found on the face; while *Demodex brevis* is commonly found over the neck and chest. They may also be found on ears, bald scalp, penis, mons veneris, buttocks, ectopic sebaceous glands in the buccal mucosa.[28] *Demodex folliculorum* occupies the hair follicle while *Demodex brevis* is found in the sebaceous and Meibomian glands. *Demodex folliculorum* assumes a head down position in the hair follicle, the tip of the abdomen protruding from the follicular orifice.[29]

Life Cycle

Female Demodex is shorter than the male mite. Both the mites have a genital opening and fertilisation is internal. Mating takes place in the follicular opening and eggs are laid inside the hair follicles or the sebaceous glands. The life cycle from eggs to larvae, nymphal stages and adult stage lasts for 10 days; the adult lives for another 10 days. After fertilisation has occurred, the female burrows down the hair follicle to the sebaceous glands where the eggs are laid. The eggs hatch, undergo moulting and the final nymphal stage emerges from the gland and enters another hair follicle where fertilisation takes place and a new life cycle begins. Demodex mites probably feed on cellular debris and ingest bacteria.[30] The dead mites decompose inside the hair follicles or sebaceous glands.

Pathogenesis

Demodex folliculorum is implicated in the pathogenesis of pityriasis folliculorum. This is characterised by diffuse facial erythema, follicular plugs and a nutmeg grater appearance of the skin of the face and was seen in females who rarely washed their faces and used multiple creams and large quantities of make-up.

The pathogenesis of demodicidosis is poorly understood. Most patients are carriers of the mite and are asymptomatic. HLA-A2 and HLA-Cw2 alleles have a role in the pathogenesis of demodicidosis; A2 allele has a

TABLE 7.18: Pathogenic mechanisms for demodicosis[35]

1. Blockage of hair follicles and sebaceous ducts by mites leading to hyperkeratosis
2. Hosts immune response (humoral and cell-mediated immunity) due to mites and their products
3. Foreign body granulomatous reaction to the mites chitinous skeleton
4. Antigenic proteins of *Bacillus oleronius* have been isolated from *Demodex folliculorum* mites which stimulate an inflammatory response in rosacea

protective role, whereas Cw2 phenotypes have increased susceptibility.[32]

Local immunosuppression may be contributory for demodicosis.[33] Primary or secondary immunosuppression due to various causes, corticosteroid therapy, malignancies, chemotherapy, HIV have been associated with the development of demodicosis.[34]

Table 7.18 gives the pathogenic mechanisms for demodicosis.

Clinical Presentations

Though cutaneous diseases caused by Demodex mites have been termed demodicosis; it is not known whether these are caused by Demodex or the increase in mite density contributes to the inflammation. The different clinical presentations of demodicosis are:

1. Burning and itching sensation over the face with diffuse erythema, follicular scales and nutmeg grater-like appearance (Fig. 7.11A)
2. Rosacea-like lesions (Fig. 7.11B)
3. Pustular eruptions around the angle of mouth
4. Perioral dermatitis like presentation
5. Blepharitis

The various cutaneous diseases in which there is increase in the density of mites are:[34]

1. Rosacea
2. Steroid-induced rosacea
3. Nonspecific facial dermatitis
4. LMDF
5. Perioral dermatitis
6. Madarosis
7. Blepharoconjunctivitis

Demodicosis is classified into primary and secondary forms based on the clinical manifestations and diagnostic criteria.[25]

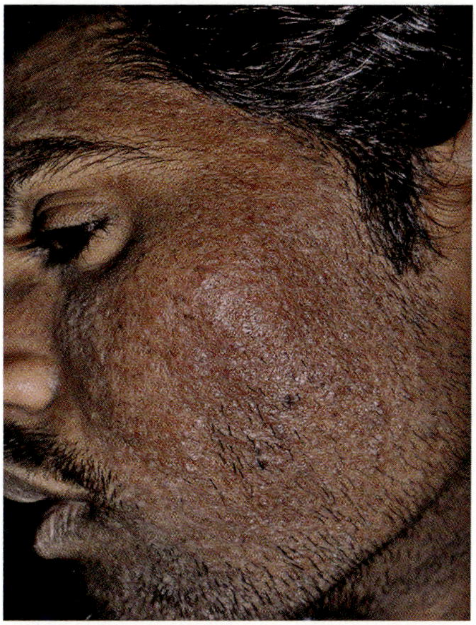

Fig. 7.11A: Diffuse erythema, follicular scales and nutmeg grater-like appearance in a case of demodicosis

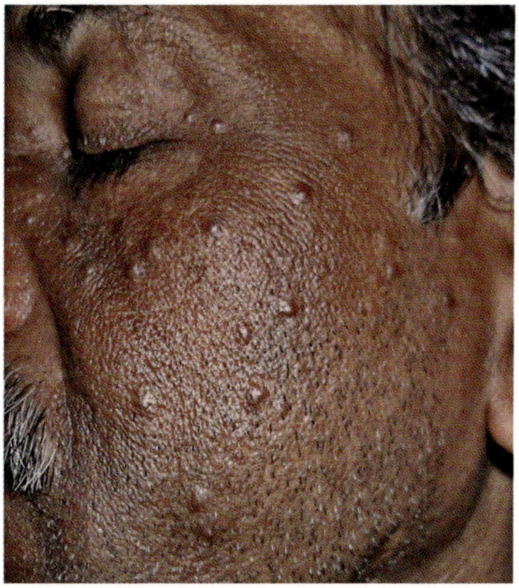

Fig. 7.11B: Papulonodular lesions of demodicosis affecting the face

Primary Demodicosis

It is characterised by late onset usually after the age of 40 years. The lesions are asymptomatic or mildly pruritic. It is characterized by:

- Absence of pre-existing or concurrent inflammatory dermatoses such as acne, rosacea or perioral dermatitis.

- Abnormal increase in mite colonisation which is identified in the active lesions.
- Remission of the disease only after the treatment with topical or systemic acaricides; but not with antibiotics having anti-inflammatory effects like tetracycline or doxycycline.

Secondary Demodicidosis

It is characterised by skin lesions associated with an abnormal increase in Demodex mites in patients with an underlying or pre-existing known cutaneous or systemic disorder. It is usually associated with immunosuppressed states like HIV, leukaemias, chronic renal failure, topical and systemic steroid treatments (Table 7.19). It may occur earlier than the primary form, have a diffuse facial and truncal involvement and is characterised by more extensive inflammation.

Diagnosis

The points for diagnosis of demodicidosis are presented in Table 7.20.

TABLE 7.19: Causes of secondary demodicidosis

1. Immunosuppressed states: HIV, leukaemias, chronic renal failure
2. Iatrogenic: Treatment with oral, topical corticosteroids, topical calcineurin inhibitors, phototherapy, EGFR inhibitors
3. Inflammatory dermatoses: Rosacea, perioral dermatitis, seborrhoeic dermatitis, mycosis fungoides

TABLE 7.20: Diagnosis of demodicidosis

History: Associated cutaneous or systemic condition, drug history

Examination: Clinical suspicion

Microscopy examination of skin scrapings, biopsy or skin surface biopsy technique (KOH preparation)–visualisation of Demodex mites (count >5 per square centimetre is diagnostic)

Dermoscopy

Demodex tails (creamy tail of the mite protruding from the follicular orifice)

Follicular openings: Round, coarse follicular openings with brown plugs and erythematous halo[36]

Treatment

The treatment of demodicidosis lacks standardisation due to lack of culture methods to evaluate the efficacy of various drugs. Various agents with anti-inflammatory and antibacterial mechanisms have been used. The therapeutic options available for the treatment of demodicidosis are enlisted in Table 7.21.

Patients are advised for regular cleansing of the face with soap and water to prevent overgrowth of mites. Topical azelaic acid 15–20% and topical metronidazole are the commonly used topical treatment modalities. Systemic agents include macrolide antibiotics including tetracycline and oral metronidazole.

TABLE 7.21: Treatment of demodicidosis

Topical	Systemic
Topical acaricides	**Oral acaricidal and anti-inflammatory**
1. Crotamiton	Ivermectin
2. Benzyl benzoate 10%	Metronidazole
3. Permethrin 5%	**Target the endosymbiotic *Bacillus oleronius* and anti-inflammatory action**
4. Precipitated sulphur 5%	Tetracyclines
Anti-inflammatory agents	
Azelaic acid 15–20%	
Metronidazole 0.75–2%	

MYIASIS

Key Points

- Myiasis is the infestation of skin and other tissues by the larvae of dipterous flies.
- The various flies causing this infection include human botflies (Dermatobia), blowflies, fleshflies, tumbu flies (*Cordylobia anthropophaga*) and screw worms.
- The treatment of choice for furuncular myiasis is surgical debridement under local anesthesia taking special precaution to avoid leaving parts of larvae inside the body.

Myiasis is the infestation of skin and other tissues by the larvae of dipterous flies. The various flies causing this infection include human botflies (dermatobia), blowflies, fleshflies, tumbu flies (*Cordylobia anthropophaga*) and screw worms. According to the organ of affection, myiasis can be classified as:

1. Ophthalmic myiasis
2. Nasopharyngeal myiasis
3. Intestinal myiasis
4. Cutaneous myiasis

Epidemiology

Myiasis is known to occur all over the world; with a higher incidence in the tropical regions of America and Africa. The flies causing myiasis prefer a warm and humid environment; frequently this infestation shows a seasonal variation with summer preponderance.

Pathogenesis

The larvae of the diptera family feed on the host's tissues, body fluids or ingested food. The most common flies causing myiasis are *Dermatobia hominis* (human botfly) and *Cordylobia anthropophaga* (tumbu fly). The routes of transmission of various fly larvae to the human hosts differ among the fly species. *D. hominis* lays its eggs on mosquitoes which are then transferred to the host; while *C. anthropophaga* lays its eggs on moist clothing and soiled blankets in sand. In wound myiasis, the flies are attracted to deposit their eggs on the raw open wounds. Once the larva makes a contact with the host, it penetrates the skin and further matures in the host tissues utilizing the host body substances. The larvae grow and mature to form adult flies within a period of 1–12 weeks.

Cutaneous myiasis can occur in the following clinical scenarios:[37]

1. Creeping eruption or creeping myiasis—larvae are seen to burrow under the surface of the skin.
2. Furuncular myiasis—boil-like lesions are produced due to infestation with the larvae.
3. Traumatic myiasis or wound myiasis—when wounds become infected with the larvae.
4. Plaque myiasis
5. Body-cavity myiasis

Myiasis may be obligatory or facultative (Table 7.22).[38]

TABLE 7.22: Differences between obligatory and facultative larvae

Obligatory larvae	Facultative larvae
Larvae have to live in a live host for at least a part of their life.	The larvae which are normally free living on dead or decaying flesh, parasitize living hosts.
Cordylobia species, *Dermatobia, Hypoderma, Gastrophilus* species	Calliphora, Lucilia, Phormia and Sacrophaga

Clinical Features

True cutaneous myiasis known as furuncular myiasis is caused by human botfly and tumbu fly and is characterised by localised boil-like lesions or migratory subcutaneous nodules associated with mild constitutional symptoms and eosinophilia. These lesions involve mainly the exposed areas like scalp, face, arms and legs and lead to discomfort and pain.

Traumatic or wound myiasis is seen in patients who neglect their wounds and ulcers.[39] These patients typically complain of chronic long-standing wound which suddenly produces pain and distress. The characteristic larvae, the maggots are seen in large numbers in the suppurating tissues. They may be visible in the superficial tissues or may be situated in deeper pockets or affect deeper structures (Fig. 7.12). Frequently, the movement of the maggots may be identified on careful close observation.

In creeping eruption (larva migrans), the mobility of the larva under the skin surface layers produce a characteristic tortuous, thread-like, red, linear lesion with a terminal vesicle. The fly larvae migrate slowly, persist for many months and are larger than the larvae of helminths causing cutaneous larva

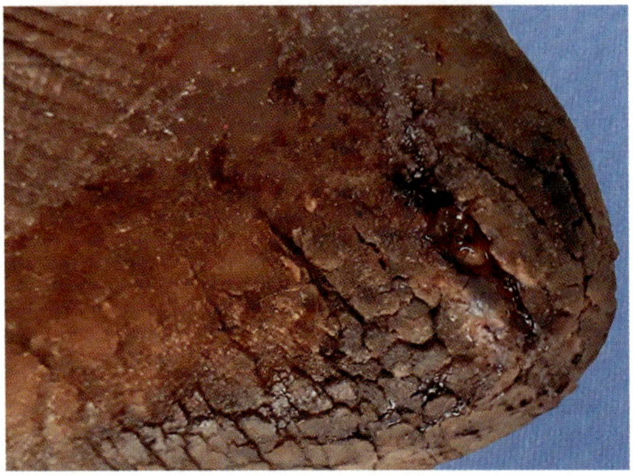

Fig. 7.12: Wound myiasis

migrans.[40] The larva is situated ahead of the vesicle in the apparently normal skin. The commonest cause of creeping eruption of myiasis is species of *Gasterophilus, G. nasalis, G. intestinalis.* Plaque myiasis typically involves many maggots and occurs after flies lay their eggs on clothing.

Diagnosis

1. Visualisation of the maggots or larvae in the suppurating wound.
2. Histopathology—superficial and deep perivascular dermatitis with lymphocytes, neutrophils, eosinophils, mast cells and plasma cells. Larvae may be visualised in cross-section.
3. Ultrasonography can help in the diagnosis, determine the size and evaluating the course of treatment.[41]

Differential Diagnosis (Table 7.23)

TABLE 7.23: Differential diagnosis of myiasis
• Furuncular myiasis: Furunculosis
• Ruptured cyst
• Abscess
• Insect bite reaction
• Tungiasis

Treatment

The treatment of choice for furuncular myiasis is surgical debridement under local anaesthesia taking special precaution to avoid leaving parts of larvae inside the body. The larvae of *Dermatobia hominis* should never be forcibly extracted through the central punctum as it has bulbous anterior end and row of spines that help it anchor to the skin and prevent simple extrusion.[42] A foreign body reaction may develop if parts of the larvae remain in the host tissues during manipulation. Other treatment modalities include occlusion or suffocation of the organisms with petroleum jelly, liquid paraffin or beeswax which causes the larvae to migrate to the surface for air; when they can be removed with the help of forceps.

Wounds infested with larvae should be treated by debridement and irrigation to completely eliminate the larvae from the wound. Myiasis may predispose a patient to tetanus and vaccination of the affected individual must be achieved. When the larvae are buried deep into the host tissues and living in sinuses, they can be forced to come out by application of open dressings of gauze soaked in turpentine. Oral ivermectin has also been used as an alternative to treat all types of cutaneous myiasis.[43]

Prevention

In endemic areas, activities which increase the risk of getting infected with larvae (e.g. wearing damp clothing, resting in sandy areas) must be avoided. Insect repellents should be used to prevent mosquitoes which harbour the human botfly larvae from coming in contact with the host.

CONCLUSION

Myiasis is not a rare infestation in elderly population. Walking barefoot, neglect and improper care of chronic wounds are the predisposing factors for myiaisis. Wounds infested with larvae should be treated by debridement and irrigation to completely eliminate the larvae from the wound.

FLEAS (SIPHONAPTERA)

Key Points

- Fleas are small insects, which do not possess wings but are unique among other ectoparasites in being laterally compressed
- Pulex irritans (human flea infestation) is rare in developed countries and occurs in areas with overcrowding and unhygienic living conditions
- Rotenone or topical pyrethrum kills fleas. Other agents like fipronil, imidacloprid, lufenuron, selamectin have been used for domestic cat and dog flea control

Introduction

Fleas are small insects (1–8 mm long) which may be a cause of infestation in humans. Fleas do not possess wings but are unique among other ectoparasites in being laterally compressed which make them easily pass between the hair and feathers of their host. A hard exoskeleton covered with strong backward directed bristles further help them to pass through the hair and prevent backward slippage. It has a characteristic method of locomotion in the form of jumps of up to 30 cm horizontally and 20 cm vertically which effectively transfers them from one particular host to another. This is possible because of its characteristically long legs which help in forward and upward propulsion.

Adult fleas feed on blood meals from the host; while larvae thrive on organic material (faeces) in the vicinity of the dwelling place of the adult fleas on the host.

The order Siphonaptera comprises three medically important families (Flowchart 7.1):
A. Family Tungidae
B. Family Pulicidae
C. Family Ceratophyllidae

Life Cycle

The adult female flea lays eggs in the debris of dwelling places. The eggs transform into elongated, slender, maggot-like larvae which live on the organic material (faeces of the adult larvae). The pupal stage then transforms into adult fleas if the temperature and humidity conditions are favourable. The pupal stage can remain dormant in its cocoon for a period of one year.

Flea Infestations in Human

Pulex irritans (human flea infestation) is rare in developed countries. It occurs in areas with overcrowding and unhygienic living conditions. Infestations with animal fleas are common and occur in individuals in contact with domestic animals. Individuals moving

Flowchart 7.1: Depicting Siphonaptera family with its medical significance

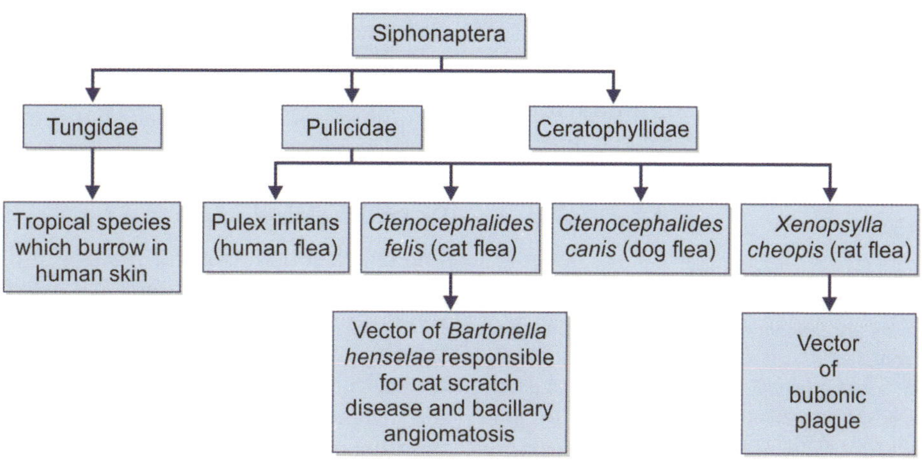

into empty premises which were previously inhabited by pet dogs or cats get severe flea infestation. Such attacks occur as the fleas do not have access to their usual hosts and remain dormant for long periods. The vibration caused by footsteps of the humans triggers the emergence of the fleas from their cocoons. Household infestations with bird flea occur from nests near the house. [44]

Clinical Features

Flea bite typically causes papular urticarial lesions in previously sensitized individuals.[45] Each lesion is morphologically described as a wheal or a papule topped with a central hemorrhagic crust. Occasionally, indurated, pustular, urticarial, bullous or erythema multiforme-like lesions may be seen. The bites may be grouped or occur in a linear configuration. The typical sites of involvement include waist, areas where clothes fit tightly. Cat and dog fleabites occur on the distal extremities.

Diagnosis

The telltale sign of flea infestation is the presence of dried concretions of flea excreta on the animals coat. This can be confirmed by microscopic examination of brushings from all the domestic pets.[46] It is important to identify the flea species responsible for the infestations so that appropriate control measures can be directed at that particular source.

Treatment

Rotenone or topical pyrethrum kills fleas. Other agents like fipronil, imidacloprid, lufenuron, selamectin have been used for domestic cat and dog flea control.[47]

TUNGIASIS

Key Points

- Tungiasis is a disease caused by sand flea *Tunga penetrans* also known as nigua, jigger or chigoe or burrowing flea
- Tungiasis was originally found in Central and South America, later spreading to Africa and Asia till the west coast of India in Maharashtra
- *Tunga penetrans* and *Tunga trimamillata* are the only sand flea species known to infect humans among all the 11 species of Tunga
- Extraction of the organism is the mainstay of treatment.

Introduction

Tungiasis is a disease caused by sand flea *Tunga penetrans* also known as nigua, jigger or chigoe or burrowing flea.[48]

Epidemiology

Tungiasis was originally found in Central and South America, later spreading to Africa and Asia till the west coast of India in Maharashtra. *Tunga penetrans* and *Tunga trimamillata* are the only sand flea species known to infect humans among all the 11 species of Tunga.[49]

Etiopathogenesis

Sand flea is one of the smallest fleas approximately 1 mm in size. The sand fleas are blood-sucking ectoparasites. They are commonly found in tropical areas of Africa and America. In India, they have been found in the coastal areas of Maharashtra. In contrast to human fleas, the sand fleas do not jump. The fertilised female sand flea burrows into the skin of the feet. The most favourable sites for burrowing are the areas with thin skin toe webs, medial side of the feet and skin under the nails.

Once the flea is embedded into the skin, its abdomen enlarges to the size of a pea and numerous eggs are produced. Eggs are then gradually extruded over 2 weeks; subsequently the female flea dies and is sloughed from the skin.

Diagnosis (Table 7.24)

The characteristic clinical feature of a white papule or nodule with a central black dot and a halo of erythema; a history of visit to a known endemic area before the appearance of the lesion is suggestive. The burrowing of the flea is asymptomatic; though occasionally pruritus or pain may be experienced by some patients. The lesion progressively evolves from a small black dot to a pearl-like white papule and subsequently transforms into a larger nodule with a well-demarcated white halo surrounding the black punctum. The morphology closely resembles a watch glass.

Dermoscopy

Dermoscopy of a lesion of tungiasis reveals a round lesion with a dark central pore which corresponds to the genital opening of the flea and a peripheral pigmented ring that corresponds to the posterior abdomen.[50] Within the papule, blue-black blotches corresponding to the eggs or the hematin in the gastrointestinal tract are seen. Some lesions show whitish oval structures linked to form chain-like structures which correspond to eggs.[51]

Histopathology

Histological examination includes hyperkeratosis, acanthosis, parakeratosis, lymphocytic and eosinophilic infiltrate. The body of the flea lies in the pseudocytic cavity at the epidermal side and the head lies in the dermis.

TABLE 7.24: Differential diagnosis of tungiasis

1. Plantar warts
2. Tick bite reactions
3. Myiasis
4. Corn
5. Cercarial dermatitis
6. Squamous cell carcinoma
7. Verruga peruana

TABLE 7.25: Complications of tungiasis[53]

S. No.	Complications
1.	Ulceration
2.	Secondary infection
3.	Lymphangitis
4.	Tetanus
5.	Gangrene
6.	Deformation or loss of nail
7.	Amputation of a digit

The histological hallmarks of tungiasis in histological sections are the findings of eosinophilic cuticle, eggs in different stages of development and tracheal rings of the parasite.[52]

Treatment

The simplest management for uncomplicated cases of tungiasis is the extraction of the entire parasite using a sterile needle. If the flea is engorged then extraction becomes difficult and surgical excision is recommended. In case of secondary infection, oral and topical antibiotics may be administered. Tetanus prophylaxis is indicated for travellers who have not received tetanus vaccine before travel.[54] No standard available drug therapy has yet demonstrated efficacy in the treatment of tungiasis. Metrifonate, thiabendazole and topical ivermectin have been reported to reduce lesions significantly in a randomised trial.[55] Oral ivermectin is reported to be effective. Tungiasis may also heal spontaneously after female sand flea dies.

Prevention

Protective measures like wearing protective clothing, socks and closed footwear can be employed to prevent infection. In addition, sweeping floors and spraying insecticides may be of help.

CONCLUSION

Infestations are commonly encountered in the geriatric age group. Early diagnosis, prompt management, appropriate counselling regarding prevention and implementation of control measures are necessary to further reduce the co-morbidity and distress caused by these infestations.

References

1. Nair BKH. Scabies a retrospect. Indian J Dermatol Venereol. 1973; 39:29–32.
2. Friedman R. The story of scabies. New York: Froben, 1947.

3. Nair BKH, Joseph A, Narayani PI. Epidemiology of scabies. Indian J Dermatol Venereol. 1973; 39: 101–05.
4. Lane AT. Scabies and head lice. Pediatric Ann. 1987; 16:51–54.
5. Marples MJ. The ecology of human skin. Springfield: CC Thomas; 1964.
6. Bartley WC, Mellanby K. The parasitology of human scabies (women and children). Parasitology 1944; 35:207–08.
7. Mellanby K. Scabies. Hampton: EW CLassey, 1972.
8. Danielssen DC, Boeck W. Traite de la Spedalsked ou Elephantiasis des Grecs. Paris: JB Bailliere, 1848.
9. Bhawan J, Milestone E, Malhotra R, et al. Scabies presenting as bullous pemphigoid-like eruption. J Am Acad Dermatol. 1991; 24:179–81.
10. Valks R, Buezo GF, Dauden E. Scabies and leucocytoclastic vasculitis in an HIV seropositive man. Int J Dermatol. 1996; 35:605–06.
11. Usha V, Gopalkrishnan Nair TV. A comparative study of oral ivermection and topical permethrin cream in the treatment of scabies. J Am Acad Dermatol. 2000; 42:236–40.
12. Rasmussen JE. The problem of lindane. J Am Acad Dermatol. 1981; 5:507–16.
13. Youssef MYM, Sadaka HAH, Eissa MM, El Ariny AF. Topical application of ivermectin for human ectoparasites. Am J Trop Med Hyg. 1995; 53:652–53.
14. Mumcuoglu KY, Barker SC, Burgess IE, Combescot-Lang C, Daldleish RC, Larsen KS, et al. International guidelines for effective control of head lice infestations. J Drugs Dermatol. 2007; 6(4):409–14.
15. Madke B, Khopkar U. Pediculosis capitis: an update. Indian J Dermatol Venereol leprol. 2012; 78(4): 429–38.
16. Burkhart CN, Burkhart CG. Head lice: scientific assessment of the nit sheath with clinical ramifications and therapeutic options. J Am Acad Dermatol. 2005; 53:129–33.
17. Gopalkrishna TV, Nair BK, Jayapalan S. Diseases caused by arthropods. In: Valia RG, Valia AR (Eds). IADVL Textbook of Dermatology, 3rd edition. India.: Bhalani Publishing House; 2008: pp. 409–13.
18. Burkhart CN, Burkhart CG, Morrell DS. Infestations. In: Bolognia JL, Joseph JL, Schaffer JV (Eds). Dermatology, 3rd edition. Philadelphia: Elsevier Saunders; 2012. pp. 1426-1430.
19. Meinking TL, Burkhart CG, Burkhart CN. Ectoparasitic diseases in dermatology: reassessment of scabies and pediculosis. In: James W (ed.). Advances in Dermatology, Vol. 15. St Louis: Mosby, 1999; 67–108.
20. Brenner S, Ophir J, Krakowski A. Pediculid—an unusal id reaction to pediculosis capitis. Demratologica. 1984; 168:189–91.
21. Mathias RG, Huggins DR, Leroux SJ, Proctor EM. Comparative trial of treatment with Prioderm lotion and Kwellada shampoo in children with head lice. Can Med Assoc J. 1984; 130:407–09.
22. Meiking TL, Taplin S, Kalter DC, Eberle MW. Comparative efficacy of treatment of pediculosis capitis infestation. Arch Dermatol. 1986; 122(3):267–71.
23. Fischer I, Morton RS. Phthirus pubis infestation. Br J Vener Dis. 1970; 46:326–29.
24. Munkvad IM, Klemp P. Co-existence of venereal infection and pediculosis pubis. Acta Derm Venereol. 1982; 62:366–67.
25. Chen W, Plewig G. Human demodicosis: revisit and a proposed classification. Br J Dermatol. 2014; 170(6):1219–25.
26. Baima B, Sticherling M. Demodicidosis revisited. Acta Derm Venereol. 2002; 82(1):3–6.
27. Forton F, Seys B. Density of *Demodex folliculorum* in rosacea: a case control study using standardised skin-surface biopsy. Br J Dermatol. 1993; 128(6): 650–59.
28. Rufli T, Mumcuoglu Y. The hair follicle mites *Demodex folliculorum* and *Demodex brevis*: biology and medical importance. A review. Dermatologica. 1981; 162(1):1–11.
29. Burns DA. Diseases caused by arthropods and other noxious animals. In: Burns T, Breathnach S, Cox N, Griffiths C (Eds). Rook's Textbook of Dermatology. 8th Edition. UK: Wiley-Blackwell; 2010. pp.11–46.
30. Spickett SG. Studies on *Demodex folliculorum*—Simon 1842. Parasitology. 1961; 51:181–92.
31. Dominey A, Tschen J, Rosen T, et al. Pityriasis folliculorum revisited. J Am Acad Dermatol. 1989; 21(1):81–84.

32. Mumcuoglu KY, Akilov OE. The role of HLA-A2 and Cw2 in the pathogenesis of human demodicosis. Dermatology. 2005; 210(2):109–14.
33. Akilov OE, Mumcuoglu KY. Immune repsonses in demodicosis. J Eur Acad Dermatol Venereol. 2004; 18(4):440–44.
34. Rather PA, Hassan I. Human Demodex mite: the versatile mite of dermatological importance. Indian J Dermatol. 2014; 59(1):60–66.
35. Hsu CK, Hsu MM, Lee JY. Demodicosis. A clinicopathological study. J Am Acad Dermatol. 2009; 60(3):453–62.
36. Segal R, Mimouni D, Feuerman H, PAgowitz O, David M. Dermoscopy as a diagnostic tool in demodicidosis. Int J Dermatol. 2010; 49(9):1018–23.
37. Alexander JOD. Arthropods and human skin. Berlin: Springer; 1984: pp. 87–113.
38. Muller R, Baker JR, Medical parasitology. London: Gower; 1990: pp. 125–8.
39. Spigel GT. Opportunistic cutaneous myiasis. Arch Dermatol. 1988; 124:1014–15.
40. McGraw TA, Turiansky GW. Cutaneous myiasis. J Am Acad Dermatol. 2008; 58:907–26.
41. Bowry R, Cottingham R. Use of ultrasound to aid management of late presentation of *Dermatobia hominis* larva infection. Emerg Med J. 1997; 14: 177–78.
42. Mohrenschlager M, Mempel M, Weichenmeier I, et al. Scanning electron microscopy of *Dermatobia hominis* reveals cutaneous anchoring features. J Am Acad Dermatol. 2007; 57:716–18.
43. McGraw TA, Turiansky GW. Cutaneous myiasis. J Am Acad Dermatol. 2008; 58:907–26.
44. Chua EC, Goh KJ. A flea-borne outbreak of dermatitis. Ann Acad Med Singapore. 1987; 16:648–50.
45. Dickey RF. Papular urticaria—hordes of fleas in the living room. Cutis 1967; 3:345–48.
46. Burns DA. The investigation and management of arthropod bite reactions acquired in the home. Clin Exp Dermatol. 1987; 12:114–20.
47. Rust MK. Advances in the control of *Ctenocephalides felis* (cat flea) on cats and dogs. Trends Parasitol. 2005; 21:232–36.
48. Londono F. Tungiasis. In: Marshall J, editor. Essays in tropical dermatology, vol 12. Amsterdam: Excerpta Medica; 1972.
49. Heukelbach J. Tungiasis. Rev Inst Med Trop Sao Paulo. 2005; 47:307–13.
50. Abarzua A, Cataldo K, Alvarez S. Dermoscopy in Tungiasis. Indian J Dermatol Venereol Leprol. 2014; 80:371–73.
51. Bakos RM, Bakos L. 'Whitish chains': A remarkable *in vivo* dermoscopic finding of tungiasis. Br J Dermatol. 2008; 159:991–92.
52. Maco V, Maco VP, Tantalean ME, Gotuzzo E. Histopathological Features of Tungiasis in Peru. Am J Trop Med Hyg. 2013; 88(6):1212–16.
53. Eisele M, Heukelback J, Van Marck E. Investigations on the biology, epidermiology, pathology and control of *Tunga penetrans* in Brazil: I. Natural history of tungiasis in man. Parasitol Res. 2003; 90: 87–99.
54. Pampiglione S, Fioravanti ML, Gustinelli A, et al. Sand flea (*Tunga* spp.) infections in humans and domestic animals: state of the art. Med Vet Entomol. 2009; 3:172–86.
55. Chen C, Haw-Yeuh T, Shiou-Hwa J. Tungiasis: a case report and review of literature. Dermatologica Sinica. 2011; 29:29–31.

CHAPTER 8

Viral Infections in the Elderly

• *Vivekananda Ittigi*

Introduction

Viral infectious diseases have a significant morbidity and mortality in elderly, even in modern era. Waning immunity and the physiologic changes that come with the ageing make elderly especially prone to infectious diseases. Cell-mediated immunity will be affected in elderly this makes them prone for viral infections. The clinical presentations of viral infections in elderly are often atypical, subtle and elusive. Sometimes this makes clinical diagnosis and treatment challenging.

HERPES SIMPLEX

Key Points

- The initial vesicular stage may not be seen in genital lesions, which present as painful ulcers or erosions. There is usually a history of preceding itching and tenderness.
- The most rapid methods of detecting virus from scrapings from the base of the ulcer are electron microscopy, immunofluorescence, or PCR. Genital herpes in a pregnant woman carries a great risk of ophthalmic infection of the infant. Caesarean section may be indicated. "Eczema herpeticum" and "Kaposi's varicelliform eruption" are terms applied to severe cutaneous and, less commonly, systemic, infection with herpesvirus in patients with atopic eczema and some other skin conditions.[1]

Epidemiology

Herpes simplex viruses have a worldwide distribution and produce primary, latent and recurrent infections. Over one-third of the world's population is thought to have the ability to transmit the virus during periods of viral shedding. Herpetic infections are often asymptomatic and of the HSV-1 type (80–90%). Analyses performed on a global basis have demonstrated HSV-1 antibodies in approximately 90% of individuals 20 to 40 years old. HSV-2 is the etiology of most genital herpes infections (70–90%), although recent studies have shown an increasing incidence attributed to HSV-1 (10–30%).[2] Antibodies to HSV-2 are rarely found prior to adolescence, due to the association of HSV-2 with sexual activity .The seroprevalence of HSV-2 has increased by more than 30% in the past two decades, with approximately 500,000 to 1,000,000 individuals acquiring primary genital HSV annually. Based upon newer serologic methods of HSV detection, the actual prevalence of genital herpes infection in the US is estimated to be between 40 to 60 million. Risk factors associated with the transmission of genital herpes include an age of 15–30 years (period of greatest sexual activity), an increased number of sexual partners, black or hispanic race, lower income levels and education, female gender, homosexuality and HIV positivity.

Etiology and Pathophysiology

Skin inoculation with herpes simplex I or II virus results in retrograde transmission of virus down the nerve, with a reservoir of virus in the ganglion and antegrade transmission of virus back to the skin during attacks. Aggravating or precipitating factors include the following—stress, sunburn (especially herpes labialis), menstrual periods, illness, immunosuppression from drugs or cancer, particularly defects in cellular immunity caused by lymphoma, leukemia, or AIDS patients with severe, progressive herpes should be examined for these underlying factors.

Clinical Features

The herpes simplex virus consists of two viral subtypes. Type I is associated with lesions on the face and fingers and sometimes genital lesions. Type II is associated almost entirely with genital infections. Recurrent episodes of infection are common; with both due to latent infection of sensory nerve ganglia. Primary herpes simplex (type I) infection usually occurs in or around the mouth, with variable involvement of the face.[9] Lesions are small vesicles which crust over and heal but there may be considerable malaise. Type II infection affects the external genitalia[9] and waist area. Recurrent infections are shorter lived, occur in the distribution of a sensory nerve on the face or genitalia, and may be triggered by a variety of stimuli from sunlight to febrile illness.

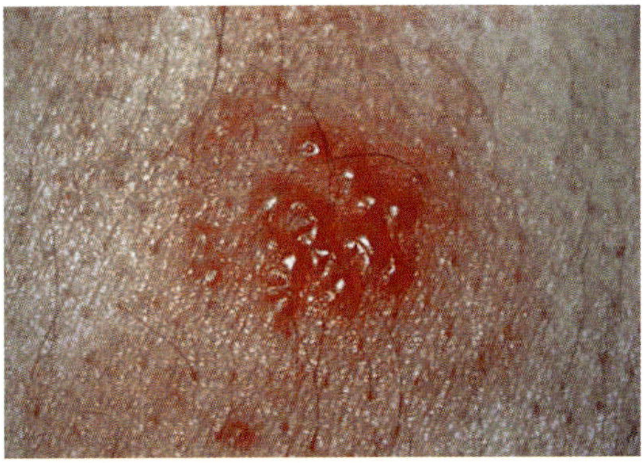

Fig. 8.1: Classical presentation of herpes simplex grouped vesicles with erythematous background

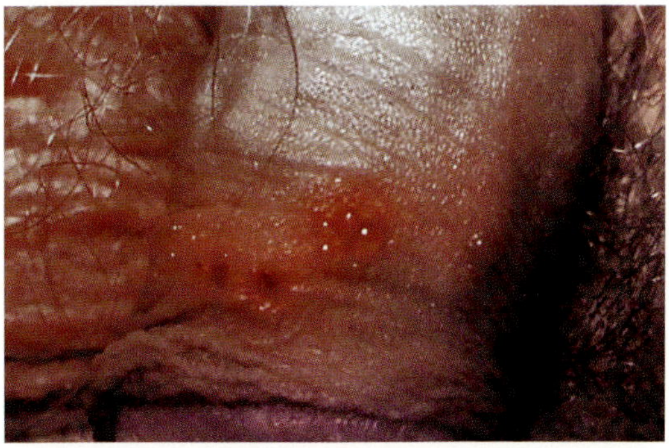

Fig. 8.2: Herpes genitalis grouped vesicles[9]

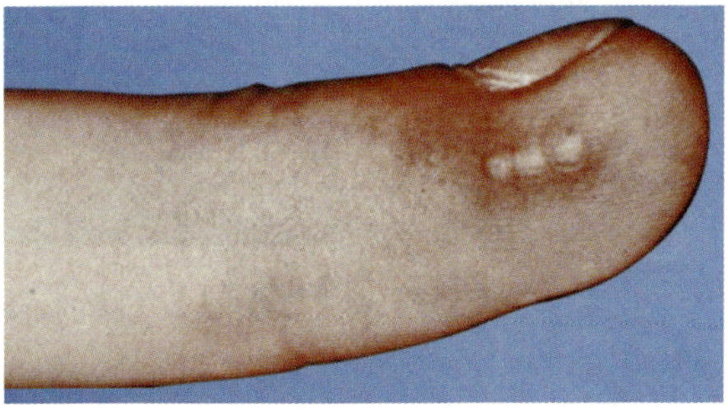

Fig. 8.3: Herpetic whitlow[9]

Histopathology

Histopathologic investigation reveals intra-epidermal reticulated vesicles with characteristic multinucleated giant cells. These may be seen by examining a Tzanck preparation (the undersides of the blister roof and blister base are scraped and visualised with modified Wright-Giemsa [Tzanck] stain).

Treatment

1. Acyclovir 200 mg orally five times daily for 5 days for severe episodes (capsule [200, 800 mg] and elixir [200 mg/5 ml]).
2. Acyclovir 800 mg orally twice daily for 5 days for severe recurrent episodes of male genital herpes.
3. Acyclovir 200 mg orally once, twice, three or four times daily for chronic long-term (1-year) suppression of frequent (twice monthly or more) episodes.
4. L-lysine and several other agents have a 30% placebo effect.

HERPES ZOSTER

Key Points

- Trigeminal zoster when affects the ophthalmic nerve (causes severe conjunctivitis), the maxillary nerve (causes vesicles on the uvula or tonsils) and the mandibular nerve (causes vesicles on the floor of the mouth and on the tongue).
- *Disseminated zoster presents with widespread lesions and visceral lesions may be accompanied by pleuritic or abdominal pain.* Extensive and haemorrhagic vesicles may develop in patients with aids.[1]

Introduction

Even in this modern era, the infectious diseases pose a significant morbidity and mortality in elderly. Immunity and the physiologic changes that accompany the ageing make elderly more prone to infectious diseases. Cell-mediated immunity will be affected in elderly this makes them prone for virus infections.

The clinical presentations viral infections in elderly often atypical, subtle and elusive. Some times this makes clinical diagnosis and treatment challenging. Synonyms for herpes simplex include cold sores, fever blisters (herpes simplex labialis), and genital herpes (herpes simplex genitalis). Herpes zoster is caused by reactivation of the VZV that causes chickenpox in children. It is primarily a disease of older adults. After acute varicella infection, VZV becomes latent in the dorsal root ganglia. An unknown triggering mechanism, possibly caused by declining or impaired cell-mediated immunity, results in a reactivation of VZV. Infection involves the ganglia and satellite cells of the affected region.

Epidemiology

Herpes zoster occurs sporadically without seasonal prevalence throughout the year. The occurrence is independent of the prevalence of varicella. There is no convincing evidence that herpes zoster can be acquired by contact with other persons with varicella or herpes zoster. Rather, the incidence of herpes zoster is determined by factors that influence the host–virus relationship. One strong risk factor is older age more than one-half of which occur in persons 60 years of age or older, and this number increases as the population ages. Another major risk factor is cellular immune dysfunction. Immunosuppressed patients have a 20 to 100 times greater risk of herpes zoster than immunocompetent individuals of the same age. HZ is associated with immunosuppressive conditions including human immunodeficiency virus GIM infection, bone marrow transplant, leukemia and lymphoma, use of cancer chemotherapy, and use of corticosteroids. This is a prominent and early "opportunistic infection" in persons infected with HIV, which is considered often the first sign of immune deficiency. Thus, in individuals who develop herpes zoster HIV infection should be considered.[7]

Etiopathogenesis

During the course of varicella, VZV from lesions in the skin and mucosal surfaces passes to the contiguous endings of sensory nerves. This is then transported centripetally up the sensory fibers to the sensory ganglia, and there the virus establishes latent infection that persists for life. Herpes zoster occurs most often in dermatomes in which the rash of varicella achieves the highest density—those innervated by the first (ophthalmic) division of the trigeminal nerve and by spinal sensory ganglia from T1 to L2.

Although the latent virus in the ganglia retains its potential for full infectivity reactivation is sporadic and infrequent, and infectious virus does not appear to be present during latency. The mechanisms involved in re-activation of latent VZV are unclear, but reactivation has been associated with immunosuppression; emotional stress; irradiation of the spinal column; tumor involvement of the cord, dorsal root ganglion, or adjacent structures; local trauma; surgical manipulation of the spine; and frontal sinusitis (as a precipitant of ophthalmic zoster). Most important, though, is the decline in VZV-specific cellular immuniry that occurs with increasing age.

VZV may also re-activate without producing overt disease. The small quantity of viral antigens released during such contained re-activations would be expected to stimulate and sustain a host immunity to VZV. When VZV-specific cellular immunity falls below some critical level, re-activated virus can no longer be contained.[11] Virus multiplies and spreads within the ganglion, causing neuronal necrosis and intense inflammation, a process that is often accompanied by severe neuralgia. 2T infectious VZV then spreads antidromically down the sensory nerve, causing intense neuritis, and is released from the sensory nerve endings in the skin, where it produces the characteristic cluster of zoster vesicles. Spread of the ganglionic infection proximally along the posterior nerve root to the meninges and cord results in local leptomeningitis, cerebrospinal fluid pleocytosis, and segmental myelitis. Infection of motor neurons in the anterior horn and inflammation of the anterior nerve root account for the local palsies that may accompany the cutaneous eruption, and extension of infection within the central nervous system (CNS) may result in rare complications of herpes zoster (e.g. meningoencephalitis, transverse myelitis).

Clinical Features

Prodrome of Herpes Zoster

Pain and paraesthesia in the involved dermatome often precede the eruption by several days and vary from superficial itching, tingling, or burning to severe, deep, burning and lancinating pain. The pain may be constant or intermittent, and it is often accompanied by tenderness and hyperaesthesia of the skin in the involved dermatome. The pre-eruptive pain of herpes zoster may simulate pleurisy, myocardial infarction, duodenal ulcer, cholecystitis, biliary or renal colic, appendicitis, prolapsed intervertebral disk, or early glaucoma, and this may lead to serious misdiagnosis and misdirected interventions.

Prodromal pain is uncommon in immunocompetent persons younger than 30 years of age, but it occurs in the majority of persons with herpes zoster over the age of 60 years. A few patients experience acute segmental neuralgia without ever developing a cutaneous eruption—a condition known as zoster sine herpete.

Herpes zoster is also known to be associated with a characteristic pain syndrome. The infected, inflamed, and damaged nerve is the source of the acute and chronic pain of herpes zoster. Zoster associated pain can be divided into the following three segments:

1. Prodromal pain is a sharp stabbing pain that occurs before the onset of rash. Depending on the affected dermatome, prodromal pain may be misdiagnosed as such conditions as myocardial infarction, appendicitis, or a gall bladder or kidney stone attack.
2. Acute pain classified as lasting throughout the course of the vesicular eruption.
3. "Post-herpes zoster pain" or PHN, also known as chronic pain, can last from months to years after the disappearance of the herpes zoster lesion.

Rash of Herpes Zoster

The most characteristic feature of herpes zoster is the distribution of the rash, which is nearly always unilateral and is generally limited to the area of skin innervated by a single sensory ganglion. The area supplied by the trigeminal nerve, particularly the ophthalmic division and the trunk from T3 to L2 are most frequently affected; the thoracic region alone accounts for more than half of all reported case. Lesions rarely occur distal to the elbows or knees. The individual lesions of herpes zoster and varicella are indistinguishable. The herpes zoster lesions tend to evolve more slowly and usually consist of closely grouped vesicles on an erythematous base, when compared to the varicella lesions which are discrete, randomly distributed. This difference reflects the intraneural spread of virus to the skin in herpes zoster. As opposed to viremic spread in varicella. Herpes zoster lesions begin as erythematous macules and papules that often first appear where superficial branches of the affected sensory nerve are given off. Vesicles form within 72 to 24 hours and evolve into pustules by the third day. These dry and crust in 7 to 10 days. The crusts generally persist for 2 to 3 weeks. In normal individuals, new lesions continue to appear for 1 to 4 days (occasionally for as long as 7 days). The rash is most severe and lasts longest in older people. Between 10% and 15% of reported cases of herpes zoster involve the ophthalmic division of the trigeminal nerve. The rash of ophthalmic zoster may extend from the level of the eye to the vertex of the skull, but it terminates sharply at the midline of the forehead. When only the supratrochlear and supraorbital branches are involved, the eye is usually spared. Involvement of the nasociliary branch, which innervates the eye as well as the tip and side of the nose, provides VZV with direct access to intraocular structures. Thus, careful attention must be given to the condition of the eye, when lesions involve the tip and the side of the nose. Nearly in 30 to 40% of patients with ophthalmic zoster there is eye involvement. When corneal sensation is severely impaired, it may lead to neurotrophic keratitis and chronic ulceration.

Herpes zoster affecting the second and third divisions of the trigeminal nerve as well as other cranial nerves may produce symptoms and lesions in the mouth, ears, pharynx, or larynx. The so-called Ramsay Hunt syndrome (facial palsy, in combination with herpes zoster of the external ear or tympanic membrane, with or without tinnitus, vertigo, and deafness) results from involvement of the facial and auditory nerves. It is not uncommon for there to be scattered lesions outside the dermatome, usually fewer than 20. In the typical case, new vesicles appear for 1–5 days, become pustular, crust, and heal. The total duration of the eruption depends on three factors: Patient age, severity of eruption, and presence of underlying immunosuppression. In younger patients, the total duration is 23 weeks, whereas in elderly patients, the cutaneous lesions of zoster may require 6 weeks or more to heal. Scarring is more common in elderly and immunosuppressed patients. Scarring also correlates with the severity of the initial eruption. Lesions may develop on the mucous membranes within the mouth in zoster of the maxillary mandibular division of the facial nerve, or in the vagina in zoster in the S2 or S3 dermatome.

Diagnosis

Tzank smear: A Tzanck smear consisting of scrapings from early lesions reveals multinucleated epithelial giant cells in the majority of herpetic lesions (75%). In biopsy specimens, ballooning of the cytoplasm of keratinocytes is one of the earliest histologic changes within the intranuclear inclusion bodies. Multinucleated giant cells form by fusion of the infected keratinocytes. Spongiosis occurs within the epidermis, and intraepidermal vesicles appear as fluid containing large quantities of virus.

Viral cultures and PCR confirms the diagnosis.

Prevention

Herpes zoster vaccine (Zostavax, Merck and Co., Inc.) was licensed and recommended in 2006 for prevention of herpes zoster among adults aged 60 years and older. In March 2011, the Food and Drug Administration (FDA) approved the use of Zostavax in adults aged 50 through 59 years. Based on a study of approximately 22,000 adults aged 50–59 years in the United States and four other countries, the FDA approved the expanded indication for Zostavax.

Complications

Most patients recover from HZ without any complications. However, in the elderly and the immunocompromised, complications are likely. The complications may be cutaneous, ocular, visceral and neurologic. The cutaneous complications include bacterial infection, scarring, zoster gangrenosum and cutaneous dissemination. The visceral complications such as pneumonitis, hepatitis, esophagitis, pericarditis, gastritis, cystitis and arthritis. Postherpetic neuralgia, meningo-encephalitis, transverse myelitis, peripheral and cranial nerve palsies, sensory loss, deafness and ocular complication are the neurological complications following HZ. Multidermatomal, disseminated or trigeminal HZ tends to have a higher complication rate.

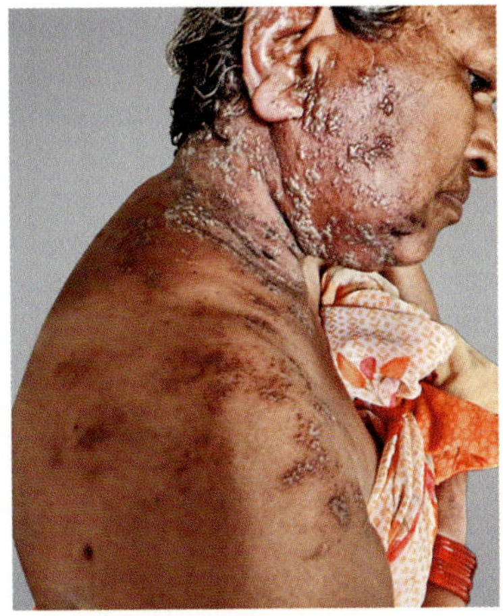

Fig. 8.4: Herpes zoster: 65-year-old female patient involving C3 and C4 dermatome

Treatment

For acute herpes zoster, the following treatment is used:

1. High-dose acyclovir 800 mg orally five times daily, for 7–10 days, reduces pain, hastens lesion healing, and may reduce the incidence of postherpetic neuralgia. Available in capsule (200, 800 mg) and elixir (200 mg/5 ml) forms, acyclovir should be taken with sufficient water to minimize the risk of crystallization in the kidney. Valacyclovir is also quite effective, when given 1 g three times daily for 10 days.
2. The use of early systemic corticosteroids to prevent PHN is controversial. In patients over 50 years of age, who have had zoster for less than 6 days, prednisone in tapering doses (60 mg, orally for 1 week, then 40 mg orally for 1 week and 20 mg orally for 1 week), or triamcinolone acetonide 40 mg IM, have been used.

Postherpetic neuralgia, when established is difficult to treat, but the following may be tried to reduce the pain:

1. Analgesics, anticonvulsants (carbamazepine), and antidepressants (amitryptyline) have been used, with varying effectiveness. These drugs must be used with great care in elderly patients because of central nervous system side effects.

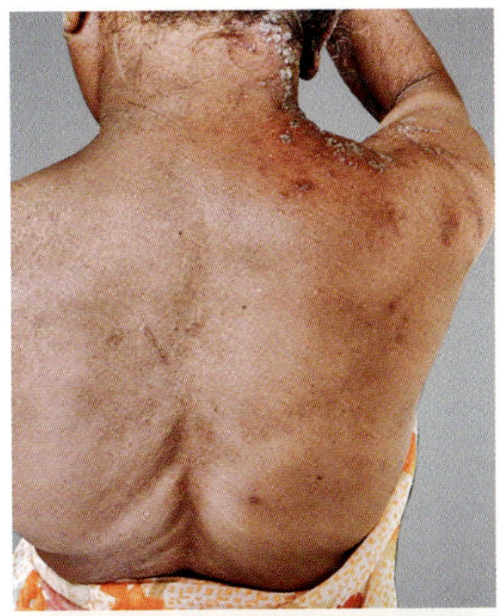

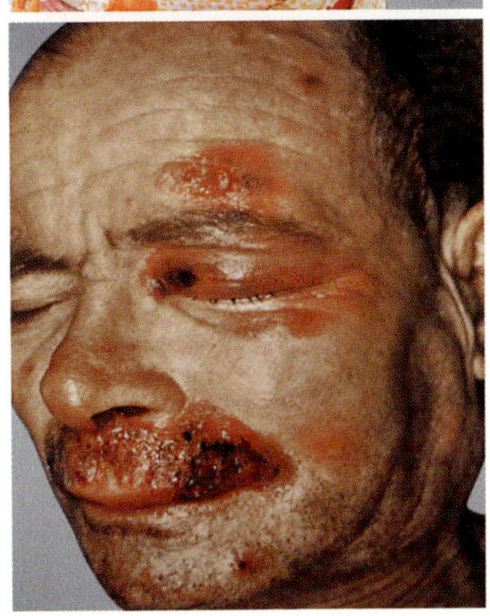

Fig. 8.5: Herpes zoster involving ophthalmic branch[9]

2. Intralesional steroids, intralesional anaesthetics (lidocaine), and a transcutaneous electrical nerve stimulation (TENS) unit may relieve pain locally.
3. Topical capsaicin cream qid depletes substance P, achemical mediator of pain.

HUMAN HERPESVIRUS TYPE 8 (HHV-8)

Introduction

HHV-8, previously called Kaposi's sarcoma-associated herpesvirus (KSHV), is a latent virus found in the vast majority of all types of Kaposi's sarcoma (KS) worldwide.

Synonym

Kaposi's sarcoma—associated herpesvirus (KSHV).

Key Points

- HHV-8 is a latent virus found in the vast majority of all types of Kaposi's sarcoma (KS) worldwide.
- The seroprevalence of HHV-8 corresponds to the incidence rates of KS and varies by geographic location.
- Primary infection with HHV-8 has not yet been identified, and its associated diseases are postulated to be a result of viral reactivation.

History

In 1872, Moriz Kaposi described a rare cutaneous neoplasm, predominantly affecting elderly men of Ashkenazi Jews and/or Mediterranean descent, that subsequently came to be known as Kaposi's sarcoma (KS). There was little medical interest in this disease until it was noticed in young, homosexual men at the onset of the AIDS epidemic. In 1994, Chang et al reported the association of KS and HHV-8 by identifying herpes-like DNA sequences in KS lesions from an AIDS patient. Associations of HHV-8 with other cancers in AIDS patients, such as Castleman's disease and body cavity-based lymphomas, were noted in 1995 and 1996.

Epidemiology

HHV-8 is found in KS lesions worldwide. The classic form of KS peaks after the sixth decade of life and typically occurs in men of Mediterranean and Ashkenazi Jews descent. HIV positive men who have sex with men are at extreme risk, developing KS at a rate 20,000 times greater than that of the general population. In Southern equatorial Africa, approximately 10% of all histologically proven malignancies are caused by African-endemic KS. This form of KS affects two distinct age groups: Young adults (mean age, 35 years) and young children (mean age, 3 years). Seroprevalence of HHV-8 varies geographically, ranging from less than 5% in North America, Britain and Northern Europe to about 10% for Southern Europe and 30 to 100% in African countries. In North America and Europe, the HHV-8 virus is present in approximately 30% of HIV-1-infected men who have sex with men.

Pathogenesis

The mechanisms of HHV-8 transmission are not well understood. Receptive anal intercourse appears to be a primary factor for transmission, as the seroprevalence of HHV-8 is higher in men who have sex with men than in HIV-infected women. The number of same-sex male partners and the presence of HIV infection may be other risk factors. Other studies have found that mother-to-child transmission occurs in about one-third of HHV-8-infected mothers in African countries. HHV-8 has been found in donated blood, and transmission by blood transfusion was recently demonstrated. KS is a vascular endothelial malignancy and the neoplastic cells are closely related to lymphatic endothelial cells. Although HHV-8 is found in the vast majority of all types of KS, there is no agreement on the exact mechanism by which HHV-8 results in the development of KS. However, studies have shown that HHV-8 can infect both lymphatic and blood vascular endothelial cells and induce transcriptional reprogramming, leading to expression of lymphangiogenic molecules.[8]

Clinical Features

The four KS types (classic, HIV/AIDS-related, immunosuppression associated, and African endemic) have somewhat different presentations and different clinical courses, although all typically evolve through stages as red, brown or violaceous papules, plaques and nodules. Oedema is often present in all types. The lesions of *classic KS* tend to have a spongy feel during the early stage of the disease and become more firm with time. Lesions initially develop as purplish-red plaques primarily on the lower legs of elderly men of Mediterranean descent and can later become brown, hyperkeratotic and/or eczematous. The oral mucosa and gastrointestinal tract are rarely involved and the disease typically has a slow[8] progression.

Treatment

Chemotherapy, in combination with ART, should be administered to patients with visceral involvement and is likely to be a useful adjunctive therapy in individuals with disseminated cutaneous KS. Liposomal doxorubicin and paclitaxel exhibit comparable response rates and progression-free survival. Liposomal doxorubicin exhibits less high-grade toxicity compared to paclitaxel, therefore, it is generally preferred as first-line therapy.[8]

CONCLUSION

In elderly population, the diagnosis and management of viral diseases of the skin are significant issues. With advances in these areas, there are new tools to combat these diseases and limit morbidity. It is important for clinicians to monitor and treat these diseases aggressively in the elderly, as these patients are susceptible for immunosuppression. Thus, further advances in antiviral therapy and the potential for the development of antiviral vaccines are necessary and will aid in the therapy of these diseases.[6]

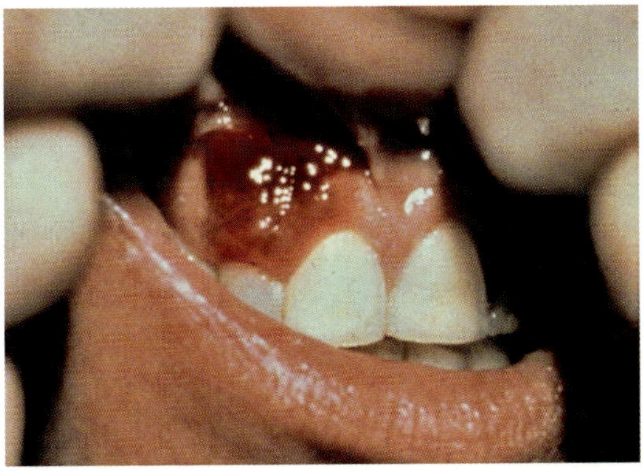

Fig. 8.6: Kaposi's sarcoma oral lesion[8]

References

1. Buxton P. ABC of Dermatology: viral infections. Br Med J (Clin Res Ed). 1988 Jan 23; 296(6617):257–61.
2. Rook's Textbook of Dermatology, viral infections, 25.2–25.92.
3. Dermatology clinics of north America journal pp. 51–60.
4. Kishore Kumar R, Max MB, Schafer SC, et al. Desipramine relieves postherpetic neuralgia. Clin Pharmacol Ther 1990; 47:305–12.
5. Beutner KR. Clinical management of herpes zoster in the elderly patient. Compr Ther. 1996; 22:183–86.
6. Skin infections in the elderly, Jeffrey M. Weinberg, MD*, Janet Vafaie, BA, Noah S. Scheinfeld, MD dermatology clinics.
7. Fitzpatrick's Dermatology in General Medicine 2008, viral infections, p. 1873.
8. Andrew's Diseases of the Skin Clinical Dermatology, viral infections, pp. 360–67.
9. Atlas of Geriatric Dermatology, Robert A Norman, Edward M Young, infections, pp. 149–57.
10. Clinical Cases in Geriatric Dermatology, Robert A Norman, Justin Endo, pp. 27–31.
11. Assefzadeh M, Ghasemi R, Naimian SH, Shahali H, Sajadi E. A 72-year-old diabetic woman with herpes zoster paresis: a case report. Iranian Journal of Clinical Infectious Diseases 2010; 5(4):239–41.
12. Bowsher D. The effects of pre-emptive treatment of postherpetic neuralgia with amitriptyline: a randomized, double-blind, placebocontrolled trial. J Pain Symptom Manage. 1997; 13(6):327–31.
13. Decroix J, Paetsch H, Gonzalez R, et al. Factors influencing pain outcome in herpes zoster: an observational study with valaciclovir. Valaciclovir International Zoster Assessment Group (VIZA). J Eur Acad Dermatol Venereol. 2000; 14(1):23–33.
14. Dworkin RH, Johnson RW, Breuer J, et al. Recommendations for the management of herpes zoster. Clin Infect Dis. 2007; 44 Suppl 1:51–526.
15. Harpaz R, Ortega-Sanchez R, Seward JF, Advisory Committee on Immunization Practices (ACIP) Centers for Disease Control and Prevention (CDC). Prevention of herpes zoster: Recommendations of the Advisory Committee on Immunization Practices (ACIP). MMWR Recomm Rep. 2008; 57(RR-S): 1–30. quiz CE2-4.

CHAPTER 9

Bacterial Infections of the Skin in Elderly

• *Asit Mittal* • *Kapil Vyas*

Key Points

- Bacteria may cause skin disease by direct invasion of tissue, through secreting toxins or through immunologic reactions.
- Skin changes with ageing specially thinning of epidermis, decreased glandular secretions, increased trauma, injuries and pressure sores and immunosuppression in older persons result in more infections of skin and soft tissues.
- Bacterial skin infections (pyodermas) are primarily caused by *Staphylococcus aureus* and *Streptococcus species*.
- Local manifestations include folliculitis, furuncle, carbuncle and impetigo while systemic reactions include staphylococcal toxic shock syndrome.
- Histopathology shows abundant neutrophilic infiltration admixed with lymphocytes.
- Treatment includes topical, oral or parenteral antibiotics considering current antimicrobial resistance patterns.
- Emergence of antibiotic resistant strains has been a major problem in treating staphylococcal infections, specially methicillin-resistant *Staph. aureus* (MRSA).

Introduction

The human skin is normally colonized by huge numbers of bacteria that live harmlessly as commensals on its surface and within its hair follicles. Overgrowth of some of these resident organisms may result into minor disease of the skin or its appendages. On the other hand, bacteria not normally found there, called pathogenic bacteria, may colonize the skin surface and lead to disease. Transient bacteria land more or less fortuitously on the skin, stay briefly in small numbers before disappearing, and are unable to multiply and thrive there. Ageing is one of the most consistently cited factors influencing morbidity and mortality.[1] A decline in the regular functions of skin is observed in ageing, including cell turnover, barrier function, sensory perception, mechanical protection, wound healing, immune responsiveness, thermoregulation, sweat and sebum production, vitamin D production, and capacity to repair DNA.[2] Superficial bacterial infections of the skin and soft tissue caused by Staphylococcus and Streptococcus are seen frequently due to alteration in ageing skin architecture and loss of barrier function caused by various physical factors, malnourishment, and nutritional deficiencies.[3]

Epidemiology

Elderly population aged 60 and above constitutes a large and rapidly growing segment exceeding 7% of Indian population. Further the geriatric population is expected to double by 2026. The reasons proposed for this are increase in life expectancy as well as decrease in birth rates.[4] Dermatoses of aged population vary from country to country. Given the variable presentation of skin and soft tissue infections (SSTIs) and also a majority of SSTIs tend to resolve within 7–10 days, an assessment of their incidence and prevalence has been difficult. A study[5] from Turkey conducted on 4099 geriatric patients found eczematous dermatitis to be the most common disorder in the population studied, followed by fungal infections, pruritus, bacterial infections, and viral infections. Bacterial infections comprised 7.3% of all the patients. A seasonal pattern was also noticed with geriatric dermatoses. Fungal and bacterial infections were common in summer. In Singapore, xerosis and asteatotic eczema were the most common disorders, followed by scabies, bacterial infections, and eczematous dermatitis.[6] The estimated incidence rate of SSTIs was 24.6 per 1000 person-years.[7] A multicentric study of skin diseases in geriatric patients observed bacterial infections comprising 8.7% of all the patients.[8] A study from Eastern India observed pyoderma in 13% of all the geriatric patients.[9] Among hospitalized patients, the estimated prevalence of SSTIs is 7–10%.[10,11] There is an increased prevalence among men (60–70% of all cases) and patients between 45 and 64 years of age. Approximately 70–75% of all cases are managed in the outpatient setting,[12] with many cases of SSTIs involving the lower leg region.[7,13] Overall, the rate of complicated cellulitis is low (erysipelas 0.09 per 1000 person-years; lymphadenitis 0.16% of all cellulitis cases; lymphangitis 0.16 per 1000 person-years and necrotizing fasciitis 0.04 per 1000 person-years).[7] A high prevalence of overall infections and infestations was seen in an Indian study (29.9%) where bacterial infections constituted 2.7% of all the patients.[14] In another Indian study prevalence rate of infections and infestations was found to be 43.5% and pyodermas as 4.2%.[15]

Risk Factors

Although aberrations of host defence mechanisms with ageing are thought to be the major risk factors for acquiring infection, other general factors, such as environmental exposure to microbes, physiological changes with ageing, associated diseases that increase susceptibility to infection, etc. may be equally important.[16] Skin changes with ageing specially thinning of epidermis and decreased glandular secretions, and increased trauma, injuries and pressure sores along with immunosuppression in older persons result in more infections of skin and soft tissues. Phagocytic function of polymorphonuclear leukocytes appears to be normal in elderly persons.[17] Cell-mediated immunity declines with ageing. Humoral immunity abnormalities with ageing have been less well defined than cell-mediated immunity. Total number of circulating B cells are unchanged with age, but there is evidence that regulatory T lymphocytes (T cells), such as suppressor and helper T cells, may play an important role in B cell responses to certain antigens such as pneumococcal polysaccharide.[18] There is also evidence that shows that ageing may affect T cells that regulate antibody response but not necessarily the antigen-specific B cells.[19]

Despite the outlined importance of an intact immune system, another crucial component is nutritional status, which in turn influences the immune system, and is compromised by malnutrition, leading to a higher risk of infection and mortality.[20]

Recent evidence suggests that bacterial infections are a relatively frequent occurrence in diabetic patients and that there may be an associated increase in morbidity and mortality.[21,22] Patients with type 2 diabetes have an increased incidence of common community acquired infections,[23,24] including lower respiratory tract infection, urinary tract infection (UTI), and skin and mucous membrane infections.[25] Also, a substantially increased susceptibility to potentially fatal infections including necrotizing fasciitis and emphysematous pyelonephritis are present, but these are rare.[21,22] In addition, diabetes has been identified as an independent risk factor for severe Gram positive blood stream infections,[24,26] and for hospital-acquired postoperative bacterial infections.[27]

The elderly are troubled with more chronic illness, thus requiring more time in hospital.

Patients 65 years or older spent approximately a third of all days in hospital in the United States.[28] On an average, the risk of acquiring a nosocomial (hospital acquired) infection is approximately 4%.[29] However, the elderly have a relative risk rate for nosocomial infection that is nearly three times that of the general population.[30] The presence of risk factors for developing an SSTI has not been shown to correlate with disease severity.[31]

Pathogenesis

Human skin serves as the first line of defence against microbial infection as a physical barrier; by secreting low pH, sebaceous fluid and fatty acids to inhibit growth of pathogens; and by possessing its own normal flora, thus deterring colonization by other pathogenic organisms.[32] Unfortunately, having penetrated the integumentary barrier, through a break in the barrier or contiguous spread, infecting organisms may incite an inflammatory response. The development of an SSTI depends on bacterial adherence to host cells, invasion of tissue with evasion of host defences and elaboration of toxins. Virulence genes, in most pathogenic bacteria, encode special proteins, such as endotoxins and exotoxins, that confer these properties and are mainly responsible for clinical disease. Endotoxins are lipopolysaccharide chains found abundantly in Gram-negative bacterial cell walls. Exotoxins, on the other hand, are actively secreted proteins that cause tissue damage or dysfunction through enzymatic reactions, cellular dysregulation or pore formation, with subsequent cell lysis. A special group of exotoxins is the superantigens. These are most notably produced by virulent *S. aureus* and *S. pyogenes* strains. These antigens bind conserved portions of T cell receptors and are, therefore, able to activate a large number of T lymphocytes resulting into massive release of cytokines causing a grossly exaggerated inflammatory response.[32]

Microbiology

The skin constantly interacts with the external environment and is colonized with a diverse population of microbes. The vast majority of colonizing flora consists of bacteria. The majority of the pyodermas are caused by either *S. aureus* or group A Streptococcus. These bacteria cause a broad clinical spectrum of infection ranging from superficial pyodermas to invasive soft tissue infections depending on the virulence of the organism and host factors. Ki and Rotstein[33] organised the distribution of flora over the body by dividing the body into two halves at the waistline. The typical organisms that colonize the skin above the waist are usually Gram-positive species such as *Staphylococcus epidermidis, Corynebacterium* species, *S. aureus* and *Streptococcus pyogenes*. The latter two species are particularly significant because they contribute to a majority of SSTIs.[34] On the other hand, the typical organisms that colonize the skin below the waist are both Gram-positive and Gram-negative species. enteric species, such as Enterobacteriaceae and *Enterococcus* species, gravitate to and colonize this area of the skin. The composition of the flora can vary drastically depending on climate, genetics, age, sex, stress, hygiene, nutrition and hospitalisation.[34]

The causative organism of SSTIs may be normal host flora transferred from the environment, community-acquired or hospital-acquired. Hospital-acquired SSTIs in North America showed an increase in more resistant organisms. Specifically, *S. aureus* (approximately 40% of all cases were methicillin resistant, MRSA), *Pseudomonas aeruginosa* (10.8%) and *Enterococcus* species (8.2%) ranked significantly higher than beta-hemolytic streptococci (2.3%), which constitute the majority of community-acquired SSTIs.[35] New evidence suggests an increase in methicillin-resistant *S. aureus* (MRSA) in community-acquired SSTIs also.[36–38] This isolate is characterised by the insertion of the staphylococcal chromosomal cassette mecA type IV and is associated with the Panton-Valentine leukocidin virulence factor.[39] The microbial flora of a chronic wound changes over time. In an early wound, Gram-positives such as *Staphylococcus aureus* and beta-hemolytic streptococci predominate. After about four weeks, Gram-negative rods, i.e. Proteus, *Escherichia coli* and Klebsiella colonize the wound. Later on anaerobes predominate and after several months the average wound may be colonized by 4–5 different organisms.[40]

Clinical Presentation

Bacterial infections of the skin produce a diversity of clinical manifestations. Typical presenting features are nonspecific and include local erythema, oedema, pain and warmth. In contrast, more severe infections may present with cytokines induced or bacterial toxin-induced systemic signs and symptoms, including hyper-/hypopyrexia, hypotension, increased heart rate, altered mental status, with a rapidly progressive course and extreme pain and vesiculobullous formations due to necrosis of the dermis.[41,42] The bacterial skin infections can be grouped on the basis of causative pathogenic bacteria rather than by morphology. However, in many cases the infectious agent will be identified by culture, and the diagnosis will be delayed till the culture results are available. In addition, in cases of impetigo, cellulitis, and necrotizing fasciitis, multiple pathogens are capable of causing the same clinical pattern and require treatment decision based on the most likely pathogens. Therefore, morphologic classification of skin lesions is still important and can guide initial diagnosis and empiric antibiotic treatment (Table 9.1).

TABLE 9.1: Classification of pyodermas

1. **Superficial pyodermas**
   a. Impetigo
   b. Folliculitis
   c. Furuncle
   d. Carbuncle
2. **Deep pyodermas**
   a. Cellulitis
   b. Erysipelas
   c. Lymphangitis/lymphadenitis
   d. Streptococcal gangrene
   e. Pyomyositis
3. **Metastatic/toxin associated pyodermas**
   a. Bacteremia/septicaemia
   b. Staphylococcal scalded skin syndrome
   c. Staphylococcal toxic shock syndrome
   d. Purpura fulminans

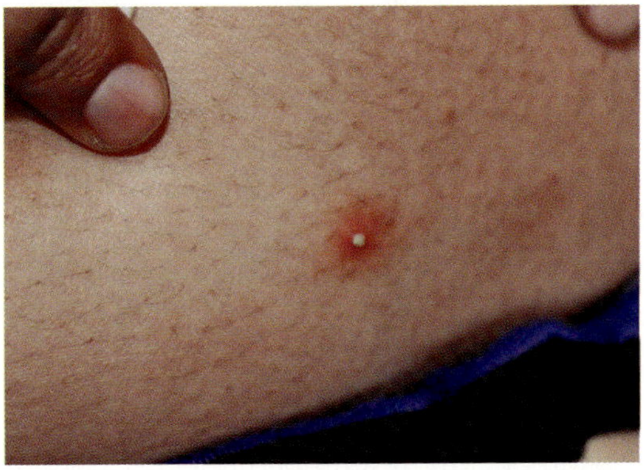

Fig. 9.1: Folliculitis: Image showing pustule with surrounding perifollicular erythema over the abdomen

FOLLICULITIS

Folliculitis is a pyoderma that begins within the hair follicle and is classified according to depth of invasion: Superficial and deep. Superficial folliculitis has also been termed follicular or Bokhart's impetigo. A small, dome-shaped pustule occurs at the ostium of a hair follicle often in the beard area, axilla or buttocks of adults that heals spontaneously without scarring (Fig. 9.1).[43] The hair shaft is frequently seen in the centre of the pustule. Systemic symptoms rarely coexist. *S. aureus* is the most likely pathogen; however, commensal organisms such as yeast and fungi occasionally appear, especially in immunocompromised patients.[44] Topical therapy with erythromycin, clindamycin, mupirocin, fusidic acid or benzoyl peroxide can be administered to accelerate the healing process. Superficial folliculitis is not always infective in origin. Physical or chemical injury to the skin may result into folliculitis, the pustules of which may be sterile or may contain coagulase-negative staphylococci. Causative bacteria will occasionally invade the deeper portion of the follicle, causing swelling and erythema with or without a pustule at the skin surface. These lesions are painful and may scar. Sycosis barbae is a deep folliculitis with perifollicular inflammation occurring in beard areas of the face and upper lip. Local topical antibiotics may be sufficient to control the infection. More extensive cases may require systemic antibiotics and include first-generation cephalosporins, penicillinase-resistant penicillins, macrolides, and fluoroquinolones. Gram-negative folliculitis affects more often the patients with a history of long-term antibiotic therapy for acne, and usually involves the face. Causative pathogens include *Klebsiella, Enterobacter*, and *Proteus* species. *Pseudomonas aeruginosa* causes "Hot tub" folliculitis, which is due to contamination of undertreated water in a hot tub or whirlpool. Within 6–72 hours after exposure, multiple pustular or papular perifollicular lesions appear on the trunk and sometimes extremities. Mild fever and malaise may occur. Lesions in the immunocompetent patient typically resolve spontaneously within a period of 7–10 days.[44]

FURUNCLES AND CARBUNCLES

A furuncle or boil is caused by *S. aureus*. It is an acute deep-seated inflammatory hard, tender, red nodule that develops around a hair follicle, usually from a preceding folliculitis and often evolving into an abscess. When ruptured there is discharge of pus and often a core of necrotic material, thus the pain surrounding the lesion subsides, and the redness and oedema diminish over several days to several weeks. Furuncles usually arise in hair-bearing areas, particularly in regions subject to friction, occlusion, and perspiration.

Carbuncles are infections of group of hair follicles that coalesce and form large, swollen, erythematous, deep, and painful masses that usually open and drain through multiple tracts. Fever, malaise and other constitutional symptoms, are commonly associated with these lesions. Gentle incision and drainage is indicated in 'pointing' fluctuant lesions. Extensive furunculosis or a carbuncle may be associated with leucocytosis. Histologic examination of a furuncle reveals dense poly-morphonuclear inflammatory infiltrate in the dermis. Loculations should be broken with a hemostat. To encourage further drainage, the wound may be packed with gauze. In severe cases, parenteral antibiotics such as cloxacillin, or a first-generation cephalosporin such as cefazolin, flucloxacillin or another penicillinase-resistant antibiotic are required.[45] If MRSA is implicated or suspected, vancomycin, 1.0 to 2.0 g intravenously daily in divided doses, is indicated.

IMPETIGO

Impetigo, although most commonly seen in children, may be seen in immunocompromised old age persons. Both bullous and non-bullous clinical forms of impetigo exist. Bullous impetigo is caused by *S. aureus* while non-bullous impetigo may be caused by both *S. aureus* and streptococci. The non-bullous type of impetigo (impetigo contagiosa) accounts for more than 70% of cases. The initial lesion is a transient thin-walled vesicle or pustule on an erythematous base that quickly evolves into a honey-coloured crusted plaque (Fig. 9.2). In bullous form, the bullae usually arise on areas of grossly normal skin. The Nikolsky sign is absent. Bullae initially contain clear yellow fluid which subsequently becomes dark and turbid. There margins are sharply demarcated without an erythematous halo. The bullae are superficial and within a day or two, they rupture forming thin light brown to golden yellow crust. Gram stain of exudates reveal Gram-positive cocci in clusters.

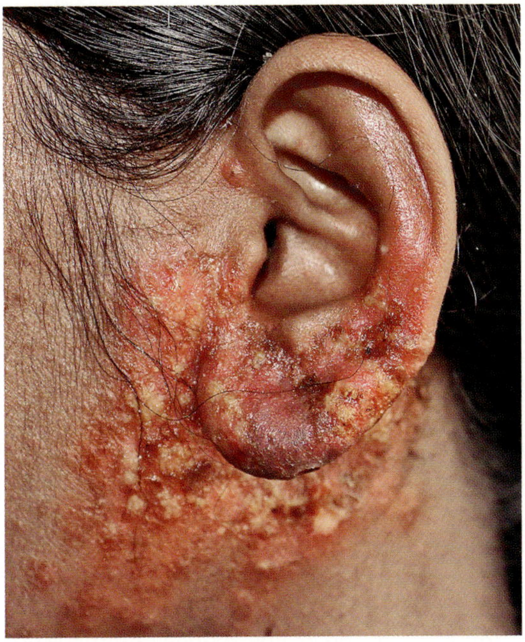

Fig. 9.2: Impetigo: Lesion over the external ear showing golden yellow crust secondary to otitis media

S. aureus phage II can be cultured from the contents of intact bullae. Histologically, the lesion of bullous impetigo shows vesicle formation in the sub-corneal or granular region. Occasional acantholytic cells, spongiosis, oedema of the papillary dermis and a mixed infiltrate of neutrophils and lymphocytes around blood vessels of the superficial plexus is seen. Regional lymphadenopathy may be present. Streptococcal impetigo accounts for the majority of cases of poststreptococcal acute glomerulonephritis (AGN).[46]

Local treatment with mupirocin ointment or cream, removal of crusts, and good hygiene is sufficient to cure most mild to moderate cases.[47] Fusidic acid is also effective against both organisms.[48] Systemic antibiotics may be required in extensive cases. Dicloxacillin or similar penicillinase resistant semi-synthetic penicillin or erythromycin 250–500 mg orally qid, should be given for 5–10 days. Azithromycin 500 mg on the first day followed by 250 mg daily on the next four days is effective and well-tolerated. Amoxicillin plus clavulinic acid 25 mg/kg/day given three times daily, cephalexin 40–50 mg/kg/day or clindamycin 15 mg/kg/day given for 10 days is equally effective alternative therapies.

ECTHYMA

Ecthyma is a bacterial infection of the skin characterised by the formation of adherent crusts, beneath which ulceration occurs. Group A streptococci were grown from all of 66 cases, and coagulase-positive staphylococci from 85% of these in one study.[49] Poor hygiene, malnutrition and minor injuries are the predisposing factors. Small bullae or pustules appear on an erythematous base surmounted by a hard crust of dried exudate, which increases in size by peripheral accretion. The base becomes indurated and a red oedematous areola may be present. When the crust is removed with difficulty, a purulent irregular ulcer is revealed. Healing occurs after a few weeks. Treatment of any underlying skin disease, nutrition and hygiene improvement are necessary. Antibiotics topical and local, active against both *Streptococcus pyogenes* and *Staphylococcus aureus* are given. Topical therapy either with sulconazole or miconazole cleared lesions satisfactorily over 1 week.[50]

CELLULITIS

Cellulitis is an infection caused by *S. aureus* and group A streptococcus usually. It is a painful, inflammation of the dermis and mainly the subcutaneous tissues, and is characterised by erythema, warmth, oedema, ill-defined, advancing borders. Escherichia coli and other Enterobacteriaceae and anaerobes are also involved in cellulitis, especially in association with old age, prolonged hospitalization, diabetes, and immunocompromised states. Patients may be febrile and may have an elevated white blood cell count. Blood culture or aspiration of the area of maximal inflammation may be useful.[50] Empiric treatment with a penicillinase-resistant penicillin, first-generation cephalosporin, amoxicillin-clavulanate, macrolide, or fluoroquinolone is appropriate.[51] More extensive disease may requires parenteral therapy. Marking the margins of erythema with ink is helpful in following the progression or regression of cellulitis. Adjunctive therapy includes cool compresses, analgesics, and immobilisation and elevation of the affected extremity.[52] A parenteral second- or third-generation cephalosporin should be considered in patients who have diabetes, immunocompromised patients and those with unresponsive infections. A plain radiograph of the area or surgical debridement to evaluate for gas gangrene, osteomyelitis, or necrotising fasciitis may be required.

ERYSIPELAS

Erysipelas is also known as St. Anthony's fire. This is an acute infection of the dermis and upper subcutaneous tissue involving the superficial dermal lymphatics, caused by beta-haemolytic group A streptococcus and is characterised by well defined, local redness, heat, swelling, and a highly characteristic raised, indurated border. It may coexist with cellulitis as, cellulitis may extend superficially and erysipelas deeply and make it impossible to differentiate. Legs and face are the common sites.[53] Frequently, polymorphonuclear leukocytosis of 20,000/mm^3 or more and lymphangitis and lymphadenopathy are seen. Fever, malaise and constitutional symptoms are seen in mild cases. Classical erysipelas starts abruptly and systemic symptoms may be acute and severe, but the response to treatment is more rapid. The incidence of erysipelas is rising, especially in young children, the elderly, persons with diabetes, alcoholic persons, and patients with compromised immune systems or lymphoedema.[52] Bacteria are present in affected tissue in small numbers, and attempts to culture them, from biopsy material, or from needle aspiration of saline injected tissue are often unsuccessful. Streptococcal serology may be helpful,[50] and immunofluorescence may identify streptococcal group antigens in biopsy specimens.[49] Erysipelas is caused almost exclusively by beta-hemolytic streptococcus and thus can be treated with standard dosages of oral or intravenous benzylpenicillin. Flucloxacillin exerts a bactericidal effect on streptococci as well as staphylococci and is used in dose of 500 mg four times daily. Clarithromycin 500 mg twice daily may be substituted in case of penicillin allergy.

ERYTHRASMA

Erythrasma is a chronic, superficial bacterial infection of the skin caused by a Gram-positive, aerobic rod, *C. minutissimum*. It is characterised by well defined, reddish brown patches occurring in intertriginous areas, most commonly in the groins, axillae and the intergluteal and submammary flexures, and toe clefts. The lesion present as well demarcated, reddish-brown, finely scaly patches. A warm, humid climate is a predisposing factor. Erythrasma may be the presenting feature in diabetics.[54] Coral-red fluorescence to coproporphyrin III with Wood's light strongly suggests erythrasma, although it does not necessarily indicate active infection. Gram or Giemsa staining shows Gram-positive rods and fine filaments. Culture on tissue culture medium 199 (without antibiotics) with 20% calf serum and 2% agar yields colonies that fluoresce coral-red under Wood's light after 18–36 h. Without treatment the condition tends to persist indefinitely, although there may be spontaneous fluctuations in severity. Topically applied benzoyl peroxide 5% gel, clindamycin 2% solution, fusidic acid and azole creams, such as clotrimazole and miconazole are effective for treatment. The duration of therapy varies, but 2 weeks is usually sufficient. For extensive lesions, erythromycin is probably the most effective approach. A 1 gm single dose of clarithromycin has been used successfully.[55] Photodynamic therapy using the porphyrin produced by the causative organisms has been tried in some patients with some benefit.[56]

SPECIAL CONSIDERATIONS

The diagnosis of most bacterial infections of the skin is based on clinical impression. Laboratory investigations help to confirm the diagnosis and elucidate characteristics of specific etiologies. Examination of a gram-stained smear of material from a suspected skin infection can rapidly guide on number and type of bacteria, as well as for the character of the inflammatory exudate and on early antibiotic therapy before a cultural diagnosis is made. Fluorescent antibody and other serologic tests in bacterial diseases of the skin are currently of limited applicability. Polymerase chain reaction technology can be applied to diagnosis of material obtained on skin punch biopsy of lesional tissue or aspirates from a vesiculobullous lesion.

Treatment of bacterial infection is determined by whether the infection is superficial or deep. Superficial bacterial overgrowth can be treated with topical agents. Deep tissue infections such as cellulitis must be treated with oral and systemic antibiotics and debridement.[57] Antibiotics are determined by Gram stain and suspicion initially and adjusted based on bacterial identification with antibiotic sensitivity. Current guidelines[58,59] recommend the use of intravenous cefazolin or ceftriaxone with or without clindamycin as the initial therapy, with cephalexin as the step-down agent of choice. In addition to the typical Gram-positive species, one needs to also consider Gram-negative or anaerobic colonisation. Chronic diabetic ulcer infections, especially with extensive necrosis, warrant anaerobic coverage.

In patients with nosocomial infections, infections secondary to specific environmental exposures, necrotising infections and colonisation with resistant organisms (e.g. MRSA), the pathogens in these infections are *S. aureus* (including MRSA), *P. aeruginosa, Enterococcus* species, *Escherichia coli* and other antibiotic-resistant Enterobacteriaceae species.[59] Guidelines recommend second- or third-generation cephalosporins as first-line agents for mild to moderate infections. With more severe or rapidly deteriorating infections, therapy should be expanded to broad-spectrum agents. In the case of MRSA, vancomycin should be added to first-line therapy.[60] Although MRSA has evolved strains with a lower susceptibility or complete resistant to vancomycin.[61,62] Linezolid, an oxazolidinone, is active against drug resistant Gram-positive bacteria. However, linezolid has been associated with hematologic adverse effects such as thrombocytopenia.[63] In addition, resistance also occurred with linezoid.[64] Avibactam, β-lactamase inhibitor with its novel reversible mechanism, is a promising agent against multidrug-resistant (MDR) Gram-negative bacteria.[65] Recently, confocal image analysis showed that silicon phthalocyanine (Pc) 4 has photodynamic antibacterial cytotoxic effects and can be effectively used to treat antibiotic-resistant strains in facultative anaerobic Gram-positive coccal bacteria, such as methicillin-resistant *Staphylococcus aureus* (MRSA).[66]

For the monitoring of antibiotic susceptibilities, it is helpful to determine the minimum growth inhibitory concentration (MIC) of antibiotics. More recently, the gene(s) responsible for the resistance, such as the staphylococcal cassette chromosome mec (SCCmec) element, have been analysed.[67] The molecular grouping technique is used to classify MRSAs into subgroup by the pulsed-field gel electrophoresis (PFGE) of the chromosomal DNA. PFGE is a useful method for genomic fingerprinting of microorganisms, and the data could be used for epidemiological study of virulent organisms. SCCmec typing is also used for the epidemiological study of MRSA.[68,69]

CONCLUSION

Management of cutaneous bacterial infections in the elderly population is quite challenging.

Treatment compliance is affected by several factors including declining cognitive status such as loss of memory and dementia, physical limitations, impaired sensory functions, comorbid conditions, and dependency on others. To maximize the efficacy and compliance, the treatment regimen should be kept as simple as possible.

References

1. Makrantonaki E. Challenge and promise: Human skin ageing. Dermatoendocrinol. 2012;4(3):225–26.
2. Norman RA, Mendez R. Structure and function of ageing skin. In: Norman RA, editor. Diagnosis of ageing skin diseases. London: Springer; 2008: p. 5–10.
3. Norman RA. Geriatric dermatology. Dermatol Ther 2003; 16:260–68.
4. Situation Analysis of Elderly in India. Central Statistics Office, Ministry of Statistics and Programme Implementation, Government of India, June 2011. Available at: http://mospi.nic.in/mospi_new/upload/elderlyinindia.pdf.
5. Yalcin B, Tamer E, Toy GG, Oztas P, Hayran M, Alli N. The prevalence of skin diseases in the elderly: analysis of 4099 geriatric patients. Int J Dermatol. 2006; 45:672–76.
6. Yap BK, Siew GM, Goh LC. Pattern of skin diseases in the elderly at the National Skin Centre (Singapore) 1990. Singapore Med J 1994; 35:147–50.
7. Ellis Simonsen SM, van Orman ER, Hatch BE, Jones SS, Gren LH, Hegmann KT, et al. Cellulitis incidence in a defined population. Epidemiol Infect. 2006; 134:293–99.
8. Souissi A, Zeglaoui F, El Fekih N, Fazaa B, Zouari B, Kamoun MR. Skin diseases in the elderly: a multicentre Tunisian study. Ann Dermatol Venereol. 2006 Mar; 133(3):231–34.
9. Chowdhury J, Das S, Roy AK. Skin diseases in elderly population from Eastern India. Journal of Pakistan Association of Dermatologists. 2016; 26(4):318–21.
10. Bilgili SG, Karadag AS, Ozkol HU, Calka O, Akdeniz N. The prevalence of skin diseases among the geriatric patients in Eastern Turkey. J Pak Med Assoc. 2012 Jun; 62(6):535–39.
11. Vinh DC, Embil JM. Rapidly progressive soft tissue infections. Lancet Infect Dis. 2005; 5:501–13.
12. Eron LJ, Lipsky BA, Low DE, Nathwani D, Tice AD, Volturo GA. Expert panel on managing skin and soft tissue infections. Managing skin and soft tissue infections: Expert panel recommendations on key decision points. J Antimicrob Chemother. 2003; 52:i3–17.
13. Björnsdóttir S, Gottfredsson M, Thórisdóttir AS, Gunnarsson GB, Ríkardsdóttir H, Kristjánsson M, et al. Risk factors for acute cellulitis of the lower limb: A prospective case-control study. Clin Infect Dis. 2005; 41:1416–22.
14. Jindal R, Jain A, Roy S, Rawat SD, Bhardwaj N. Skin disorders among geriatric population at a Tertiary Care Center in Uttarakhand. J Clin Diagn Res 2016; 10:6–8. doi:10.7860/JCDR/2016/17015.7500.
15. Grover C, Narasimhaul CRV. A clinical study of skin changes in geriatric population. Indian J Dermatol Venereol Leprol. 2009;75:305–06.
16. Yoshikawa TT. Important infections in elderly persons. West J Med. 1981; 135:441–55.
17. Phair JP, Kauffman CA, Bjornson A, Gallagher J, Adams L, Hess EV. Host defences in the aged: Evaluation of components of the inflammatory an immune responses. J Infect Dis. Jul 1978; 138:67–73.
18. Baker PJ, Amsbaugh DF, Stashak PW, Caldes G, Prescott B. Regulation of the antibody response to pneumococcal polysaccharide by thymus derived cells. Rev Infect Dis. Mar-Apr 1981; 3:332–41.
19. Makinodan T, Kay MMB: Age influence on the immune system, In Dixon FJ, Kunkel HG (Eds): Advances in Immunology, New York, Academic Press, 1980; 29:287–330.
20. Atiyeh BS, Al-Amm CA. Immunology of Burn Injury—An Overview. Ann Burns Fire Disasters. 2001; 14:78–84.
21. Shah BR, Hux JE. Quantifying the risk of infectious diseases for people with diabetes. Diabetes Care 2003; 26:510–13.
22. Peleg AY, Weerarathna T, McCarthy JS, Davis TM. Common infections in diabetes: pathogenesis, management and relationship to glycaemic control. Diabetes Metab Res Rev 2007; 23:3–13.
23. Davis TM, Weerarathne T, Foong Y, Mason C, Davis WA. Community acquired infections in type 2 diabetic patients and their nondiabetic partners. The Fremantle Diabetes Study. J Diabetes Complications. 2005; 19:259–63.

24. Thomsen RW, Mor A. Diabetes and risk of community-acquired respiratory tract infections, urinary tract infections, and bacteremia. The Open Infectious Diseases Journal 2012; 6(Suppl 1: M2): 27–39.
25. Muller LM, Gorter KJ, Hak E, Goudzwaard WL, Schellevis FG, Hoepelman AI, et al. Increased risk of common infections in patients with type 1 and type 2 diabetes mellitus. Clin Infect Dis 2005; 41: 281–88.
26. Thomsen RW, Riis AH, Kjeldsen S, Schonheyder HC. Impact of diabetes nd poor glycaemic control on risk of bacteraemia with haemolytic streptococci groups A, B, and G. J Infect 2011; 63:8–16.
27. Guvener M, Pasaoglu I, Demircin M, Oc M. Perioperative hyperglycemia is a strong correlate of postoperative infection in type II diabetic patients after coronary artery bypass grafting. Endocr J 2002; 49:531–37.
28. Rossman I: Environments of geriatric care, Chap 38, In Clinical Geriatrics, 2nd Ed. Philadelphia, JB Lippincott Co, 1979; pp. 668–80.
29. Chow AW: Nosocomial infections, In: I Yoshikawa TT, Chow AW, Guze LB (Eds): Infectious Diseases—Diagnosis and Management. Boston, Houghton Mifflin, 1980; pp. 262–73.
30. Freeman J, McGowan JE Jr: Risk factors for nosocomial infection. J Infect Dis. 1978; 138:811–19.
31. Baddour LM. Epidemiology, clinical features, and diagnosis of cellulitis. <http://www.utdol.com/utd/content/topic.do?topicKey=skin.inf/11185 and selectedTitle=1150 and source=searc_result 2008> (Version current at February 12, 2008).
32. McAdam AJ, Sharpe AH. Infectious diseases—bacterial infections. In: Kumar V, Abbas AK, Fausto N, eds. Robbins and Cotran, Pathologic Basis of Disease. Philadelphia: Elsevier Inc. 2005; pp. 371–96.
33. Ki V, Rotstein C. Bacterial skin and soft tissue infections in adults: A review of their epidemiology, pathogenesis, diagnosis, treatment and site of care. Can J Infect Dis Med Microbiol 2008; 19(2): 173–84.
34. Todar K. The bacterial flora of humans. http://textbookofbacteriology.net/normalflora.html (Version current at February 12, 2008).
35. Rennie RP, Jones RN, Mutnick AH; SENTRY Program Study Group (North America). Occurrence and antimicrobial susceptibility patterns of pathogens isolated from skin and soft tissue infections: Report from the SENTRY Antimicrobial Surveillance Program (United States and Canada, 2000). Diagn Microbiol Infect Dis. 2003; 45:287–93.
36. King MD, Humphrey BJ, Wang YF, Kourbatova EV, Ray SM, Blumberg HM. Emergence of community-acquired methicillin resistant *Staphylococcus aureus* USA 300 clone as the predominant cause of skin and soft tissue infections. Ann Intern Med. 2006; 144:309–17.
37. Frazee BW, Lynn J, Charlebois ED, Lambert L, Lowery D, Perdreau-Remington F. High prevalence of methicillin-resistant *Staphylococcus aureus* in emergency department skin and soft tissue infections. Ann Emerg Med. 2005; 45:311–20.
38. Eady EA, Cove JH. Staphylococcal resistance revisited: Community-acquired methicillin—resistant *Staphylococcus aureus*—an emerging problem for the management of skin and soft tissue infections. Curr Opin Infect Dis 2003; 16:103–24.
39. Moroney SM, Heller LC, Arbuckle J, Talavera M, Widen RH. Staphylococcal cassette chromosome mec and Panton-Valentine leukocidin characterization of methicillin-resistant *Staphylococcus aureus* clones. J Clin Microbiol 2007; 45:1019–21.
40. Schultz GS, Sibbald RG, Falanga V, Ayello EA, Dowsett C, Harding K, et al. Wound bed preparation: a systemic approach to wound management. Wound Repair Regen, 2003; 11(Suppl 1):S1–S28.
41. Stevens DL, Bisno AL, Chambers HF, Dellinger EP, Goldstein EJ, Gorbach SL, et al. Practice guidelines for the diagnosis and management of skin and soft tissue infections: 2014 update by the Infectious Diseases Society of America. Clin Infect Dis. 2005; 41:1373–406.
42. Vinh DC, Embil JM. Rapidly progressive soft tissue infections. Lancet Infect Dis. 2005; 5:501–13.
43. Jaworsky C, Gilliam AC. Immunopathology of the human hair follicle. Dermatol Clin 1999; 17:561–68.
44. Sadick NS. Current aspects of bacterial infections of the skin. Dermatol Clin. 1997; 15:341–49.
45. Stone SP. Unusual, innovative, and long-forgotten remedies. Dermatol Clin 2000; 18:323–38.
46. Berrios X, Lagomarsino E, Solar E, Sandoval G, Guzmán B, Riedel I. Post-streptococcal acute glomerulonephritis in Chile—20 years experience. Pediatric Nephrol 2004; 19:306–12.
47. Gisby J, Bryant J. Efficacy of a new cream formulation of mupirocin: Comparison with oral and topical

agents in experimentals kin infections. Antimicrob Agents Chemother. 2000; 44:255.

48. Koning S, van Suijlekom-Smit LW, Nouwen JL, Verduin CM, Roos M D Bernsen RMD, et al. Fusidic acid cream in the treatment of impetigo in general practice: double blind randomised placebo-controlled trial. BMJ. 2002; 324:203–07.
49. Bernard P, Bedane C, Mounier M, Denis F, Catanzano G, Bonnetblanc JM. Streptococcal cause of erysipelas and cellulitis in adults. Arch Dermatol. 1989; 125:779–82.
50. Leppard BJ, Seal DV, Colman G, Hallas G. The value of bacteriology and serology in the diagnosis of cellulitis and erysipelas. Br J Dermatol 1985; 112: 559–67.
51. Gilbert DN, Moellering RC, Sande MA. The Sanford guide to antimicrobial therapy 2000. 30th ed. Hyde Park, Vt.: Antimicrobial Therapy, 2000; 39.
52. Trubo R, Bisno AL, Hacker SM, Roaten SP Jr. Today's strategies for bacterial skin infections. Patient Care 1997; 31:78–94.
53. Chartier C, Grosshans E. Erysipelas: an update. Int J Dermatol. 1996; 35:779–81.
54. Leopoldo F, Montes LF, Dobson H, Dodge BG, Knowles WR. Erythrasma and diabetes mellitus. Arch Dermatol. 1969; 99:674–78.
55. Wharton JR, Wilson PL, Kincannon JM. Erythrasma treated with single-dose clarithromycin. Arch Dermatol. 1998; 134(6):671–72. doi:10.1001/archderm.134.6.671
56. Darras-Vercambre S, Carpentier O, Vincent P, Bonnevalle A, Thomas P. Photodynamic action of red light for treatment of erythrasma: preliminary results. Photodermatol Photo 2006; 22:153–56.
57. Sibbald RG, Williamson D, Orsted HL, Campbell K, Keast D, Krasner D, et al. Preparing the wound bed—debridement, bacterial balance, and moisture balance. Ostomy Wound Manage. 2000; 46:14–22.
58. Fung HB, Chang JY, Kuczynski S. A practical guide to the treatment of complicated skin and soft tissue infections. Drugs 2003; 63:1459–80.
59. Rosser WW, Pennie RA, Pila NJ; The Anti-infective Review Panel. Anti-infective Guidelines for Community-acquired Infections. Toronto: MUMS Guideline Clearinghouse, 2005. https://www.ti.ubc.ca/wordpress/wp-content/uploads/2010/08/5.pdf
60. Van Hal SJ, Fowler VG, Jr. Reply to parra-ruiz. Clin. Infect. Dis. 2013; 57:1219–1220. doi: 10.1093/cid/cit460.
61. Sievert DM, Rudrik JT, Patel JB, McDonald LC, Wilkins MJ, Hageman JC. Vancomycin-resistant *Staphylococcus aureus* in the United States, 2002–2006. Clin Infect Dis 2008; 46:668–674. doi: 10.1086/527392.
62. Tenover FC, Weigel LM, Appelbaum PC, McDougal LK, Chaitram J, McAllister S, et al. Vancomycin-resistant *Staphylococcus aureus* isolate from a patient in Pennsylvania. Antimicrob Agents Chemother. 2004; 48:275–80.
63. Attassi K, Hershberger E, Alam R, Zervos MJ. Thrombocytopenia associated with linezolid therapy. Clin Infect Dis. 2002; 34:695–698. doi: 10.1086/338403.
64. Pillai SK, Sakoulas G, Wennersten C, Eliopoulos GM, Moellering RC, Jr, Ferraro MJ, et al. Linezolid resistance in *Staphylococcus aureus*: Characterization and stability of resistant phenotype. J. Infect. Dis. 2002; 186:1603–1607. doi: 10.1086/345368.
65. Drawz, SM, Papp-Wallace KM, Bonomo RA. "New β-lactamase Inhibitors: A Therapeutic Renaissance in an MDR World." Antimicrobial Agents and Chemotherapy 58.4 (2014): 1835–1846. PMC. Web. 5 Dec. 2017.
66. Dimaano M, Rozario C, Nerandzic M, Donskey C, Lam M, Baron E. The photodynamic antibacterial effects of silicon phthalocyanine (Pc) 4. Int. J. Mol. Sci. 2015;16:7851–7860. doi: 10.3390/ijms16047851.
67. 18. Katayama Y, Ito T, Hiramatsu K. A new class of genetic element, staphylococcal cassette chromosome *mec*, encodes methicillin resistance in *Staphylococcus aureus*. Antimicrob. Agents Chemother. 2000; 44:1549–55.
68. Wu D, Wang Q, Yang Y, Geng W, Wang Q, Yu S. Epidemiology and molecular characteristics of community-associated methicillin-resistant and methicillin-susceptible *Staphylococcus aureus* from skin/soft tissue infections in a children's hospital in Beijing, China. Diagn Microbiol Infect Dis. 2010; 67:1–8.
69. Center for Diseases Control and Prevention (CDC). Community-associated methicillin-resistant and *Staphylococcus aureus* infection among healthy newborns. Morb Mortal Wkly Rep. 2006; 55: 329–32.

CHAPTER 10

Fungal Infections in the Elderly

• *Shital Poojary* • *Krishna Bhalala*

Key Points

- There is a definite increased risk of fungal infections in elderly patients especially with concomitant diabetes mellitus and obesity.
- Azoles are either contraindicated or to be used with caution in concomitant diseases such as cardiac diseases.
- Interactions of commonly used drugs in elderly with oral antifungals (especially azoles) are to be closely monitored and decide the choice of antifungals in elderly.

Introduction

Elderly patients have a definite increased risk of infections, including fungal infections. Both superficial and deep fungal infections may occur in the elderly. The degenerative changes in the skin, depression of cell-mediated immunity coupled with systemic comorbid metabolic conditions and polypharmacy in the elderly can make treatment of fungal infections in the elderly a therapeutic conundrum.

Classification

I. Superficial fungal infections:
- Dermatophytosis
- Candidiasis
- Pityrosporum infections
- Tinea nigra
- Piedra

II. Subcutaneous fungal infections:
- Mycetoma
- Sporotrichosis
- Chromoblastomycosis
- Subcutaneous zygomycosis
- Subcutaneous phaeohyphomycosis
- Rhinosporidiosis

III. Systemic fungal infections:
- Cryptococcosis
- Mucormycosis
- Histoplasmosis
- Penicilliosis
- Coccidioidomycosis
- Paracoccidioidomycosis

FACTORS CONTRIBUTING TO INCREASED INCIDENCE OF FUNGAL INFECTIONS IN THE ELDERLY[1–3]

i. Degenerative skin damage due to intrinsic aging and external environmental factors increases the fragility of the skin. As a result, breaks in the skin on minor trauma serve as a portal of entry for microorganisms such as fungi.

ii. Immune senescence with depression of cell-mediated immunity increases predisposition to fungal infections.

An experimental study showed significant lower levels of IL-6 and TNF-α in aged mice when stimulated with ligands for TLR 1, 2 and 6, TLR3, TLR4, TLR5, and TLR9 when compared with those from young mice. This causes decline in adaptive as well as innate immune response due to reduction in TLR expression and function and inflammatory responses. TLR2 and IL-6 are especially related to immune response to fungi. TLR2 and TLR4 involvement has been reported in chronic dermatophytosis.

iii. Metabolic disorders such as diabetes mellitus: Diabetes is a definite risk factor for cutaneous fungal infections.[4] Elderly patients with diabetes mellitus tend to have more extensive and recurrent fungal infections.[5] Diabetic patients with tinea pedis are more likely to develop tinea ungium. Superficial fungal infections is the second most common dermatological condition in elderly diabetics.[6,7] Candidiasis is often a presenting marker of diabetes mellitus. Dermatophytosis is however more common than candidiasis, with onychomycoses and intertriginous tinea pedis being the most common dermatophytosis in elderly diabetics. Persistent hyperglycemia, impaired peripheral microcirculation (microangiopathy), impaired immune response are responsible for increased fungal infections in diabetics.

iv. Underlying conditions such as anaemia (due to poor nutrition), renal disease, lymphoproliferative disorders, malignancies, chemotherapy also lead to an increased risk of fungal infections.

v. Peripheral vascular disease increases the risk of dermatophyte infections of the feet especially tinea unguium.

vi. Physical factors such as use of dentures can increase risk of oral candidiasis.

vii. Incontinence, lack of bladder and bowel control especially in unconscious patients can result in fungal infections especially candidiasis.

viii. Non-compliance with drug therapy due to cognitive impairment and physical immobility.

ix. In post-menopausal women, pH of vagina increases with increased chances of infection. Estrogen deficiency also increases risk of candidal vulvovaginitis.[8]

x. Special situations such as renal transplant/bone marrow transplant with attendant immunosuppression can increase risk of opportunistic fungal infections including histoplasmosis, aspergillosis and cryptococcosis.

DRUGS AND FUNGAL INFECTIONS IN ELDERLY[9–11]

Polypharmacy and its Impact on Fungal Infections in the Elderly

Table 10.1 depicts the interactions of commonly used antifungals with other drugs. Itraconazole is a potent CYP3A4 inhibitor, while fluconazole is potent CYP2C9 inhibitor and moderate CYP3A4 inhibitor

i. Presence of comorbid conditions in elderly often result in polypharmacy.

ii. Polypharmacy leads to increased incidence of drug reactions.

iii. Drug interactions can lead to decreased efficacy of antifungal drugs.

iv. Patients who are on life-saving medication for their comorbid conditions (e.g. warfarin, digoxin, oral hypoglycemics, cyclosporine). These patients would have a restricted choice of antifungals as antifungals (especially azoles) alter the blood levels of these drugs. Else, a close monitoring of these drug levels (e.g. cyclosporine) or their effects (blood sugar levels in oral hypoglycemics, coagulation parameters in warfarin) is required.

v. Itraconazole/fluconazole is should be cautiously used in patients who are on statins as rhabdomyolysis can occur.

Concomitant Diseases and Impact on Drug Usage in Elderly

i. Impaired renal function can preclude use of nephrotoxic drugs such as amphotericin B in deep and systemic mycosis.

TABLE 10.1: Drug interactions of commonly used antifungals

	Itraconazole	Terbinafine	Fluconazole
Drugs increasing the plasma antifungal level	Erythromycin, clarithromycin, ritonavir, indinavir	Fluconazole, cyclosporine	
Drugs decreasing the plasma antifungal level	Isoniazid, rifabutin, rifampicin, carbamazepine, phenytoin, phenobarbital, nevirapine, H2 receptor antagonist, proton pump inhibitors, antacids *Action:* Avoid nevirapine, H2 receptor antagonist, proton pump inhibitors, antacids	Rifampicin	Phenobarbital, rifampicin *Action*: Increase in dosage of antifungal required
Antifungal increases the plasma drug level	Rifabutin, verapamil, digoxin, atorvastatin, cerivastatin, warfarin, saquinavir, indinavir, ritonavir, cyclosporine, sirolimus, tacrolimus, budesonide, fluticasone, methylprednisolone, oral hypoglycemics *Action:* Monitor dosage carefully: Warfarin, digoxin, cyclosporine Monitor sugar levels if concomitant hypoglycemics	Tricyclic antidepressants (amitriptyline, doxepin), beta blockers, flecainide, propafenone, anticoagulants *Action:* Careful drug monitoring, reduction of drug dosage	Oral hypoglycemics *Action*: Monitor sugar levels Amitriptyline: Monitor drug dosage Losartan: BP monitoring required Warfarin: Monitoring required
Antifungal decreases the plasma drug level		Cyclosporine	

ii. Terbinafine clearance is reduced by approximately 50% in patients with renal impairment (creatinine clearance <50 ml/min) compared to normal volunteers; terbinafine may not be a suitable choice for patients with renal impairment; or dose adjustment is required.

iii. Liver diseases: Terbinafine and itraconazole are not recommended in acute/chronic liver disease. Griseofulvin is contraindicated in liver failure.

Pharmacokinetics of Antifungals in Elderly

i. Gastric acid is an essential factor for absorption of itraconazole. Elderly patients have a higher risk of achlorhydria, thereby affecting the absorption of itraconazole.

ii. H2 blockers, antacids and proton pump inhibitors should not be administered along with itraconazole as its absorption is impaired.

Adverse Effects/Contraindications of Antifungals and their Relevance in Elderly

i. Itraconazole is contraindicated in patients with ventricular dysfunction, cardiac failure and in patients on antiarrhythmic drugs/cardiac drugs. Itraconazole causes prolongation of QT interval, torsades de pointes, ventricular tachycardia and cardiac arrest.

ii. A relatively less common side effect of itraconazole, which occurs most frequently in elderly, is the triad of hypertension, oedema, and hypokalaemia. This side effect warrants stoppage of the drug.

Important Point to Remember while Prescribing Oral Antifungals in Elderly

Terbinafine is the preferred oral drug in elderly (including diabetics) in view of fewer side effects and drug interactions. However, in the present epidemic of dermatophytosis there have been reports of decreased responsiveness to terbinafine; this indicates at least extension of standard duration of 2–4 weeks therapy.

SUPERFICIAL FUNGAL INFECTIONS[12–14]

Epidemiology

Superficial fungal infections constitute a large proportion of cutaneous disorders in the elderly with both dermatophyte and candidal infections being more common in elderly as compared to younger age groups.

Incidence of superficial fungal infections has ranged from 5.6 to 37.5% in Indian studies with dermatophytosis being more common than candidal infections.[5,15–20] Amongst dermatophytosis, tinea corporis, tinea pedis and onychomycosis have been reported commonly.

Dermatophytosis

The three genera Microsporum, Trichophyton, and Epidermophyton cause superficial infection of skin, hair and nails. Commonest causative organism is *Trichophyton rubrum* in India. However, in the present scenario of recurrent and recalcitrant dermatophytosis, the proportion of *T. mentagrophytes* as the causative organism has gradually increased.[21]

Tinea corporis is dermatophyte infection of the glabrous skin. Commonest causative organism is *T. rubrum* followed by *T. mentagrophytes.*

Clinical features: Tinea corporis is characterised by annular, scaly, sharply marginated plaques with central clearing. Large geographic lesions can occur in cases of immunosuppression as also in cases of prior prolonged topical steroid usage. Vesicles and pustules can predominate in the more inflammatory variants caused by *T. mentagrophytes*. Other atypical variations in clinical presentation include: (i) Ill-defined lesions with barely perceptible scaling, (ii) psoriasiform lesions, (iii) deep nodular lesions, (iv) lichenified plaques (especially in chronic lesions). The recently unfolding epidemic has resulted in several cases of extensive tinea indecisiva especially in obese elderly patients (Fig. 10.1).

Differential diagnosis of tinea corporis in elderly includes nummular eczema, lichenified eczema, psoriasis and eczema craquele.

Tinea capitis is extremely uncommon in elderly with only sporadic cases being reported.[22] Causative organisms include *M. canis, T. schoenleinii, T. tonsurans, T. rubrum* and *T. violaceum.*[23]

Clinical features: Types of tinea capitis in elderly include the classical grey patch, black dot type and kerion. Tinea capitis in the elderly

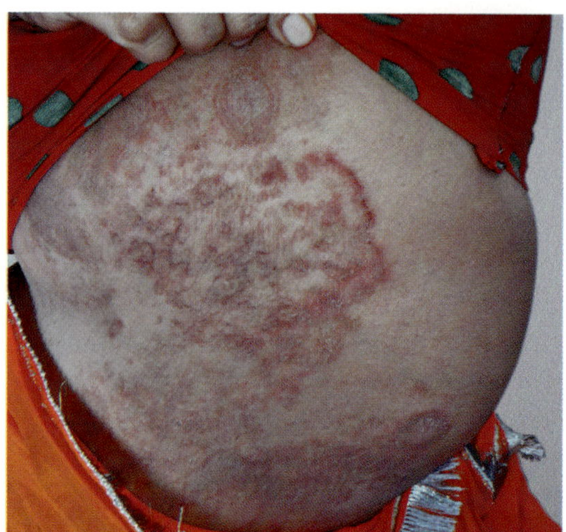

Fig. 10.1: Tinea recidivans in an elderly obese female with prior history of application

can be morphologically unique with lesions resembling psoriasis, seborrhoeic dermatitis and lichen planopilaris. It often presents as asymptomatic indolent disease with hair loss, mild perifollicular scaling and little inflammation especially in *T. tonsurans* infection. Also the classical black dots may not be evident in elderly due to white hair. Lack of diagnosis is also of concern as they can then be asymptomatic carriers who can transmit infection especially in the setting of old age homes.

Favus has been reported from an elderly female from Kashmir while an unusual case of black dot type tinea capitis due to *T. schoenleinii* has been reported from Pune, Maharashtra.[24,25] In the elderly, tinea capitis is more common in females; possible explanation being reduced sebaceous gland function due to estrogen withdrawal at menopause.[26]

Differential diagnosis of tinea capitis includes bacterial folliculitis which can mimic kerion, alopecia areata, lichen planopilaris, psoriasis, seborrhoeic dermatitis.[27]

Tinea barbae: Dermatophyte infection of the moustache and beard area is uncommon in elderly. Common causative organisms are *T. mentagrophytes* and *T. verrucosum*. *T. violaceum* and *T. rubrum* are occasional causes.[28]

Clinical features: Tinea barbae can be inflammatory or non-inflammatory. The inflammatory type is more common and resembles kerion. Occasionally, the lesions may be less inflammatory presenting as scaly plaques of alopecia with lustreless broken hair stubs. Rare cases of sycosiform *T. barbae* due to *T. rubrum* have been described.[28]

Differential diagnosis includes bacterial folliculitis, pseudofolliculitis (inflammatory) and alopecia areata (non-inflammatory type).

Tinea faciei is dermatophyte infection of glabrous skin of face. *T. rubrum* and *T. mentagrophytes* are the commonest organisms.

Clinical features: Tinea faciei presents as annular, circinate erythematous plaques. Tinea faciei is often misdiagnosed or diagnosed late as: (i) Lesions may be very subtle, ill-defined scaly plaques, (ii) symptoms of burning and exacerbation may be present after sun exposure.

Differential diagnosis includes seborrhoeic dermatitis, psoriasis, discoid lupus erythematosus, polymorphous light eruption and contact dermatitis.

Tinea cruris is dermatophytic infection of the groins. *T. rubrum* is the commonest causative organism, followed by *T. mentagrophytes*. It is more common in males than in females. Also obesity is a risk factor.

Clinical features: Tinea cruris presents as scaly, erythematous annular plaques in the crural folds sometimes extending to the thighs and the buttocks. In the present epidemic of dermatophytosis, often the thighs and buttocks are extensively involved and it may extend even to the anterior abdominal wall up to the umbilicus (Fig. 10.2). It can also extend to the penile skin. Specific risk factors in elderly include lack of bladder/bowel control, unconscious state often leading to hygiene issues and retention of moisture.

Differential diagnosis: Candidiasis is a common differential diagnosis; but the characteristic

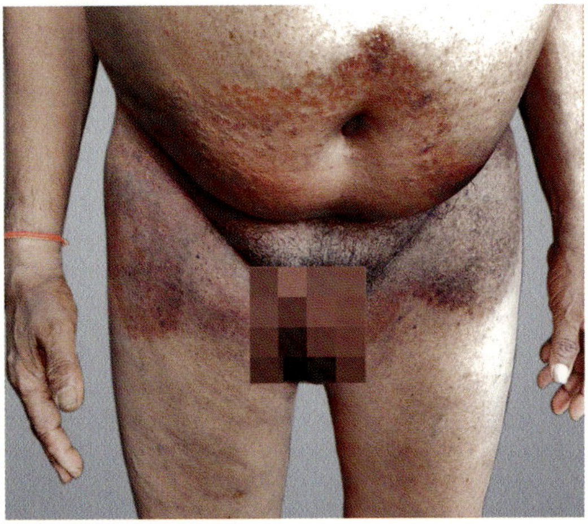

Fig. 10.2: Extensive tinea cruris extending to thighs and lower abdomen in an elderly diabetic male

satellite pustules and absence of central clearing in candidiasis are helpful in diagnosis

Tinea manuum is dermatophyte infection of the palmar surfaces of the hands. Commonest organism is *T. rubrum* followed *T. mentagrophytes*.

Clinical features: Tinea manuum presents as diffuse scaling of the palms extending to the palmar surface of the fingers. Similar to young adults, occupational factors such as prolonged exposure to moisture may still play a role in elderly females and even in males with occupations like farming, pottery

Differential diagnosis: Contact dermatitis, psoriasis can be mostly ruled out due to the unilateral nature of tinea manuum.

Tinea pedis is dermatophyte infection localised to the feet and interdigital spaces. It is more common in elderly males than females.[29] Common causative organisms are *T. rubrum*, *T. interdigitale* and *Epidermophyton floccosum*.

Clinical features: Tinea pedis can present in four clinical variants: (1) Moccasin, (2) interdigital, (3) inflammatory (vesiculobullous), and (4) ulcerative. Tinea pedis is often associated with tinea unguium, most often with *T. rubrum* and *T. interdigitale* infection. Deformities of the feet (especially toes) due to arthritis (especially rheumatoid arthritis) can predispose to intertriginous tinea pedis.

Early tinea pedis is often asymptomatic and the minimal scaly lesions may be mistaken for dryness by the elderly. Secondary infection leading to cellulitis and also diabetic foot can occur. Hence, early detection and treatment of tinea pedis is very important in the elderly.

Differential diagnosis: Hyperkeratotic plantar eczema, palmoplantar pustular psoriasis or dyshidrotic eczema, candidial intertrigo and soft corn are important differential diagnosis of different types of tinea pedis.

Tinea unguium is dermatophyte infection of nails. Commonest organism is *T. rubrum* followed by *T. mentagrophytes*. The white superficial type is most often caused by *T. mentagrophytes*. *Candida albicans* and non-dermatophyte molds are other causes of onychomycosis.

Clinical features: Types of onychomycosis are distal subungual onychomycosis, proximal subungual onychomycosis, white superficial onychomycosis and total dystrophic onychomycosis. Distal subungual onychomycosis is the commonest type. Thickened nails can cause discomfort to the extent of causing limited mobility in the elderly. A yellow or white streak in the nail is suggestive of a dermatophytoma, which is a walled off mass of fungus. This requires surgical excision as it does not respond to oral and topical antifungal therapy.

Risk factors for onychomycosis include male gender, increasing age, use of immunosuppressive drugs, diabetes mellitus, peripheral vascular disease, recurrent trauma and pre-existing tinea pedis/tinea manuum. Also to be noted, the rate of nail growth decreases by 0.5% each year from 25 to 100 years of age.[30] In males, the slowing of the growth rate is more pronounced from sixth to eighth decades while in females it is more pronounced till the sixth decade. Occasionally, prior dystrophic nail may be secondarily invaded, e.g. onychogryphosis which is common in elderly.

Differential diagnosis of tinea unguium includes: (i) Psoriasis: Presence of nail pits and also oil spots are diagnostic of nail psoriasis, (ii) nail lichen planus: Characteristic ridging and thinning of nail plate, (iii) nail changes secondary to eczema; eczematous changes in the periungual skin and an irregularly buckled nail are classical features.

Nondermatophyte molds such as *Scopulariopsis brevicaulis*, *Hendersonula toruloidea* and *Scytalidium hyalinum*, Aspergillus (*A. niger*, *A. flavus*, *A. fumigatus*) can also cause onychomycosis (Figs 10.3 and 10.4). In a study from Libya, NDM outnumbered dermatophytes and Candida as causative organism of onychomycosis.[31]

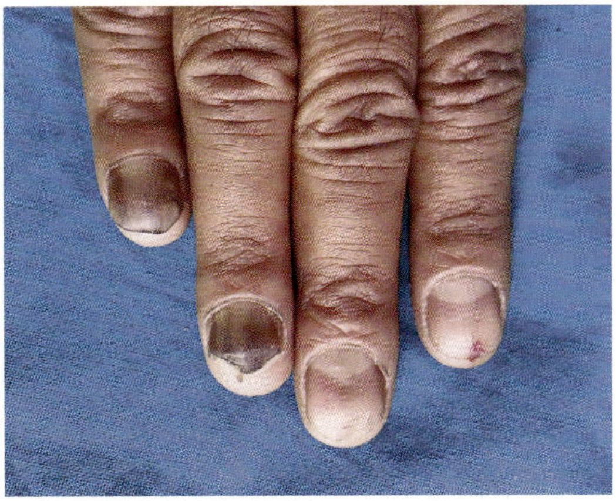

Fig. 10.3: Onychomycosis caused by *Aspergillus flavus*

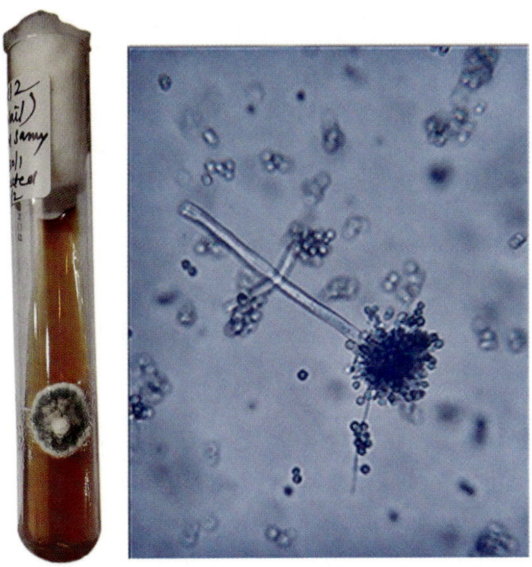

Fig. 10.4: *Aspergillus flavus:* Typical yellow-green colonies on Sabouraud's agar with radiate conidial heads on LCB mount (inset)

Diagnosis of Dermatophytosis

***Microscopic examination*:** KOH mount of skin scrapings, hair mount or nail clippings: Demonstration of branched hyphae and spores.

***Culture*:** On Sabouraud's dextrose agar with lactophenol cotton blue mount of the colonies for identification of the species.

Treatment of dermatophytosis[10–12, 14, 32–35]

- Few general measures for prevention and treatment of dermatophyte infections:
  i. To wear loose cotton clothes, avoid tying *saree/dhoti* too tightly
  ii. Washing clothes in hot water (at least 60°C) or drying clothes in sunlight
  iii. Avoid sharing clothes, combs, shoes
  iv. Use talcum powder to keep feet dry
  v. Avoid contact with stray animals
- Topical antifungals alone are recommended in following cases in elderly patients with dermatophytosis
  i. Localised infections
  ii. Patients with underlying systemic conditions, e.g. hepatic disorders wherein all three primary oral antifungals, i.e. terbinafine, griseofulvin and itraconazole would be contraindicated.
  iii. Patients with multiple comorbidities and polypharmacy where the risk of drug-drug interactions is extremely high.

Topical antifungals are also helpful as an adjuvant all types of dermatophytosis including tinea unguium.[36] (Topical antifungals are listed in Table 10.2.)

- Oral antifungals with dosages and duration of therapy in dermatophyte infection are enumerated in Table 10.3.

Candidiasis

Candidiasis is caused by the yeast of the genus Candida, most commonly *Candida albicans*. Other species of Candida (nonalbicans species) include *C. tropicalis*, *C. dubliniensis*, *C. parapsilosis*, *C. guilliermondii*, *C. krusei*, *C. pseudotropicalis*, *C. lusitaniae* and *C. glabrata* are occasional causes; more often seen in immunocompromised patients. Chronic and recurrent cutaneous candidiasis can be a marker of diabetes, immunocompromised state such as HIV infection or malignancy.

TABLE 10.2: Topical antifungals

Type of antifungal	Drug name	Concentration and dosage*
Azoles		
Imidazoles	Clotrimazole	1% cream/lotion twice daily for 4–6 weeks
	Ketoconazole	2% cream/gel once daily
	Econazole	1% cream twice daily for 2–4 weeks
	Miconazole	2% cream/gel twice daily for 4–6 weeks
	Oxiconazole	1% cream/lotion once daily for 4–6 weeks
	Sertaconazole	2% cream twice daily for 4 weeks
	Luliconazole	1% cream once daily for 2–4 weeks
	Eberconazole	1% cream twice daily for 2–4 weeks
Allylamines	Terbinafine	1% cream twice daily for 4 weeks
Morpholines	Amorolfine	5% nail lacquer once/twice a week for 6–12 months for onychomycosis 0.25% cream once daily for 4–6 weeks
Hydroxypyridinones	Ciclopirox 8%	Nail lacquer 1% cream once/twice daily for up to 48 weeks
Others	Whitfield's ointment	Once a day on alternate days; short contact time Avoid on intertriginous areas
	5–10% salicylic acid solution	Once a day on alternate days; short contact time Avoid on intertriginous areas

*Topical antifungals can be continued for 2 weeks after complete clearance to avoid recurrence.

TABLE 10.3: Oral antifungals for dermatophyte infection

Type of tinea	Antifungal	Dosage and duration
Tinea corporis/cruris	Itraconazole	100–200 mg/day for 2–4 weeks
	Griseofulvin	500 mg–1 gm/day for 4 weeks
	Terbinafine	250 mg OD for 2–4 weeks
	Fluconazole	150–300 mg/week for 2–4 weeks
Tinea pedis	Itraconazole	200 mg/day for 2–4 weeks
	Griseofulvin	250 mg TDS for 4–8 weeks
	Terbinafine	250 mg OD for 2–6 weeks
	Fluconazole	150 mg/week for 2–6 weeks
Tinea barbae	Itraconazole	200 mg/day for 4–6 weeks
	Griseofulvin	250 mg TDS for 4–8 weeks
	Terbinafine	250 mg OD for 4–6 weeks
	Fluconazole	150 mg/week for 4–6 weeks
Tinea faciei	Itraconazole	200 mg/day for 3–4 weeks
	Griseofulvin	250 mg TDS for 4–6 weeks
	Terbinafine	250 mg OD for 3–4 weeks
	Fluconazole	150 mg/week for 3–4 weeks

(contd.)

TABLE 10.3: Oral antifungals for dermatophyte infection (*contd.*)

Type of tinea	Antifungal	Dosage and duration
Tinea unguium	Itraconazole	200 g/day for 12 weeks for toe nails Pulse therapy 400 mg/day for 1 weeks/month Finger nails: Monthly for 2–3 months Toe nails: Monthly for 3–4 months
	Griseofulvin	1 gm/day Fingernail: 4–8 months Toenail: 9–12 months
	Terbinafine	250 mg/day Fingernail: 6 weeks Toenail: 12 weeks
	Fluconazole	150–300 mg once a week Fingernail: 3–6 months Toenail: 9–12 months

Types of Candidiasis

Cutaneous intertriginous candidiasis is common in the elderly especially in patients who are diabetic or obese.

Clinical features: Include well defined erythema with satellite pustules which leave behind collarette of scales and maceration of skin. Other risk factors include immobility (e.g in patients with stroke) and lack of bladder/ bowel control leading to exposure of skin to prolonged moisture, urine and faeces. Common sites apart from groin include axilla, inframammary folds, natal cleft and inter-digital areas.

Differential diagnosis of intertriginous candidiasis includes tinea, seborrhoeic dermatitis, bacterial intertrigo, flexural psoriasis.

Oral candidiasis. Pseudomembranous candidiasis is seen in elderly especially in immunocompromised patients. Other risk factors include dry mouth, impaired dentition, usage of oral steroids, corticosteroid sprays. It is seen as whitish plaques overlying areas of erythema on the tongue, buccal, palatal, or oropharyngeal mucosa (Fig. 10.5). In chronic hyperplastic oral candidiasis, unresponsive to treatment, a biopsy should be done to rule out leukoplakia. Chronic erythematous candidiasis is associated with denture usage. Acute erythematous/acute atrophic type is characterised by denuded, erythematous areas on the dorsum of the tongue (Fig. 10.6).

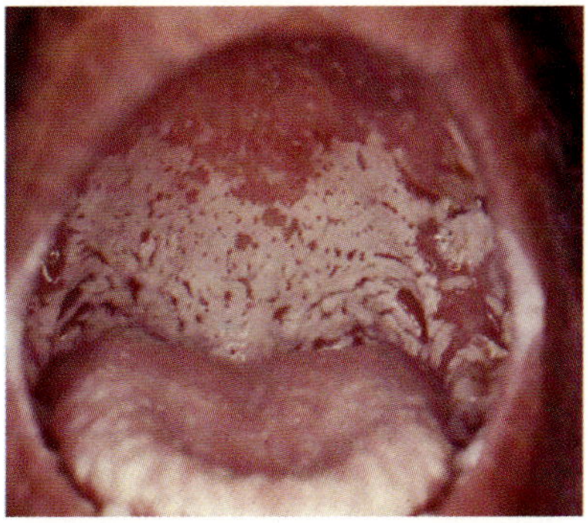

Fig. 10.5: Pseudomembranous oral candidiasis (*Courtesy:* Dr JK Maniar)

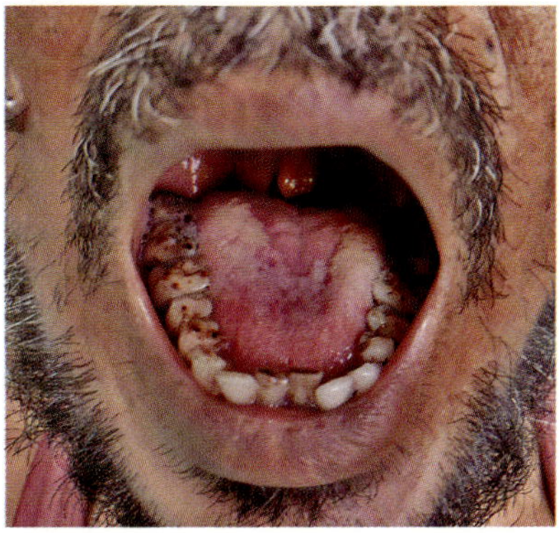

Fig. 10.6: Acute erythematous/atrophic candidiasis in an elderly male

Perlèche (angular cheilitis): Angular cheilitis can be associated with denture stomatitis and is an infection of the angles of the mouth. It presents as maceration and fissuring at the angles of the mouth. Patients with this condition are often edentulous and have a collection of saliva in this area because of redundant skin folds and drooling.

Candidal paronychia: Presents as red, edematous, boggy, painful swelling along proximal and lateral nail folds. In chronic cases, multiple transverse ridges may be seen in the nail plate. Often there may be superadded bacterial infection.

Erosio interdigitalis blastomycetica: Commonly seen in the 3rd webspace on the hand and sometimes in the feet. Repeated exposure to water, detergents, etc. leads to breakdown of skin barrier resulting in colonization and growth of Candida. This condition is common in diabetics.

Candidal balanitis: More often seen in diabetic elderly males. It initially begins as tiny pustules, later a glazed appearance and fissure appear on the prepucial skin.

Candidal vulvovaginitis: It is seen in elderly women possibly as a result of estrogen deficiency. Diabetes and usage of long-term antibiotics are also risk factors. It presents as erythema of the vaginal mucosa and the vulval skin, with curdy white discharge and associated dyspareunia (Fig. 10.7). The lesions can extend to the perineum and groins. In elderly patients, the infection may become chronic with a glazed and atrophic vagina.

Candidal onychomycosis: Distal and lateral subungual onychomycosis (DLSO) associated with paronychia may occur.

Management of Candidiasis

General measures

i. For oral candidiasis: Antiseptic mouth washes, maintaining denture hygiene.

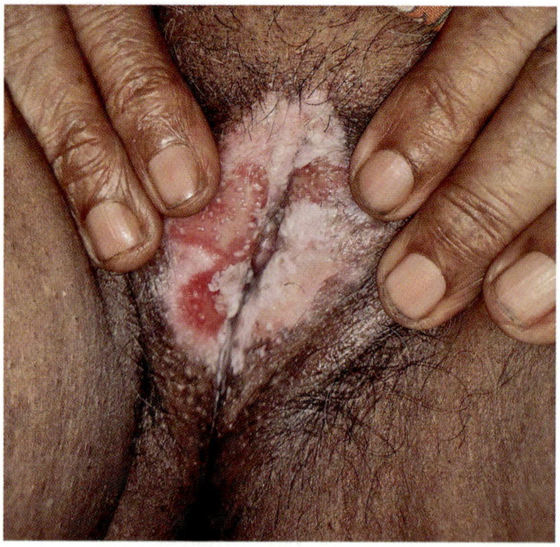

Fig. 10.7: Vulvovaginal candidiasis in an elderly female

ii. Intertriginous candidiasis: Keeping area dry, usage of powders to absorb moisture, maintenance of hygiene and regular nursing care in unconscious patients, use of open footwear.

iii. Candidal paronychia/onychomycosis: To avoid frequent contact with water and detergents.

Topical treatment

i. Azoles: Imidazoles: Clotrimazole, miconazole, econazole. Clotrimazole vaginal pessaries can be used for vaginitis.

ii. Nystatin: One of the older antifungals is still effective against Candida.

Systemic antifungals for candidiasis:

i. Fluconazole: Very effective for candidiasis. Dosage: (100–200 mg/day) for 2 weeks. A single dose of 150 mg for vaginal candidiasis is effective. There are occasional strains of *C. albicans* and nonalbicans species such as *C. krusei*, *C. dubliniensis* and *C. glabrata* which may be resistant to fluconazole.

ii. Itraconazole (100–200 mg/day) for 2 weeks. Single dose of 600 mg is effective in vaginal candidiasis.

iii. Candidal paronychia requires longer duration of treatment: Up to 4 weeks.
iv. Amphotericin B, newer antifungals such as voriconazole, posaconazole in systemic candidiasis/esophageal candidiasis (in immunocompromised patients).

Pityrosporum Infections

Pityriasis versicolor: Caused by *Malassezia furfur* is not common in elderly.

Clinical features are similar to that in young adults with hypopigmented/hyperpigmented/erythematous macules and patches with typical fine scaling mainly on upper trunk. Diagnosis can be confirmed with demonstration of hyphae and spores on KOH mount alone or with special stains such as CSB.[37]

Treatment: Topical antifungals; azoles such as ketoconazole are the first line of treatment. Oral antifungals; fluconazole 400 mg single dose or itraconazole 200 mg daily for 5 days are useful in extensive or recalcitrant cases.

Seborrhoeic dermatitis: Though in elderly patients, sebocyte turnover decreases, seborrhoeic dermatitis is not infrequently seen in elderly. It often presents as dry scalp and scaly erythematous patches on face (eyebrows, nasolabial fold, forehead).

Treatment: Ketoconazole 2% shampoos are helpful for scalp involvement. Mild topical steroids (hydrocortisone 2.5%) and topical antifungals (ketoconazole, miconazole) can be used for lesions on face.

Pityrosporum folliculitis: It is infrequently seen in elderly. But may be seen in patients who are diabetic, or those who have used broad-spectrum antibiotics/corticosteroids.

Clinical features: It presents as intensely pruritic papules and pustules on the back.

Treatment: Itraconazole 200 mg OD for 2weeks, fluconazole 150 mg weekly for 2–4 weeks. Ketoconazole shampoo can be used as an adjunct.

Tinea nigra: It is a rare superficial infection of the palms caused by *Exophiala werneckii*. KOH mount shows brown, branched, closely septate hyphae with elongated budding cells.

Clinical features: Tinea nigra is characterised by darkly pigmented, nonscaly patches on the palm, rarely on neck, trunk or soles.

Treatment: Topical azoles; ketoconazole, clotrimazole.

Piedra: Two types of piedra; Black piedra and white piedra have been described. They can be seen in elderly females, especially those who follow the cultural practice of tying hijab.

Ketoconazole shampoo and oral terbinafine are effective in treatment.

Subcutaneous mycoses are caused due to direct inoculation of fungi into deep dermis and subcutaneous tissue. Although not particularly common in elderly, certain occupations or habits may make them prone to develop these infections, e.g in farmers or elderly patients who pursue gardening as a hobby. Also because of the inherent immunosuppression in the elderly, occasionally the infections may be widespread or may disseminate.

Direct examination of the discharging pus (KOH mount), culture and histopathological examination (with special stains; GMS, PAS stains) are essential to make an appropriate diagnosis.

Mycetoma: Eumycetomas are caused by the fungi, *Madurella mycetomatis, Madurella grisea,* Fusarium, Acremonium (Sarocladium), *Leptosphaeria senegalensis, Cochliobolus lunata. Madurella mycetomatis* is the commonest reported organism in India. Although eumycetoma is more common in the age group of 21–40 years, it can be seen in elderly especially in the lower socio-economic strata, rural settings and in endemic areas.[40]

Clinical features: Eumycetoma is characterised by a gradually progressive indurated swelling

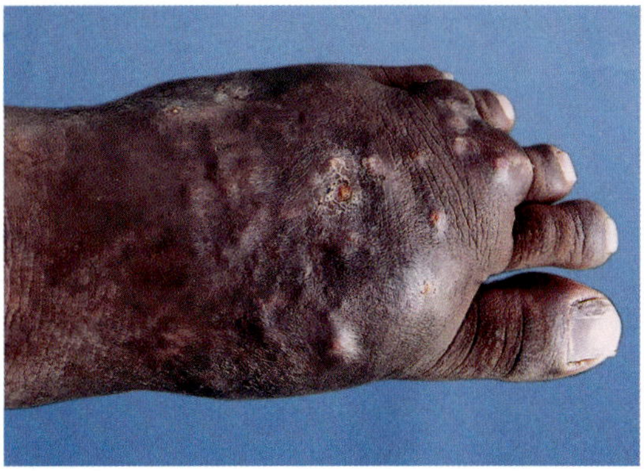

Fig. 10.8: Eumycotic mycetoma in an elderly male farmer

with discharging sinuses and grains (Fig. 10.8). Bone involvement is present with multiple punched out lytic areas with no bone reaction. Extensive tissue fibrosis over a prolonged period can lead to elephantiasis.

Diagnosis: Diagnosis can be confirmed by microscopic examination of grains and histopathological examination. Presence of thick walled septate hyphae and chlamydospores differentiates eumycetoma from actinomycetoma. Ultrasonography and CT scan be used to demarcate the exact extent of the lesions and bony involvement.

Treatment: Itraconazole 400 mg/day and terbinafine 500 mg BD/day have been used for 9 months up to one year with variable results. Posaconazole 800 mg/day and voriconazole 400–600 mg/day have given 80% to complete cure in 16–20 months.[41] Post-medical therapy, the shrunken lesions can be excised surgically for a better therapeutic outcome.

Sporotrichosis: It is caused by the dimorphic fungus *Sporothrix schenkii*. Other causative species described include *S. braziliensis*, *S. mexicana* , *S. globosa* and *S. lurei*.

Clinical features: Two commonest clinical types are lymphatic and fixed type (Fig. 10.9). Dissemination to other organs like bones, joints and rarely central nervous system can occur in immunosuppressed (HIV) patients.

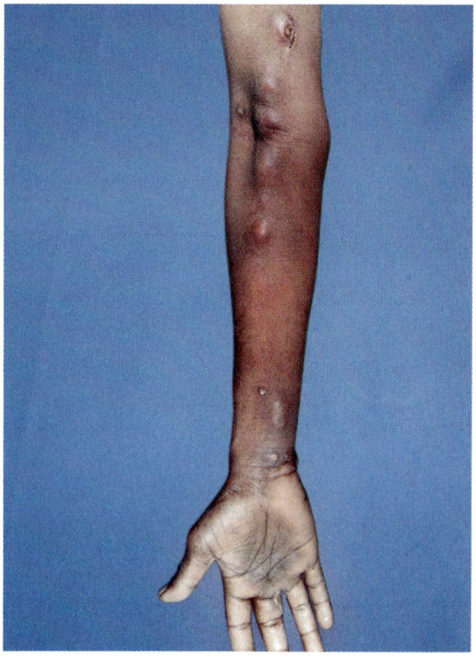

Fig. 10.9: Lymphatic type of cutaneous sporotrichosis

Diagnosis: Histopathology shows suppurative granulomas with characteristic asteroid bodies.

Treatment: Itraconazole 200–400 mg/day, terbinafine 250 mg/day for at least 3 months are effective in treatment of sporotrichosis. Saturated solution of potassium iodide is also equally effective. IV Amphotericin B can be used in systemic dissemination.

Chromoblastomycosis: It is a chronic subcutaneous fungal infection caused by pigmented fungi; phialophora verrucosa, *Fonsecaea pedrosoi*, *F. compacta* and *Cladophialophora carrionii*.

Clinical features: It is characterised by gradually progressive hypertrophic, verrucous lesions predominantly on exposed areas such as legs.

Diagnosis: Histopathology characteristically shows suppurative granulomas with septate thick walled yellow brown sclerotic bodies.

Treatment: Itraconazole 200–400 mg/day and terbinafine 250–500 mg/day for 6–12 months.

Posaconazole has also been reported to be effective. Cryotherapy is helpful in long-standing hypertrophic lesions.

Subcutaneous zygomycosis: It is caused by the Entomophthorales group of fungi.[38,39] It is of two types; basidiobolomycosis and conidiobolomycosis caused by the genera Conidiobolus and Basidiobolus respectively. The common causative species include *C. coronatus*, *C. incongruous*, and *B. ranarum*. Infection due to Basidiobolus is uncommon in adults and old individuals. Mode of transmission is via nasal inhalation of spores where it can implant on traumatised nasal mucosa.

Clinical features: Rhinoentomophthoromycosis (conidiobolomycosis) is characterised by woody hard swelling of the rhinofacial region initially starting from the inferior turbinate region. Nasal stuffiness/obstruction is a common symptom.

Diagnosis: KOH mount of the nasal smear and skin biopsy reveal nonseptate/sparsely septate hyphae branching at right angles. CT scan will demarcate the entire extent of the lesion.

Treatment: Oral itraconazole (200 to 400 mg/day), ketoconazole (200 to 400 mg/day) and potassium iodide for 3–5 months are effective in treatment. Treatment is recommended to be continued 1–2 months after disease subsidence.

Subcutaneous phaeohyphomycosis/pheomycotic cyst: Infection of subcutaneous tissue/intramuscular tissue (rare) caused by pigmented (dematiaceous) fungi; *Exophiala jeanselmei, E. dermatitidis* , *Bipolaris* spp., *Alternaria alternata, Cladophialophora bantiana, Phialophora* spp.

Clinical features: The disease presents as well defined cystic lesions of gradually increasing size most commonly on the extremities.

Diagnosis: FNAC and skin biopsy reveal pigmented hyphae, pseudohyphae and yeasts. Pattern of inflammation can be a suppurative granuloma or a foreign body granuloma around a wooden splinter.

Treatment: Surgical excision is the treatment of choice. Pre- and postoperative therapy with antifungals is recommended especially in immunocompromised patients and in recurrent cases; itraconazole 200 mg/day, flucytosine 150 mg/kg/day, IV amphotericin B. Intralesional amphotericin B has also been found to be efficacious.

Rhinosporidiosis: It is caused by *Rhinosporidium seeberi*. It is endemic in Kerala, Tamil Nadu and Chhattisgarh. Often bathing in the same ponds as animals in villages has been reported as risk factor.

Clinical features: Rhinosporidiosis presents most commonly as polypoid tumors of nose, eyes and larynx. Cutaneous lesions are much rarer and presents as tumorous growths/nodules.

Diagnosis: Histopathology is characterised by granulomatous infiltrate with thick walled large sporangia (100–450 μm) of rhinosporidium.

Treatment: Surgical excision is the treatment of choice. Recurrences are however common. Dapsone has been shown to prevent recurrences.

Systemic mycoses: Endemic mycoses are histoplasmosis, blastomycosis, coccidioidomycosis, paracoccidioidomycosis and infection caused by Penicillium (current name; *Talaromyces marneffei*). Endemic mycoses are relatively uncommon in India. Opportunistic mycoses occur only in the setting of immunosuppression; these include cryptococcosis, systemic candidiasis, aspergillosis, zygomycosis and penicilliosis.

Cryptococcosis: It is primarily a systemic mycosis affecting central nervous system and lungs with secondary involvement of skin. Infection is by inhalation of the fungus. It is caused by *C. neoformans* and *C. gattii*. It is predominantly associated with immunosuppressed states (HIV infection), malignancies (lymphoma) and following renal transplantation. It has been reported occasionally in diabetics. Treatment with corticosteroids, renal failure, liver dysfunction and chronic obstructive pulmonary disease are also risk factors for cryptococcosis in the elderly. In 20% cases, there may not be any risk factor except old age.

Clinical features: Cutaneous cryptococcosis occurs in 10–15% of cases of disseminated cryptococcosis and can present as molluscoid lesions, subcutaneous nodules or abscesses. Primary cutaneous cryptococcosis is extremely rare. Cutaneous lesions can be a presenting feature or can be accompanied by neurological symptoms. Dementia can often be the only presenting symptom of cryptococcosis in the elderly without any other neurological symptoms. Clinical outcome of disseminated cryptococcosis tends to be worse in the elderly as compared to younger adults. Primary cutaneous cryptococcosis although rare tends to be more common in elderly as compared to younger age groups.[42–44]

Diagnosis: Demonstration of cryptococci from skin smears, sputum, urine, CSF by simple India ink preparation or Gram stain is useful. Histopathology of the skin shows 2 patterns of inflammation: Gelatinous and granulomatous. Mucicarmine stain is specific for Cryptococcus (Fig. 10.10). Detection of cryptococcal antigen from serum, CSF and body fluids by latex agglutination test and ELISA is useful for diagnostic and prognostic purposes.

Treatment: First line treatment is IV amphotericin B 0.7–1 mg/kg/day combined with flucytosine 100 mg/kg/day for 2 weeks followed by fluconazole 400 mg/day for 4 weeks. In patients with no evidence of systemic manifestations, fluconazole 400–600 mg/day or itraconazole 400 mg/day for 6–8 weeks is effective.[45] Long-term suppressive treatment with oral fluconazole 400 mg/day is required in HIV seropositive patients.

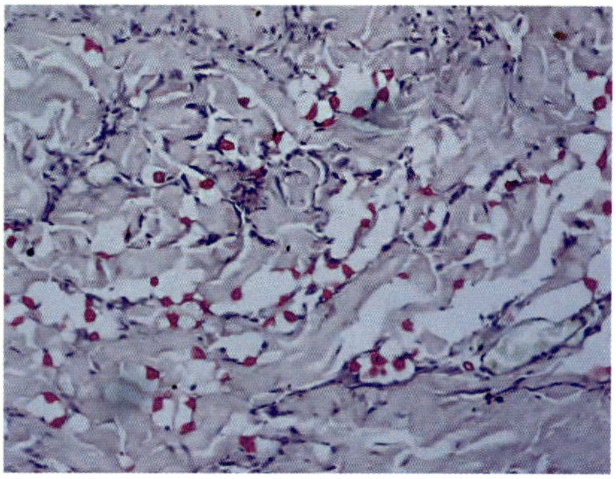

Fig. 10.10: Mucicarmine stain showing typical budding capsulated spores of *Cryptococcus neoformans*

Mucormycosis: Mucormycosis has been described in elderly diabetic patients often with rhinocerebral involvement.[46–47] Other underlying risk factors include associated neutropenia, renal disease, renal transplant and lymphoma, malnutrition and chronic corticosteroid therapy. It is caused by species of Rhizomucor, Lichtheimia (earlier named Absidia) and Rhizopus. Primary mode of infection is via inhalation of spores or it can occur via traumatic inoculation of mucous membranes/skin.

Clinical features: Mucormycosis is characterised by acute, rapidly progressive, angioinvasive infection. The most common form is rhinocerebral involving the nose, paranasal sinuses, orbits and central nervous system. It often presents to the dermatologist as periorbital, perinasal oedema/cellulitis, which rapidly progresses to necrosis and eschar formation and can be fatal.

Diagnosis: It is by demonstration of broad and generally nonseptate hyphae on smears and histopathology.

Treatment: IV amphotericin B is the treatment of choice oral posaconazole 400 mg BD/day for 6 weeks is also effective.

Histoplasmosis: It predominantly involves reticuloendothelial system and is caused by

Histoplasma capsulatum, a dimorphic fungus. Skin lesions are more common with the duboisii variant, but duboisii variant is seen only in Africa. Skin lesions are also more common on the background of HIV infection as compared to other patient groups.

Clinical features: It is seen in immunocompromised patients (lymphoma, HIV infection) and occasionally in diabetic patients. Mucocutaneous manifestations include oropharyngeal ulcers, umbilicated (Molluscoid) papules and nodules on the skin (Fig. 10.11). Systemic manifestations include fever, weight loss, hepatosplenomegaly, anaemia, leucopenia and thrombocytopenia (due to bone marrow involvement).

The specific type of histoplasmosis that has been described in older adults is chronic progressive disseminated histoplasmosis. There is extensive parasitization of the reticuloendothelial system. Patients present with fever, night sweats, anorexia, weight loss, fatigue, pancytopenia, mucocutaneous ulcerations and pustular lesions. Elevated alkaline phosphatase level is common. Diffuse adrenal involvement leads to Addison's disease, which should be suspected if there is weakness, orthostatic hypotension, hyperkalaemia, and hyponatraemia.

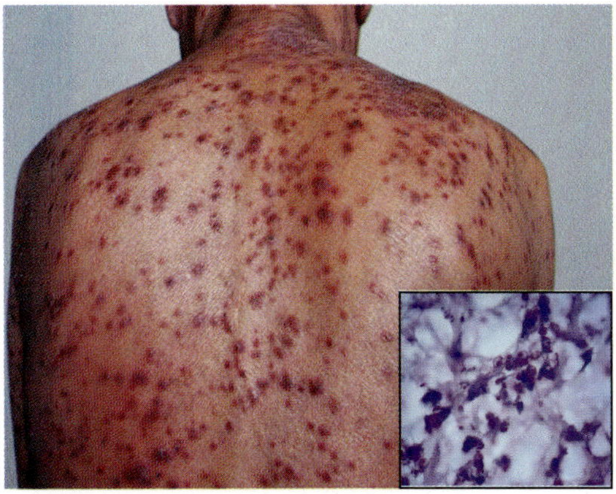

Fig. 10.11: Disseminated histoplasmosis in an HIV seropositive male, inset: Small intracellular yeast cells of Histoplasma (*Courtesy:* Dr JK Maniar)

Diagnosis: Skin histopathology/sputum/bone marrow aspirate/specimens show small, oval yeast cells with narrow necked budding within macrophages as well extracellularly. Serological tests such as complement fixation test, latex agglutination test are also useful in diagnosis as well as assessing prognosis. RT PCR, a real time, rapid method is useful for direct detection of organism from clinical specimens.

Treatment: Itraconazole 200–400 mg/day is effective and is to be continued until clinical remission. In severe infections, amphotericin B 0.5–1 mg/kg daily (or liposomal amphotericin B 3 mg/kg daily) for 2 weeks may be preferred. Posaconazole is effective in patients refractory to itraconazole.

Penicilliosis, coccidioidomycosis and paracoccidioidomycosis have been rarely reported in India. Penicilliosis has been reported from the North Eastern state of Manipur. Coccidioidomycosis and paracoccidioidomycosis have been reported only sporadically in India.

CONCLUSION

Elderly patients have a definite risk of fungal infection; both superficial as well as systemic infections especially in the setting of concomitant diabetes mellitus and immunosuppression as well as a varied clinical picture which may delay diagnosis. Choice of antifungal depends on the nature/severity of infection, concomitant diseases, concomitant drug therapy in the context of adverse drug effects and drug interaction.

References

1. Chopra A, Kullar J, Chopra D, Dhaliwal S R. Cutaneous physiological and pathological changes in elderly. Indian J Dermatol Venereol Leprol 2000; 66:274.
2. Renshaw M, Rockwell J, Engleman C, Gewirtz A, Katz J, Sambhara S. Cutting edge: impaired Toll-like receptor expression and function in aging. J Immunol. 2002; 169(9):4697–701.

3. Jafferany M, Huynh TV, Silverman MA, Zaidi Z. Geriatric dermatoses: A clinical review of skin diseases in an aging population. Int J Dermatol. 2012; 51:509–22.
4. Timshina DK, Thappa DM, Agrawal A. A clinical study of dermatoses in diabetes to establish its markers. Indian J Dermatol. 2012; 57:20–5.
5. Patange S V, Fernandez R J. A study of geriatric dermatoses. Indian J Dermatol Venereol Leprol. 1995; 61:206–8.
6. Nair PA, Vora R. Association of Systemic Diseases with Cutaneous Dermatosis in Elderly Population: Preliminary Observation at a Rural Tertiary Care Centre. J Family Med Prim Care. 2015; 4(1):74–78.
7. Asokan N, Binesh VG. Cutaneous problems in elderly diabetics: A population-based comparative cross-sectional survey. Indian J Dermatol Venereol Leprol. 2017; 83:205–11.
8. Nair PA. Dermatosis associated with menopause. J Mid-life Health 2014; 5:168–75.
9. Shivanna R, Rajesh. Management of dermatophytosis in elderly and with systemic comorbidities. Clin Dermatol Rev. 2017; 1:S38–41.
10. Gupta AK. Systemic antifungals In Wolverton SE. Ed. Comprehensive Dermatologic Drug Therapy, 3rd ed, Elsevier Saunders, Edinburgh 2013; 98–119.
11. Rengasamy M, Chellam J,Ganapati S. Systemic therapy of dermatophytosis: Practical and systematic approach. Clin Dermatol Rev. 2017; 1:S19–23.
12. Hay RJ, Ashbee HR. Fungal Infections. In Griffiths CEM, Barker J, Bleiker T, Chalmers R, Creamer D. Eds. Rook's Textbook of Dermatology. 9th ed ,Wiley Blackwell, Oxford, UK, 2016; 1:32.1–32.96.
13. Scheinfeld N. Infections in the elderly. Dermatol Online J. 2005;11(3):8.
14. Varade RS, Burkemper NM. Cutaneous fungal infections in the elderly. Clin Geriatr Med. 2013; 29(2):461–78.
15. Thapa DP, Jha AK, Kharel C, Shrestha S. Dermatological problems in geriatric patients: A hospital based study. Nepal Med Coll J. 2012; 14:193–5.
16. Grover S, Narasimhalu CR. A clinical study of skin changes in geriatric population. Indian J Dermatol Venereol Leprol. 2009; 75:305–6.
17. Scheinfeld NS. Skin Disorders in Elderly Persons: Identifying Fungal Infections. Infect Med. 2007; 24:509–515.
18. Dhumale SB, Khyalappa R. Study of cutaneous manifestations in geriatrics. Int J Res Med Sci. 2016; 4(5):1343–1346.
19. Ali YS, Reddy GS, Sravanthi P. A clinical study of dermatological manifestations in geriatric patients in Shadan Institute of Medical Sciences and Teaching Hospital and Research Centre, Hyderabad, Telangana, India. Indian Journal of Clinical and Experimental Dermatology. 2017; 3(1):24–28.
20. Jindal R, Jain A, Roy S, Rawat SDS, Bhardwaj N. Skin Disorders Among Geriatric Population at a Tertiary Care Center in Uttarakhand. Journal of Clinical and Diagnostic Research. 2016; 10(3): WC06–WC08.
21. Poojary SA. Epidemiological transformation of dermatophytes in India—mycological evidence (microbiology and culture based). In: Sardana K, Khurana A, Poojary SA, Eds. IADVL Manual of Dermatophytes, CBS Publishers 2018, in print.
22. Auchus IC, Ward KM, Brodell RT, Brents MJ, Jackson JD. Tinea capitis in adults. Dermatol Online J. 2016; 22(3).
23. Rallis E, Koumantaki-Mathioudaki E, Papadogeorgakis H. Microsporum canis tinea capitis in a centenarian patient. Indian J Dermatol Venereol Leprol 2011; 77:626.
24. Hassan I, Rather PA, Sajad P. Favus in an elderly Kashmiri female: A rare occurrence. Indian J Dermatol. 2013; 58(5):411.
25. Ghadgepatil SS, Sharma YK, Misra R, Dash KN, Patvekar MA, Deo KS. An unusual case of tinea capitis caused by *Trichophyton schoenleinii* in an elderly female. Indian Dermatol Online J. 2015; 6(1):49–50.
26. Cervetti O, Albini P, Arese V, Ibba F, Novarino M, Panzone M. Tinea Capitis in Adults. Advances in Microbiology, 2014; 4:12–14.
27. Ahmad SM, Wani GM, Khursheed B. Kerion mimicking bacterial infection in an elderly patient. Indian Dermatol Online J 2014; 5:494–6.
28. Furlan KC, Kakizaki P, Chartuni JCN, Valente NYS. Sycosiform tinea barbae caused by *Trichophyton rubrum* and its association with autoinoculation An Bras Dermatol. 2017; 92(1):160–1.

29. Hahnel E, Blume-Peytavi U, Trojahn C, et al. Prevalence and associated factors of skin diseases in aged nursing home residents: a multicentre prevalence study. BMJ Open 2017; 7:e018283.

30. Singh G, Haneef NS, Uday A. Nail changes and disorders among the elderly. Indian J Dermatol Venereol Leprol. 2005; 71(6):386–92.

31. Bridan W, Baiu S, Kalfa H. Non-dermatophyte as Pathogens of Onychomycosis among Elderly Diabetic Patients. J Microbiol Exp 2017; 5(4): 00157.

32. Poojary SA. Topical antifungals: A review and their role in current management of dermatophytoses. Clin Dermatol Rev. 2017; 1:S24–9.

33. Sahoo AK, Mahajan R. Management of tinea corporis, tinea cruris, and tinea pedis: A comprehensive review. Indian Dermatol Online J. 2016 Mar-Apr; 7(2):77–86.

34. Kaul S, Yadav S, Dogra S. Treatment of Dermatophytosis in Elderly, Children, and Pregnant Women. Indian Dermatol Online J. 2017; 8(5):310–318.

35. Shemer A. Update: Medical treatment of onychomycosis. Dermatol Ther. 2012; 25:582–593.

36. Shemer A, Gupta AK, Kamshov A et al. Topical antifungal treatment prevents recurrence of toenail onychomycosis following cure. Dermatologic Therapy. 2017; 30: e12545.

37. Lodha N, Poojary SA. A novel contrast stain for the rapid diagnosis of pityriasis versicolor: A comparison of Chicago Sky Blue 6B stain, potassium hydroxide mount and culture. Indian J Dermatol. 2015; 60:340–4.

38. Thomas MM, Bai SM, Jayaprakash C, Jose P, Ebenezer R. Rhinoentomophthoromycosis. Indian J Dermatol Venereol Leprol. 2006; 72:296–9.

39. Dutta S, Sarkar S, Linka U, Dora S. Conidiobolomycosis: A case report of rare fungal infection from the Eastern India. Indian Dermatol Online. J 2015; 6:393–5.

40. Wadal A, Elhassan TA, Zein HA, Abdel-Rahman ME, Fahal AH (2016) Predictors of Postoperative Mycetoma Recurrence Using Machine-Learning Algorithms: The Mycetoma Research Center Experience. PLoS Negl Trop Dis. 10(10):e0005007.

41. Welsh O, Al-Abdely HM, Salinas-Carmona MC, Fahal AH Mycetoma Medical Therapy. PLoS Negl Trop Dis. 2014; 8(10):e3218.

42. Werchniak, AE and Baughman, RD. Primary cutaneous cryptococcosis in an elderly man. Clinical and Experimental Dermatology. 2004; 29:159–160.

43. Lu Y, Wu C, Hong C. Primary cutaneous cryptococcosis in an immunocompetent man: A case report Dermatologica Sinica. 2013; 31:90–93.

44. Oliveira EV, Almeida MT, Turatti A, Gomes CM, Roselino AM. Paracoccidioidomycosis and cryptococcosis with localized skin manifestations: report of two cases in the elderly. An Bras Dermatol. 2016; 91(2):243–4.

45. Landucci G, Farinelli P, Zavattaro E, Giorgione R, Gironi LC, et al. Complete Remission of Primary Cutaneous Cryptococcosis in an Immunosuppressed Patient after Fluconazole Treatment. J Infect Dis Ther. 2017; 5:326.

46. Nilesh K, Malik NA, Belgaumi U. Mucormycosis in a healthy elderly patient presenting as oro-antral fistula: Report of a rare incidence. J Clin Exp Dent. 2015; 7(2):e333–5.

47. Yamaguchi S, Okubo Y, Katano A, Sano A, Uezato H, Takahashi K. Primary cutaneous mucormycosis caused by Mucor irregularis in an elderly person. The Journal of Dermatology, 2015; 42:210–214.

CHAPTER 11

Genital Dermatoses and Sexually Transmitted Infections (STIs) in Elderly

• *Shital Poojary* • *Krishna Bhalala*

STIs include a variety of infectious sexually transmitted conditions with varied clinical manifestations. STIs have major impact on sexual and reproductive health. Significant proportion of these STIs is common in developing countries like India.

STIs IN ELDERLY

Most researchers on STIs have focused on younger patients as STIs are believed to be common among them. STIs in elderly are often overlooked by patients and also by healthcare providers. However, surveillance data from various studies demonstrate that rates of STIs in patients aged 50 and over may be increasing.[1] A national survey done in United States found that majority of older adults engaged in intimate relationships and considered sexuality as an important part of their lives.[2]Although, sexual activity declined with age but not sufficient enough to immune them from STIs.

Data from nationwide surveys suggest that many older patients remain sexually active well into their eighth decade of life.[3] According to recent CDC (centre for disease control and prevention) data, over 6 new cases of STD per 10,000 patients were elderly, which is almost 50% increase since 1996.

It is important to understand that STIs do occur in elderly in significant proportion and it is essential to know how their manifestations differ in elderly. It is also essential for elderly and more importantly their caregivers to get educated about the risk of STIs. If STIs are undiagnosed or left untreated, they can cause significant effect on health like depression or social withdrawal.

FACTORS CONTRIBUTING TO INCREASED STIs IN ELDERLY

Since this population differs from younger individuals in their lifestyle including sexual practice, the factors responsible are also different.

1. Numerous physiological and pathological changes in elderly puts them at higher risk of acquiring STIs. Immune system may not be as robust as that of younger adults and thus are more susceptible to the infections and show less favourable response to treatment.
2. Older adults potentially may have co-existent illnesses requiring polypharmacy. This increases the chance for adverse health events and may impact treatment effectiveness.
3. Elderly patients feel inhibited to disclose their sexual concerns to the physician due to fear of social embarrassment and prejudices. Patients may attribute their symptoms of genital tract to age-related changes leading to delay in diagnosis.
4. Availability of drugs for erectile dysfunction and use of hormone replacement

therapy enables them to engage in sexual activity by restoring their libido and correcting sexual problems.Use of hormonal lubricating creams by elderly women takes care of the associated discomfort due to dry vagina encouraging them to indulge in sex.

5. For older women, decreased estrogen leads to physiological changes such as thinning and increased dryness of the vaginal mucosa. Such an environment makes the vagina more likely to have abrasions and tears during sexual intercourse and a greater chance of entry of organism. Also, the added decline in progesterone may lead to more vaginal infections.
6. Elderly are looking for partners as the rate of divorce in the middle years of life. The sexual activity is likely to be resumed with new/unknown partner.
7. Psychosocial changes, such as demise of spouse promote activities like online dating, which also play a role in acquiring STIs.
8. Elderly population comprising of postmenopausal women and men indulge in free sex uninhibitedly due to false sense of protection as they are no longer in the reproductive age group. This is supported by the fact that seniors are one-sixth time less likely to use condoms than people in their twenties.[4,5]
9. Sexual preference plays an important role in the transmission of STIs as well. Disproportionately greater rates of STIs occur in men having sex with men (MSM) with respect to multiple partners and unprotected anal-genital, oral-genital and oral-anal intercourse.[6]

IMPORTANCE OF STIs IN ELDERLY

Data on sexual behaviour and STIs in elderly are concerning because of the morbidity associated with it. Possible contributing factors for this are:

1. They are likely to receive diagnosis when it is too late partly due to lack of caregivers to bring them to healthcare facility.
2. Asymptomatic infections are common with many STIs. Patients are diagnosed late when it may not be amenable to treatment or the sequelae have already occured.[1,4]
3. STIs can be present in elderly who are no longer sexually active. For example, syphilis may present later owing to its long incubation period and asymptomatic nature in early stage. Pelvic inflammatory disease, PID, a complication of gonorrhoea/Chlamydia which may have been contracted during active sexual life can present later in life and may cause significant morbidity, for example, chronic pelvic pain.
4. STIs have long-term and short-term issues like risk of HIV transmission and economic burden on healthcare system.

COMMON STIs AND RESPECTIVE ORGANISMS

Discussion of each STI in detail is beyond the scope of this chapter. Common STIs and their classical clinical features are tabulated in brief in Table 11.1.

RECOMMENDATIONS FOR SCREENING FOR SEXUALLY TRANSMITTED INFECTIONS AMONG OLDER ADULTS—CDC 2006-2007

- Adults who are sexually active should talk to their healthcare provider about STI testing and which tests may be right for them.
- All adults should be tested at least once for HIV.
- All sexually active older women with risk factors such as new or multiple sex partners should be screened annually for chlamydia and gonorrhoea.
- Trichomoniasis screening should be conducted at least annually for all women with HIV.
- Screening is recommended at least once per year for syphilis, chlamydia, gonorrhoea, and HIV for all sexually active bisexual men, and other men who have sex with men (MSM).

TABLE 11.1: Important STIs, causative agents and their salient features

STIs	Causative organisms	Clinical features
Bacterial		
Syphilis	*Treponema pallidum*	Primary chancre (Fig. 11.1)/mucocutaneous manifestation of secondary syphilis/gumma of tertiary syphilis
Chancroid	*Haemophilus ducreyi*	Painful, multiple ulcers with undermined margin, ragged border, tender and suppurative lymphadenopathy
Gonorrhoea	*Neisseria gonorrhoeae*	Can present as urethritis/cervicitis as purulent/mucopurulent urethral/cervical discharge, burning micturition, urethral/cervical inflammation (Fig. 11.2)
Lymphogranuloma venereum	*Chlamydia trachomatis*	Superficial or deep painless ulcer, tender and suppurative loculated lymphadenopathy
Granuloma inguinale	*Klebsiella granulomatis*	Single/multiple beefy red painless ulcer that bleed easily with pseudobubo
Viral		
Anogenital wart	Human papillomavirus (HPV)	Macular, popular, pedunculated growth. It can be pigmented /skin colored depending on their location
Genital herpes	Herps simplex virus 1 and 2	Grouped vesicle/erosion on erythematous base, with or without prior prodrome (Fig. 11.3)
Molluscum contagiosum	Molluscum contagiosum virus	Usually multiple, pearly white papule with central umbilication
Protozoal		
Trichomoniasis	*Trichomonas vaginalis*	Epididymitis, urethritis, prostatitis Diffuse, malodorous, yellow greenish vaginal discharge
Arthropod		
Genital scabies	*Sarcoptes scabiei*	Multiple itchy papules/nodules on external genitalia, nocturnal itching, positive family/partner history can be supportive

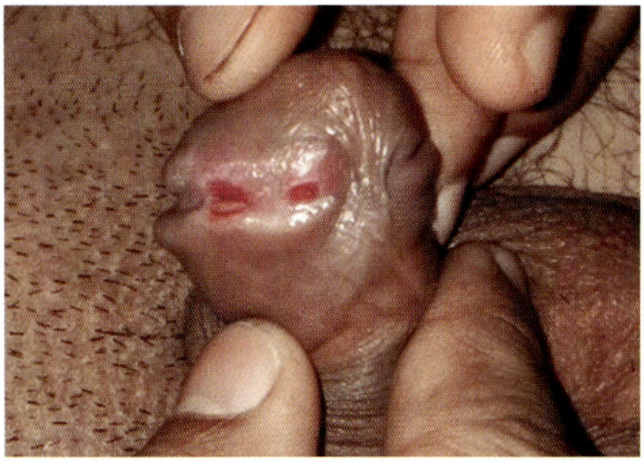

Fig. 11.1: Hard chancre on coronal sulcus, patient also had bilateral discrete, firm, painless inguinal lymphadenopathy and showed positive serology for syphilis

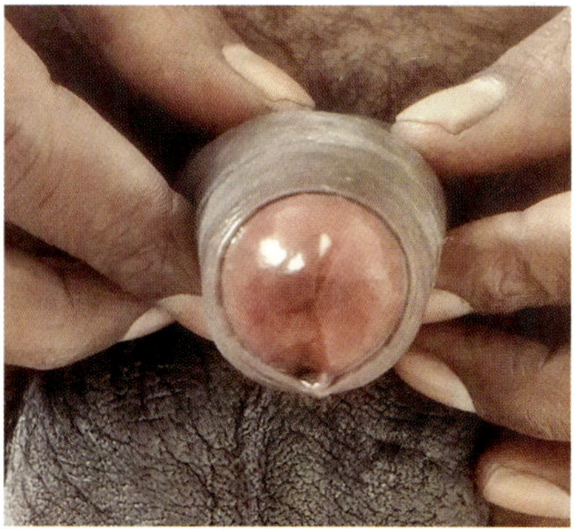

Fig. 11.2: Frank purulent discharge at the urethral meatus in a patient of gonococcal urethritis

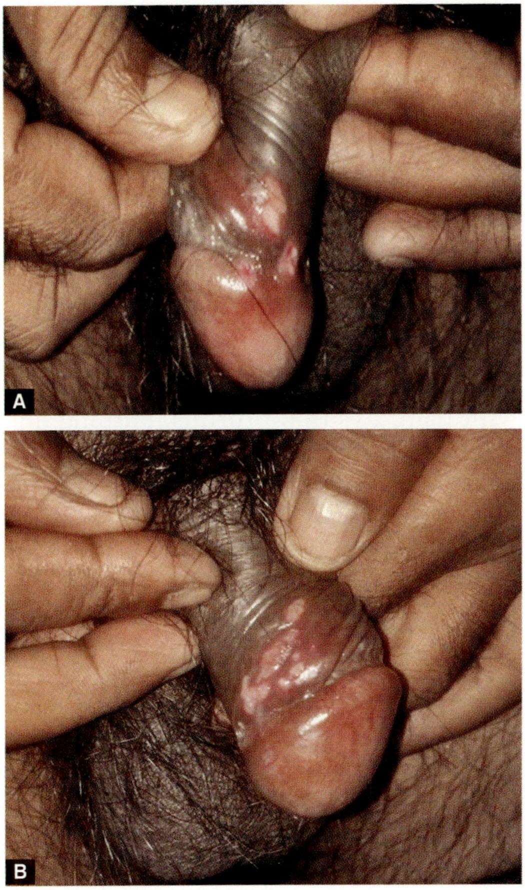

Fig. 11.3A and B: Multiple erosions with polycyclic margins in a patient of herpes genitalis

- More frequent screening (3–6 monthly) should be done for MSM with anonymous partner, history of illicit drug use in patients or in their partner.

Points to remember while taking history in elderly

- Eliciting sexual history might be difficult as it is a sensitive issue. One should gain the confidence of the patient before eliciting sexual history. Moreover, elderly are less likely to unravel their contact history especially the extramarital contact history or history of homosexual intercourse.
- For "partners," the initial questions include "Are you currently sexually active?" and, if no, "Have you been sexually active in the past?" and related questions, instead of directly asking about partners.

Treatment of STIs

It is beyond the scope of this chapter to cover CDC and NACO guidelines of all the STIs. Readers should refer to corresponding websites for complete details regarding management. Treating doctor should make treatment changes accordingly in case of renal and hepatic impairment and should consider drug interaction wherever appropriate, to ensure safe and effective.

CONCLUSION

STIs are primarily a health issue of young people, both in terms of incidence and health sequel. However, the population globally is ageing and rapidly increasing numbers of people are living long and healthy. There is enough evidence showing increase in incidence of STIs among elderly attributed to potentially active sexual life. Elderly are more likely to remain sexually active in the ongoing times hence there is a greater chance of diagnosing sexually transmitted infections in them. Sexual health should be considered as an important aspect of older peoples' lives. Preparation through education, use of safe sex practices, discussion with partner(s) about sexual risks, STI testing, awareness about age-related physiological or bodily changes affecting sexuality of older men and women, and seeking assessment and treatment promptly if an STI is suspected can enhance sexual health.

NON-SEXUALLY TRANSMITTED GENITAL DERMATOSES GENITAL DERMATOSES

Not all the genital lesions are sexually transmitted. Caregivers/physicians should be familiar with these lesions as they are a cause of concern to the patients because they might be considered as STI/malignancy by the patient.

Classification is shown in Table 11.2. A few important non-sexually transmitted genital dermatoses have been discussed below.

TABLE 11.2: Non-sexually transmitted infections and genital dermatoses

Non-sexually transmitted infections and genital dermatoses	Generalised dermatoses with genital predilection	Specific to genitalia
Herpes zoster	Psoriasis	Zoon's balanitis/vulvitis
Candidiasis	Immunobullous disease	Lichen simplex
Tinea cruris		Lichen sclerosus
Intertrigo		Bowen's disease
Fournier gangrene		Atrophic vaginitis
		Bowenoid papulosis, erythroplasia of Queyrat

ZOON'S BALANITIS/PLASMA CELL BALANITIS AND ZOON'S VULVITIS[8]

It is an idiopathic chronic, benign, inflammatory mucositis affecting glans, prepuce and vulva, commonly seen in middle aged-elderly individuals.

Disturbed preputial ecology has been proposed to result in the development of this condition.

Other factors implicated include infection with *M. smegmatis*, HPV (human papilloma virus) infection, and disturbed local circulation. Histopathologically it resembles lichen aureus, hence it has also been likened to have a vasculitic component. It is also postulated to be due to immediate hypersensitivity reaction to yet unknown antigens. It is also suggested to be a type of extramedullary plasmocytic infiltration since plasma cells are the predominant cells seen in the infiltrate. Other lesser known causes include trauma, friction, heat and rubbing.

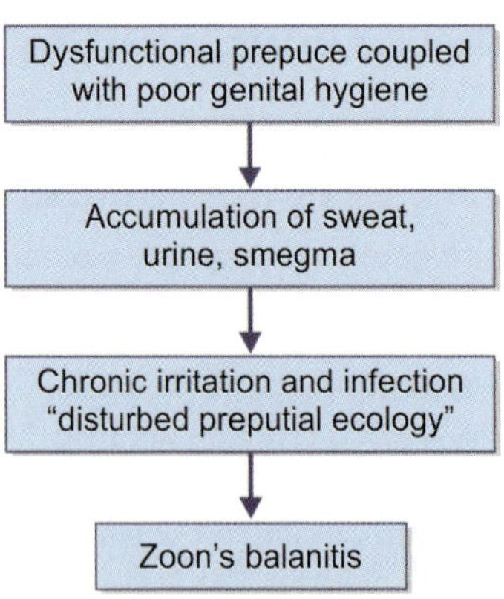

Patient can be asymptomatic or can present with pain, dysuria, pruritus, burning and dyspareunia. On examination, solitary, well-defined, shiny, glazed erythematous plaque over glans can be seen (Fig. 11.4). Multiple pinpoint, bright red spot over the lesion are observed which are due to punctate haemorrhage. Analogous lesion if present over vulva is called Zoon's vulvitis. Rarely erosive and vegetative types can be seen.

Histopathology reveals acanthosis, parakeratosis, spongiosis, necrotic keratinocytes, and lozenge-shaped ketainocytes being a characteristic feature. Dermis shows lichenoid infiltrate, out of which >50% is composed of plasma cells. Dermis also shows red blood cell extravasation, supporting its association with vasculitic process. It also shows hemosiderin

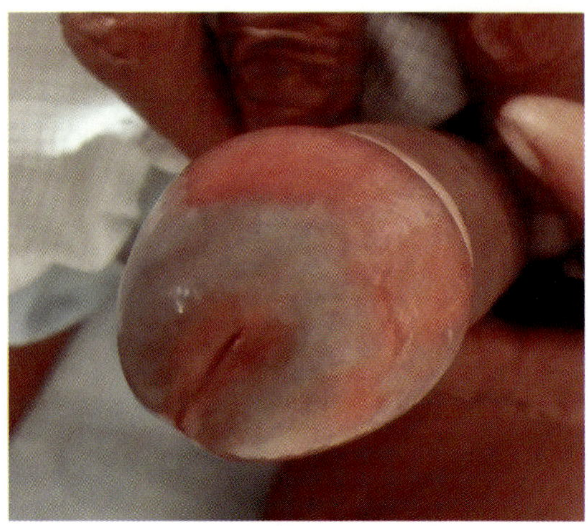

Fig. 11.4: Zoon's balanitis showing well-defined erythematous erosive lesion over glans penis

deposition, proliferating and dilated capillaries.

Treatment

General measures are of utmost importance. Patients should be emphasized about promotion of local hygiene. Topical modalities like corticosteroids, calcineurin inhibitors, 5% imiquimod can be used. Circumcision is the treatment of choice as removes the prepuce and hence prevents the accumulation of sweat, urine, smegma but this surgical option is to be considered when other modalities fail and is culturally appropriate. Follow-up of the patients is necessary as rare cases of conversion into premalignant conditions like erythroplasia and frank malignancy have been reported.

PREMALIGNANT LESIONS OF MALE GENITALIA[9]

Differentiating premalignant penile lesions from benign penile dermatoses present aunique challenge due to the rarity of these conditions. There is a tendency for delayed presentation, often due to long-term self-management or unsuccessful treatment, which can result in progression to an invasive carcinoma.

Risk factors can be classified as HPV-related and non-HPV-related. Infection with HPV is one of the most important and widely studied risk factors in penile cancer development, with HPV DNA found in approximately 50% of all penile squamous cell carcinomas. High-risk HPV 16, 18 are implicated in majority of the cases. Non-HPV-related factors include presence of a foreskin, phimosis, poor hygiene, smoking, chronic inflammation and having multiple sexual partners. Important conditions are listed in Table 11.3.

Carcinoma *in situ* (CIS) includes 2 eponyms, erythroplasia of Queyrat (EQ) and Bowen's disease (BD). Both are essentially the same histological premalignant condition, differing primarily only in location. The vast majority of cases occur in uncircumcised men with phimotic foreskin. Exact incidence of these conditions is less well-established than malignant conditions.

TABLE 11.3: Pre-malignant lesions of male genitalia

HPV-related	Non-HPV-related
Carcinoma *in situ* (erythroplasia of Queyrat and Bowen's disease)	Lichen sclerosus
Bowenoid papulosis, BP	Cutaneous horn
Giant condyloma accuminata	Leukoplakia
PeIN, penile intraepithelial neoplasia	Differentiated PeIN

Erythroplasia of Queyrat

EQ arises from mucosa, such as the inner surface of prepuce and glans. Lesions in EQ are usually asymptomatic sharply defined plaques, which have a smooth, velvety, bright red appearance, surface may show erosions. The risk of malignant transformation is variable in different studies, in one of the studies it has been reported to be up to 30%, if left untreated.[10]

Bowen's Disease

BD is essentially considered the same pathological process as EQ affecting the skin of the penile shaft. In BD lesions are usually solitary, well defined, scaly, dull-red plaques, often with areas of crusting. Lesions may also be heavily pigmented. Occasionally, they may have associated leukoplakic, nodular, or ulcerated changes.

Bowenoid Papulosis

BP occurs primarily in young sexually active men in their 30s but may occur in elderly. Lesions occur mainly on the penile shaft or mons, although they can also occasionally arise on the glans and prepuce. They are usually multiple, red, velvety, maculopapular lesions, which can coalesce to form larger plaques, can be associated pigmentation. They often cause pruritus or discomfort. BP is commonly associated with HPV 16 similar EQ and BD. However, BP shows moderate dysplasia and runs a more benign course unlike the severe dysplasia of the two conditions mentioned earlier.

Treatment of Premalignant Conditions

Treatment options include topical chemotherapy/immunotherapy with 5-fluorouracil and imiquimod, ablative or nonablative lasers like CO_2 or Nd:YAG, cryotherapy, photodynamic therapy. Surgical excision/Moh's microscopic surgery of the lesion is also an option, which ensures the complete removal of the lesion. Circumcision can also be considered if the general condition permits the surgery.

GENITAL LICHEN SCLEROSUS (LS)/BALANITIS XEROTICA OBLITERANS (BXO)

This is an idiopathic, chronic, progressive inflammatory process. This is the most important non-HPV-related premalignant condition.[9] It is six to ten times more common in women than in men.[13]

Pruritus, pain and burning are common symptoms. As the disease advances dysuria, dyspareunia can set in. The lesions are noted as ivory coloured, plaques over labia majora, minora, introitus and the perianal area. It can form a figure of 8 configuration. The skin becomes atrophic and papery thin with formation of telangiectasia, ulcers, excoriations, erosions and bleeding. Long-term complications include stenosis of introitus, atrophy of labia and clitoris. Squamous cell carcinoma is a long-term complication. Stenotic labia can make the intercourse uncomfortable. It may also interfere with medical examination, if speculum is to be used. It also exhibit the phenomenon of koebnarisation.[15]

Balanitis xerotica obliterans (BXO) is considered as the male genital variant of LS. It primarily affects the glans penis and prepuce of uncircumcised men, and in advanced cases it can involve the urethral meatus and anterior urethra. Lesions classically appear as pale, atrophic, sclerotic plaques, which may coalesce causing phimosis and meatal stenosis.[9]

Although European guidelines consider LS to be a premalignant condition, whether it truly represents a premalignant process remains controversial.[11] In the largest series to date, squamous cell carcinoma was found in 2.3% of 522 patients diagnosed with LS.[12] In this study, all cases epithelial dysplasia and LS were found adjacent to tumour foci, indicating possible histological progression from chronic inflammation to dysplasia and eventually to malignant transformation.[12] For the same reason, lesions showing atypical morphology and not responding to conventional treatment, biopsy should be considered.[16]

Treatment

General measures/patient education are important. Patient should be educated to avoid scratching which may exacerbate the lesion by koebnarisation, wear loose and breathable clothes (cotton, silk), avoiding tight underwear use at night. Sedative antihistamines, topical anaesthetics, lubricants and emollients are given for symptomatic relief. Tricyclic antidepressants (amitriptyline, desipramine, nortriptyline) can be considered, if no relief is obtained with above measures. One should consider to treat associated urinary incontinence and secondary infections if any (Candida, herpes). Super potent topical corticosteroids are the first line of management. It should be applied once a day for 4 weeks, followed by alternate day for 4 weeks followed by twice a week for next 4 weeks. Topical tacrolimus 0.03% can be used as steroid sparing agent. Its use should be limited to steroid non-responsive cases. Systemic therapies like retinoids, methotrexate, immunosuppressants should be considered only in exceptional cases. Intralesional triamcinolone, PUVA, photodynamic therapy can be tried.

Follow-up

The first visit after beginning the treatment of LS should be no later than 3 months and the following visit not longer than 6 months. The risk of malignant transformation remains elevated throughout the life. Thus, follow-up must be kept indefinitely, at least every 6–12 months. Some authors are of the opinion that in older age group, the monitoring should be more intensified.[17]

ATROPHIC VAGINITIS

It is a physiological change in female genitals as a part of postmenopausal change causing significant morbidity and discomfort. With natural menopause, ovarian production of estrogen gradually falls, and hormonal support of estrogen-dependent tissues wanes. These effects are seen early and more severely in those who undergo premature menopause by surgical/medical oophorectomy or as a result of chemotherapeutics.[18]

Genital Changes Associated with Estrogen Loss

Estrogen receptors, alpha and beta, are expressed throughout the squamous epithelium, connective tissue and smooth muscle of the vulva, vagina and urogenital mucosa.[19]As a result, with the loss of estrogen stimulation, profound changes occur within the vulvovaginal mucosa. In the dermal layer, collagen fibers fuse and undergo hyalinization, whereas the elastin fibers fragment. The result of these changes is an overall loss of mucosal elasticity.[20] Concentrations of hygroscopic, intercellular acid mucopolysaccharide and hyaluronic acid within the dermis decrease, which reduce mucosal hydration.[21] The vagina loses its rugae, and there is a shortening and narrowing of the vagina. The mucosa of the vagina, introitus, and labia minora becomes thin and pale.[22] With menopause there is a loss of vascular support, the volume of vaginal secretions also decreases making the mucosa dry. There is a marked reduction in the lactobacillus population, leading to higher vaginal pH, which makes it more prone for bacterial infection.[23]

Clinical Features

Although genital changes occur in most women with loss of estrogen support, the extent to which women become symptomatic varies. When arises, it includes spectrum of symptoms. More commonly, the diagnosis of atrophic vaginitis is applied to a spectrum of symptoms including painful intercourse, vulvovaginal dryness, itching or pain, recurrent urinary tract infections, as well as, abnormal vaginal discharge. With decreased endogenous lubrication and narrowing of the hymenal diameter, women often complain of postcoital friction induced inflammation of the labia minora, fissuring of the introitus and fourchette, and postcoital painand spotting. Thinning of epithelium coupled with dryness produces itching, soreness.[24] Urethral discomfort during voiding, urinary frequency, haematuria, dysuria, urge incontinence and recurrent urinary tract infections are also seen.[25]

On examination, pubic hair would be grey and sparse. The subcutaneous fat within the mons pubis and labia majora decreases, and there is a reduction in labia minora volume. The introitus appears pale, shiny, and dry and shows petechiae. Sometimes dryness is severe enough to produce fissures or it can be a result of coitus through narrow in elastic introitus. There is atrophy of introitus and vagina. pH of the vaginal is increased to >5, which is a sign if estrogen deficiency.[26]

Based on the pathophysiology, it is clear that the most effective therapy for reducing the symptoms of atrophic vaginitis is the administration of estrogen, local or systemic. Although systemic hormonal replacement therapy, using oral or transdermal estrogen formulations, will also improve vulvovaginal symptoms, many women prefer local, directed therapy, which avoids higher systemic estrogen exposures.[27]

CANDIDAL BALANOPOSTHITIS AND VULVOVAGINAL CANDIDIASIS (CBP & VVC)

Balanitis describes inflammation of the glans penis and posthitis means inflammation of the prepuce. In practice, both areas are often affected together, and the term balanoposthitis then used. This descriptive term is a collection of separate conditions with distinct etiology. Clinical presentation can be similar, certain clinical feature may be suggestive of specific etiology but not completely pathognomonic.[28]

Balanitis is common in uncircumcised men as a result of poor hygiene and aeration or because of irritation by smegma and in many cases preputial dysfunction is a causal or contributing factor. Balanitis and vulvovaginitis may be more severe in the presence of some underlying medical conditions like immunosuppression or diabetes mellitus (DM).[29] Causes of balanoposthitis and vulvovaginitis are listed in Table 11.4.

Out of all the causes, since candidal etiology is quite commonly seen in elderly due to associated comorbidities like diabetes and higher proportion of men being uncircumcised.

Predisposing conditions for candida balanoposthitis include DM, HIV infection, antibiotic misuse, hormone replacement therapy (HRT). Acquired balanoposthitis can be the first clinical sign of diabetes. In one of the study from Britain, 26% of adult patients with an acquired phimosis were found to suffer from type II diabetes. The diagnosis of DM was made for the first time in 8% of these patients which means that candidal balanoposthitis in an apparently healthy male is a cutaneous marker of DM.[30] Late diagnosis, irregular monitoring of blood sugar, and infrequent follow-up by the physician are also contributory. Balanoposthitis is less common in circumcised men.[31]

TABLE 11.4: Causes of balanoposthitis and vulvovaginitis

Causes
Fungal: Candidal
Bacterial: Aerobic and anaerobic infection, *Treponema pallidum*
Protozoal: Trichomonas vaginalis
Viral: Herpes simplex virus, human papillomavirus

Patient presents with itching as the predominant symptom along with soreness, burning, external dysuria, raw area, fissured skin. Fissures that are seen in this condition are explained by the accumulation of advanced glycation end-products (AGEs) in the skin. AGEs content is increased by inadequate glycemic control in diabetics. AGEs impair production of collagen and extracellular organization, which in turn causes deleterious effects such as a greater impairment and alteration of biomechanical properties of the skin, namely, elasticity and hydration.[32]

On examination, moist area, erythema, diffuse/blotchy, with thick white, odour free, cottage cheese-like deposits over the affected area can be seen (Fig. 11.5). Vertical preputial fissures/fissures over inner aspect of labia majora are the characteristic feature (Fig. 11.7A and B). KOH (potassium hydroxide) scraping of the lesion show budding yeast cells of Candida (Fig. 11.6). Investigations to rule out immunosuppression like HIV and diabetes should be done.[28] The condition is treated according to CDC guidelines depending on the severity and frequency. Control of underlying hyperglycaemia is of paramount importance.

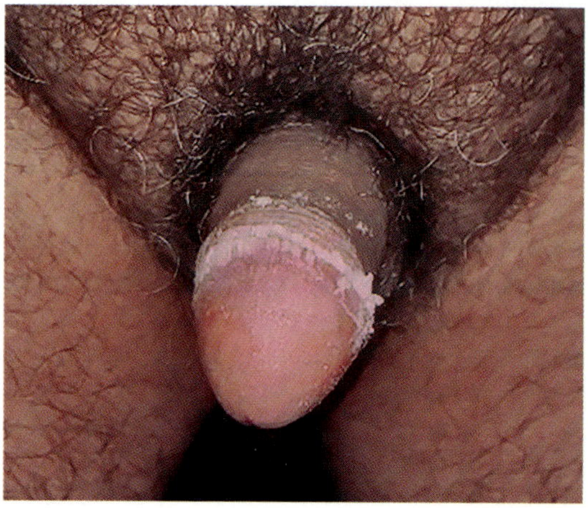

Fig. 11.5: Cottage cheese-like deposits in a patient of CBP

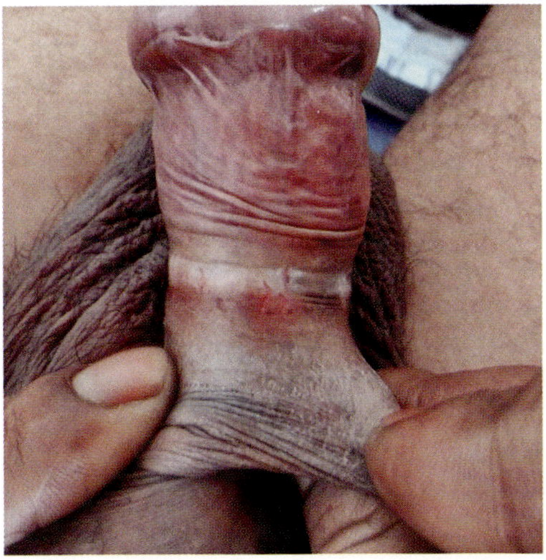

Fig. 11.6: Multiple fissures in a patient of CBP

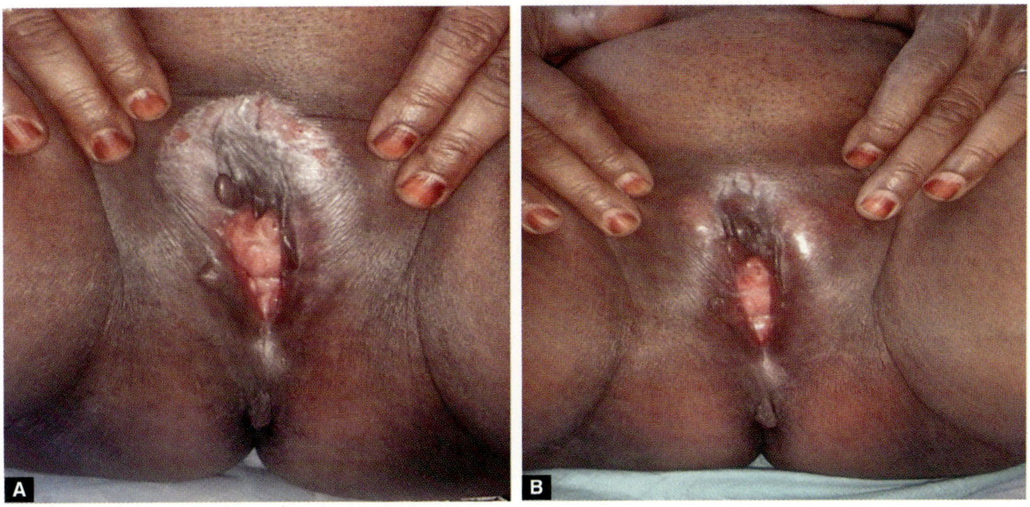

Fig. 11.7A and B: (A) Similar findings in a female patient with VVC, (B) same patient after single dose of fluconazole 150 mg

References

1. Minichiello V, Rahman S, Hawkes G, Pitts M. STI epidemiology in the global older population: emerging challenges. Perspect Public Health 2012; 132:178–81.
2. Lindau ST, Schumm LP, Laumann EO, Levinson W, O'Muircheartaigh CA, Waite LJ. A study of sexuality and health among older adults in the United States. N Engl J Med 2007; 357:762–74.
3. Stall R, Catania J. AIDS risk behaviors among late middle-aged and elderly Americans. The National AIDS behavioral Surveys. Arch Intern Med 1994; 154:57–63.
4. Zagaria ME. Sexually transmitted diseases in older patients. US Pharm 2003; 23(12):26–9.
5. Letvak S, Schoder D. Sexually Transmitted Diseases in the Elderly: What You Need to Know. Geriatric nursing 1996; 156–60.

6. Beers MH, Berkow R. The Merck Manual of Geriatrics. 3rd ed. Whitehouse Station, NJ: Merck and Co 2000;1357-59,1378-82.
7. Johnson BK. Sexually transmitted infections and older adults. Journal of Gerontological Nursing 2013; 53–60.
8. Dayal S, Sahu P. Zoon balantis: a comprehensive review. Indian J of sexually transmitted disease and AIDS 2016; 129–38.
9. Shabbir M, Minhas S, Muneer A. Diagnosis and management of premalignant penile lesions. TherAdvUrol 2011; 151–58.
10. Wieland U, Jurk, S, Weissenborn S, Krieg T, Pfister H, Ritzkowsky A. Erythroplasia of Queyrat: Coinfection with cutaneous carcinogenic human papillomavirus type 8 and genital papillomaviruses. J Invest dermatol 2000; 115(3):396–401.
11. Algaba, F, Horenblas S, Pizzocaro G, Solsona E, Windahl T. EAU guidelines on penile cancer. EurUrol 2002; 199–203.
12. Depasquale I, Park AJ, Bracka A. The treatment of balanitis xerotica obliterans. BJU Int 2000; 459–65.
13. Meffert JJ, Davis BM, Grimwood RE. Lichen sclerosus. J Am Acad Dermatol 1995; 32(3):393–416.
14. Vieira-Baptista P, Lima-Silva J, Cavaco-Gomes J, Beires J, Martinezde-Oliveira J. What differentiates symptomatic from asymptomatic women with lichen sclerosus? Gynecol Obstet Invest 2015; 79:263–68.
15. López FRP, Baptista PV. Lichen sclerosus in female: A review. Climacteric 2017; 339–47.
16. Neill SM, Lewis FM, Tatnall FM, Cox NH. British Association of Dermatologists' guidelines for the management of lichen sclerosus. Br J Dermatol 2010; 672–82.
17. Bleeker MC, Visser PJ, Overbeek LI, van Beurden M, Berkhof J. Lichen sclerosus: incidence and risk of vulvar squamous cell carcinoma. Cancer Epidemiol Biomarkers Prev 2016; 1224–30.
18. Stika CS. Atrophic vaginitis. Dermatil Ther 2010; 514–22.
19. Onnis A, Nardelli GB, Lamaina V, Mozzanega B, Becagli L, Fais GF. Hormonal receptors in vulvar tissues. Eur J Gynaecol Oncol 1985; 6(2):125–28.
20. Castelo-BrancoC, Cancelo MJ, Villero J, Nohales F, Julia MD. Management of postmenopausal vaginal atrophy and atrophic vaginitis. Maturitas 2005; S46–52.
21. Oriba HA, Elsner P, Maibach HI. Vulvar physiology. Semin Dermatol 1989; 8(1):2–6.
22. Pandit L, Ouslander JG. Postmenopausal vaginal atrophy and atrophic vaginitis. Am J Med Sci 1997; 314(4):228–31.
23. Caillouette JC, Sharp CF, Jr, Zimmerman GJ, Roy S. Vaginal pH as a marker for bacterial pathogens and menopausal status. Am J Obstet Gynecol 1997; 176(6):1270–5.
24. Pandit L, Ouslander JG. Postmenopausal vaginal atrophy and atrophic vaginitis. Am J Med Sci 1997; 314(4):228–31.
25. Notelovitz M. Estrogen therapy in the management of problems associated with urogenital ageing: a simple diagnostic test and the effect of the route of hormone administration. Maturitas 1995; S31–3.
26. Erickson KL, Montagna W. New observations on the anatomical features of the female genitalia. J Am Med Womens Assoc 1972; 27(11):573–81.
27. Suckling J, Lethaby A, Kennedy R. Local oestrogen for vaginal atrophy in postmenopausal women. Cochrane Database Syst Rev 2006; 1–12.
28. Pandya I, Shinojia M, Vadukul D, Marfatia YS. Approach to balanitis/balanoposthitis: Current guidelines. Indian J Sex Transm Dis AIDS 2014; 35(2): 155–57.
29. Edwards S. Balanitis and balanoposthitis: A review. Genitourin Med. 1996; 72(3):155–59.
30. Bromage SJ, Crump A, Pearce I. Phimosis as a presenting feature of diabetes. BJU Int 2008; 338–40.
31. Verma SB, wollina U. Looking through the cracks of diabetic candidal balanoposthitis! Int J Gen Med 2011; 4:511–13.
32. Ye X, Tong Z, Dang Y, *et al*. Effects of blood glucose fluctuation on skin biophysical properties, structure and antioxidant status in an animal model. Clin Exp Dermatol 2009; 80–2.

CHAPTER 12

Cutaneous Adverse Drug Reactions in Elderly Patients

• *Lalit Gupta*

Key Points

- Adverse drug reactions (ADRs) form an important subset of diseases affecting the elderly population.
- Increasing life expectancy, presence of multiple medical illnesses and consumption of multiple drugs for these, coupled with reduced renal and hepatic clearance of drugs make elderly population a vulnerable group to develop ADRs.
- Age-related physiological, pharmacodynamic and pharmacokinetic alterations, comorbidities and polypharmacy make this age group not only susceptible to CADR, but also make the management challenging.
- Urticaria and maculopapular rash are the commonest CADR, as in general population.
- Antihypertensives, anti-diabetic, lipid lowering agents, antipsychotics, cancer chemotherapeutics are the drugs which are more commonly consumed by this subset of population and hence common culprits for ADRs.

Introduction

An adverse drug reaction (ADR) is defined as an undesirable clinical manifestation resulting from administration of a drug; this includes reactions due to overdose, predictable side effects and non-predictable adverse manifestations. ADRs are one of the major preventable health problems. Skin is a common and most easily observed target organ of ADRs. It has been estimated in one study that 14% of adverse drug reactions in hospital care are cutaneous or allergic in nature.[1]

With increasing life expectancy and changing lifestyles, the prevalence of multiple comorbidities is on the rise, with hypertension, diabetes mellitus, hyperlipidemia, cardiovascular disorders, mental disorders, musculoskeletal diseases and cancer being more common.[2] This increases the risk of polypharmacy and drug interactions. Self-medication with alternative medication further worsens the condition.[3]

Although CADR can affect any age group; fraility, pharmacodynamic and pharmacokinetic changes in body, associated systemic diseases or multiple morbidities and polypharmacy make elderly patients more susceptible. For the same reason, management is difficult and prognosis is poor in geriatric age group.

EPIDEMIOLOGY

Adverse drug reactions (ADRs) are very common in elderly individuals, mainly comprising of delirium, falls, sedation, etc. which are usually type A reactions, i.e. they are attributable to a predictable known pharmacological effect of a drug. Globally, the prevalence rate of ADRs is highly variable and is influenced by the care setting. In a retrospective study comprising of 30,195 hospitalized patients in New York, adverse drug reactions were the most common single type of adverse event (19%), 14% of these reactions were cutaneous/allergic in nature.[1] In a study by Bigby et al on 15,438 consecutive in patients, the overall cutaneous ADR rate was 2.2%.[4]

Indian studies have reported an incidence rate of 2–5% in admitted patients.[5–9] Patel et al in their systematic review of 3671 cases from 18 prospective studies, reported the incidence of CADRs as 82.59/1000 and 8.72/1000 in inpatient and outpatient settings respectively.[8] In an earlier study by Chatterjee et al., the incidence of CADRs was found to be 2.6% (i.e. 26/1000) in a dermatology outpatient setting.[9]

CADRs are most common in second and third decades of life. In the study by Patel et al.,[8] majority of patients (54.42%) belonged to 21–39 years age group, and 7.96% fell in >60 years age group. In a retrospective study where 4-year data of 4099 geriatric patients was analyzed to determine the frequencies of dermatologic conditions in geriatric population, the prevalence of CADR was found to be 1.4%.[10] Most of the studies focusing on elderly patients suggest that the prevalence of CADR in this age group is not different from general population.[10–14] It was reported in one study that the SCAR such as SJS/TEN (Stevens-Johnson syndrome/toxic epidermal necrolysis), DRESS (drug-related eosinophilia and systemic symptoms) and anaphylaxis are less common in elderly in comparison to non-elderly patients.[15]

ETIOPATHOGENESIS

1. Factors Predisposing Elderly Patients to ADR

There are various factors which make geriatric population predisposed to cutaneous adverse drug reactions (Box 12.1). The major factors are discussed as follows:

Box 12.1: Factors predisposing to ADRs in elderly patients

- Age-related changes in pharmacodynamics and pharmacokinetics
- Presence of comorbidities/multimorbidity
- Polypharmacy
- Problems due to compliance/adherence
- Other risk factors[35]
  - Advanced age (≥85 years)
  - Female sex
  - Lower socio-economic status
  - Lives alone
  - Lower body weight
  - History of prior drug reactions
  - Regular use of alcohol
  - Prior ADR
  - Recent hospitalization
  - Dementia
  - Hepatic or renal insufficiency (creatinine clearance <50 ml/min)
  - Multiple prescribers
  - Long duration of use

i. Age-related changes in pharmacodynamics and pharmacokinetics: Ageing is the sum of cumulative local effects on molecular, cellular and tissue level and is associated with time-related loss of functional units. Physiological changes in body lead to pharmacokinetic and alterations, like changes in drug distribution volumes, metabolism and clearance of drugs which can prolong the half-life, increase potential for drug toxicity and the risk of adverse drug reactions.[16] In addition, there are alterations in receptor responsiveness which causes pharmacodynamic alterations. Inter-individual variability in the pharmacological response also increases with age.

Tables 12.1 and 12.2 illustrate the various physiological changes associated with ageing and their pharmacokinetic and pharmacodynamic implications.[16]

ii. Presence of comorbidities/multimorbidity: Where comorbidity refers to occurrence of medical conditions additional to an 'index disease', multimorbidity refers to co-occurrence of any two or more medical conditions, which may or may not directly interact with each other in an individual.[19] A systematic review of 39 studies from 12 different countries found that 95.1% of the people aged 65 years and above were multimorbidity.[20] Hypertension and osteoarthritis

TABLE 12.1: Pharmacokinetic implications of age-related physiological changes

Age-related physiological changes		Pharmacokinetic (pK) and practical implications	Drugs affected
Renal	• Reduction in renal mass • Reduced renal plasma flow • Reduced glomerular filtration rate (GFR)	• Reduced clearance of drugs • No concomitant increase in plasma creatinine due to reduced renal mass, hence serum creatinine is not a reliable indicator of GFR[17]	Drugs with narrow therapeutic index (e.g. lithium, aminoglycosides, digoxin) are likely to have serious adverse effects
Hepatic	• Progressive reduction in liver volume and blood flow • Moderate alteration in hepatic structure and enzymatic functions • Decrease in cytochrome p-450 activity	• Reduction in first-pass metabolism • Activation of prodrugs is slowed and reduced • Clearance of drugs with high extraction ratio (dependent upon the metabolizing capacity of liver) is reduced	Bioavailability of drugs with extensive first pass metabolism increases (e.g. proparanol and labetolol) Activation of prodrugs (enalapril and perindopril) affected
Gastrointestinal	• Reduction in hydrochloric acid and pepsin secretion • Reduced absorption in small intestine • Enzyme levels (lipase and trypsin) decrease dramatically	• Reduction in the absorption of various drugs	Absorption of levodopa is increased due to reduced amount of dopadecarboxylase in gastric mucosa[18]
Neuroendocrine responses	• Damage or loss of hippocampal neurons	• Impaired feedback inhibition of HPA axis suppression • Increased secretion of glucocorticoids • Learning and memory impairment	Side effects of steroids tend to be more frequent and dose regulation is important
Body composition	• Progressive reduction in total body water and lean body mass • Relative increase in body fat	• Water soluble drugs have smaller volume of distribution (*V*) resulting in higher serum levels • The reduction in *V* for water-soluble drugs tends to be balanced by a reduction in renal clearance (CL) • Fat soluble drugs have higher *V*, which leads to prolongation of half-life	Gentamicin, digoxin, ethanol, theophylline, and cimetidine are water-soluble drugs. Diazepam and amitriptyline are examples of fat-soluble drugs

TABLE 12.2: Changes in the pharmacodynamic effect for selected drugs with age[16]

Drug	Pharmacodynamic effect	Age-related change
Diazepam	Sedation	Increases
	Postural hypotension	
Diphenhydramine	Postural sway	No significant change
Furosemide	Peak diuretic effect	Decreases
Morphine	Analgesic effect	Increases
	Respiratory depression	No significant change
Propranolol	Antagonism of chronotropic effects of isoproterenol	Decreases
Heparin	Anticoagulant effect	No significant change
Warfarin	Anticoagulant effect	Increases

was the most frequent combination, followed by different combinations of cardiovascular conditions. In India, the prevalence of morbidity in elderly has been recorded as ranging from 70 to 99.5% in various studies.[21–25] Eye problems, including visual impairment and refractory errors was the most common chronic medical condition in a community based cross-sectional study in North India.[24] This was followed by hypertension and acid-peptic disease. Some studies have pointed to musculoskeletal diseases as the commonest.[26,27]

Elderly individuals vary greatly from younger population in terms of health, disability and physiologic reserves, which makes management of these chronic diseases difficult. Clinical trials designed to formulate management guidelines often exclude older and co-morbid people from the studies,[28,29] hence the extrapolation of evidence and the practicality of these guidelines is limited in this age group.

Increase in multimorbidity increases the burden of drug prescription, drug–drug interactions and the risk of adverse drug reactions. Moreover, the drugs which are commonly prescribed for the treatment of various CADRs become contraindicated or require careful monitoring due to associated comorbidities. SCARs, in particular, pose difficulties in terms of the complications associated with these reactions as well as the treatment instituted.

iii. Polypharmacy: Polypharmacy has been consistently identified as an individual risk factor in the development of adverse drug reactions. The precise minimum number of medications used to define "polypharmacy" is variable, but generally ranges from 5 to 10.[30] While polypharmacy most commonly refers to prescribed medications, it is important to also consider over-the-counter and herbal/ supplements used.

It has been estimated that 20% of medicare beneficiaries have five or more chronic conditions and 50% receive five or more medications.[29] In one study including ambulatory older adults with cancer, 84% were receiving five or more and 43% were receiving 10 or more medications.[31]

The risk of ADRs increases from 13% in a person taking two medicines to 58% when taking five and 82% when taking seven or more.[32] Field et al found the number of regular prescribed medications correlated with risk of adverse drug events, those taking five to six medicines Odds Ratio (OR) 2 [95% confidence interval (CI)1.2, 3.2], seven to eight medicines 2.8 (95% CI 1.7, 4.7) and nine or more medicines OR 3.3 (95% CI 1.9, 5.6), respectively.[33]

iv. Problems due to compliance/adherence: In a study on 312 outpatients in Boston, 545 discrepancies in the use of medications were found in 76% patients; 51% were the result of patients taking medications which were not recorded, 29% due to intake of non-recorded medications and 20% due to difference in dosage.[34] The possible reasons attributing to these are cognitive and memory impairments, lack of understanding, barriers to communication, complex regimen, changes in dosage, inconvenient scheduling, lack of perceived need, adverse events, cost and social isolation. These discrepancies further increase the risk of developing ADRs which is already higher because of multimorbidities and polypharmacy and make the assessment of causative drug(s) difficult.

2. Drugs Commonly Responsible for CADRs in Elderly

Although many of the drugs responsible for CADR in general population can also affect the elderly, there are some drugs liable to cause CADRs more frequently. These include drugs used in diseases which are more prevalent in this age group, like hypertension, diabetes mellitus, cardiovascular disorders, diseases of joints, mental illnesses and cancers. Antimicrobials, anticoagulants, diuretics, hypoglycemic agents, antineoplastic agents, nonsteroidal anti-inflammatory drugs, cardiovascular medicines, and analgesics were responsible for more than a half of the ADRs occurring in the hospital.[36–38] Antimicrobials account for approximately 20–42% of ADRs.[11,38–40]

CLINICAL PRESENTATION

The most common cutaneous adverse drug reactions described in elderly in one study were maculopapular rash and urticaria.[11] In a retrospective study over a period of 16 years, of all the adverse drug reactions observed, 68.2% were cutaneous with maculopapular rash being commonest (30.4%), followed by isolated pruritus (12.7%%) and photodermatoses (10.9%).[40] Other CADRs include psoriasiform, lichenoid, fixed drug eruption (FDE), vasculitic and drug induced autoimmune reactions, including pemphigus, bullous pemphigoid and lupus erythematosus. The common CADRs, causative agents and their clinical features are shown in Table 12.3 and described below.

TABLE 12.3: Characteristics of major cutaneous adverse drug reactions

Type of CADR	Morphology	Mucous membrane involvement	Time of onset	Commonly implicated drugs	Special comments in relation to elderly patients
Exanthematous rash	Erythematous maculopapular generalized	Absent	4–14 days	Antibiotics, antiepileptics, allopurinol, NSAIDs	Commonest cause of new onset rash inpatients
Fixed drug eruptions	One or more round, well circumscribed, erythematous, edematous plaques Sometimes central bullae, usually heals with hyperpigmentation (Fig. 12.1)	First exposure: 1–2 weeks Re-exposure: <48 hours, usually within 24hours	Cotrimoxazole (trimethoprim/ sulfamethoxazole) NSAIDs Tetracyclines Pseudoephedrine		
Urticaria	Wheals pruritus	Absent	Minutes to hours	Penicillins Opioids Aspirin/NSAIDs Sulfonamides Radiocontrast media	Urticaria could be the first manifestation of diseases like diabetes, dysthyroidism, autoimmune diseases and malignancies in the geriatric age. Possibility of bullous pemphigoid and dermatitis herpetiformis should be kept in mind
Angioedema	Swollen deep dermal and subcutaneous tissue (Fig. 12.3)	Present or absent	Minutes to hours	Angiotensin-converting-enzyme (ACE) inhibitors Aspirin/NSAIDs	ACE inhibitors induced angioedema often does not remit even after discontinuation of the drug

(contd.)

TABLE 12.3: Characteristics of major cutaneous adverse drug reactions (*contd.*)

Type of CADR	Morphology	Mucous membrane involvement	Time of onset	Commonly implicated drugs	Special comments in relation to elderly patients
Lichenoid drug eruption	Pruritic, flat-topped violaceous papules and plaques more generalized (Fig. 12.4) than idiopathic lichen planus (LP), often photo distributed (Fig. 12.5) and sparing the classical sites of LP	Rare	1 month to 2 years	Gold, NSAIDs, ACE inhibitors, antimicrobials, and antiarthritics	Age of onset is 10 years later than LP, i.e. in 6th or 7th decade
Psoriasiform drug reaction	Limited or generalized erythematous plaques with thick, large, silvery scales, pustular lesions, or erythroderma (Fig. 12.6)	Absent	Weeks to years	β-blockers, lithium, synthetic antimalarials, NSAIDs, and tetracyclines	Needs to be differentiated from late-onset psoriasis
Drug-induced cutaneous vasculitis	Palpable purpura Vesicles and bullae, urticaria, and splinter haemorrhages may also be seen	May be present	Days to months	Antimicrobials, NSAIDs, allopurinol, anticonvulsants, Antihypertensives	May be complicated by visceral by visceral involvement, including gastrointestinal, joint and renal manifestations
Erythroderma	Erythematous and pruritic patches involving >90% of the cutaneous surface	Absent	2 weeks to several months	β-blockers, trimethoprim, sulfamethoxazole, ketoconazole, griseofulvin, nifedipine	
Acute generalized exanthematous pustulosis	Nonfollicular, sterile pustules, arising on background of edematous erythema (Fig. 12.7)	Present or absent	<4 days	β-lactam antibiotics Macrolides Calcium channel blockers	
Drug-induced hypersensitivity syndrome	Severe exanthematous rash	Infrequent	1–6 weeks	Anticonvulsants Sulfonamides Allopurinol	

(*contd.*)

TABLE 12.3: Characteristics of major cutaneous adverse drug reactions (*contd.*)

Type of CADR	Morphology	Mucous membrane involvement	Time of onset	Commonly implicated drugs	Special comments in relation to elderly patients
SJS/TEN	SJS: Atypical targets <10% body surface area (Fig. 12.8) TEN: Confluent and extensive epidermal detachment >30% body surface area (Fig. 12.9)	Present	7–21 days	Anticonvulsants Sulfonamides Allopurinol NSAIDs	Age >40 years, presence of malignancy, blood urea nitrogen (BUN) >28 mg/dL and blood glucose >252 mg/dL are important prognostic parameters in the severity-of-illness score of TEN (SCORTEN), and the likelihood of these being present in elderly are higher than other age groups, hence increasing the mortality rate. Elderly age is also associated with increased risk of complications and delayed wound healing.

Source: Modified from D'souza, et al.[41]

CADR: Cutaneous adverse drug reaction; ACE: Angiotensin converting enzyme; NSAIDs: Non-steroidal anti-inflammatory drugs

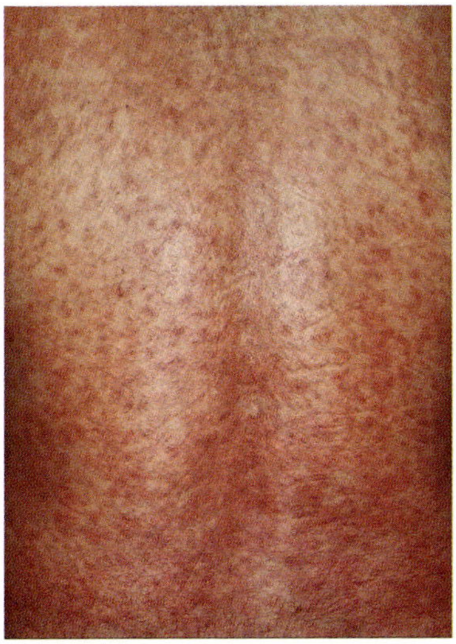

Fig. 12.1: Discrete maculopapular rash over back, due to nevirapine

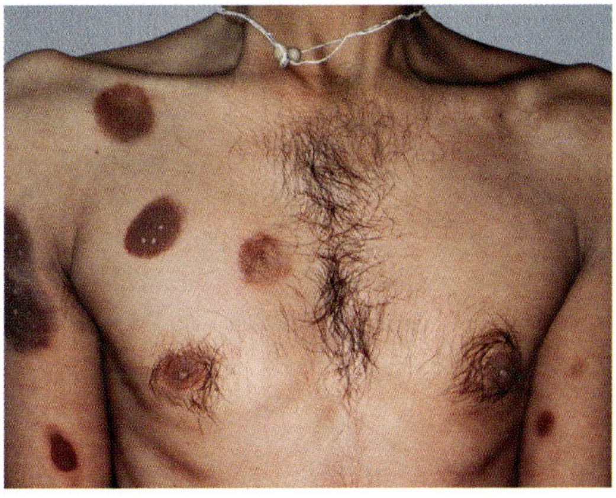

Fig. 12.2: Multiple lesions of fixed drug eruption with central erosion and pigmentary changes from ornidazole

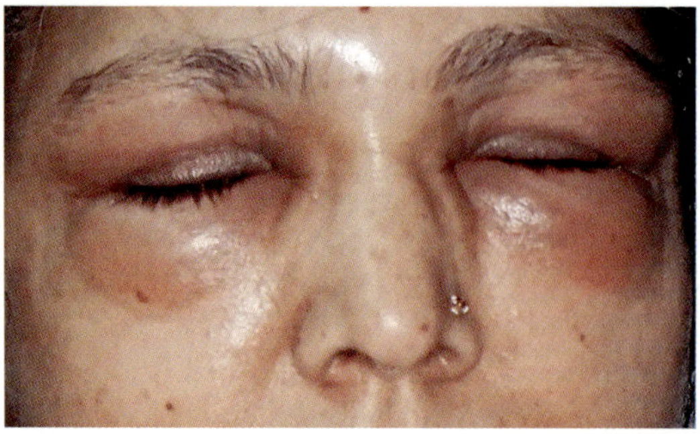

Fig. 12.3: Drug-induced angioedema due to ramipril

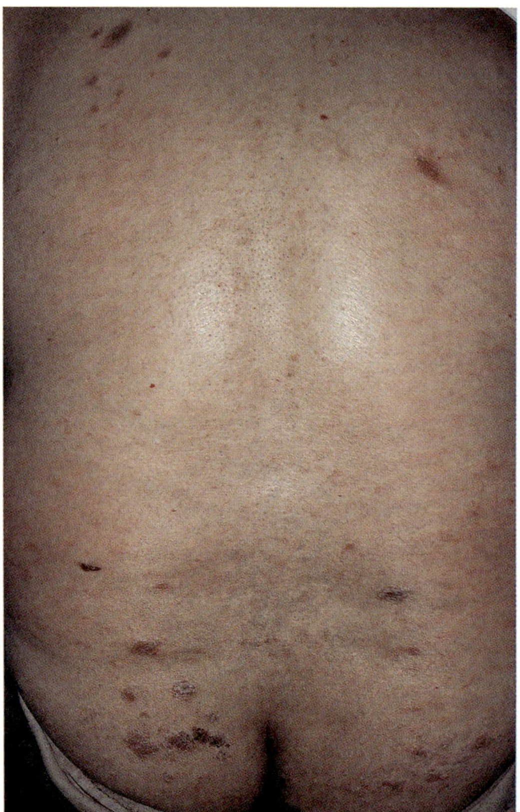

Fig. 12.4: Lichenoid rash in a patient taking amlodipine for 3 months

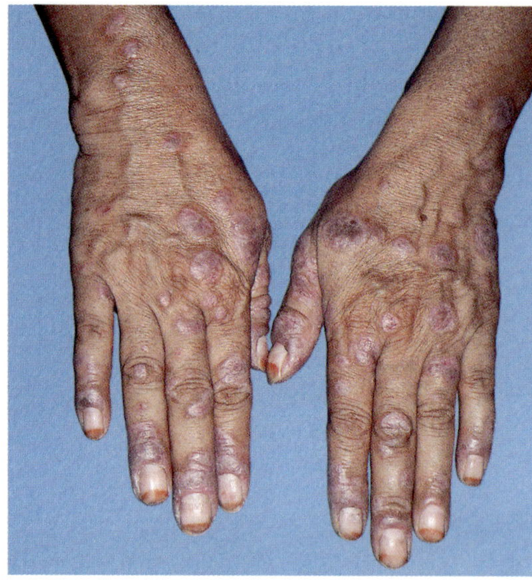

Fig. 12.5: Lichenoid rash in photodistribution due to griseofulvin

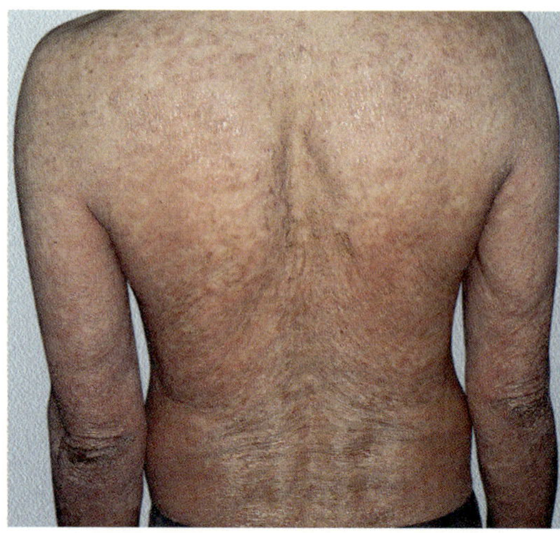

Fig. 12.6: Psoriasiform drug reaction undergoing erythroderma in a patient on lithium

1. Xerosis and Pruritus

Aging skin is susceptible to xerosis and pruritus due to the cumulative effect of the physiological changes occurring in skin, like decrease in skin surface lipids, reduced hydration, loss of sweat and sebaceous glands, loss of collagen, impaired immune system responses, impaired blood circulation, increased neurotransmitters and impaired function of skin as a barrier to pathogens.[42] Underlying metabolic conditions and systemic

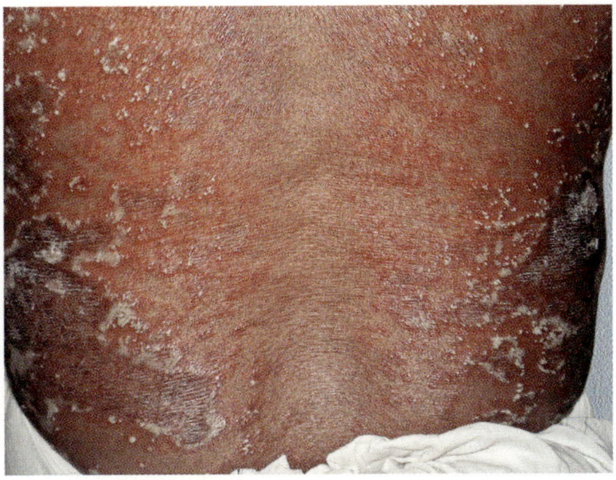

Fig. 12.7: AGEP over trunk induced by terbinafine

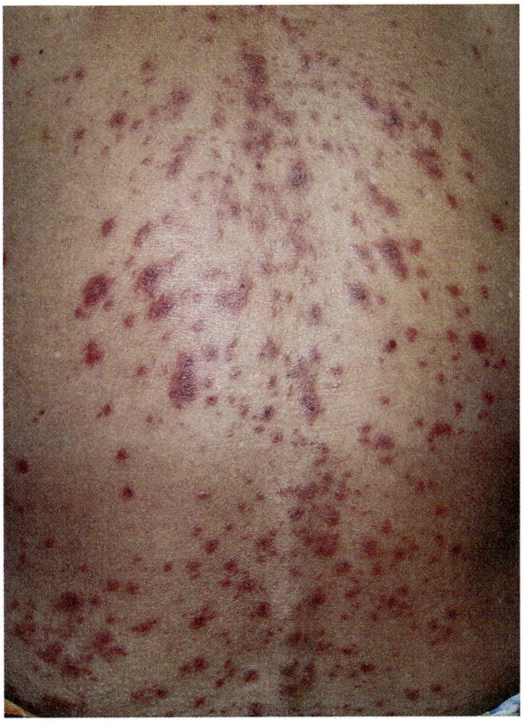

Fig. 12.8: Atypical target lesions of SJS over trunk due to carbamazepine

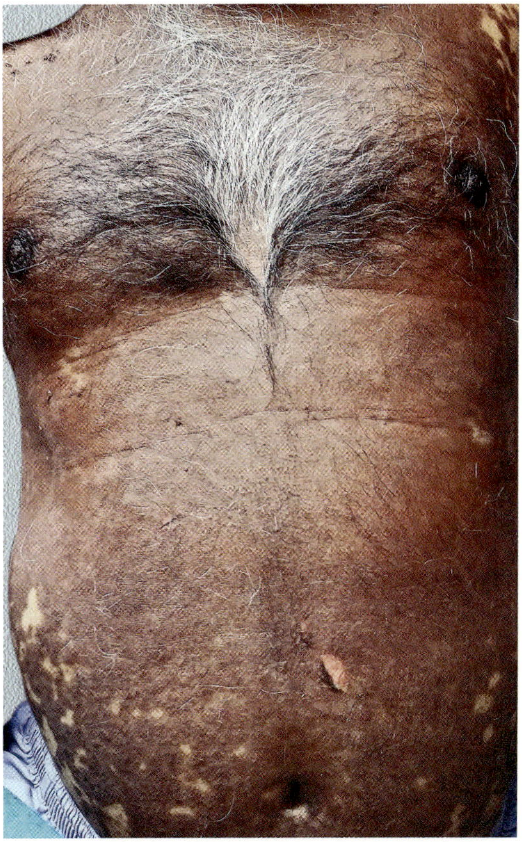

Fig. 12.9: Sheets of skin loss in TEN

diseases like renal failure, chronic liver disease, HIV, diabetes mellitus, thyroid disease, parathyroid disease, hypervitaminosis A, iron deficiency anaemia, neuropathy and malignancy can also cause pruritus and xerosis. Among drugs, anti-androgen therapy, diuretics and statins are frequently associated with precipitation and exacerbation of xerosis.[43]

Some medications like angiotensin receptor blockers (ARBs) and angiotensin converting enzyme (ACE) inhibitors result in pruritus by mediating the release of bradykinins.[43] Although opioids can cause degranulation of mast cells and release of histamine resulting in urticarial rash, primary opioid induced pruritus appears to involve binding of the drug to central opioid pain receptors in the medullary dorsal horn. Serotonin and dopamine D2 receptors, spinal inhibitory pathways and prostaglandins have also been implicated in opioidinduced pruritus. Other drugs which can result in primary drug-induced pruritus are cytokines (IL-2),

Box 12.2: List of drugs causing xerosis and pruritus

Drugs causing xerosis	Drug-induced pruritus
Anti-androgen drugs	ARBs
Diuretics	ACE inhibitors
Statins	Opioids
	Cytokines (IL-2)
	SSRIs
	Sulphonylurea derivatives
	Anti-malarials

serotonin selective receptor inhibitors (SSRIs), sulphonylurea derivatives and anti-malarials. Drugs causing xerosis and pruritus are listed in Box 12.2.

2. Dermatitis

Chronic Eczematous Eruptions

The possible association between eczema and antihypertensive drugs was first reported by Morin et al[44] in 2002. Subsequently, Joly et al[45] showed that chronic use of calcium channel blockers (CCBs) was significantly associated with chronic eczematous eruptions in elderly [adjusted odds ratio (OR) of 2.5 (95% confidence interval)]. This was supported by drug withdrawal and re-challenge test. In 2013, Summers, et al[46] provided further evidence to support the association of eczema in elderly with chronic use of CCBs [matched ORs 4.21, 95% confidence interval (CI) 1.77–9.77] and thiazides [matched OR 2.07, 95% CI 1.08-3.96]. There are some case reports and case series which implicate ACE inhibitors, ARBs and statins in drug-induced eczema; the association, however, is not very strong.[47,48]

Drug-induced chronic eczematous eruptions are difficult to distinguish from endogenous eczema because of long latent period and insidious onset. The lesions are symmetrically distributed, with preferential localization to sun-exposed areas.[46] The latency period for CCBs varies from 1 month to 10 years (median 3 months).[45]

The pathogenesis of drug-related eczema is poorly understood. The epidermal calcium gradient (very low at stratum basale → high at stratum corneum) is lost with ageing. It has been postulated that CCBs further disrupts the calcium homeostasis, resulting in impaired skin barrier function.[49] Similarly, sodium channels in the skin have role in epidermal differentiation and use of hydrochlorthiazide blocks sodium-chloride co-transporter which may affect the skin barrier function.[49] Statins causes xerosis and eczematous reactions by disruption of the skin barrier due to their effects on cholesterol biosynthesis.[48]

Prick testing, patch test and intracutaneous tests are seldom useful. Drug withdrawal and rechallenge is the gold standard for confirmation.

Contact Dermatitis

Allergic contact dermatitis (ACD) is common in elderly and may arise from contact or ingestion of offending allergens. Although elderly people have somewhat decreased cell-mediated immunity and may be harder to sensitize under experimental conditions, they have had many years to acquire allergic responses, and, therefore, develop contact dermatitis frequently.[50] The two most common allergens detected in this population with patch testing nickel and fragrance or balsam of Peru. Another common allergen is para-phenylenediamine, which is used in hair dyes.[51] Stasis dermatitis and venous ulcers are associated with increased susceptibility to develop ACD due to long-term application of various topical medications and dressings. In addition, contact allergy to dental prostheses and medications used to treat ocular disease are common in the elderly as a result of increased usage and exposure.[50] Patch testing is a valuable tool to diagnose contact allergy and should be used often in the elderly, particularly in patients at high risk of contact dermatitis.

Systemically reactivated ACD, i.e. ACD upon ingestion or other systemic exposure to a contact allergen in an already sensitized person, is less common than topical sensitization.

Risk of irritant contact dermatitis (ICD) declines with advancing age, due to decrease in (a) percutaneous absorption and (b) microciculatory efficiency, which results in decreased inflammatory response.[52] Several studies are conducted to elucidate the age-relationship to ICD, but the results are conflicting. While majority of reports demonstrated a delayed and decreased susceptibility to sodium laurel sulphate (SLS)-induced irritation,[53–57] few suggest no significant difference and increased susceptibility.[58–60] Site-related changes have also been observed. A stronger reaction is observed over forehead, cheek, chin and naso-labial folds due to higher stratum corneum turnover rate on these sites.[59,60] In postmenopausal women, age-related differences in irritation were found to be more apparent on the forearm, but not on vulva.[53–55] Despite the observations from various studies on SLS-induced irritation, marketed transdermal formulations, tested in clinical populations of varying ages, have failed to reveal any significant age-related differences in the irritation response.[52] The common irritants in elderly include antiseptics (chlorhexidine), diclofenac, lidocaine, nicotine, fentanyl, estradiol, testosterone, buprenorphine, clonidine and capsaicin.

3. Chemotherapy Related Cutaneous Reactions

Cancer is a major public health problem worldwide. In India, more than 1 million new cases of cancer are diagnosed every year. Ageing is a risk factor of cancer, of which lung, colorectal, breast, prostate and stomach cancers are among the most common.[61] Significant advances have been made in the field of cancer chemotherapy which have resulted in the management of many cancers and have increased the survival rate and life expectancy. The past several decades have seen the advent and rapidly expanding use of biological agents and targeted therapeutic agents in the treatment cancer. The classification of anticancer drugs and the common CADRs associated are given in Table 12.4. The CADRs which are more frequently and specifically associated with chemotherapeutic agents are described as follows:

TABLE 12.4: Classification of anticancer agents and common cutaneous adverse drug reactions reported with them[62–66]

Class	Subclass	Drugs	Common CADRs reported
Cytotoxic agents	Alkylating agents	Nitrogen mustards (cyclophoshamide, chlorambucil, melphalan), thiotepa, busulfan, carmustine, lomustine, dacarbazine, procarbazine	Hyperpigmentation, alopecia, urticaria, neutrophilic eccrine hidradenitis, porphyria cutanea tarda, radiation recall
	Platinum compounds	Cisplatin, carboplatin, oxaloplatin alopecia, radiation recall	Hyperpigmentation, hypersensitivity
	antimetabolites	Fludarabine, cladribine, 5-FU, gemcitabine, capecitabine, pemetrexed	Hand-foot syndrome (HFS), maculopapular rash, photosensitivity, hyperpigmentation, alopecia, stomatitis, pyogenic granuloma, cutaneous lupus erythematosus, pyogenic granuloma, granulomatous septic panniculitis
	Microtubule inhibitors	Vincristine, vinblastine, docetaxel, paclitaxel	HFS, nail changes, alopecia, hypersensitivity, maculopapular rash, erythema multiforme like lesions
	Topoisomerase inhibitors	Etoposide, topotecan, irinotecan	Alopecia, hypersensitivity, HFS, paronychia, perianal irritation
	antibiotics	Actinomycin, doxorubicin, daunorubicin, bleomycin, mitomycin C	HFS, follicular rash, intertrigo-like eruptions, melanotic macules, radiation recall, flagellate pigmentation, Raynaud's phenomenon, fibrosis

(contd.)

TABLE 12.4: Classification of anticancer agents and common cutaneous adverse drug reactions reported with them[62–66] *(contd.)*

Class	Subclass	Drugs	Common CADR(s) reported
	Miscellaneous	Hydroxyurea, L-asparaginase, tretinoin, arsenic trioxide	Hyperpigmentation, alopecia, xerosis, photosensitivity, LE, lichenoid reaction, urticaria, anaphylaxis
Targeted drugs	BCR-ABL tyrosine kinase inhibitors	Imatinib, nilotinib	Facial oedema, morbilliform rash, hyper- or hypopigmentation, pruritus, acne
	Multikinase inhibitors	Sorafenib, sunitinb	HFS, seborrhoeic dermatitis, transient yellow discoloration of skin, subungual splinter haemorrhages, alopecia
	EGF receptor inhibitor	Erlotinib, gefitinib	Papulopustular rash/ acneiform reaction, xerosis, nail changes, photosensitivity, hyperpigmentation, mucositis, radiation recall, HFS
	Angiogenesis inhibitor	Bevacizumab	Mucocutaneous haemorrhage, exfoliative dermatitis
	Proteasome inhibitor	Bortezomib	Erythematous to violaceous morbilliform rash with desquamation, cutaneous vasculitis
	Pi3K-AKT-mTOR pathway inhibitors	Rapamycin, temsirolimus	Stomatitis, maculopapular rash, acneiform eruptions, eczematous reaction, xerosis and pruritus
	Hedgehog signaling pathway inhibitors	Vismodegib	Alopecia, dysgeusia, keratoacanthoma
Hormonal drugs	Glucocorticoids	Prednisolone	Acne, cutaneous thinning and atrophy, telangiectasia, striae distensae, purpura, ecchymosis, hypertrichosis, impaired wound healing, pigmentary alterations, cushingoid features
	Estrogens	Ethinyl estradiol, fosfesterol	Urticaria, eczema, premenstrual exacerbation of papulovesicular eruptions, generalized pruritus, spider naevi, acanthosis nigricans
	Selective estrogen receptor modulators	Tamoxifen	Hirsutism, alopecia, xerosis
	Selective estrogen receptor downregulators	Fulvesterant	Cutaneous vasculitis
	Aromatase inhibitors	Letrozole, anastrozole	Leukocytoclastic vasculitis, erythema nodosum, SCLE, rashes
	Antiandrogens	Flutamide	
	5α-reductase inhibitors	Finasteride	Erythema annulare centrifugum
	GnRH analogues	Nafarelin, Triptorelin	Injection site granuloma
	Progestins	Medroxyprogesterone acetate	Pigmented purpura, skin necrosis at injection site

HFS: Hand-foot syndrome; LE: Lupus erythematosus, SCLE: Subacute cutaneous lupus erythematosus

i. **Hand–foot syndrome:** Classic HFS has been described with the use of various chemotherapeutic agents, including sunitinib, cabozantinib, sorafenib, regorafenib, cytarabine, capecitabine, doxorubicin hydrochloride and fluorouracil.[67,68] It generally starts with prodromal symptoms of tingling and numbness on the palms and soles, and sometimes a painful sensation induced upon touching hot objects, hence also known as palmo-plantar erythrodysesthesia. This is followed by three phases: The inflammatory phase, characterized by erythema (Fig. 12.10A), desquamation and blisters with a perilesional erythematous rim; the hyperkeratotic phase (Fig. 12.10B), marked by the appearance of new lesions that become hyperkeratotic and development of pain in the older, hyperkeratotic areas; and the resolution phase, typified by clearing of the lesions as a result of dose modification or drug termination.[69]

ii. **Acneiform eruptions:** This is the most common CADR associated with EGFR inhibitors (>75%)[65] and it has been variously described as papulopustular rash, acneiform rash, maculopapular rash, and monomorphic pustular rash in different reports.[68] It typically starts within the first 2 weeks of starting treatment. Follicular erythematous papules and pustules start in the seborrhoeic areas of head and trunk and gradually become generalized, sparing palms and soles. Unlike acne, comedones are characteristically absent and the rash is pruritic.[68,70] It evolves in a dose-dependent manner and clears completely in a few weeks of stopping treatment. Histology shows predominantly neutrophilic folliculitis and perifolliculitis with hyperkeratosis and ectatic infundibula.[64,68] The monoclonal antibodies are more commonly associated with severe rash than the small molecule TKI inhibitors.[71]

iii. **Alopecia:** It is the most common cutaneous adverse reaction to chemotherapeutic agents. It usually manifests as anagen effluvium, which occurs due to interruption of mitotic activity in the hair matrix cells that are rapidly dividing. This leads to cessation of hair shaft formation or produces a weakened hair shaft that is prone to breakage. Anagen effluvium manifests as sudden diffuse hair loss that starts within 7–10 days of initiation of chemotherapy and peaks around 2 months. Hair in the

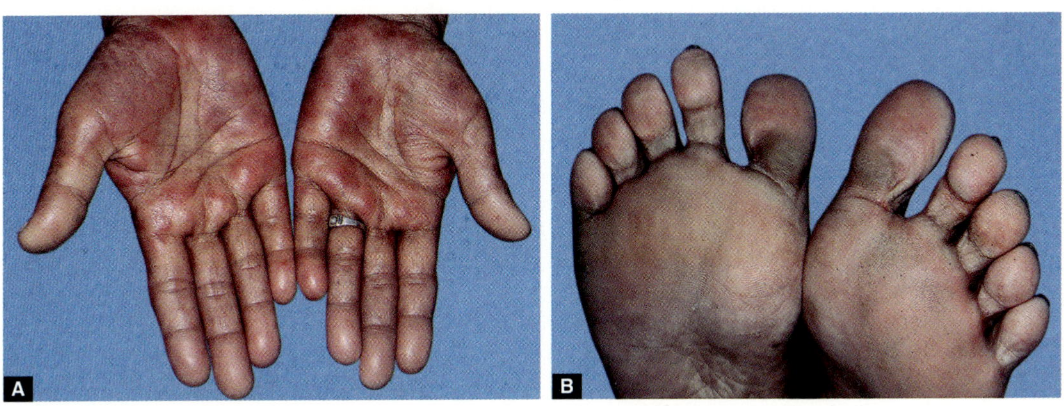

Fig. 12.10: Sorafenib-induced hand–foot syndrome: (A) Erythematous plaques over palms involving the pressure-bearing area with sparing of central, non-pressure-bearing region, (B) hyperkeratotic plaques over metatarsophalangeal area and sides of sole

resting phase are spared leading to incomplete hair loss which may become complete with repeated exposures. Long-term therapy can also affect anagen hair in other body parts.[72] Chemotherapy-induced hair loss is usually reversible after cessation of drug. However, the hair colour or texture may change.

iv. **Flagellate erythema and pigmentation:** Flagellate erythema is a distinctive morphologic presentation of linear, whiplash-like pattern, red streaks on the skin which usually leaves residual postinflammatory hyperpigmentation behind. It has been described with antineoplastic agents including bleomycin (most commonly), bendamustine, docetaxel, peplomycin and trastuzumab.[73–77] Other conditions which may lead to flagellate dermatoses include chikungunya fever, parvovirus B19 infection, hypereosinophilia syndrome, inflictions and abuse, phytophotodermatitis, paederous dermatitis, toxin induced (mushroom, shiitake) and rheumatologic conditions (SLE, dermatomyositis, adult onset Still's disease).[77]

v. **Radiation recall:** A previously irradiated site may become inflamed on administration of a chemotherapeutic agent. This is known as radiation recall. Causative agents include doxorubicin, dactinomycin, hydroxyurea, methotrexate, etoposide, vinblastine, 5-flurouracil, melphalan, cyclophosphamide, cytarabine. The reaction can occur within days to years of radiation therapy but generally occurs within hours to days. It is characterized by erythema, desquamation, oedema, and vesiculation with or without pain or ulceration. The reaction is usually cutaneous but in rare cases organ involvement may occur.
There are several factors that affect the severity of reaction:
1. Period between radiotherapy and chemotherapy: Short interval correlates with severe radiation recall reactions.
2. Dose of irradiation used: Higher dose correlates with severe reactions.

It usually subsides within hours to weeks of withdrawal of chemotherapy.

DIAGNOSIS

The diagnosis of CADR is essentially clinical, mainly based on a meticulous history of all the prescriptional as well as OTC and alternative medications taken by the patients, establishing a temporal correlation between drug intake and appearance of rash, effect of reduction/withdrawl of drug (dechallenge) and reappearance of rash upon reintroduction of the drug (rechallenge). A thorough clinical examination to look for the morphological pattern of rash and ruling out confounders and other clinical mimics is important from management view point. It is important to delineate whether the rash is simple or limited to skin or is complex/multisystemic in nature so as to assess the overall prognosis of the case. No specific, reliable and validated laboratory investigations are helpful in confirming CADR.

Haematological and biochemical investigations are sometimes required to ascertain the diagnosis (as in DRESS); to differentiate from idiopathic counterparts (like systemic lupus erythematosus); to assess the severity, systemic affection and to calculate the severity score (especially in SJS/TEN); and to decide the management option. Histopathological examination is particularly helpful in lichenoid drug reactions, pustular drug eruptions and drug induced psoriasis. To identify the culprit agent, a trial of drug elimination, *in vitro* and *in vivo* diagnostic tests including challenge by re-exposure are often used. Rechallenge should, however be avoided in patients with SCARs. Figure 12.11 illustrates the algorithm that can be helpful in the diagnosis of suspected CADR and to identify the causative drug.

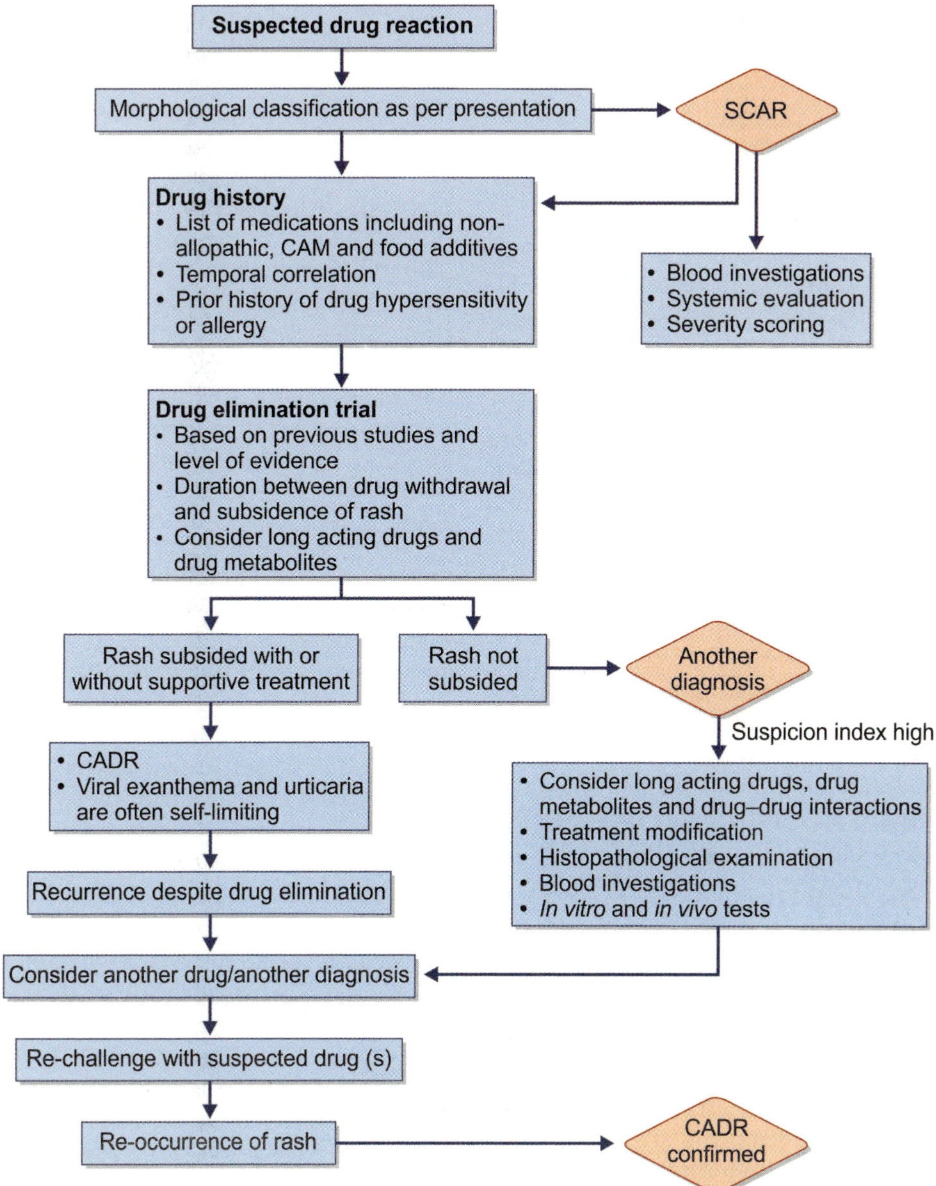

CAM: Complementary and alternative medicines

Fig. 12.11: Algorithm for approaching a case of suspected CADR

1. **Blood investigations:** Eosinophilia is seen in urticaria, angioedema, anaphylaxis and DRESS. Leukocytosis and atypical lymphocytosis are features suggestive of DRESS. Hepatic and renal function tests are carried out to assess systemic involvement and to decide the line of treatment. If facilities exist, test for viral reactivation (herpes group) may be carried out.
   Blood urea nitrogen, glucose and bicarbonate levels are used as prognostic indicators of SJS/TEN.

Antinuclear antibody profile is carried out in cases of vasculitis and autoimmune reactions.

Findings which are specific to some reaction patterns are as follows:

i. Elevated serum tryptase concentration: Anaphylactic reaction
ii. Elevated plasma and urine histamine level: Anaphylactic reaction
iii. Low C4 levels: Angioedema (no urticaria)
iv. Antibodies to single stranded DNA/ histone: Drug-induced lupus

2. ***Histopathology:*** Certain drug reactions present with several inflammatory histological patterns that overlap with other dermatological disorders (i.e. psoriasiform, spongiotic, and interface vacuolar), whereas others are quite characteristic for a particular drug, and a skin biopsy undertaken at an appropriate time can, toa large extent, sort out the diagnosis and differentiate it from its close mimickers.

The histological features which are helpful in differentiating CADR from their idiopathic counterparts and close mimickers are illustrated in Table 12.5.

3. ***In vitro tests:*** *In vitro* tests are apparently safer than *in vivo* tests.[79] However, they are not freely available and practically are largely research tools at present. The list of *in vitro* tests is given in Box 12.3.

In vivo test: *In vivo* tests include skin testing [skin prick test (SPT) and intradermal test (IDT)], patch testing and provocation or rechallenge test. Intradermal and skin prick tests are used for the diagnosis of IgE medicated Type I hypersensitivity reactions (HSR). In both of these skin tests, the allergen introduced into the dermis binds to IgE antibodies to cause mast cell degranulation and subsequent release of histamine from mast cells. Whereas, drug patch tests are based on delayed HSR and help in assessing the culpability of the drug without increasing the risk of precipitation of a reaction. Drug provocation is the administration of drug(s) in a controlled setting, in order to establish the diagnosis of CADR or in some cases also to provide a list of alternative drugs that can be safely taken by the patient. The details of these tests and procedures are summarized in Table 12.6.

Box 12.3: *In vitro* tests for CADR

- Histamine release test
- Basophil degranulation test
- Passive haemagglutination
- Leukocyte and macrophage migration inhibition factor tests
- Lymphocyte transformation test
- Lymphocyte toxicity assay

Special consideration and limitations of diagnostic tests in elderly: The immune system undergoes an involution process with consequent decline in immunoglobulin production, including IgE and IgG. The skin undergoes atrophy with fewer cell layers, decreased collagen, vascularity and a reduction in mast cells. Hence, there are some differences in the responsiveness of elderly skin to the diagnostic tests used for CADR and they are enumerated as follows:

1. There is age associated reduction in skin reactivity of the elderly to histamine and allergens. Skassa-Brociek et al[86] demonstrated a decrease in skin tests reactivity to histamine after 50 years of age, reaching a plateau after the age of 60. A wheal to histamine was reported in all subjects aged over 70 years, but flare was difficult to detect in a proportion of subjects. Hence, it was suggested that in geriatric age the intensity of the skin response should be expressed as the ratio between allergen and histamine induced wheals.
2. Skin reactivity varies in different body regions, and back was found to be more reactive than the forearm, and this difference was greater for allergen than for histamine skin tests.[87]

TABLE 12.5: Histopathological features of CADR

Type of CADR	Histological features
Maculopapular/Morbiliform rash	Spongiosis (most common), focal basal cell degeneration, lymphocytic and neutrophilic exocytosis, necrotic keratinocytes, papillary dermal oedema. Eosinophilia, basal cell vacuolar degeneration and positive FasL binding are more common in drug induced MP rash than viral exanthema.[78]
Urticaria, angioedema and anaphylaxis	Dermal oedema, mild perivascular and interstitial mononuclear cell infiltrate admixed with eosinophils. Complement mediated urticaria demonstrates neutrophilic infiltrate Urticarial vasculitis has fibrinoid necrosis of vessel wall, neutrophilic infiltrate, karyorrhexis and RBC extravasation
Psoriasiform drug reaction	Most of the features resemble classic psoriasis. A helpful feature distinguishing drug-induced psoriasis from idiopathic psoriasis is the absence of tortuous papillary dermal capillaries and suprapapillary epidermal thinning.
Lichenoid drug reaction	The findings that favor LDR over LP include focal parakeratosis, apoptotic/dyskeratotic keratinocytes in the upper layers of epidermis, presence of eosinophils within the lichenoid dermal infiltrate, exocytosis of lymphocytes into the upper epidermis, and sometimes a deep perivascular infiltrate.
Fixed drug eruption	Interface lichenoid tissue reaction, marked pigment incontinence, mixed cell infiltrate in superficial and deep dermis
Vasculitic drug reactions	Leukocytoclastic changes with eosinophilic infiltrate (difficult to differentiate from nondrug-induced vasculitis)
SJS/TEN	Keratinocyte necrosis, partial to full thickness necrosis of epidermis, moderate-to-dense dermal infiltrate with lymphocyte predominance
DRESS	Dermal oedema, dense perivascular eosinophilic and lymphocytic (including atypical lymphocytes) papillary dermal infiltrate along with extravasated erythrocytes
Papulopustular eruptions	Superficial perifolliculitis and florid neutrophilic suppurative folliculitis are the two major histopathologic patterns. Superficial perifolliculitis is characterized by neutrophilic infiltrate around the dilated and plugged follicular infundibulum, whereas florid neutrophilic suppurative folliculitis presents with rupture of the follicular epithelium and subsequent perifollicular granuloma formation.
Hand–foot syndrome	Parakeratosis and dyskeratosis with band-like areas of necrotic keratinocytes, superficial telangiectasia and a mild perivascular lymphohistiocytic infiltrate. Dysmorphic eccrine cells with scant cytoplasm and cystic changes can be observed in sweat glands.

TABLE 12.6: Summary of various *in vivo* tests

Test	Procedure	Interpretation	Uses	Limitations	Other comments
SPT	Allergen in solution form is applied on the surface of skin and a small prick using lancet or needle is given at the site. Histamine solution (10 mg/mL) is used as positive control.	Wheal diameter more than 3 mm in comparison to control and an associated flare after 20 minutes.	Type I HSR like urticaria, angio-edema and anaphylaxis.	Not useful for reactions due to non-allergic mechanism.	Multiple allergens can be tested in the same setting. Easier to perform, relatively safe and less painful. Less sensitive than IDT
IDT	A small amount of allergen, i.e. 0.02–0.05 mL in solution form is injected directly into the dermis of volar fore-arm with the help of a tuberculin or insulin syringe to raise a bleb of 3 mm diameter. Normal saline is used as control.	Wheal diameter more than 3 mm in comparison to control and an associated flare after 20 minutes.	Type I HSR like urticaria, angio-edema and anaphylaxis	Not useful for reactions due to non-allergic mechanism. Testing multiple allergen is cumbersome and inconvenient to patient. More chances of irritant and false positive reactions.	Less easy to perform, less safe and more painful. More sensitive than SPT
Patch testing	Test is performed on the unaffected and untreated skin over the upper back using Finn chambers or an equivalent and fixed with hypo-allergic tape.	Reading after 20 min, day 2, 4 and 7 (as per ESCD) for erythema, infiltration, papules and vesicles	Type IV delayed type HSR including MPR, FDE, eczematous reaction, DRESS, SDRIFE, SJS/TEN	Variable positivity rate (9–25% in SJS/TEN[80-82] to 40–87% in FDE[83,84]) False negative and false positive reactions are common.	Best performed 3–6 weeks after the CADR has subsided.
Drug provocation test	Drug is administered (as whole and sometimes in graded manner), under medical supervision with availability of emergency resuscitation facilities round the clock, preferably by the same route of administration as during the reaction and should be started with a placebo	Timing of drug administration and development of signs and symptoms is noted. Photographic documentation is helpful.	Non-serious CADR. There is case series where patients of TEN have safely underwent provocation testing.[85]	Lack of uniform protocols, difficult to standardize the procedure.	Considered the gold standard to confirm or to refute the diagnosis of CADR.

SPT: Skin prick test, IDT: Intradermal test, HSR: Hypersensitivity reaction, ESCD: European Society of Contact Dermatitis, MPR: Maculopapular rash, FDE: Fixed drug eruption, DRESS: Drug-related eosinophilia and systemic symptoms, SDRIFE: Symmetrical drug-related intertriginous and flexural exanthema, SJS: Stevens-Johnson syndrome, TEN: Toxic epidermal necrolysis

3. Atrophic or photo changes at the site of skin prick test may influence the response to allergens and give false negative results.[88]
4. Medications such as antihistamines and antidepressants affect the response to skin test negatively.
5. There also exists the possibility that older subjects are no longer exposed to specific allergens they were positive to, and this may greatly reduce the skin test responses.
6. The overall sensitization rate to patch testing decreases with age and is lowest among patients >70 years age (34.9%). The rate of positive reactions to nickel and thimerosal was reported to decrease with age, while fragrance mix and metallic mercury stayed at the same level through all age groups.[89]
7. Elderly patients with severe comorbidities such as uncontrolled asthma, cardiac, hepatic, renal or other organ specific or systemic diseases; which can be worsened or activated if the hypersensitivity reaction is provoked by oral drug provocation test; are at higher risk of developing adverse/unintended reactions.[90]

MANAGEMENT

A possibility of drug reaction should always be considered in a patient who suddenly develops a rash that is itchy and symmetrical. All the drugs, usually consumed by the patient in last 2 months should be suspected as possible causal agents. However, it should be remembered that all the drugs being taken by the patient, even beyond 2 months may be responsible for some reactions like angioedema, lichenoid reactions and pseudolymphomatous drug reactions.

Once diagnosis of CADR is established and the offending drug identified, it is imperative to discontinue it immediately, particularly in serious drug reactions (SCARs), to prevent further progression of the CADR. If the agent cannot be identified with certainty, which is often the case, then ideally all drugs being taken by the patient should be withheld. This is easier said than done as some of the patients are on critical lifesaving drugs, the withdrawal of which could endanger their lives. In such a situation the advice should be to withdraw all nonessential drugs and if possible substitute the essential drugs with alternate medications of different pharmacological groups having similar pharmacologic action and used for same indication.

Sometimes, in a simple or uncomplicated rash, a *"carry through approach,"* with continuation of suspected medication(s) may be adopted, with a close observation on progression of the rash. However, in patients with suspected SCARs, like angioedema, SJS-TEN, DHS/DRESS and erythroderma it is essential to hospitalise the patients in a well-equipped setup with immediate institution of supportive and specific measures.

Symptomatic treatment with anti-histamines, emollients and topical steroids may be all that may be sufficient in a milder, pure cutaneous drug reaction. Specific treatment with corticosteroids and other immunomodulatory agents may be required in serious reactions like SJS/TEN and DRESS. A multidisciplinary approach of management is imperative in such cases. Corticosteroids should however be instituted at an early stage and for a short period, ranging from 7 to 10 days in SJS/TEN. In contrast, corticosteroids for a fairly prolonged period, ranging from 3 to 6 months are generally required to treat patients with DHS/DRESS. Cyclosporine A (CsA) should be used cautiously in elderly as the drug clearance decreases with age and a significantly larger proportion of whole blood CsA concentration is achieved at the site of action (within T lymphocytes).[91] Polypharmacy also has specific relevance for elderly patients treated with CsA as this agent is a substrate of both CYP3A and P-glycoprotein, both of which are important in the elimination of many commonly used drugs. Intravenous immunoglobulin (IVIg) should not be used to treat elderly with SJS/TEN as it is associated with many potential side effects, including acute renal failure.[92]

Reporting CADR to Appropriate Authorities

All the CADRs, particularly the severe ones should be reported to the competent authorities. Recording and reporting of CADR has always been a weak link in the chain of measures to tackle the issue of ensuring future drug safety. This is because most CADRs are mild and tolerable and so are conveniently ignored both by patients as well as physicians. This neglect may have a high price later, as reactions on re-exposure with the same drug can be severe and endanger life. The importance of pharmacovigilance therefore cannot be overstated. Post-marketing surveillance networks, observational studies, and registries to identify adverse events are required if we want to have a safe pharmaceutical milieu for our patients.

Prevention of CADR

Situations involving higher risk for drug reactions need to be identified and preventive action undertaken. It is necessary to assess risk based on the drug and use a safer alternative. For example, phenytoin and carbamazepine have higher incidence of drug reactions in comparison to sodium valproate in epilepsy. Likewise, avoid ampicillin in patients with EBV infection. In patients with renal dysfunction avoid Gadolinium contrast media as this can cause scleromyxedema. Avoidance of abacavir in Africans and Europeans with HLA-B*5701, carbamazepine in Han Chinese and Indians with HLA-B*1502 are also such examples of ensuring drug safety.

A practice called "Brown bag reviews" is well established in United States for some years, where patient is asked to bring all their medications, including over-the-counter drugs and alternative medicines to an appointment with a community pharmacist.

Extreme care should also be taken to treat patients or even relatives with past history of CADR specially the severe ones. Patients with ADRs should be educated to always carry ***drug alert card*** with them whenever they need medical care and show it to their treating physician.

CONCLUSION

Ageing population is increasing globally. Clinicians should execute extreme caution while prescribing medications in elderly due to a higher propensity in them to develop adverse drug reactions and drug interactions. This is attributed to age-related skin changes, pharmacokinetic and pharmacodynamic alterations, presence of multiple comorbidities and thus need for multiple drugs to treat them and increased tendency to self-medication. Like in other population, urticarial, MP rash and FDE are the common reaction patterns in elderly, as are eczematous reactions. The drugs commonly causing CADRs are the ones used to treat multiple comorbidities and include antibiotics, anti-hypertensive, antidiabetics, anti-rheumatic and chemotherapeutic agents. The management of serious drug reactions like TEN and DRESS may also pose difficulty in elderly due poor tolerance of aggressive therapies like corticosteroids and immunosuppressive agents, thereby enhancing mortality. Likewise, provocation test are relatively contraindicated in elderly due to higher prevalence of hepatic, renal and cardiac impairment.

References

1. Leape LL, Brennan TA, Laird N, *et al.* Results of the Havard Medical Practice study II. N Eng J Med 1991; 324:377.
2. Schäfer I, Hansen H, Schön G, *et al.* The influence of age, gender and socioeconomic status on multimorbidity patterns in primary care. First results from the multicare cohort study. BMC Health Serv Res 2012; 12:89.
3. Jerez-Roig J, Medeiros LF, Silva VA, *et al.* Prevalence of self-medication and associated factors in an elderly population: a systematic review. Drugs Aging 2014; 31:883–96.

4. Bigby M, Jick S, Jick H, Arndt K. Drug-induced cutaneous reaction. A report from the Boston collaborative drug surveillance programme on 15,438 consecutive inpatient, 1975 to 1981. JAMA 1986; 256:3358–63.

5. Nayak S, Acharya B. Adverse cutaneous drug reaction. Indian J Dermatol 2008; 53:2–8

6. Jhaj R, Uppal R, Malhotra S, Bhargava V K. Cutaneous adverse reactions in in-patients in a tertiary care hospital. Indian J Dermatol Venereol Leprol 1999; 65:14–7

7. Pudukadan D, Thappa DM. Adverse cutaneous drug reactions: Clinical pattern and causative agents in a tertiary care center in South India. Indian J Dermatol Venereol Leprol 2004; 70:20–4.

8. Patel TK, Thakkar SH, Sharma DC. Cutaneous adverse drug reactions in Indian population: A systematic review. Indian Dermatol Online J 2014; 5, Suppl S2:76–86.

9. Chatterjee S, Ghosh AP, Barbhuiya J, Dey SK. Adverse cutaneous drug reactions: A one year survey at a dermatology outpatient clinic of a tertiary care hospital. Indian J Pharmacol 2006; 38:429–31.

10. Yalc¸in B, Tamer E, Toy GG, *et al*. The prevalence of skin diseases in the elderly: analysis of 4099 geriatric patients. Int J Dermatol 2006; 45:672–6.

11. Tuchinda P, Chularojanamontri L, Sukakul T, *et al*. Cutaneous adverse drug reactions in the elderly: a retrospective analysis in Thailand. Drugs Aging 2014; 31:815–24.

12. Fiszenson-Albala F, Auzerie V, Mahe E, *et al*. A 6-month prospective survey of cutaneous drug reactions in a hospital setting. Br J Dermatol 2003; 149:1018–22.

13. Andriole VT, Haverstock DC, Choudhri SH. Retrospective analysis of the safety profile of oral moxifloxacin in elderly patients enrolled in clinical trials. Drug Saf 2005; 28:443–52.

14. Ball P, Mandell L, Patou G, *et al*. A new respiratory fluoroquinolone, oral gemifloxacin: a safety profile in context. Int J Antimicrob Agents 2004; 23: 421–9.

15. Chng HH, Leong KP, Cheng YK, *et al*. Elderly inpatients have drug allergy manifestations and outcome similar to the nonelderly but serious reactions are less common: results of a 9-year prospective study. Allergy 2008; 63 (Suppl 88):379.

16. Mangoni A, Jackson S. Age-related changes in pharmacokinetics and pharmacodynamics: basic principles and practical applications. Br J ClinPharmacol 2004; 57: 6–14.

17. Swedko PJ. Serum creatinine is an inadequate screening test for renal failure in elderly patients. Arch Intern Med 2003; 163: 356–60.

18. Klawans HL. Emerging strategies in Parkinson's disease. Neurology 1990; 40(Suppl 3): 1–76.

19. Van den Akker M, Bunhx F, Knottnerus JA. Comorbidity or multimorbidity: what's in a name? A review of the literature. Eur J Gen Pract 1996; 2: 65–70.

20. Violan C, Foguet-Boreu Q, Flores-Mateo G, Salisbury C, Blom J, Freitag M, Glynn L, Muth C, Valderas JM. Prevalence, determinants and patterns of multimorbidity in primary care: A systematic review of observational studies. PLoS One 2014; 9: 102149.

21. Sharma D, Mazta S, Parashar A. Morbidity pattern and health-seeking behavior of aged population residing in Shimla hills of North India: A cross-sectional study. J Fam Med Primary Care 2013; 2(2):188–93.

22. Joshi K, Kumar R, Avasthi A. Morbidity profile and its relationship with disability and psychological distress among elderly people in Northern India. Int J Epidemiol 2003; 32(6):978–87.

23. Ghosh A, Singh A. Health status of elderly in a rural area of north east region of India. Nat J Community Med 2014; 5(2):236–39.

24. Shankar R, Tondon J, Gambhir I, *et al*. Health status of elderly population in rural area of Varanasi district. Indian journal pf public health [Internet] cited Jan 6 2016, 2007; 51(1):56–8.

25. Gupta A, Girdhar S, Chaudhary A, *et al*. Patterns of multimorbidity among elderly in an urban area of North India. J. Evolution Med. Dent. Sci. 2016; 5(19):936–41.

26. Khokhar A, Mehra M. Life style and morbidity profile of geriatric population in an urban community of Delhi. Indian J Med Sci 2001; 55(11):609–15.

27. Srinivas PJ, Manjubhashini S. A study on morbidity profile among elderly population in Visakhapatnam

District, Andhra Pradesh. Journal of Dental and Medical Sciences 2014; 13(9):21–5.

28. Van Spall HG, Toren A, Kiss A, Fowler RA. Eligibility criteria of randomised controlled trials published in high-impact general medical journals: a systematic sampling review. JAMA 2007; 297: 1233–40.
29. Tinetti ME, Bogardus ST, Agostini JV. Potential pitfalls of disease-specific guidelines for patients with multiple conditions. N Engl J Med 2004; 351: 2870–74.
30. Ferner RE, Aronson JK. Communicating information about drug safety. BMJ 2006; 333:143.
31. Nightingale G, Hajjar E, Swartz K, Andrel-Sendecki J, Chapman A. Evaluation of a pharmacist-led medication assessment used to identify prevalence of and associations with polypharmacy and potentially inappropriate medication use among ambulatory senior adults with cancer.JClinOncol. 2015 May; 33(13):1453–9.
32. Prybys K, Melville K, Hanna J, Gee A, Chyka P. Polypharmacy in the elderly: Clinical challenges in emergency practice: Part 1: Overview, etiology, and drug interactions. Emerg Med Rep 2002; 23:145–53.
33. Field TS, Gurwitz JH, Avorn J, McCormick D, Jain S, Eckler M, Benser M, Bates DW. Risk factors for adverse drug events among nursing home residents. Arch Intern Med 2001; 161:1629–34.
34. Bedell SE, Jabbour S, Goldberg R, et al. Discrepancies in the use of medications: their extent and predictors in an outpatient practice. Arch Intern Med 2000; 160:2129–3.
35. Hajjar ER, Hanlon JT, Artz MB, *et al*. Adverse drug reaction risk factors in older outpatients. *Am J Geriatr Pharmacother*. 2003; 1:82–9.
36. Mannesse CK, Derkx FH, de Ridder MA, Man in 't Veld AJ, van der Cammen TJ. Adverse drug reactions in elderly patients as contributing factor for hospital admission: cross sectional study. Br Med J 1997; 315:1057–8.
37. Lazarou J, Pomeranz BH, Corey PN. Incidence of adverse drug reactions in hospitalized patients: a meta-analysis of prospective studies. JAMA 1998; 279:1200–5.
38. Routledge PA, O'Mahony MS, Woodhouse KW. Adverse drug reactions in elderly patients. Br J ClinPharmacol 2004; 57:121–6.
39. Faulkner CM, Cox HL, Williamson JC. Unique aspects of antimicrobial use in older adults. ClinInfec Dis 2005; 40:997–1004.
40. Charfi R , ElAidli S , Zaiem A , Kastalli S , Srairi S , Daghfous R, *et al*. Adverse drug reactions in older adults: A retrospective study from pharmacovigilance. Therapie. 2012; 67(5):471–6.
41. D'Souza P, Jaiswal P, Dhali T, Choudhary S, *et al*. Approach to a suspected drug reaction. In: Gupta LK, Martin AM, D'souza P, Pande S, editors. IADVL's textbook on Cutaneous Adverse Drug Reaction- A comprehensive guide. 1st ed. Mumbai: Bhalani Publishing House; 2018. p 54–63.
42. Cohen RK, Frank J, Salbu RL, Israel I. Pruritus in the elderly: clinical approaches to the improvement of quality of life. P T. 2012 Apr; 37(4): 227–232, 236–9.
43. Davies E, O'Mahony M. Adverse drug reactions in special populations–the elderly. Br J ClinPharmacol 2015; 80:796–807.
44. Morin C, Joly P, Courville P, *et al*. Chronic eczematiform eruption in the elderly [in French]. Ann DermatolVenereol 2002; 129:19–22.
45. Joly P, Benoit-Corven C, Baricault S, *et al*. Chronic eczematous eruptions of the elderly are associated with chronic exposure to calcium channel blockers: results from a case-control study. J Invest Dermatol. 2007; 127(12):2766–71.
46. Summers EM, Bingham CS, Dahle KW, *et al*. Chronic eczematous eruptions in the aging: further support for an association with exposure to calcium channel blockers. J Am Med AssocDermatol 2013; 149:814–8.
47. Vena GA, Cassano N, Coco V, De Simone C. Eczematous reactions due to angiotensin-converting enzyme inhibitors or angiotensin II receptor blockers. ImmunopharmacolImmunotoxicol 2013; 35:447–50.
48. Kerasovec M, Elsner P, Burg G. Generalized eczematous skin rash possibly due to HMG-CoA reductase inhibitors. Dermatology 1993; 186: 248–52.
49. Heng YK, Lim YL. Cutaneous drug reactions in the elderly. CurrOpin Allergy ClinImmunol. 2015 Aug; 15(4):300–7.

50. Nedorost ST, Stevens SR. Diagnosis and treatment of allergic skin disorders in the elderly. Drugs Aging 2001; 18:827–35.
51. Carneiro SC, Azevedo-e-Silva MC, Ramos-e-Silva M. Drug eruptions in the elderly. ClinDermatol. 2011 Jan-Feb; 29(1):43–8.
52. Zhai H, Meier-Davis SR, Cayme B, Shudo J, Maibach H. Irritant contact dermatitis: effect of age. CutanOculToxicol. 2012 Jun;31(2):138–43.
53. Elsner P, Wilhelm D, Maibach HI. Sodium lauryl sulfate induced irritant contact dermatitis in vulvar and forearm skin of premenopausal and post-menopausal women. J Am Acad Dermatol 1990; 23:648–52.
54. Elsner P, Wilhelm D, Maibach HI. Irritant effect of a model surfactant on the human vulva and forearm. Age-related differences. J Reprod Med 1990; 35:1035–39.
55. Elsner P, Wilhelm D, Maibach HI. Effect of low-concentration sodium lauryl sulfate on human vulvar and forearm skin. Agerelated differences. J Reprod Med 1991; 36:77–81.
56. Schwindt DA, Wilhelm KP, Miller DL, Maibach HI. Cumulative irritation in older and younger skin: a comparison. ActaDermVenereol 1998; 78:279–83.
57. Robinson MK. Population differences in acute skin irritation responses. Race, sex, age, sensitive skin and repeat subject comparisons. Contact Derm 2002; 46:86–93.
58. Bowman JP, Kligman AM, Stoudemayer T, Nicholson J. Effects of age on human cumulative irritation responses. J Cosmet Sci 2005; 56:213–8.
59. Marrakchi S, Maibach HI. Sodium lauryl sulfate-induced irritation in the human face: regional and age-related differences. Skin Pharmacol Physiol 2006; 19:177–80.
60. Marrakchi S, Maibach HI. Functional map and age-related differences in the human face: non-immunologic contact urticaria induced by hexyl nicotinate. Contact Derm 2006;55:15–9.
61. Ferlay J, Soerjomataram I, Dikshit R, *et al*. Cancer incidence and mortality worldwide: sources, methods and major patterns in GLOBOCAN 2012. Int J Cancer 2015; 136:E359–E386.
62. Reyes-Habito CM, RohEk. Cutaneous reactions to chemotherapeutic drugs and targeted therapy for cancer. Part I: conventional chemotherapeutic drugs. J Am Acad Dermatol. 2014 Aug; 71(2):203.e1-203.e12; quiz 215–6.
63. Reyes-Habito CM, RohEk. Cutaneous reactions to chemotherapeutic drugs and targeted therapy for cancer. Part II: targeted therapy. J Am Acad Dermatol. 2014 Aug;71(2):217.e1-217.e11; quiz 227–8.
64. Macdonald JB, Macdonald B, Golitz LE, LoRusso P, Sekulic A. Cutaneous adverse effects of targeted therapies: Part I: Inhibitors of the cellular membrane. J Am AcadDermatol. 2015 Feb; 72(2): 203–18.
65. Macdonald JB, Macdonald B, Golitz LE, LoRusso P, Sekulic A. Cutaneous adverse effects of targeted therapies: Part II: Inhibitors of intracellular molecular signaling pathways. J Am AcadDermatol. 2015; 72(2):221–36.
66. Hammond-Thelin LA. Cutaneous reactions related to systemic immunomodulators and targeted therapeutics. Dermatol Clin 2008; 26:121–159.
67. Strumberg D, Awada A, Hirte H, Clark JW, Seeber S, Piccart P, *et al*. Pooled safety analysis of BAY 43-9006 (sorafenib) monotherapy in patients with advanced solid tumours: is rash associated with treatment outcome? Eur J Cancer 2006; 42:548–56.
68. Susser WS, Whitaker-Worth DL, Grant-Kels JM. Mucocutaneous reactions to chemotherapy. J Am Acad Dermatol 1999; 40:367–98.
69. Autier J, Escudier B, Wechsler J, Spatz A, Robert C. Prospective study of the cutaneous adverse effects of sorafenib, a novel multikinase inhibitor. Arch Dermatol 2008; 144:886–892.
70. Belloni B, Schonewolf N, Rozati S, Goldinger SM, Dummer R. Cutaneous drug eruptions associated with the use of new oncological drugs. Chem Immunol Allergy 2012; 97:191–202.
71. Lacouture ME, Anadkat MJ, Bensadoun RJ, Bryce J, Chan A, Epstein JB, *et al*. MASCC Skin Toxicity Study Group: Clinical practice guidelines for the prevention and treatment of EGFR inhibitor-associated dermatologic toxicities. Support Care Cancer 2011; 19 (8):1079–95.
72. Pillans P, Woods D. Drug-associated alopecia. Int J Dermatol 1995; 34:149–58.

73. Biswas A, Chaudhari PB, Sharma P, Singh L, Julka PK, Sethuraman G. Bleomycin induced flagellate erythema: revisiting a unique complication. J Cancer Res Ther 2013; 9:500–503.
74. Mahmoud BH, Eide MJ. Bendamustine-induced “flagellate dermatitis” Dermatol Online J. 2012; 18(11):12.
75. Tallon B, Lamb S. Flagellate erythema induced by docetaxel. Clin Exp Dermatol. 2008; 33:276–7.
76. Araki Y, Tamura K, Seita M. Side effects of peplomycin. GanTo Kagaku Ryoho. 1986; 13:2446–50.
77. Cohen PR. Trastuzumab-associated flagellate erythema: Report in a woman with metastatic breast cancer and review of antineoplastic therapy-induced flagellate dermatoses. DermatolTher (Heidelb). 2015; 5(4):253–64.
78. Wang ECE, Lee JSS, Tan AWH, Tang MBY. Fas-ligand staining in non-drug- and drug-induced maculopapular rashes. J CutanPathol 2011; 38(2):196–201.
79. Nigen S, Knowles SR, Shear NH. Drug eruptions: Approaching the diagnosis of drug-induced skin diseases. J Drugs Dermatol 2003 June; 2(3):278–99.
80. Wolkenstein P, Chosidow O, Fletchet ML, Robbiola O, Paul M, Dume L, *et al*. Patch testing in sever cutaneous adverse reactions, including Stevens-Johnson syndrome and toxic epidermal necrolysis. Contact Dermatitis 1996; 35:234–6.
81. Barbaud A. Skin testing in delayed reactions to drugs. Immunol Allergy Clin North Am 2009; 29:517–35.
82. Barbaud A, Collet E, Milpied B, Assier H, Stoumont D, Avenel-Audran M.A multicentric study to determine the value and safety of drug patch tests for the three main classes of severe cutaneous adverse drug reactions. Br J Dermatol 2013; 168:555–62.
83. Kavoussi H, Rezaei M, Derakhshandeh K, *et al.* Clinical features and drug characteristics of patients with generalized fixed drug eruption in the West of Iran (2005–2014). Dermatol Res Pract 2015; 2015: 236703.
84. Lee E. Topical provocation in 31 cases of fixed drug eruption: Change of causative drugs in 10 years. Contact Dermatitis 1998; 38:258–60.
85. Pasricha JS, Khaitan BK, Shantharamam R, Mittal A, Girdhar M, *et al*. Toxic epidermal necrolysis. Int J Dermatol 1996; 35: 523–7.
86. Skassa-Brociek W, Manderscheid JC, Michel FB, Bousquet J. Skin test reactivity to histamine from infancy to old age. Journal of Allergy and Clinical Immunology 1987; 80:711e6.
87. Nelson HS, Knoetzer J, Bucher B. Effect of distance between sites and region of the body on results of skin prick tests. Journal of Allergy and Clinical Immunology 1996; 97:596e601.
88. King MJ, Lockey RF. Allergen prick-puncture skin testing in the elderly. Drugs Aging 2003; 20:1011e7.
89. Wohrl S, Hammer W, Focke M, Gotz M, Jarisch R. Patch testing in childrens, adults and elderly: influence of age and sex on sensitization patterns. Pediatr Dermatol 2003; 20(2):119–23.
90. Kowalski ML, Ansotegui I, Aberer W, *et al*. Risk and safety requirements for diagnostic and therapeutic procedures in allergology: World Allergy Organization Statement. The World Allergy Organization Journal. 2016; 9(1):33.
91. Falck P, Asberg A, Byberg KT, bremer S, Reubsaet JL, Midvedt K. Reduced elimination of cyclosporine in elderly (>65 years) kidney transplant recipients. Transplantation. 2008 Nov 27; 86(10):1379–83
92. Katz U, Achiron A, Sherer Y, Shoenfeld Y. Safety of intravenous immunoglobulin (IVIG) therapy. Autoimmun Rev 2007; 6:257–9.

CHAPTER 13

Environmental Dermatoses in Elderly

• *Pratik Gahalaut*

Key Points

1. A lifetime exposure of various exogenous entities, combined with intrinsic changes in the dermal structures, predisposes geriatric individual to a wide variety of environmental dermatoses.
2. Majority of these environmental dermatoses are not terminal, but they are characterized by high morbidity and significant decrease in the quality of life among elderly.
3. Research in geriatric environmental dermatoses is in nascent stage presently.
4. There are no widespread appropriate, evidence-based, well accepted guidelines for managing these dermatoses among elderly.
5. The objective of this chapter is to highlight common environmental cutaneous problems associated with aging skin and provide appropriate advice for managing these.

Introduction

Skin is an interface between man and his environment.[2] The literal dictionary meaning of word environment is 'the surroundings or conditions in which a person, animal, or plant lives'.[2] Ageing results in numerous inevitable degenerative and metabolic changes throughout the skin layers, i.e. intrinsic or natural skin ageing.[3] Occurrence of skin diseases may be due to macroclimate or microclimate.[4] Macroclimate constitutes the environmental factors like geography, temperature, rainfall, and humidity of a given area.[5] Microclimate refers to the individual and his or her ecological and socio-economic environment.[4] While various environmental factors may influence or accentuate this chronological skin ageing, these same exogenous physical entities may result in a specific subset of skin diseases, termed environmental dermatoses (ED).[6] ED may be broadly classified as those occurring or modified by the moisture, temperature, weather, ultraviolet radiation exposure, contact allergens or irritants (Flowchart 13.1).[6] Discussion regarding each of these entities is not warranted here and hence only few relevant entities pertaining to geriatric population are being discussed henceforth.

SKIN AND MOISTURE

1. Dry Skin or Xerotic Eczema[7,8]

- Characterized by pruritic, dry, cracked and fissured skin with scaling.
- Varied prevalence up to 99.5% has been reported among geriatric population from India and worldwide.
- Susceptibility to xerosis increases in elderly due to concomitant medications, nutritional deficiencies, thyroid disorders, pre-existing malignancies, end-stage renal disease.
- Occurs most commonly in elderly on the anterolateral lower limbs, back, flanks, abdomen, waist, arms and spares the groin, axilla, face and scalp.
- While fissuring of skin increases the risk of contact dermatitis and secondary infections.

Flowchart 13.1: Etiological classification of environmental dermatoses among elderly

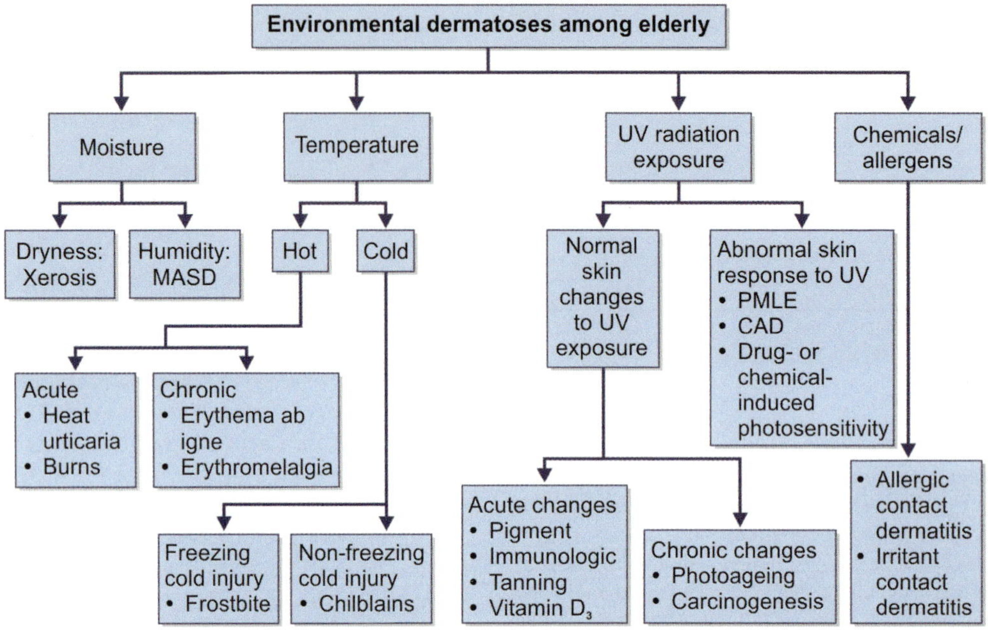

- Cold, dry weather or air conditioning worsens xerosis.
- Keratolytics, moisturisers with or without steroids and antipruritics are the main stay of treatment along with minimal usage of soap and hot water during bathing.

2. Moisture Associated Skin Damage (MASD)

- An ensemble of skin problems that arise from barrier dysfunction which is caused by prolonged exposure to moisture in an occluded environment.[9]
- MASD is most often related to incontinence associated dermatitis (IAD), intertrigo, ostomy leakage and peri-wound skin.[10]
- IAD, also referred to as perineal dermatitis, affects up to 50% of nursing home residents and between 10 and 35% of community-dwelling elders.[9]
- Diaper dermatitis (DD) can occur in adults and the elderly admitted in ICU, confined to bed or having mental disorders like Alzheimer's disease.[11]
- In elderly skin wrinkling or folding results in free hanging, overlapping skin which predisposes to peristomal dermatitis or intertrigo.[12]
- Other predisposing factors include obesity, diabetes, chronic bedrest, inadequate personal hygiene, and the use of broad-spectrum antibiotics, all more in geriatric age group.
- IAD can be controlled by changing diapers regularly, especially newer hypoallergenic, superabsorbent (sodium polyacrylate) diapers.[11,13]
- Fungal superinfection warrants appropriate antimycotics for 7–10 days. Low-potency steroids (hydrocortisone) are recommended for short time in absence of any bacterial or mycotic infections.[11,14]
- Barrier creams with zinc formulations or emollients such as petrolatums and lanolin can also be used.[11,15]
- Systemic antifungal medications should be used with caution in elderlies because of polypharmacy, drug interactions and their potential side effects.[16]

- An optimal skin care regimen enabling frequent washing without compromising skin barrier function is the mainstay to prevent MASD-related problems.[9]
- A body wash such as syndet with a neutral pH or a cleanser combined with an emollient has therapeutic, practical, and economic advantages.[17]

SKIN AND TEMPERATURE

Extreme temperature exposure may cause burns and freezing and/or non-freezing cold injuries. Abnormal reactions to moderate degrees of heat and cold can cause erythema ab igne and chilblains respectively. Cold or heat may precipitate cryoglobulinemia, cold panniculitis, and erythromelalgia. Physical urticarias like heat urticarial are also temperature-dependent.[18] Heat has been implicated in various heat cancers and infrared elastosis.

Acute Adverse Effects of Heat

- Ageing reduces heat conduction due to the diminished skin blood flow, decreased dermal thickness, increased subcutaneous fat thickness.[19]
- Geriatric population has general diminution of senses, decreased environmental awareness, and delayed reaction time; all of which decrease the heat tolerance.[19]
- Ageing also decreases cellular and humorally mediated immune responses, which further increases the likelihood of wound infection.[20]
- Hence older individuals are susceptible to skin damage, burns, and show slower healing.

Chronic Adverse Effects of Heat

1. Erythema ab igne (EAI)

- Itoccurs due to repeated or prolonged exposure to heat, insufficient toproduce a burn.[18,21]
- Occurs over legs and inner thighs of elderly women sitting in proximity to heaters, fires, or stoves; lumbar region in patients applying hot water bottles or heating pads for chronic backache; face in bakers or silversmiths, and others who work over near heat source (Fig. 13.1).

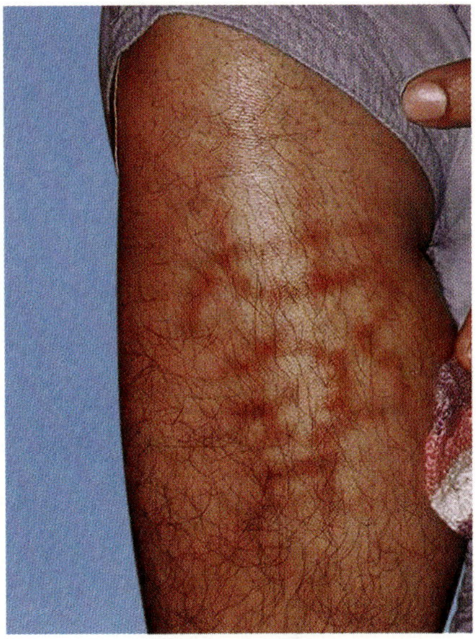

Fig. 13.1: Erythema ab igne—reticulate hyperpigmentation with erythema (*Courtesy:* Dr Nitin Mishra, SRMSIMS, Bareilly)

- A transient, blanchable, reticulated erythema develops in the starting after exposure to moderate IR.[22]
- Repetitive and prolonged thermal exposure causes fixed reticulate hyperpigmentation, erythema, epidermal atrophy, scaling and telangiectases followed by infrequent transformations to squamous or Merkel cell carcinoma after decades of IR exposure.[21]
- The most important treatment for erythema ab igne is immediate removal of the source of infrared radiation.[21,22]
- Presently, there are no effective medical therapies available and treatment is symptomatic. While topical tretinoin, hydroquinone and low fluence Q-switch Nd:YAG lasers have been tried for persistent hyperpigmentation.[21] Treatment with topical fluorouracil or imiquimod may be useful in countering keratinocyte dysplasia.[23]

2. Heat Urticaria (HU)

- It is an immediate-type reaction in which characteristic wheals develop at the sites of contact within a few minutes of exposure to temperature >38°C due to either hot water, hot car seats, hot air, or hot fire places.[24]
- It is a rare form of urticaria seen more in females which starts in early adulthood usually and rarely persists into geriatric age group.[24]
- Treatment of HU is usually symptomatic. Avoidance of the precipitating agents and the intake of antihistamines, just like other physical urticarias, are advocated.[25]

3. Erythromelalgia

- Characterised by paroxysmal attacks of erythema, heat and burning pain on extremities, usually legs.[26] Lesions can be reproduced by raising the skin temperature to the critical range of 32° to 36°C.[27]
- Though it is more frequent among young adults, secondary adult onset thrombocytosis related type due to myeloproliferative disorders usually occurs in late sixth decade.[26]
- Elevation and/or cooling of the extremity provides symptomatic relief.[26]
- In absence of an universal treatment consensus while NSAID, SSRI, calcium channel antagonists are helpful in thrombocythemic diseases, the response of erythromelalgia to treatment of the underlying myeloproliferative disease has been variable.[26,28]

SKIN REACTIONS TO COLD

Exposure to cold may cause freezing or non-freezing injuries.

1. Freezing Cold Injury

- Frost bite occurs acutely at temperatures below the freezing point (–2° to 0°C).[29]
- It affects exposed soft tissues such as the nose, ear lobes, cheeks, fingers, and toes.
- Old age, children, alcohol or nicotine consumption, vasoconstrictive drug abuse, impaired mental state, previous frostbite, peripheral vascular disease, tight constrictive or inadequate clothing and immobility are predisposing risk factors.[25]
- Additionally, environmental factors strong winds, high altitude, and contact with cold metals or water may accentuate cold induced damage.[25]
- A cold numbness with accompanying sensory loss in the extremities, "like a block of wood", may be felt.[30] Thawing and reperfusion is often intensely painful and pain may persist for weeks or months, even after tissue demarcation.[29] Residual tingling sensation starting after one week has been described and may be due to an ischaemic neuritis.
- Frostbite injury has been classified as either mild/superficial (no tissue loss) or severe/deep (with loss of tissue).[30] The severity of frostbite injuries can now be assessed with triple phase bone scanning.[30]
- The treatment of frostbite is initially conservative and depends on the extent of damage and the full depth of viable tissue. Rapid return of skin warmth, sensation, erythema, oedema, and vesicles containing clear fluid are good prognostic signs.[30]
- Main stay of treatment is rapid rewarming of affected areas in warm water at 37°–39°C (99°–102°F) for 15–30 mins or until thawing is complete.[29] Early hyperbaric oxygen therapy appears to improve outcome and the use of intravenous drugs such as synthetic prostaglandin analogues infusions and tissue plasminogen activator have shown a reduced amputation rates.[29]

2. Non-freezing Cold Injuries (NFCI)

- Chilblains (CB, perniosis) are localized inflammatory lesions due to maladaptive vascular response precipitated by exposure to damp non-freezing cold temperatures where there are periods of temperatures between 16°C (60°F) and 0°C (32°F).[25,31]

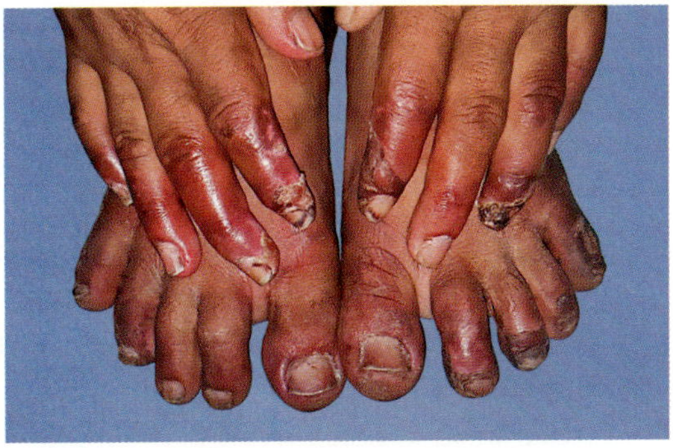

Fig. 13.2: Perniosis—oedema with erythematous plaques and scales on toes and fingers

- Elderly people, children, smokers, women and relatives of affected patients are more susceptible.[31]
- Presents as erythematous or violaceous edematous papules, patches, or plaques classically involving the hands (fingers), feet (toes), or face (nose, ear lobes) associated with tenderness or burning usually between late fall and early spring season (Fig. 13.2). Occasionally, other exposed areas, such as the thighs, hips, or abdomen, may be affected.[31]
- Lesions are usually self-limited, resolving over 2 to 3 weeks, but they may become chronic, especially in elderly people who suffer from peripheral vascular or systemic disease.[32]
- In elderly men, they may be the early manifestation of underlying leukaemia.[32]
- The mainstay of treatment is prevention by using warm clothing and proper heating along with rest. The calcium channel blocker nifedipine, 20 mg tds, is beneficial in the treatment and prophylaxis of this condition.[31]

SKIN AND ULTRAVIOLET RADIATIONS

Though solar radiation spectrum is broad, only about 2–3% of ultraviolet radiations (UVR), approximately 32% of visible light, and slightly <66% of infrared light reaches the Earth's surface.[33] The harmful effects of sunlight on biological systems including skin are due almost entirely to radiation within the ultraviolet spectrum of the sun's emission.[34]

- The cutaneous changes in reactivity on exposure to UVR can be considered in two categories: Those that occur in normally ageing skin, either acute or chronic; and those that are the result of photosensitivity disorders or photodermatoses.[35]

1. Acute and Subacute Effects of UVR on Normal Skin

Include erythema, pigment darkening, delayed tanning, epidermal hyperplasia, immunologic changes and decreased vitamin D_3 synthesis.[36]

2. Chronic Effects of UVR on Normal Skin (Fig. 13.3)

- Result in photoageing and photocarcinogenesis.[36]
- Photoageing occurs due to extrinsic factors like UV light, lifestyle influence, smoking, nicotine use and chemicals mainly on sun-exposed areas of the body such as the neck, decollete, face, forearms and hands.[37]

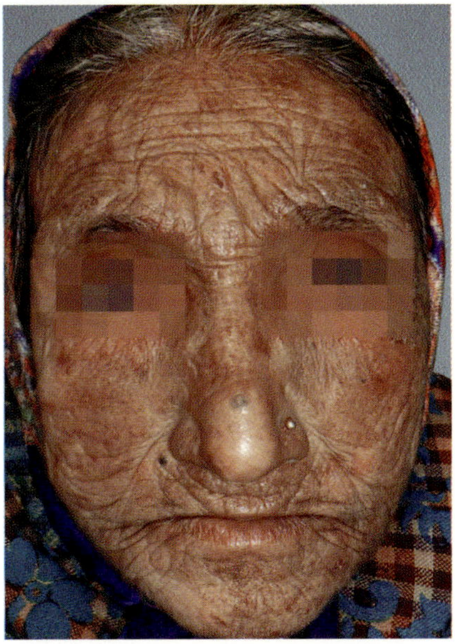

Fig. 13.3: Facial skin changes due to chronic UVR exposure

- Photoageing is characterized by wrinkles, laxity, a leathery skin appearance, increased fragility, blister formation, impaired wound healing, irregular freckling, lentigines, diffuse hyperpigmentation, guttate hypomelanosis, stellate pseudoscars, fine nodularity, telangiectasia, venous lakes, purpura, comedones, sebaceous hyperplasia, citrine skin (Milian), cutis rhomboidalis nuchae (Jadassohn), nodular elastoidosis with cyst and comedones (Favre-Racouchot), diffuse elastoma (Dubreuilh), elastic nodule of ear, acrokeratoelastoidosis marginalis, striated beaded lines, actinic granuloma and actinic comedonal plaque.[38]
- Compared to chronological ageing, photoageing affects mainly the fair skinned individuals and it is less common in Asian skin type IV (dark skinned).[38]

3. Photodermatoses

- These are a group of disorders wherein there is an abnormal tissue response to UVR resulting in visible changes on sun-exposed skin.[39]
- The distinct photosensitive cutaneous conditions can be classified into four main categories: Immunologically mediated photodermatoses; drug- and chemical-induced photosensitivity; defective DNA nucleotide excision repair disorders; and photoaggravated dermatoses.[34]
- Roelandts has stressed that chronic actinic dermatitis, drug-induced photosensitivity and photoaggravated dermatoses are the predominant photodermatoses where symptoms first occur in geriatric age group, although other photodermatoses may also persist into geriatric population.[40]

a. Polymorphic light eruption (PMLE)

- It is the most common endogenous photodermatosis which affects men and women of all ages including elderly.[41]
- It has been reported that 11% of patients developed PMLE after the age of 50 years.[42]
- It occurs commonly in fair skinned individuals having Fitzpatrick skin types I–IV.[42]
- Though the exact pathogenesis of PMLE is not known, a delayed-type hypersensitivity immune reaction to UVR-induced neoantigens of the skin plays a role.[41] The action spectrum is most commonly UV rays (290–365 nm) and rarely visible light.[39]
- It manifests as nonscarring erythematous pruritic papules, vesicles, pinpoint papules, papulovesicles, plaques, and nodules that erupt usually within a few hours to 2 days of sun exposure on photo-exposed parts commonly.[43]
- For an individual patient, though the lesions may be polymorphic, the same morphology is usually present with each eruption.[39] Pinpoint papules are more commonly seen in patients with darker skin[44] (Fig. 13.4).
- In temperate climates, the eruption worsens in early summer or spring and improves as the sunny season progresses.[43]
- Photoprotection is the mainstay of treatment in all photodermatoses.[34] This may be achieved by avoiding sun exposure (change of lifestyle may be warranted); use of protective clothing and regular applications of broad-spectrum physical sunscreens.[39]

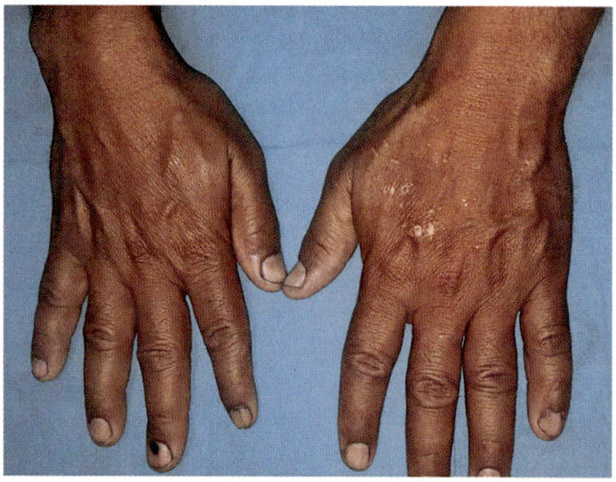

Fig. 13.4: Papular PMLE with koebnerisation

- Short-term systemic steroids (prednisone 1 mg/kg/1) for 1 to 2 weeks can be initiated for acute and severe exacerbations of the condition.[34]
- Hardening or controlled exposure to sunlight or artificial UVR sources may be tried as preventive UV phototherapy and/or psoralen plus UVA (PUVA) therapy[61,68] hardening may be accomplished with either UVA or/and UVB.[39] The treatment is usually initiated during spring and an average of 15 sessions is usually sufficient to induce hardening.[34]

b. Chronic actinic dermatitis

- It is a rare chronic photodermatosis of sun-exposed and, to a lesser extent, covered skin.[39]
- Chronic actinic dermatitis (CAD) presents at any time after the fourth decade.[36]
- It usually affects men aged 40–80 years, although 10–22% of affected persons are women. The precise incidence of this photosensitivity disorder is uknown.[36]
- CAD is a contact-allergy like delayed type hypersensitivity against endogenous, photo-induced cutaneous allergen(s).[35,36,39] In India, patients with CAD exhibit contact sensitivity to a range of contact allergens, especially parthenium hysterophorus, oleoresins from a weed of Compositae family, and to alesser extent to phosphorus sesquisulfide, colophony, rubber, metals, and allergens used in medicaments, perfumes, and sunscreens.[39,45] Parthenium and oleoresins from Compositae plants might play a role in inducing photoaggravation of CAD.[39]
- Clinically CAD is a pruritic dermatitis with widespread persistent eczematous changes, often with scaly lichenification or infiltrated plaques, particularly on the sun-exposed skin with a sharp cut-off at the lines of clothing.[36,46] Nevertheless about half of all patients have non-exposed site involvement at some point in their lives.[36] Infiltration of the skin results in accentuation of skin markings on the face and rarely leonine facies may occur in severe cases.[46] Skin furrows, upper eyelids, skin within the hair bearing scalp, under the chin and behind the ear lobes is usually spared (Fig. 13.5).[36] Palmar, plantar and other eczemas may occur in up to 90% of these patients.[36,46] Though CAD usually remains static, occasional spontaneous remissions or progression to erythroderma is possible.[35] Resolution occurs in 10% over 5 years, 20% over 10 years and 50% over 15 years.[43,47]
- Patch tests are frequently positive to one or more exogenous allergens, often airborne or in frequent contact with widespread body areas (including sunscreens).[35,39] Even if photosensitivity resolves, any accompanied contact allergy usually persists. Severe UVB photosensitivity and the presence of 2 or

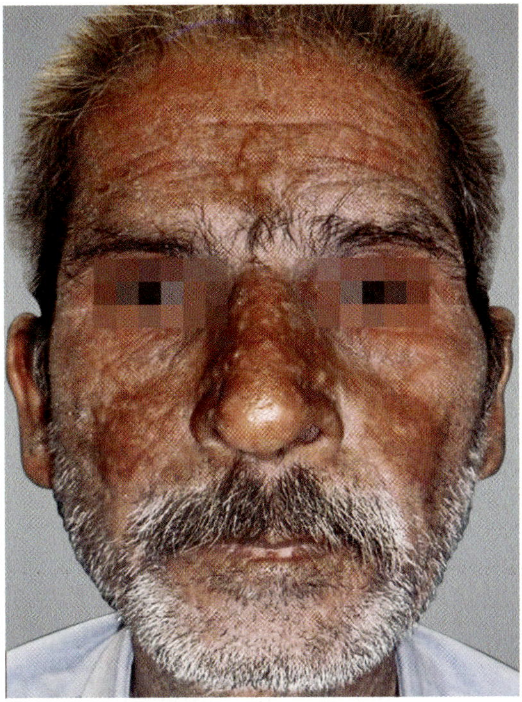

Fig. 13.5: Erythrodermic parthenium dermatitis

greater contact allergens are poor prognostic indicators.[43]

- The diagnosis of CAD is suggested by patients history and clinical appearance aided by histological features if necessary (done to rule out cutaneous lymphoma), presence of normal antinuclear antibodies, and normal blood, urine and stool porphyrin concentrations.[48]
- Strict photoprotection including visible light, if indicated, and avoidance of contact allergens, if any, are the mainstay for managing CAD.[39] Short course of topical steroids with emollients and systemic steroids is effective during flares. In refractory cases, azathioprine (1–2.5 mg/kg/day), mycophenolate mofetil (25–50 mg/kg/day), low-dose PUVA helps.[39] Though cyclosporine (3.5–5 mg/kg/day) is usually effective caution is warranted in elderly due to its side effect profile.[36,49]Azathioprine is moderately to extremely effective after 1 month of initiating treatment in approximately two-thirds of patients with CAD and some patients remain free of the disease after cessation of treatment.[46] Patients of CAD managed with systemic immunosupressants might be expected to be at a true increased risk of developing lymphomas.[36]
- Treatment has to be long-term as relapses appear when treatment is stopped.[49]

c. Drug- and chemical-induced photosensitivity

- Exposure to UV or visible light can alter topical and systemic agents into potent photosensitizers.[43]
- Photosensitivity from various exogenous industrial, cosmetic or therapeutic agents can be classified into phototoxicity or photoallergy.[46]
- The exact prevalence of exogenous drug-induced photosensitivity is not known but phototoxicity is commoner than photoallergy.[50]

i. Drug-induced phototoxic reactions are non-allergic cutaneous responses induced by a variety of topical and systemic agents.[39] Drug-induced phototoxic reactions are dose dependant; require a greater substance exposure; do not require prior sensitization and occur minutes to hours after sunlight exposure.[51] Clinically, a phototoxic reaction resembles a sunburn, manifested as painful erythema, blistering, scaling, eczematoid, lichenoid eruptions and slate-grey hyperpigmentation confined to sun-exposed sites, after a moderate sun exposure that would not be sufficient to produce an actual one.[36,43] It can theoretically occur in everyone in the presence of the activating radiation and adequate doses of the phototoxic agent.[36]

   Dose reduction may reduce photosensitivity, especially in phototoxic reactions.[52] Discontinuation of a phototoxic drug is the treatment per se. Sometimes, it is possible that with sun avoidance, sunscreens, and local supportive measures, a necessary photosensitizing medication can be continued.[52]A phototoxic reaction usually resolves with desquamation and hyperpigmentation within a few days, or in a few, very rare instances after a few months.[35]

ii. Drug-induced photoallergic reactions are delayed hypersensitivity immune reaction and not dependent upon the dose of either medication or radiant energy. Reaction requires prior sensitization and develops 24 hours or more after the initial exposure even after a relatively minimal exposure to the photosensitizing medication.[51]

   It occurs as an eczematous dermatitis that may spread beyond the sun-exposed skin and may be provoked by molecularly similar medications (so-called crossreacting medications).[51]

Discontinuation of offending drug is pertinent in treating photoallergy. If lesions are severe, a course of systemic steroids is warranted.[39]

ED due to various chemicals, allergens and insect bites will be discussed elsewhere in separate chapter on contact dermatitis and hence not discussed here.

CONCLUSION

Though ED are a distinct subset of skin diseases occurring not so infrequently in elderlies, epidemiological data regarding the same in geriatric age group is inadequate. Current research is investigating the dermatological problems associated with the loss of cutaneous function in ageing. Future research should focus on developing appropriate, evidence based protocols, encompassing both medical treatment and basic skin-care strategies, for managing various ailments among geriatric population.

References

1. Amer M, Metwalli M. Environmental Dermatology: An Overview. Clin Dermatol 1998; 16:23–5.
2. Cambridge Advanced Learner's Dictionary and Thesaurus. Environment Meaning in the Cambridge English Dictionary [Internet]. Dictionary.cambridge.org 2018 [cited 26 February 2018]. Available from: https://dictionary.cambridge.org/dictionary/english/environment.
3. Smith E, Fleischer A, Feldman S. Demographics of ageing and skin disease. Clin Geriatr Med 2001; 17(4):631–41.
4. Lober CW, Fenske NA. Photoageing and the skin: Differentiation and clinical response. Geriatrics 1990; 45:36–42.
5. Smith DR, Leggat PA. Prevalence of skin disease among the elderly in different clinical environments. Australas J Ageing 2005; 24(2):71–6.
6. Meffert JJ. Environmental skin diseases and the impact of common dermatoses on medical readiness. Dermatol Clin 1999; 17(1):1–17.
7. Norman RA. Xerosis and pruritus in the elderly: recognition and management. Dermatol Ther 2003; 16:254–9.
8. Durai PC, Thappa DM, Kumari R, Malathi M. Ageing in Elderly: Chronologival versus Photoageing. Indian J Dermatol 2012; 57(5):343–52.
9. Humbert P, Dréno B, Krutmann J, Luger TA, Triller R, Meaume S, Seite S. Recommendations for managing cutaneous disorders associated with advancing age. Clin Interv Ageing 2016;11:141–8.
10. Voegeli D. Moisture-associated skin damage: aetiology, prevention and treatment. Br J Nurs 2012;21:517–518, 520–521. DOI: 10.12968/bjon.2012.21.9.517
11. Bonifaz A, Saldaña M, Escandón-Pérez S and Tirado-Sánchez A. Diaper Dermatitis in Elderly. J Dermatitis 1:1. Available from https://pdfs.semanticscholar.org/f497/852fac447efcbb6610c0746572ce077149c3.pdf. Last accessed on February 25th, 2018.
12. Turnbull GB. Minding the gap: the art of manageing peristomal topography. Ostomy Wound Manage 2006; 52:11–12.
13. Klunk C, Domingues E, Wiss K. An update on diaper dermatitis. Clin Dermatol 2014; 32:477–87.
14. Bonifaz A, Rojas R, Tirado-Sánchez A, Chávez-López D, Mena C, Calderon L, *et al.* Superficial mycoses associated with diaper dermatitis. Mycopathologia 2016; 181:671–679.
15. Haugen V. Perineal skin care for patients with frequent diarrhea or fecal incontinence. Gastroenterol Nurs 1997; 20:87–90.
16. Varade RS, Burkemper NM. Cutaneous Fungal Infections in the Elderly. Clin Geriatr Med 2013; 29:461–78.
17. Beeckman D, Schoonhoven L, Verhaeghe S, Heyneman A, Defloor T. Prevention and treatment of incontinence-associated dermatitis:literature review. J Adv Nurs 2009; 65:1141–54.
18. Page EH, Shear NH. Temperature-dependent skin disorders. J Am Acad Dermatol 1988; 18(5):1003–19.
19. Petrofsky JS, McLellan K, Bains GS, Prowse M, Ethiraju G, Lee S, *et al.* The influence of ageing on the ability of the skin to dissipate heat. Med Sci Monit, 2009; 15(6):CR261–8.
20. Jerred DA, Cappadoro K. Burns in the elderly patient. Emerg Med Clin North Am 1990; 8(2):421–8.
21. Kim J, Seo H, Kim Y, Lee J, Lee S, Park J, *et al.* Treatment of Erythema ab igne with Combination of Topical Hydroquinone and 1,064-nm Q-switched

Neodymium-Doped Yttrium Aluminum Garnet Laser with Low Fluence. Med Laser 2013;2(2):73–75. Doi:10.25289/ML.2013.2.2.73.

22. Beleznay K, Humphrey S, Au S. Erythema ab igne. CMAJ 2010;182(5):E228. DOI:10.1503/cmaj.081216.
23. Sahl W, Taira JW. Erythema ab igne: Treatment with 5-fluorouracil cream. J Am Acad Dermatol 1992; 27:109-10. Doi:10.1016/S0190-9622(08) 80818-3.
24. Zuberbier T, Maurer M. Urticaria: Current Opinions about Etiology, Diagnosis and Therapy. Acta Derm Venereol 2007; 87:196–205.
25. Kibbi AG, Tannous Z. Skin Diseases Caused by Heat and Cold. Clin Dermatol 1998; 16:91–8.
26. Tang Z, Chen Z, Tang B, Jiang H. Primary erythromelalgia: a review. Orphanet J Rare Dis 2015 10:127. Doi:10.1186/s13023-015-0347-1.
27. Kligman LH, Kligman AM. Reflection on heat. Br J Dermatol 1984; 110:369–75.
28. Buttaci CJ. Erythromelalgia: A Case Report and Literature Review. Pain Med 2006; 7(6):534–8.
29. Imray C, Grieve A, Dhillon S. Cold damage to the extremities: frostbite and non-freezing cold injuries. Postgrad Med J 2009;85:481–8. doi:10.1136/pgmj.2008.068635.
30. Grieve AW, Davis P, Dhillon S, Richards P, Hillebrandt D, Imray CHE. A Clinical Review of the Management of Frostbite. J R Army Med Corps 2011; 157(1): 73-78. doi: 10.1136/jramc-157-01–13.
31. AlMahameed A, Pinto DS. Pernio (Chilblains). Curr Treat Options Cardiovasc Med 2008, 10:128–35.
32. Kelly JW, Dowling JR. Pernio: A possible association with chronic myelomonocytic leukemia. Arch Dermatol 1985; 121:1048–52.
33. Wolf R. Photodermatoses. Clin Dermatol 1998; 16:41–57.
34. Bylaite M, Grigaitiene J, Lapinskaite GS. Photodermatoses: classification, evaluation and management. British J Dermatol 2009; 161(Suppl.3): 61–68. doi: 10.1111/j.1365-2133.2009.09451.x.
35. Hawk JLM. Photosensitivity in elderly. Br J Dermatol 1999; 122:29–41.
36. Trakatelli M, Charalampidis S, Novakovic LB, Patsatsi A, Kalabalikis D, Sotiriadis D. Photodermatoses with onset in the elderly. British Journal of Dermatology 2009; 161 (Suppl. 3):69–77.
37. Farage MA, Miller KW, Elsner P, Maibach HI. Intrinsic and extrinsic factors in skin ageing: a review. Int J Cosmet Sci 2008; 30:87–95.
38. Durai PC, Thappa DM, Kumari R, Malathi M. Ageing in Elderly: Chronological versus Photoageing. Indian J Dermatol 2012;57(5):343-52. Doi: 10.4103/0019-5154.100473.
39. Srinivas CR, Sekar CS, Jayashree R. Photodermatoses in India. Indian J Dermatol Venereol Leprol 2012; 78:1–8.
40. Roelandts R. The diagnosis of photosensitivity. Arch dermatol 2000; 136:1152–7.
41. Hanigsmann H. Polymorphous light eruption. Photodermatol Photoimmunol Photomed 2008; 24:155–61.
42. Jansén CT: The natural history of polymorphous light eruptions. Arch Dermatol 1979; 115:165–9.
43. Santoro FA, Lim HW. Update on photodermatoses. Semin Cutan Med Surg 2011; 30:229–38.
44. Kontos A, Cusack C, Chaffins M, *et al.* Polymorphous light eruption in African-Americans: Pinpoint papular variant. Photodermatol Photoimmunol Photomed 2002; 18:303–6.
45. Somani VK. Chronic actinic dermatitis-A study of clinical features. Indian J Dermatol Venereol Leprol 2005; 71:409–13.
46. Millard TP, Hawk JLM. Photodermatoses in the elderly. Clin Geriatr Med 2001; 17:691–714.
47. Dawe RS, Crombie IK, Ferguson J. The natural history of chronic actinic dermatitis. Arch Dermatol 2000; 136:1215–20.
48. Hawk JLM. Chronic actinic dermatitis. Photodermatol Photoimmunol Photomed 2004; 20:312–314. doi:10.1111/j.1600-0781.2004.00129.x.
49. Stinco G, Codutti R, Frattasio A, *et al.* Chronic actinic dermatitis treated with cyclosporin -A. Eur J Dermatol 2002; 12:455–7.
50. Selvaag E. Clinical drug photosensitivity. A retrospective analysis of reports to the Norwegian Adverse Drug Reactions Committee from the years 1970–1994. Photodermatol. Photoimmunol. Photomed. 1997;13(1-2):21 -23. doi:10.1111/j.1600-0781.1997.tb00103.x.
51. Stein KR, Scheinfeld NS. Drug-induced photoallergic and phototoxic reactions. Expert Opin Drug Saf 2007; 6(4):431–43.
52. Moore DE. Drug-induced cutaneous photosensitivity: incidence, mechanism, prevention and management. Drug Saf 2002; 25:345–72.

CHAPTER 14

Papulosquamous Diseases in the Elderly

• Najeeba Riyaz • Faiz Riyaz Arakkal • Roshin Anish

Introduction

Dermatologic diseases are very common in geriatric patients but there are very few studies on geriatric dermatoses.[1]

Normal ageing process along with other factors like ultraviolet radiation, irritants, allergens, temperature, humidity and xerosis of skin may lead to the development of various geriatric dermatoses.[2] Though there are several studies in the West on dermatoses in the elderly, there is a scarcity of Indian studies.[2,3] The published data on papulosquamous diseases in the elderly are also very little.

Papulosquamous diseases include:

- Psoriasis
- Lichen planus and lichenoid eruptions
- Pityriasis rubra pilaris

The incidence of papulosquamous diseases among geriatric patients has been found to be about 10–12% in various studies.[2-5]

PSORIASIS

Key Points

- Psoriasis is a T cell mediated multisystem inflammatory disorder with multiple comorbidities like obesity, hypertension, diabetes, metabolic syndrome and psychiatric illness.
- The incidence in the elderly ranges from 1 to 11%.
- The psychosocial impact of psoriasis may be out of proportion to the severity of disease.
- Treatment of psoriasis has to be tailor-made.
- Careful monitoring is essential while giving systemic medications in elderly.
- Apremilast, a phosphodiesterase 4 inhibitor, is a new oral drug that inhibits production of multiple cytokines involved in the pathogenesis of psoriasis.

Introduction

Psoriasis, which affects about 3% of the population, is a chronic T cell mediated papulosquamous inflammatory disease with a genetic predisposition.

Epidemiology

Psoriasis affects both genders almost equally. The incidence in the elderly ranges from 1 to 11.2% in various studies.[1-5] Type I or early onset psoriasis is seen between 16 and 22 years and type II or late onset psoriasis (LOP) between 57 and 62 years.[6]

Etiopathogenesis

Variations in the interleukin genes IR1 and IL-B may be associated with LOP.[7] A different Langerhans cell pathophysiology, immunological profile and a higher anxiety level have been described in LOP.[8]

Clinical Features

LOP tends to be less extensive than early onset disease.[6] Family history of psoriasis is rare in LOP. Chronic plaque psoriasis is the most common clinical type in the elderly characterised by typical well defined erythematous plaques with silvery white scales affecting mainly the extensor aspects of extremities, elbows, knees and scalp (Figs 14.1 and 14.2). Generalized plaques, an overlap of psoriasis with seborrhoeic dermatitis of the scalp (Fig. 14.3), face and retroauricular area, and inverse and erythrodermic psoriasis (Fig. 14.4) may also be seen.[9]

Guttate and generalized pustular psoriasis are rare.[6] The latter can be severe and occasionally life-threatening.

Nail changes like pitting, subungual hyperkeratosis, oil-drop sign, onycholysis, onychomadesis, yellowish discolouration and dystrophy may be seen.

Arthritis may be found in about one-third of patients with psoriasis. Skin lesions usually develop first, although in about 15% arthritis may precede skin lesions. It may be associated with severe nail lesions.

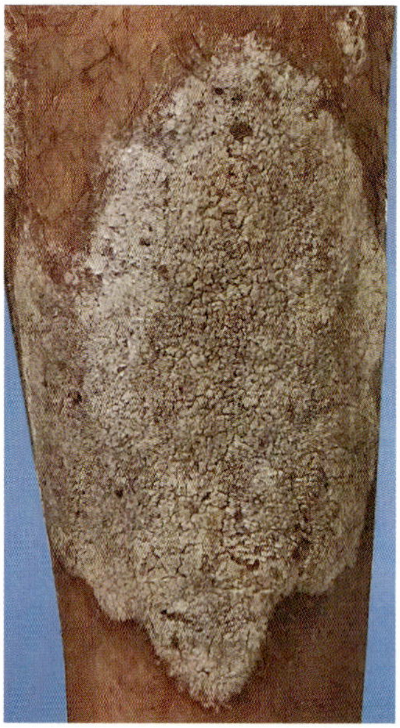

Fig. 14.2: Classical psoriatic plaque with silvery-white scales

Prognosis

Psoriasis is characterised by remissions and exacerbations. The severity of the disease can improve or worsen over time and can be controlled with treatment.

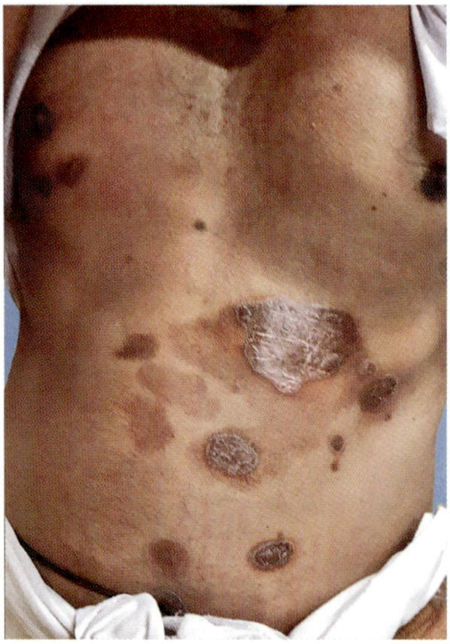

Fig. 14.1: Chronic plaque psoriasis

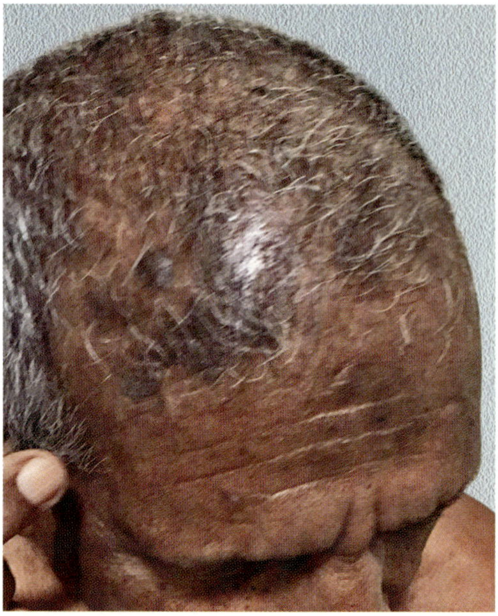

Fig. 14.3: Sebopsoriasis

Diagnosis

Psoriasis is diagnosed by the typical clinical findings and confirmed by skin biopsy.

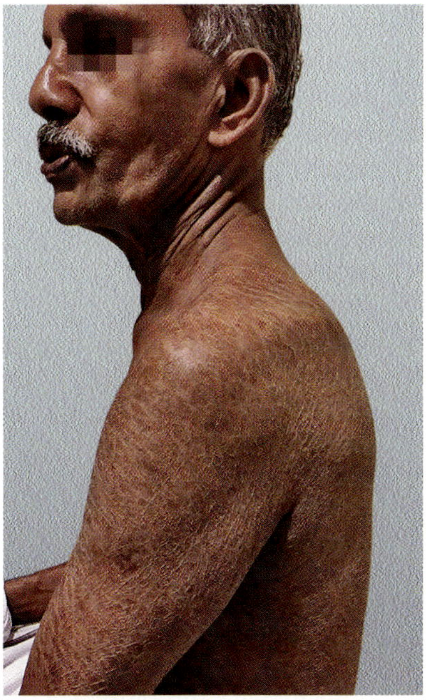

Fig. 14.4: Psoriatic erythroderma

Differential Diagnosis

The differential diagnoses include pityriasis rosea, seborrhoeic dermatitis, pityriasis rubra pilaris, lichen simplex chronicus, dermatophytosis and candidiasis, especially in the flexures. Drug eruptions are also an important differential diagnosis in the elderly as they take more medications.

Complications

Though psoriasis is a benign disease, there may be associated life threatening co-morbidities irrespective of the severity or duration of disease like hypertension, dyslipidaemia, cardiovascular diseases and type 2 diabetes, resulting in metabolic syndrome. This may be due to the proinflammatory cytokines and adipokines on lipid status, endothelial function and glucose regulation.[10,11]

The increased production of angiotensin II in visceral fat, free radicals and serum endothelin-1 may be responsible for the associated hypertension.[12] However, the exact mechanism remains uncertain. Hence, it is important to screen all psoriatics for cardiovascular risk factors at diagnosis itself. Nonalcoholic fatty liver disease which has a direct correlation with severity of the disease and vice versa, should also be ruled out.

Low serum levels of adiponectin in psoriatics can be used as a marker of disease severity irrespective of the presence of metabolic syndrome. There may be a therapeutic role for adiponectin in psoriasis. Elderly psoriatics with metabolic syndrome tend to have a higher incidence of obstructive sleep apnoea.[13] Depression and anxiety are found to be more in psoriatics.

Treatment

Psoriasis being a systemic inflammatory disease associated with increased risk for multiple disorders, a comprehensive approach to the management is essential. It includes topical and systemic therapy.[14] Treatment of psoriasis in the elderly should be tailor-made.[9]

Topical Therapy

Emollients

Liquid paraffin and white petrolatum are the most commonly used emollients. Urea and salicylic acid containing creams give additional keratolytic effect.

Topical Corticosteroids

Mild to moderate steroids like hydrocortisone, betamethasone valerate and mometasone furoate are used for facial, flexural, genital and scalp psoriasis.

Vitamin D_3 Analogues

Calcipotriene and calcitriol are effective but expensive topical agents which can be safely used in elderly without much side effects.

Vitamin A analogues like **tazarotene** are also effective.

Tar preparations are very useful and are available in various forms like ointments, oils, lotions and shampoos, and can be combined with phototherapy.

Anthralin, being an irritant, a short contact therapy for 10 to 30 minutes/day is used. It may cause yellowish staining of skin and clothing.

Topical calcineurin inhibitors like tacrolimus and pimecrolimus have been tried with variable effect for facial and flexural psoriasis.

Phototherapy

Narrow band UVB is a good option for elderly psoriatics. PUVA therapy is better avoided due to the possible hepatotoxicity.

Systemic Therapy[9,14]

Methotrexate is used in resistant types of elderly psoriatics with careful monitoring of liver and renal functions as well as haemogram. It may cause severe drug interactions with diuretics, macrolides, NSAIDs, etc. As elderly patients may be on multiple drugs, drug interaction is a possibility. Folic acid 1 mg daily or leucovorin (folinic acid) 5 mg weekly is recommended to reduce adverse effects like agranulocytosis.

Retinoids

Acitretin is used for severe recalcitrant psoriasis. Patient may improve within one month, although the full effect may take up to 3–6 months.

Side effects include cheilitis, xerosis, diffuse alopecia, arthralgia, depression, and elevated levels of triglycerides and liver enzymes which may be monitored regularly.

Apremilast, a phosphodiesterase 4 inhibitor, is a new oral drug that inhibits multiple cytokine production involved in its pathogenesis. It is started with 10 mg daily and increased to 60 mg within a week. In severe renal disease half the dose is given.[15] Side-effects include diarrhoea, nausea and headache.

Cyclosporine, an immune modulator, is used in acute exacerbation of psoriasis.[16]

Biologicals

Biologicals may be beneficial in the treatment of resistant psoriasis.[17] These include **infliximab, adalimumab, etanercept, ustekinumab, secukinumab, ixekizumab, brodalumab, guselkumab and tildrakizumab**. The adverse effects are comparable. Due to the high cost and potential side effects, they are generally reserved for severe refractory psoriasis only.

Biologicals should not be used in patients with serious infections like tuberculosis which should be ruled out before starting treatment.

CONCLUSION

Psoriasisis common in elderly, the chronic plaque type being the commonest. The management is similar to that in younger patients but careful monitoring is required while giving systemic medications. Apremilast, a phosphodiesterase 4 inhibitor, is a new oral drug for psoriasis.[15]

References

1. Yalcin B, Tamer E, Toy GG, Oztas P, Haryan M, Alli N. The prevalence of skin diseases in the elderly: Analysis of 4099 in geriatric patients. Int J of Dermatol. 2006; 45:672–6.
2. Raveendra L. A clinical study of geriatric dermatoses. Our Dermatol Online. 2014; 5:235–9.
3. Patange VS, Fernandez RJ. A study of geriatric dermatoses. Ind J Dermatol Venerol Leprol. 1995; 61:206–8.
4. Sahoo A, Singh PC, Pattnaik S, Panigrahi RK. Geriatric Dermatoses in Southern Orissa. Indian J Dermatol. 2000; 45:66–8.
5. Darjani A, Mohtasham-Amiri Z, Mohammad Amini K, Sadre-Eshkevari S, Alizade N. Skin disorders among elder patients in a referral center in Northern Iran. Dermatology Research and Practice 2013. Article ID 193205 http://dx.doi.org/10.1155/2013/193205)
6. Henseler T , Christophers E . Psoriasis of early and late onset: characterization of two types of psoriasis vulgaris. J Am Acad Dermatol 1985; 13:450–6.
7. Hebert HL, Bowes J, Smith RL, McHugh NJ, Barker JN, Griffiths CEM, Barton A, Warren RB. Polymorphisms

in IL-1 B distinguish between psoriasis of early and late onset. J Invest Dermatol 2014; 134:1459–62.
8. The Theodorakopoulou E, Yiu ZZN, Bundy C. Early- and Late-onset psoriasis: A cross-sectional clinical and immunocytochemical investigation. BR J Dermatol 2016; 175:1038–44.
9. Scheinfeld NS. Psoriasis: the "nuts and bolts" of management. *Consultant*. 2005; 45:798–807.
10. Gerdes S, Rostami-Yazdi M, Mrowietz U. Adipokines and psoriasis. Exp Dermatol 2011; 20:81.
11. Armstrong AW, Harskamp CT, Armstrong EJ. Psoriasis and the risk of diabetes mellitus: a systematic review and meta-analysis. JAMA Dermatol 2013; 149:84.
12. Armstrong AW, Harskamp CT, Armstrong EJ. The association between psoriasis and hypertension: a systematic review and meta-analysis of observational studies. J Hypertens 2013; 31:433.
13. Shalom G, Dreiher J, Cohen A. Psoriasis and obstructive sleep apnea. Int J dermatol 2016, 55, e579–e584.
14. Strober BE, Siu K, Menon K. Conventional systemic agents for psoriasis. A systematic review. J Rheumatol 2006; 33:1442.
15. Schafer PH, Parton A, Gandhi AK, L.Capone, M Adams, L Wu, *et al.* Apremilast, a cAMP phosphodiesterase-4 inhibitor, demonstrates anti-inflammatory activity *in vitro* and in a model of psoriasis. Br J Pharmacol 2010; 159:842.
16. Sandhu K, Kaur I, Kumar B, Saraswat A. Efficacy and safety of cyclosporine versus methotrexate in severe psoriasis: a study from north India. J Dermatol 2003; 30:458.
17. Signorovitch JE, Betts KA, Yan YS, LeReun C, Sundaram M, Wu EQ, *et al.* Comparative efficacy of biological treatments for moderate-to-severe psoriasis: a network meta-analysis adjusting for cross-trial differences in reference arm response. Br J Dermatol 2015; 172:504.

LICHEN PLANUS

Key Points

- Lichen planus(LP) is a common papulosquamous disorder possibly of autoimmune aetiology.
- The incidence in the elderly is about 4–5%.
- It may affect the skin, nails, or mucous membranes.
- Cutaneous LP typically presents as pruritic, polygonal, violaceous papules and/or plaques with an overlying white lines, Wickham's striae (WS).
- The association with hepatitis C infection is still controversial.
- Topical corticosteroids are the mainstay of treatment for localized forms.
- Generalized LP may require systemic steroids.

Introduction

Lichen planus is a common papulosquamous disorder seen in the elderly. It is a chronic inflammatory disease possibly autoimmune in nature, associated with multiple factors like bacterial and viral infections, psychic stress, drug intake, etc.

Epidemiolgy

Lichen planus affects less than 1% of the population.[1] It is most commonly seen between 30 and 60 years.[1,2] The incidence is 4–5% in various studies.[3,4] Both sexes are equally affected.

Precipitating Factors

Lichen planus is precipitated by several factors:

- Psychological stress
- Focus of infection like dental caries
- Trauma
- Drugs—beta blockers, calcium channel blockers, ACE inhibitors, methyl dopa, NSAIDs, heavy metals, etc.
- Hepatitis C (HC): The association of HC with LP is controversial, and a cause and effect relationship is uncertain.[5] Its prevalence with oral LP varies widely from 0 to 62%.[6]

Aetiopathogenesis

The exact aetiology is unknown. An immune-mediated mechanism involving activated T cells, especially CD8+ T cells, directed against basal keratinocytes has been proposed.[7]

Upregulation of intercellular adhesion molecule 1 and cytokines associated with a Th1 immune response like interferon gamma, tumour necrosis factor alpha, IL-1 alpha, IL-6, and IL-8, may also play a role.[7,8]

Clinical Features

Lichen planus may affect the skin, mucous membranes, scalp, nails, and genitalia.[1] It may be localized or generalized.

The classic features are intensely **p**ruritic, **p**lane topped, **p**urple, **p**olygonal, **p**apules and **p**laques (the 6 **P**s).

Rare zosteriform[10–12] and inverse (intertriginous)[2] patterns of cutaneous LP have been observed in the elderly. Koebner reaction is common. Asymptomatic eruptions are rare and lesions often heal with significant post-inflammatory hyperpigmentation.

Morphological types of LP include[2]

- Atrophic
- Annular
- Actinic
- Bullous
- Hypertrophic
- Inverse
- Lichen planus pigmentosus
- Lichen planopilaris
- Lichen planus pemphigoides
- Lichen planus-lupus erythematosus overlap syndrome.

Oral LP may be isolated or associated with cutaneous lesions. In Thappa's study, oral LP was found in 2.7% of geriatric patients. The typical lesions are white lace like on the buccal mucosa, gums, palate and tongue, followed by pigmented and atrophic lesions. Erosive lesions may turn malignant.[13]

Genital LP presents with violaceous papules on the glans or the vulva. The vulvovaginal lesions are relatively resistant to treatment.[14]

Esophageal LP presents with dysphagia or odynophagia.[15] The endoscopic findings are pseudomembranes, friable and inflamed mucosa, submucosal papules, lacy white plaques, erosions and strictures. Associated oral, genital or cutaneous lesions may be present.[15]

Diagnosis

Diagnosis is mainly clinical which can be confirmed by skin biopsy. The characteristic histopathologic findings are:

- Hyperkeratosis
- Wedge-shaped hypergranulosis
- Irregular acanthosis
- Vacuolization of the basal layer
- "Saw-tooth" shaped rete ridges
- **Civatte bodies** (apoptotic keratinocytes) in the lower epidermis
- **Max-Joseph spaces**—clefts at the dermal-epidermal junction
- Pigment incontinence
- Band-like lymphocytic infiltrate in the upper dermis
- **Colloid bodies** (apoptotic keratinocytes) in the papillary dermis

Dermoscopy may show white crossing lines suggestive of WS on a dull red background and peripheral arrangement of vessels.[16] Friedmann has observed white pearly structures corresponding to WS with arboriform projections of "fern leaf" pattern and erythematous globules at their edges.[17]

Differential Diagnosis

Lichenoid eruption: Cutaneous lesions are more pruritic, inflammatory and eczematous with intense post-inflammatory pigmentation (Fig. 14.5). The history of drug intake and a skin biopsy help to differentiate it from idiopathic LP. Histopathology shows a patchy lymphoid infiltrate with abundant eosinophils unlike the band-like and monomorphic lymphoid infiltrate in idiopathic LP.

Chronic graft-versus-host disease causes a lichenoid eruption which is clinically and histopathologically similar to LP. The history of haematopoietic cell transplant helps in the differentiation.

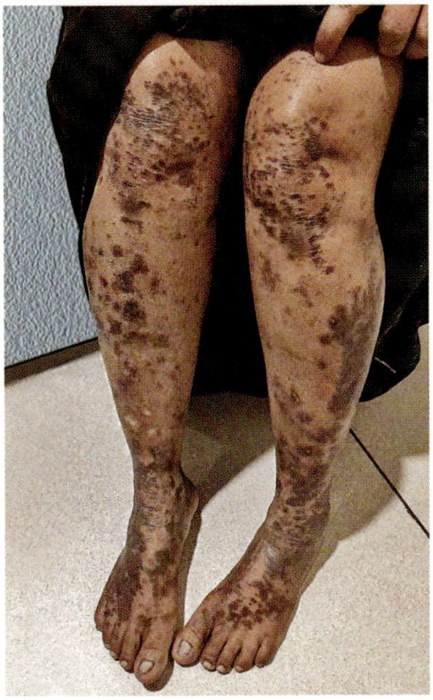

Fig. 14.5: Lichenoid eruption due to amlodipine

Diseases like psoriasis, lichen simplex chronicus, subacute cutaneous LE, DLE, pityriasis rosea, secondary syphilis, and prurigo nodularis can be differentiated from LP by the typical clinical findings and histopathology.

Complications

Erosive oral LP may rarely turn malignant. Dyslipidemia has also been reported.[18,19]

Treatment

Treatment depends on the type of LP, whether localized or generalized.

Topical corticosteroids are the mainstay of treatment for localized LP. Moderate to high potency steroids like betamethasone dipropionate 0.05%, mometasone or clobetasol are commonly used.[1,20] Intralesional triamcinolone acetonide is used for hypertrophic lesions. A short course of systemic steroids, 30–60 mg daily for 4–6 weeks with weekly tapering, is useful in widespread lesions.

Lower doses and shorter courses have also been tried. For generalised or eruptive LP systemic steroids are required for a period of 8–12 weeks.

Alternative treatments include acitretin and narrowband UVB.[20]

CONCLUSION

Lichen planus is a common papulosquamous disorder of autoimmune aetiology. Its association with HC is still unproven. It may be associated with dyslipidaemia. Dermoscopy may aid in diagnosis. Treatment includes topical and systemic steroids.

References

1. Le Cleach L, Chosidow O. Clinical practice. Lichen planus. N Engl J Med 2012; 366:723.
2. Wagner G, Rose C, Sachse MM. Clinical variants of lichen planus. J Dtsch Dermatol Ges 2013; 11:309.
3. Raveendra L. A clinical study of geriatric dermatoses. Our Dermatol Online. 2014; 5:235–9.
4. Sahoo A, Singh PC, Pattnaik S, Panigrahi RK. Geriatric Dermatoses in Southern Orissa. Indian J Dermatol. 2000; 45:66–8.
5. Shengyuan L, Songpo Y, Wen W, Wenjing T, Haitao Z, Binyou W. Hepatitis C virus and lichen planus: a reciprocal association determined by a meta-analysis. Arch Dermatol 2009; 145:1040.
6. Chainani-Wu N, Lozada-Nur F, Terrault N. Hepatitis C virus and lichen planus: a review. Oral Surg Oral Med Oral Pathol Oral Radiol Endod 2004; 98:171.
7. Lehman JS, Tollefson MM, Gibson LE. Lichen planus. Int J Dermatol 2009; 48:682.
8. Hussein MR. Evaluation of angiogenesis in normal and lichen planus skin by CD34 protein immunohistochemistry: preliminary findings. Cell Biol Int 2007; 31:1292.
9. Chen X, Liu Z, Yue Q. The expression of TNF-α and ICAM-1 in lesions of lichen planus and its implication. J Huazhong Univ Sci Technolog Med Sci 2007; 27:739.
10. Perry D, Fazel N. Zosteriform lichen planus. Dermatol Online J 2006; 12:3.
11. Shemer A, Weiss G, Trau H. Wolf's isotopic response: a case of zosteriform lichen planus on the site of healed herpes zoster. J Eur Acad Dermatol Venereol 2001; 15:445.

12. Ghorpade A. Wolf's isotopic response—lichen planus at the site of healed herpes zoster in an Indian woman. Int J Dermatol 2010; 49:234.
13. Durai PC, Thappa DM, Kumari R, and Malathi M. "Aging in elderly: chronological versus photo-aging." Indian Journal of Dermatology 2012; 57: 343–52.
14. Eisen D. The vulvovaginal-gingival syndrome of lichen planus. The clinical characteristics of 22 patients. Arch Dermatol 1994; 130:1379.
15. Fox LP, Lightdale CJ, Grossman ME. Lichen planus of the esophagus: what dermatologists need to know.J Am Acad Dermatol 2011; 65:175.
16. Lallas A, Kyrgidis A, Tzellos TG.Accuracy of dermoscopic criteria for the diagnosis of psoriasis, dermatitis, lichen planus and pityriasis rosea. Br J Dermatol 2012; 166:1198.
17. Friedman P, Sabban EC, Marcucci C, Peralta R, Cabo H. Dermoscopic findings in different clinical variants of lichen planus. Is dermoscopy useful? Dermatol Pract Concept 2015; 5:51.
18. Arias-Santiago S, Buendía-Eisman A, Aneiros-Fernández J, Giron–Prieto MS,Guttierrrez–Salmeron MT, Mellado VG et alCardiovascular risk factors in patients with lichen planus. Am J Med 2011; 124:543.
19. Dreiher J, Shapiro J, Cohen AD. Lichen planus and dyslipidaemia: a case-control study. Br J Dermatol 2009; 161:626.
20. Lehman JS, Tollefson MM, Gibson LE. Lichen planus. Int J Dermatol 2009; 48:682.

PITYRIASIS RUBRA PILARIS

Key Points

- PRP is a papulosquamous disease characterised by erythematous, follicular hyperkeratotic papules and plaques with islands of normal skin, diffuse scaling of scalp and 'keratodermic sandals' of hands and feet.
- There are 6 clinical types, the most common in elderly being type I.
- Type V PRP is considered an autoinflammatory disease caused by *CARD14* mutations.
- A rare variant of *CARD14* is implicated in the pathophysiology of other forms of PRP.
- Diagnosis is based on clinical features and histopathology.
- The important differential diagnoses are psoriasis and drug eruptions.
- Systemic retinoids are effective, methotrexate being an alternative drug.
- Cyclosporine, azathioprine and biologicals may be effective in resistant PRP.

Introduction

PRP is a chronic papulosquamous disorder of unknown aetiology. It has a diverse clinical picture characterised by follicular erythematous hyperkeratotic papules and scaly psoriasiform plaques, with islands of normal skin, diffuse scaling of scalp and palmoplantar hyperkeratosis.

Epidemiolgy

In the study by Darjani et al, the prevalence of pityriasis rubra pilaris was 1.1%.[1]

Both sexes are almost equally affected.

Etiopathogenesis

The exact etiology is still unknown. Several immunodeficient states, autoimmune disorders and malignancies are associated with it suggestive of immune dysfunction.[2]

Type V PRP is considered an autoinflammatory disease caused by *CARD14* mutations, and a rare variant of *CARD14* is implicated in the pathophysiology of other forms of PRP.[3]

Clinical Features

According to **Griffith's classification,** there are 6 clinical subtypes.[3]

Type 1 (classical adult) is the most common form seen in the elderly. A cephalocaudal progression of lesions is seen. The characteristic findings are follicular, erythematous, hyperkeratotic, papules and plaques with fine and powdery scales with islands of normal skin, and diffuse hyperkeratosis of the palms and soles. It generally has a favourable prognosis as almost 80% of patients achieve spontaneous remission within three years.[4]

Type II (atypical adult) classical cephalo-caudal progression is not seen. The most striking features are thick scaly plaques mainly on the lower extremities and prominent palmoplantar hyperkeratosis. The prognosis is less favourable as it has a protracted course of several years, and less than 20% achieve clinical resolution within three years.[5]

Type III (classical juvenile) the clinical manifestations are similar to type I.

Type IV (circumscribed juvenile) is seen in prepubertal children and young adults.

Type V (atypical juvenile) is relatively uncommon, representing around 5% of cases.

Type VI associated with HIV infection is characterised by extensive erythematous follicular keratotic papules and inflammatory plaques.[6] Erythroderma is a frequent complication.[4] It may occur along with other disorders of follicular occlusion like acne conglobata, hidradenitis suppurativa and lichen spinulosus.[7] Oral mucosal involvement is rare and may appear as white papules or plaques **(frost glass appearance)** on the palate, buccal mucosa and tongue. Ocular lesions include cicatricial ectropion and peripheral ulcerative keratitis.

Diagnosis

The diagnosis of PRP depends on the typical clinical and histopathologic features.

Histopathology

The typical features are hyperkeratosis with patchy parakeratosis, alternating orthokeratosis and parakeratosis in vertical and horizontal directions; surrounding follicular ostia resembling checkerboard, irregular acanthosis, normal granular layer and mild perivascular lymphohistiocytic infiltrate in the dermis. Mild spongiosis and focal acantholytic dyskeratosis may also be seen.

Differential Diagnosis

Psoriasis is the most important differential diagnosis.

Both may present with scaly erythematous plaques. Follicular keratotic papules and plaques with fine scales and keratodermic sandals of palms and soles are characteristic of PRP while sharply demarcated non-follicular erythematous papules and plaques with silvery white scales suggest psoriasis. Typical nail changes of psoriasis also help in differentiation.

Prognosis

The prognosis is variable and depends on the clinical type and associations.

Treatment

Topical therapeutic agents include emollients, keratolytics like salicylic acid and urea, coal tar preparations, topical steroids, calcipotriene, cacipotriol, topical tretinoin and tazarotene.[8,9]

Systemic Treatment

Retinoids are the first-line drugs.[10] Isotretinoin in a dose of 1 mg/kg/day and acitretin 0.5 mg/kg/day are used.

Adverse effects of retinoid therapy include dryness of skin and mucosae, hyperlipidaemia, transaminase elevations and visual or bone changes.[11]

Methotrexate is an alternative agent. Dose is 5–25 mg/week for patients who fail to respond to systemic retinoids, or if retinoids are contraindicated.[11,12] For non-responders to methotrexate, cyclosporine and azathioprine may be used.

Biologic Agents

TNF-alpha inhibitors like etanercept, infliximab and adalimumab may be useful in resistant cases. **Ustekinumab**, a human monoclonal antibody that targets IL-12 and IL-23, has been tried in type I and familial PRP. One patient with refractory PRP responded to **secukinumab**, an anti-IL-17A antibody.[13,14]

Reactivation or exacerbations of infections are potential side effects of these biologic agents.

Phototherapy NBUVB has been found to be effective.

Apremilast (oral phosphodiesterase 4-inhibitors) is a new addition in the treatment of refractory PRP.[15]

CONCLUSION

PRP is a papulosquamous inflammatory dermatosis occasionally encountered in elderly. The typical clinical features include follicular hyperkeratotic plaques, islands of normal skin and palmoplantar hyperkeratosis. Immune dysfunction may have an etiologic role.

Systemic retinoids, biologic agents, immunosuppressants and PDE4 inhibitors like apremilast may be tried for refractory cases.

Papulosquamous diseases are rather rare in the elderly. History taking, diagnosis and management may be challenging in them due to various factors like declining cognitive status such as loss of memory, dementia, impaired sensory functions and physical limitations. To maximize the efficacy and compliance, the treatment regimen should be kept as simple as possible.

References

1. Darjani A,Mohtasham-Amiri Z, Mohammad Amini K, Sadre-Eshkevari S, Alizade N. Skin disorders among elder patients in a referral center in Northern Iran. Dermatology Research and Practice 2013. Article ID 193205.
2. Garretson CB, Machan ML, Krejci-Manwaring J, Aires D, Tonkovic-Capin V.Letter: Adenocarcinoma of the lung associated with pityriasis rubra pilaris. Dermatol Online J 2011; 17:14.
3. Takeichi T, Sugiura K, Nomura T, Sakamoto T,Ogawa Y,Oiso N et al. Pityriasis Rubra Pilaris Type V as an Autoinflammatory Disease by CARD14 Mutations. *JAMA Dermatol.* 2017; 153:66–70. doi:10.1001/jamadermatol. 2016.3601
4. De D, Dogra S, Narang T, Radotra BD, Kanwar AJ. Pityriasis rubra pilaris in a HIV-positive patient (Type 6 PRP). Skinmed 2008; 7:47.
5. Blasdale C, Turner RJ, Leonard N, Ong ELC, Lawrence CM. Spontaneous clinical improvement in HIV-associated follicular syndrome. Clin Exp Dermatol 2004; 29:480.
6. Griffiths WA. Pityriasis rubra pilaris. Clin Exp Dermatol 1980; 5:105.
7. Klein A, Landthaler M, Karrer S. Pityriasis rubra pilaris: a review of diagnosis and treatment. Am J Clin Dermatol 2010; 11:157.
8. Eastham AB, Femia AN, Qureshi A, Vleugels RA. Treatment options for pityriasis rubra pilaris including biologic agents: a retrospective analysis from an academic medical center. JAMA Dermatol 2014; 150:92.
9. Ross NA, Chung HJ, Li Q, Andrews JP, Keller MS, Uitto J. Epidemiologic, Clinicopathologic, Diagnostic, and Management Challenges of Pityriasis Rubra Pilaris: A Case Series of 100 Patients. JAMA Dermatol 2016; 152:670.
10. Patton TJ, Zirwas MJ, Wolverton SE. Systemic retinoids. In: Comprehensive Dermatologic Drug Therapy, 2nd ed, Wolverton SE (Ed), Elsevier, Philadelphia 2007. p.275.
11. van Dooren-Greebe RJ, van de Kerkhof PC. Extensive extraspinal hyperostoses after long-term oral retinoid treatment in a patient with pityriasis rubra pilaris. J Am Acad Dermatol 1995; 32:322.
12. Durairaj VD, Horsley MB. Resolution of pityriasis rubra pilaris-induced cicatricial ectropion with systemic low-dose methotrexate. Am J Ophthalmol 2007; 143:709.
13. Petrof G, Almaani N, Archer CB,Griffiths WA, Smith CH. A systematic review of the literature on the treatment of pityriasis rubra pilaris type 1 with TNF-antagonists. J Eur Acad Dermatol Venereol 2013; 27:e131.
14. Feldmeyer L, Mylonas A, Demaria O.Interleukin 23-Helper T Cell 17 Axis as a Treatment Target for Pityriasis Rubra Pilaris. JAMA Dermatol 2017; 153:304.
15. Krase IZ, Cavanaugh K, Curiel-Lewandrowski C. Treatment of Refractory Pityriasis Rubra Pilaris With Novel Phosphodiesterase 4 (PDE4) Inhibitor Apremilast. JAMA Dermatol 2016; 152:348.

CHAPTER 15

Connective Tissue Diseases in Elderly

• *Angoori Gyaneswari*

Introduction

Connective tissue disorders are the diseases in which the basic pathology lies in the connective tissue. Lupus erythematosus, systemic sclerosis, dermatomyositis, rheumatoid arthritis and Sjögren's syndrome are included in connective tissue disorders.

LUPUS ERYTHEMATOSUS

Key Points

- Uncommon in elderly
- Female predominance not very conspicuous
- Malar rash, renal manifestations less frequent
- Lung involvement, pericarditis, sicca syndrome seen

Systemic lupus erythematosus (SLE) is a multisystem disorder whose spectrum runs from benign, self-limiting cutaneous eruptions to severe, often fatal, systemic disease.

Epidemiology

The prevalence of SLE in elderly population ranges from 4 to 18%[1] and the female to male ratio being 1.1:1.[2] Lesser predominance of female population in elderly group is due to lack of hormonal influence (estrogens) which is the most important factor in pathogenesis of SLE. Estrogens modulate T cell function, cytokine production and various other immunological pathways in women, hence SLE is more common in women in the child-bearing age group.

Etiopathogenesis

It is postulated that SLE is an autoimmune disease. Genetic, environmental and hormonal factors play an important role in initiation and aggravation of autoimmune response. Drugs known to precipitate SLE are hydralazine, procainamide, minocycline and isoniazid.

The pathological changes of SLE are fibrinoid necrosis, collagen sclerosis, necrosis and basophilic body formation, with vascular endothelial thickening.

Clinical Features

Gillian classified cutaneous lupus into three major forms:

1. Acute cutaneous lupus erythematosus
2. Subacute cutaneous lupus erythematosus
3. Chronic cutaneous lupus erythematosus

Acute Cutaneous Lupus Erythematosus (ACLE)

Acute presentation of lupus may be first detected on the skin. Classically the acute eruption of SLE may present as a photosensitive 'butterfly rash', consisting of erythema across the malar cheeks and nose[3] (Fig. 15.1).

Classic malar rash is less prevalent among elderly people in whom the frequent manifestations include sicca syndrome, pericarditis or lung involvement.[4,5] Renal manifestations are less prevalent in late onset SLE. Other cutaneous

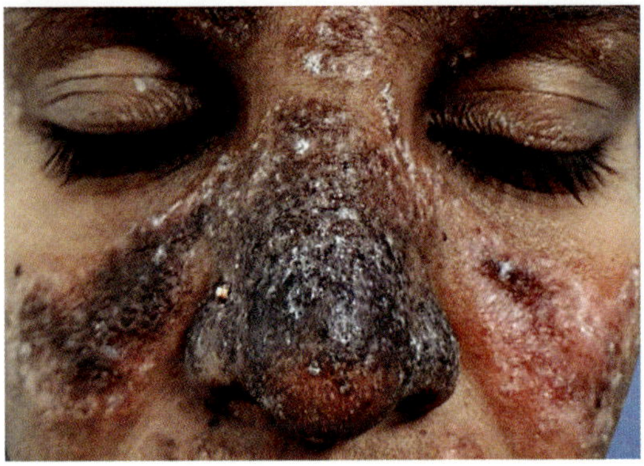

Fig. 15.1: Malar rash

manifestations may include oral or nasal ulcerations, periungual telangiectasia, and diffuse and nonspecific alopecia (Box 15.1).

Subacute Cutaneous Lupus Erythematosus (SCLE)

SCLE presents in two forms: Annular and psoriasiform.[6] Both forms tend to present on the sun-exposed skin of the face, arms, upper chest and back. The annular form presents with erythematous rings of scaling and central clearing. The psoriasiform variant presents with more uniformly erythematous and scaly plaques, similar to psoriasis, but not involving only extensor surfaces. SCLE is more commonly associated with Sjögren's syndrome.

Chronic Cutaneous Lupus Erythematosus (CCLE)

CCLE also known as DLE (discoid lupus erythematosus), tends to involve the photo-exposed areas of the head, neck and upper trunk. Presence of lesions below the neck are seen in generalized DLE which has a higher risk of systemic involvement. Classically, DLE presents with indurated, erythematous, and scaly plaques that are associated with follicular plugging and central hypopigmentation with peripheral hyperpigmentation. The disease often first becomes apparent in the conchal bowls of the ear (Shuster's sign).

Box 15.1: Clinical manifestations of SLE in patients with late-onset disease

Common
- Nonspecific symptoms (fatigue, weakness, etc.)
- Serositis
- Lung involvement
- Sjögren's syndrome
- Cytopenias
- Cognitive dysfunction

Infrequent
- Seizures
- Psychosis
- Renal involvement
- Integument manifestations
- Arthritis

Diagnosis

By SLICC—systemic lupus erythematosus international collaborating clinic criteria.

≥4 criteria (at least one clinical and one laboratory criteria) or biopsy proven lupus nephritis with positive ANA or anti-DNA.

Clinical Criteria

1. **Acute cutaneous lupus or subacute cutaneous lupus**
   - *Acute cutaneous lupus:* Lupus malar rash (do not count if malar discoid), bullous lupus, toxic epidermal necrolysis variant of SLE, maculopapular lupus rash, photosensitive lupus rash (in the absence of dermatomyositis).
   - *Subacute cutaneous lupus:* Non-indurated psoriasiform and/or annular polycyclic lesions that resolve without scarring, although occasionally with postinflammatory dyspigmentation or telangiectasia.
2. **Chronic cutaneous lupus**
   - Classic discoid rash localized (above the neck) or generalized (above and below the neck), hypertrophic (verrucous) lupus, lupus panniculitis (profundus), mucosal lupus, lupus erythematosus tumidus, chilblain lupus, discoid lupus/lichen planus overlap.

3. **Oral ulcers or nasal ulcers:**
   - Oral: Ulcers on palate (Fig. 15.2), buccal mucosa and tongue.
   - Nasal ulcers.
   - In the absence of other causes, such as vasculitis, Behçet's disease, infection (herpesvirus), inflammatory bowel disease, reactive arthritis, and acidic foods.
4. **Non-scarring alopecia:** Diffuse thinning or hair fragility with visible broken hairs, in the absence of other causes such as alopecia areata, drugs, iron deficiency, and androgenic alopecia.
5. **Synovitis involving 2 or more joints:**
   - Characterized by joint swelling or effusion.
   - Tenderness in 2 or more joints and at least 30 minutes of morning stiffness.
6. **Serositis:**
   - Typical pleurisy for more than one day or pleural effusions or pleural rub.
   - Typical pericardial pain (pain with recumbency improved by sitting forward) for more than one day or pericardial effusion or pericardial rub or pericarditis by electrocardiography.
   - In the absence of other causes, such as infection, uraemia, and Dressler's pericarditis.

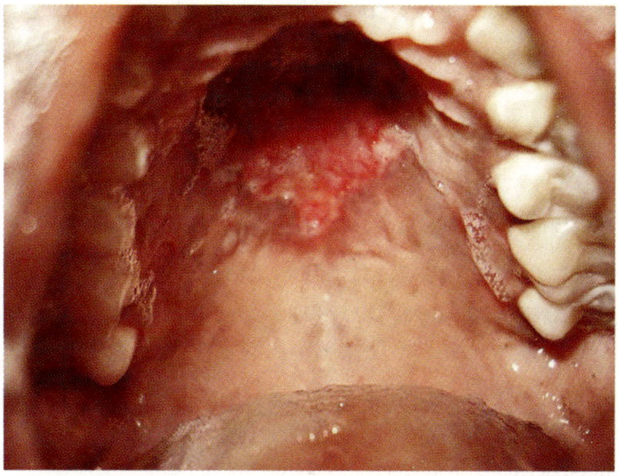

Fig. 15.2: Ulcers on palate

7. **Renal** Urine protein-to-creatinine ratio (or 24-hour urine protein) representing 500 mg protein/24 hours or red blood cell casts.
8. **Neurologic:** Seizures, psychosis, mononeuritis multiplex (in the absence of other known causes such as primary vasculitis), myelitis, peripheral or cranial neuropathy (in the absence of other known causes such as primary vasculitis, infection, and diabetes mellitus), acute confusional state (in the absence of other causes, including toxic/metabolic, uraemia, drugs).
9. **Hemolytic anaemia**
10. **Leukopenia (<4000/cubic mm) or lymphopenia (<1000/cubic mm):**
    - Leukopenia at least once: In the absence of other known causes such as Felty's syndrome, drugs, and portal hypertension.
    - Lymphopenia at least once: In the absence of other known causes such as corticosteroids, drugs, and infection.
11. **Thrombocytopenia (<100,000/mm^3):**
    - At least once in the absence of other known causes such as drugs, portal hypertension, and thrombotic thrombocytopenic purpura.

Immunologic Criteria

1. ANA level above laboratory reference range.
2. Anti-dsDNA antibody level above laboratory reference range (or 2-fold the reference range if tested by ELISA).
3. Anti-Sm: Presence of antibody to Sm nuclear antigen.
4. Antiphospholipid antibody positivity, as determined by:
   - Positive test for lupus anticoagulant
   - False-positive test result for rapid plasma reagin
   - Medium- or high-titer anticardiolipin antibody level (IgA, IgG, or IgM)
   - Positive test result for anti-2-glycoprotein I (IgA, IgG, or IgM).

5. Low complement (C3, C4, or CH50).
6. Direct Coombs' test (in the absence of haemolytic anaemia).

A. Patients with late-onset lupus may exhibit a different autoantibody profile compared to patients with younger-onset disease. Lower frequency of anti-dsDNA,[7,8] anti-RNP,[7,9] anti-Sm[10,11] antibodies are found in SLE of late-onset. Higher frequency of rheumatoid factor,[12] anti-Ro and anti-La antibodies[13] are found which correlate with the increased frequency of Sjögren's syndrome in the elderly patients.

B. Skin biopsy may reveal vacuolar alterations of the basal layer of keratinocytes, dermal mucin accumulation, and superficial, deep, and periadnexal inflammatory infiltrate. Overlying hyperkeratosis and follicular plugging are prominent in case of DLE.

Complications

1. Diffuse alveolar haemorrhage with haemoptysis
2. Severe neurological impairment
3. Systemic vasculitis
4. Rapidly progressive glomerulonephritis
5. Malignancy and skin scarring. Some studies have found increased association of SLE with thyroid cancers. Hodgkin and non-Hodgkin lymphomas.

Treatment

The basic principles of photoprotection like long-sleeved clothes, shirts that button high on the chest, broad-brimmed hats, and broad-spectrum (UVA and UVB blocking) sunscreens remain the same regardless of the age of patient, but it is necessary to take into account the pharmacokinetics of dugs which might be altered in elderly people. Antimalarial agent, hydroxychloroquine (HCQS) can be prescribed safely in elderly. Glucocorticoids and immunosuppressants such as cyclophosphamide, azathioprine and mycophenolate mofetil are indicated in systemic involvement; renal, respiratory, haemopoietic or central nervous system. As these drugs are needed for prolonged periods, judicious usage is imperative in order to avoid potential risk of life-threatening infections and malignancy. Since most geriatric individuals have comorbidities like diabetes mellitus and hypertension and are on polypharmacy, treating physician need to be vigilant while treating these patients. Moreover, careful dose titration is required to lessen the burden on liver and kidneys. Since DLE is not usually associated with systemic involvement, treatment is primarily aimed at preventing and controlling symptoms. An initial workup for systemic lupus is warranted for a patient with newly diagnosed DLE. Sunscreens, high-potency topical and intralesional steroids are the mainstay of treatment.

The prognosis of SLE in the elderly is better than that of younger population. If corticosteroid therapy is required, the use of smaller doses may be sufficient to treat the more severe component of the disease.

SYSTEMIC SCLEROSIS IN ELDERLY (Synonyms: Scleroderma; Progressive Systemic Sclerosis)

Key Points

- Majority of cases seen before 65 years. Digital ischaemia is less common
- May have higher prevalence of anticentromere antibodies
- Late onset disease has higher prevalence of pulmonary artery hypertension, cardiac and renal involvement.

Introduction

Systemic sclerosis (SSc) is an uncommon autoimmune connective tissue disease of unknown aetiology that affects the skin, blood vessels (obliterative vasculopathy) and internal organs. The term scleroderma is derived from the Greek word *skleros* (hard or indurated).

Classification

It encompasses two clinical variants, limited and diffuse.

Limited systemic sclerosis (LSSc) represents fibrotic changes limited to fingers, hands and face and includes CREST syndrome.

Diffuse systemic sclerosis (dSSc): Here, fibrotic changes are more generalised usually starting from fingers and hand but spread to forearms, arms, trunk, face and lower extremities.

Diffuse SSc is more frequently associated with early onset (within 5 years of disease onset) of internal organ involvement compared to limited disease.

Systemic sclerosis sine scleroderma denotes condition with serological positivity and Raynaud's phenomenon without skin lesions.[14]

Epidemiology

Usually more common between ages of 30 and 50 years but can occur in children and elderly.[14] True incidence in elderly is believed to be under reported as specialist consultations are less frequent. Moreover, disease pattern might be slightly different and symptoms might mimic other chronic age-related disorders.[15] Most of the elderly onset SSc patients develop SSc before 65 years of age whereas LSSc is more common in elderly after the age of 75 years.[17] SSc occurs more frequently in women compared to men. Predictors for worst prognosis are male sex, black race, older age,[4] internal organ involvement, fibrosis of trunk and elevated ESR.[14]

Etiopathogenesis

Basic pathology includes:[14]

1. Microvascular injury and damage
2. Immune activation with autoantibody production
3. Tissue fibrosis with deposition of collagen and extracellular matrix proteins.

Criteria for Diagnosis

The ACR-EULAR Criteria

These criteria are applicable to any patient considered for inclusion in a SSc study.

1. These criteria are not applicable to: (a) Patients having a SSc-like disorder better explaining their manifestations, such as: nephrogenic sclerosing fibrosis, generalised morphea, eosinophilic fasciitis, scleroderma diabeticorum, scleromyxedema, erythromyalgia, porphyria, lichen sclerosis, graft-versus-host disease, and diabetic cheiropathy. (b) Patients with *'skin thickening sparing the fingers'*.

Cutaneous features: Early phase of SSc is represented by edematous phase with possible pitting oedema of digits followed by phases of induration and atrophy consecutively. Apart from fibrosis, dyspigmentation is very common in form of hyperpigmentation and localized depigmentation sparing the perifollicular areas giving rise to characteristic 'salt and pepper' appearance (Fig. 15.3). Matted or squared-off telangiectasia is seen most often on lips and palms. SSc is a common cause of secondary Raynaud's phenomenon. Individuals with late onset SSc usually exhibit Raynaud's phenomenon at around 65 years of age. Capillary changes in proximal nail folds, calcinosis cutis (usually on joints and distal extremities), cutaneous ulcers, stellate scars (Fig. 15.4) (due to ischaemia, fibrosis and trauma) and dryness (loss of hair follicles and sebaceous glands) form rest of the cutaneous manifestations.[14] Digital ischaemia is less frequent in late-age onset compared to younger onset SSc.[16]

Manifestations of systemic involvement include: Pulmonary artery hypertension (PAH), restrictive lung disease, cardiac disease, digital ischaemia, severe gastrointestinal involvement, renal involvement, muscle weakness. PAH is the most significant health concern among elderly SSc patients. In late onset SSc risk of PAH is twice that of

Items	Sub-items	Weight/score
Skin thickening of the fingers of both hands extending proximal to the metacarpophalangeal joints *(sufficient criterion)*		9
Skin thickening of the fingers	Puffy fingers	2
	Sclerodactyly of the fingers (distal to metacarpophalangeal joints (MCP) but proximal to the proximal interphalangeal joints (PIP)	4
Fingertip lesions *(only count the highest score)*	Digital tip ulcer	2
	Fingertip pitting scars	3
Telangiectasia		2
Abnormal nailfold capillaries		2
Pulmonary arterial hypertension and/or Interstitial lung disease* (*Maximum score is 2)	Pulmonary artery hypertension (PAH) Interstitial lung disease (ILD)	2
Raynaud's phenomenon		3
Scleroderma related antibodies** (any of anti-centromere, anti-topoisomerase I, anti-RNA polymerase III) (**Maximum score is 3)		3

*Patients having a total score of 9 or more are being classified as having definite systemic sclerosis.
**Add the maximum weight (score) in each category to calculate the total score.
(*Adapted from* classification criteria for systemic sclerosis: An ACR-EULAR collaborative initiative).

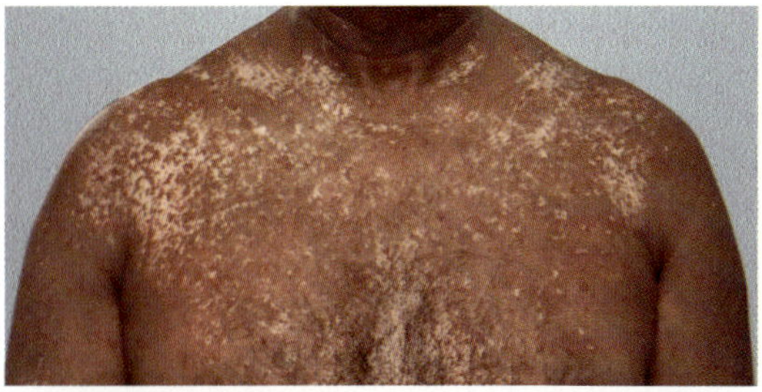

Fig. 15.3: Salt and pepper dyspigmentation

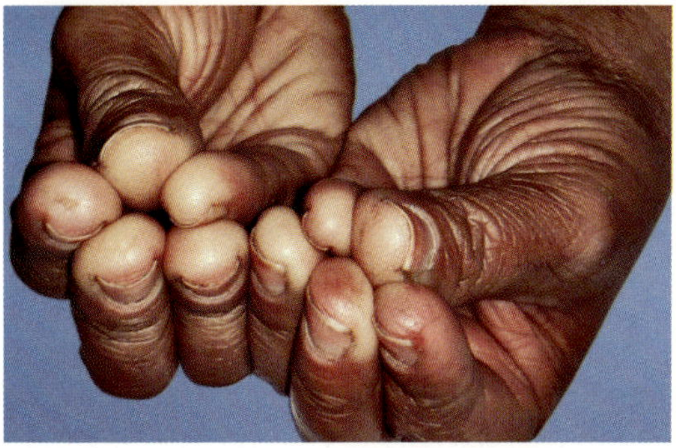

Fig. 15.4: Stellate scars

younger onset. Patients with long-term, active interstitial lung fibrosis, long standing gastro-oesophageal reflux disease and extensive skin fibrosis have higher risk of development of late lung, skin or oesophageal cancers.[18]

Scleroderma-like paraneoplastic syndrome (SPS) can occur in elderly patients suffering from cancers and must be differentiated especially in elderly patients with SSc symptoms. SPS can be differentiated from late onset SSc by positive family history of malignancies and oncogenic exposures earlier in life, asymmetric skin fibrosis, absence or asymmetric Raynaud's phenomenon, lack of abnormalities typical for SSc on capillaroscopy, absence of antibody characteristic for scleroderma, absence of fever and weight loss, poorer response to treatment and disappearance of symptoms after successful treatment of underlying malignancy.[19]

Possible Clinical Features of Systemic Sclerosis

Skin manifestations	Diffuse oedema—hands and feet, progressive skin tightening, sclerodactyly, calcinosis, telangiectasia, digital ulcers and stellate scars, hyper- and hypopigmentation of skin with salt and pepper appearance, and characteristic facies
Vascular features	Raynaud's phenomenon, nail fold capillary changes, digital ischaemia, ulcers, vasculitic leg ulcers
Pulmonary changes	• Interstitial lung disease, including alveolitis and interstitial fibrosis, pulmonary hypertension • Recurrent aspiration pneumonitis caused by oesophageal reflux and dysmotility, chest wall restriction (decreased thoracic compliance), respiratory muscle weakness
Cardiac	• Cardiomyopathy (systolic and diastolic dysfunction): Congestive heart failure, conduction defects • Septal infarction pattern, ventricular conduction abnormalities, arrhythmias, heart blocks, pericarditis or pericardial effusion (impending renal crisis)
Renal	Scleroderma renal crisis (hypertension, renal failure MAHA)?
Muscular	• Arthralgia, tendon friction rubs (relatively specific for diffuse scleroderma), inflammatory arthritis, erosive arthropathy (rare) myopathy, myositis
Gastrointestinal	• Gastroesophageal reflux, esophageal dysmotility, aperistaltic esophagus, esophageal stricture • Adenocarcinoma arising in Barrett's esophagus (occasionally), watermelon stomach (gastric antral vascular ectasia—GAVE): Iron-deficiency anaemia, decreased peristalsis throughout the GI tract, leading to bloating, early satiety, stasis, and pseudo-obstruction, bacterial overgrowth and malabsorptive diarrhoea, alternating diarrhoea and constipation, megacolon (rare), colonic wide-mouth diverticuli (usually asymptomatic), pneumatosis cystoides intestinalis, primary biliary cirrhosis, anal incontinence
Neurological	• Carpal tunnel syndrome, trigeminal neuralgia

Autoantibodies in Systemic Sclerosis

Serologically SSc is characterized by several autoantibodies against nucleus, cytoplasm and extracellular autoantigens. ANAs are detected in more than 90% of patients with SSc. Autoantibodies participate in disease pathogenesis and can precede the clinical manifestation and have prognostic value also. Anti-centromere antibodies (ACA), anti-DNA topoisomerase I antibodies, and anti-RNA polymerase III antibodies are representative ANAs found in patients with SSc.[20] Late onset SSc patients tend to have more ACA, but less anti-U1RNP antibodies than those with younger-age onset disease.[17]

Treatment of Systemic Sclerosis

The updated EULAR recommendations for treatment of systemic sclerosis, according to the organ involvement.

ACE, angiotensin converting enzyme; ERA, endothelin receptor antagonist; EULAR: European league against rheumatism; GERD: Gastroesophageal reflux disease; HSCT: Haematopoietic stem cell transplantation; ILD: Interstitial lung disease; PAH: Pulmonary arterial hypertension; PDE-5: Phosphodiesterase type 5; PPI: Proton pump inhibitors; RCT: Randomized controlled trial; SRC: Scleroderma renal crisis; SSc: Systemic sclerosis; SSc-RP: Raynaud's phenomenon in patients with systemic sclerosis.

Organ involvement	Recommendation
I. SSc-RP	Dihydropiridine-type calcium antagonists, usually oral nifedipine, should be considered for first-line therapy for SSc-RP. PDE-5 inhibitors should also be considered in treatment of SSc-RP. Intravenous iloprost should be considered for severe SSc-RP. Experts recommend that intravenous iloprost should be used for treatment of SSc-RP attacks after oral therapy. Fluoxetine might be considered in treatment of SSc-RP attacks.
II. Digital ulcers in patients with SSc	Intravenous iloprost should be considered in the treatment of digital ulcers in patients with SSc PDE-5 inhibitors should be considered in the treatment of digital ulcers in patients with SSc Bosentan should be considered for reduction of the number of new digital ulcers in SSc, especially in patients with multiple digital ulcers despite use of calcium channel blockers, PDE-5 inhibitors or iloprost therapy
III. SSc-PAH	ERA, PDE-5 inhibitors or riociguat should be considered to treat SSc-related PAH. Intravenous epoprostenol should be considered for the treatment of patients with severe SSc-PAH (class III and class IV). Prostacyclin analogues should be considered for the treatment of patients with SSc-PAH.
IV. Skin and lung disease	Methotrexate may be considered for treatment of skin manifestations of early dSSc. In view of the results from two high-quality randomized controlled studies and despite its known toxicity, cyclophosphamide should be considered for treatment of SSc-ILD, in particular for patients with SSc with progressive ILD. HSCT should be considered for treatment of selected patients with rapidly progressive SSc at risk of organ failure. In view of the high risk of treatment-related side effects and of early treatment-related mortality, careful selection of patients with SSc for this kind of treatment.
V. SRC	Experts recommend immediate use of ACE inhibitors in the treatment of SRC Blood pressure and renal function should be carefully monitored in patients with SSc treated with glucocorticoids.
VI. SSc-related gastrointestinal disease	Proton pump inhibitors should be used for the treatment of SSc-related gastro-oesophageal reflux and prevention of oesophageal ulcers and strictures. Prokinetic drugs should be used for the management of SSc-related symptomatic motility disturbances (dysphagia, GERD, early satiety, bloating, pseudo-obstruction, etc). Intermittent or rotating antibiotics should be used to treat symptomatic small intestine bacterial overgrowth in patients with SSc.

DERMATOMYOSITIS

Key Points

- Late onset (>60 years) is associated with risk of internal malignancies
- Higher probability of cardiac involvement, bacterial pneumonia and bowel infarction

Classic dermatomyositis (DM) is an autoimmune connective tissue disease that may affect multiple systems along with skin.

Epidemiology

Incidence rates of dermatomyositis (DM) are bimodal, peaking in childhood and then again in adults with mean age of 45–64 years.[21] The mean age is higher (60 years) for those with malignancy-associated myositis, and conversely, the elderly individuals with DM have a higher incidence of malignancy.[22]

Etiopathogenesis

It is believed to result from an immune-mediated process triggered by various factors such as malignancy, drugs and infectious agents in genetically predisposed individuals. Here the autoantigens activate the immune process in which complement is deposited in capillaries, resulting capillary necrosis, leading to ischaemia.

Clinical Features

1. Proximal muscle weakness: Insidious onset (3–6 months) marked by exacerbations and remissions
2. Muscle atrophy and tenderness
3. Contractures
4. Heliotrope rash: A lilac discolouration of upper eyelids
5. Periorbital oedema
6. Gottron's sign: Scaly, erythematous eruption over knuckles, elbows, knees, medial malleoli, neck, face, and upper chest
7. Periungal erythema
8. Sclerodactyly
9. Raynaud's phenomenon
10. Arthralgias
11. Systemic: Fever, anorexia, weight loss, fatigue, malaise
12. Cardiac: Arrhythmias, congestive failure
13. Pulmonary: Interstitial lung disease

There were no differences in the duration of symptoms among elderly prior to diagnosis, or in frequencies of myositis diagnosed, Raynaud's phenomenon, dysphonia, cardiac impairment, interstitial lung disease, and peripheral neuropathy when compared with younger age group. However, higher incidence of oesophageal dysfunction and bacterial pneumonia are seen in elderly group. There is increased frequency of malignancy[23] in elderly onset dermatomyositis.

Diagnosis

Bohan and Peter criteria for diagnosis of polymyositis and dermatomyositis

1. Symmetrical proximal muscle weakness
2. Elevated serum muscle enzymes
3. Myopathic EMG
4. Muscle biopsy abnormality

The diagnosis of polymyositis is complete, if all four criteria are met. The diagnosis of dermatomyositis is complete, if three of the criteria plus a characteristic skin rash are identified.

Laboratory features of polymyositis/ dermatomyositis

1. Elevation of serum muscle enzymes, CPK, and aldolase in 98% of patients.
2. ESR variable; not specific.
3. Anaemia: Normochromic, normocytic; usually mild.
4. ANA levels are increased and anti-Jo-1 antibodies are found in approximately 20% of adults with dermatomyositis.

Complications

Malignancy is most common complication in patients with DM of late onset particularly ovarian and gastric cancer. Other complications include cardiomyopathy, cardiac conduction defects, diffuse interstitial pneumonitis, large bowel infarction, muscle atrophy and ocular complications.

Treatment

1. Bedrest
2. Mobilization and physical therapy
3. Patient education
4. Prednisone, 20 mg/day for at least 6 months, sometimes for as long as 5 years; no proven efficacy.
5. Immunosuppressive agents like methotrexate, IVIG and azathioprine if treatment fails with prednisone.

The response to therapy and outcome of elderly patients with PM–DM is poorer than that in younger adults.[24] Poor prognostic factors in DM include old age, presence of malignancy, gender, disease severity, dysphagia, bacterial pneumonia, delay in initiating therapy, and resistance to therapy.

SJÖGREN'S SYNDROME

Key Points

- Late onset disease more common in males
- Dry mouth and dry eyes are common symptoms
- Arthralgias are also frequent
- Anti-Ro antibody, parotitis, vasculitis–less common

Sjögren's syndrome is a progressive systemic autoimmune disease that affects primarily the exocrine system. The disease is characterized by lymphocytic infiltration causing exocrine gland dysfunction, resulting in mucosal dryness and other complications.

Epidemiology

Although Sjögren's syndrome can occur at almost any age, women in their fourth to sixth decades of life are most likely to be diagnosed with the disease. The estimated prevalence of Sjögren's syndrome in the general adult population is thought to be around 2–3%.[25]

Etiopathogenesis

Pathogenesis of Sjögren's syndrome is believed to be multifactorial. It is known to be autoimmune, but studies suggest that the disease process has genetic, environmental (Epstein-Barr virus/hepatitis C virus) and hormonal (associated with high prevalence in women especially estrogen) components.

Clinical Features

It is characterized by xerostomia (dry mouth), xerophthalmia (dry eyes), and lymphocytic infiltration of the exocrine glands. Cutaneous manifestation includes dryness and scaling of the skin, partial or complete anhidrosis, dry, sparse, and brittle hair leading to diffuse alopecia.

Erythema of the nose and cheeks may be present. Annular erythematous and scaling rash on the face and neck. Sjögren's vasculitis occurs (a form of leukocytoclastic vasculitis), typically on the lower legs (formerly Waldenstrom purpura).

Patients with Sjögren's syndrome have overlapping and/or associated acute systemic lupus erythematosus, subacute cutaneous lupus erythematosus, scleroderma or mixed connective tissue disease, and rheumatoid arthritis.

Elderly onset Sjögren's syndrome patients may be more likely to be male, have less parotid gland enlargement, articular involvement, cutaneous vasculitis, anti-Ro antibodies, and higher prevalence of peripheral neuropathy, interstitial pneumonitis, and hepatitis.[26]

Diagnosis

Criteria proposed by the American–European Consensus Group include six features:[27]

1. Ocular symptoms
2. Oral symptoms
3. Ocular signs (positive Schirmer's test or rose Bengal score)
4. Histopathology of minor lip salivary gland biopsy (greater or equal to one lymphocyte focus of 50 lymphocytes per 4 square mm of glandular tissue)
5. Salivary gland involvement (unstimulated salivary flow or parotid sialography)
6. Autoantibodies to Ro (SSA) or La (SSB) antigen.

Classified as having primary Sjögren's syndrome if four of the six criteria are met, including either positive histopathology or serology.

Complications

- Rheumatoid arthritis
- B cell non-Hodgkins lymphoma
- Raynaud's phenomenon

Treatment

Treatment depends on the severity of the disease. Artificial tear and saliva products are available to help with chronic dryness. The skin will often require repeated use of thick moisturizers, such as petrolatum. Systemic therapy includes hydroxychloroquine, steroids and cytotoxic therapy. Newer therapy includes anti-B cell monoclonal antibodies for glandular and extraglandular manifestations.

RHEUMATOID ARTHRITIS

Key Points

- 2% of prevalence among elderly onset rheumatoid arthritis (EORA)
- No female predominance when compared to younger onset rheumatoid arthritis (YORA)
- Large joints involvement and acute onset is seen in EORA
- Associated with malignancy

Rheumatoid arthritis (RA) is a progressive, systemic inflammatory disease that targets synovial tissues.

Epidemiology

The prevalence[27] of rheumatoid arthritis among persons 60 years of age and older has been estimated at around 2%. It is the most common inflammatory arthritis in adults, with a peak age of onset between 40 and 60 years of age.

Etiopathogenesis

RA is T cell driven disease. Activated T helper cells release several inflammatory mediators (chemokines and cytokines) which cause synovial and vascular proliferation resulting in pannus formation.[28] Secretion of enzymes like matrix metalloproteinases (MMPs from the activated T cells) results in damage to the articular cartilage and adjacent bone.[29]

Clinical Features

Late onset RA develops *de novo* after 60 years as an acute onset arthritis of joints of upper extremities and is seen as pain and stiffness of the shoulder joints. This is known as elderly onset rheumatoid arthritis (EORA).[30–32]

RA developing before 60 years of age can persist into old age and this variant is known as younger onset rheumatoid arthritis (YORA). EORA patients have acute onset of RA with high ESR in contrast to YORA.[33,34] Males are more commonly affected in EORA.[35]

The spectrum of disease in EORA ranges from inactive with bony deformities and rheumatoid nodules signifying earlier active disease to a full range of articular and systemic manifestations that are symptoms of ongoing active disease. Acute-onset RA has been noted in elderly patients who present with a GI malignancy.

Diagnosis

The most important characteristics in the elderly include joint pain, swelling, and tenderness. In addition, morning stiffness lasting longer than 30 minutes is an important distinguishing feature and may often be the earliest diagnostic finding. Associated laboratory findings may include an anaemia of chronic disease, elevated erythrocyte sedimentation rate (ESR), and a positive rheumatoid factor. The ESR is often mildly elevated in the elderly and as such is neither sensitive nor specific in the diagnosis of RA. The diagnosis of RA is a complex one made largely on the basis of clinical presentation.

Complications

- Joint deformities
- Systemic involvement—lung and heart involvement
- Osteoporosis
- Carpal tunnel syndrome

Treatment

- Patient education
- Rest: Although rest is an important component of therapy, it is essential that the older individual maintain a baseline activity

level. Prolonged bedrest may result in an overall decline in function, reduced muscle mass, negative calcium balance, and an increased susceptibility to infections.

- Salicylate therapy
- Non-steroidal anti-inflammatory drugs (NSAIDs)
- Aggressive therapy including the use of gold salts, systemic steroids administration, antimalarial agents, penicillamine, and low-dose methotrexate are controversial in elderly persons with RA and should be used cautiously if at all.

References

1. Catoggio LJ, Skinner RP, Smith G, Maddison PJ. Systemic lupus erythematosus in the elderly: clinical and serological characteristics. J Rheumatol 1984; 11(2):175–81.
2. Pu SJ, Luo SF, Wu YJ, Cheng HS, Ho HH. The clinical features and prognosis of lupus with disease onset at age 65 and older. Lupus 2000; 9(2):96–100.
3. Vila L M, Alarcón G S, McGwin G, Friedman A, Bastian BA, Fessler BJ, *et al*. "Early clinical manifestations, disease activity and damage of systemic lupus erythematosus among two distinct US Hispanic subpopulations". Rheumatology 2003; 43(3):358–363.
4. Mak SK, Lam EK, Wong AK. Clinical profile of patients with late-onset SLE: not a benign subgroup. Lupus 1998; 7:23–8.
5. Ho CT, Mok CC, Lau CS, Wong RW. Late onset systemic lupus erythematosus in southern chinese. Ann Rheum Dis 1998; 57:437–40.
6. Parodi A, Caproni M, Cardinali C, *et al*. Clinical, histological and immunopathological features of 58 patients with subacute cutaneous lupus erythematosus: a review by the Italian group of immunodermatology. Dermatology 2000; 200:6–10.
7. Boddaert J, Huong DL, Amoura Z, Wechsler B, Godeau P, Piette JC: Late-onset systemic lupus erythematosus: a personal series of 47 patients and pooled analysis of 714 cases in the literature. Medicine Baltimore 2004; 83(6), 348–59.
8. Font J, Pallares L, Cervera R, *et al*. Systemic lupus erythematosus in the elderly: Clinical and immunological characteristics. Ann Rheum Dis 1991; 50:702–5.
9. Catoggio LJ, Skinner RP, Smith G, Maddison PJ. Systemic lupus erythematosus in the elderly: clinical and serological characteristics. J Rheumatol 1984; 11(2):175–181.
10. Bertoli AM, Alarcon GS, Calvo-Alen J, Fernandez M, Vila LM, Reveille JD. Systemic lupus erythematosus in a multiethnic US cohort. XXXIII. Clinical [corrected] features, course, and outcome in patients with late-onset disease. Arthritis Rheum 2006; 54(5):1580–87.
11. Costallat LT, Coimbra AMV. Systemic lupus erythematosus: Clinical and laboratory aspects related to age at disease onset. Clin Exp Rheumatol 1994; 12(6):603–7.
12. Padovan M, Govoni M, Castellino G, Rizzo N, Fotinidi M, Trotta F. Late onset systemic lupus erythematosus: no substantial differences using different cut-off ages. Rheumatol Int 2007; 27(8):735–41.
13. Mak SK, Lam EK, Wong AK. Clinical profile of patients with late-onset SLE: not a benign subgroup. Lupus 1998; 7(1):23–8.
14. Bolognia Van den Hoogen F Khanna D, Fransen J, Johnson SR, Baron M, Tyndall A, Pope. Classification Criteria for Systemic Sclerosis: An ACR-EULAR Collaborative Initiative. Arthritis and Rheumatism, 2013; 65(11):2737–47.
15. Systemic sclerosis in old age. Br Med J 1979; 2:1313–14.
16. Rebecca L. Manno, Fredrick M. Wigley, Allan C Gelber, and Laura K. Hummers, Late-age onset scleroderma. J Rheumatol 2011; 38(7):1317–25.
17. Mayes MD, Lacey JV Jr, Beebe-Dimmer J, Gillespie BW, Cooper B, Laing TJ, Schottenfeld D. Prevalence, incidence, survival, and disease characteristics of systemic sclerosis in a large US population. Arthritis Rheum 2003; 48(8):2246–55.
18. Onishi A, Sugiyama D, Kumagai S, Morinobu A. Cancer incidence in systemic sclerosis. Arthritis Rheum 2013; 65:1913–21.
19. Marek Mand Rudny R.Scleroderma of geriatric age and scleroderma-like paraneoplastic syndrome–description of two cases. Rheumatologia 2016; 54(2):91–4.

20. Hamaguchi Y. Autoantibodies in Systemic Sclerosis. In: Takehara K, Fujimoto M, Kuwana M. (eds) Systemic Sclerosis. Springer, Tokyo The updated EULAR recommendations for treatment of systemic sclerosis, according to the organ involvement (adapted from Kowal-Bielecka O, Fransen J, Avouac J EUSTAR Coauthors, *et al*. Update of EULAR recommendations for the treatment of systemic sclerosis. Annals Rheum Dis 2017; 76:1327–1339.
21. Medsger TA, Dawson WN, Masi AT. The epidemiology of polymyositis. Am J Med 1970; 48:715.
22. Love LA, Leff RL, Fraser DD, *et al*. A new approach to the classification of idiopathic inflammatory myopathy: myositis-specific autoantibodies define useful homogeneous patient group. Medicine 1991; 70:360.
23. Marie I, Hatron PY, Levesque H, *et al*. Influence of age on characteristics of polymyositis and dermatomyositis in adults. Medicine 1999; 78:139.
24. Whaley K, Williamson J, Wilson T, McGavin DD, Hughes GR, Hughes H, *et al*. Sjogren's syndrome and autoimmunity in a geriatric population. Age Ageing 1972; 1:197–206.
25. García-Carrasco M, Cervera R, Rosas J, Ramos-Casals M, Morlá RM, Sisó A, *et al*. Primary Sjögren's syndrome in the elderly: clinical and immunological characteristics. Lupus 1999; 8:203.
26. Rasch EK, Hirsch R, Paulose-Ram R, Hochberg MC. Prevalence of rheumatoid arthritis in persons 60 years of age and older in the United States: effect of different methods of case classification. Arthritis Rheum 2003; 48:917–26.
27. Vitali C, Bombardieri S, Jonsson R, Moutsopoulos HM, Alexander EL, Carsons SE, *et al*. Classification criteria for Sjogren's syndrome: a revised version of the European criteria proposed by the American-European Consensus Group. Ann Rheum Dis. 2002; 61:554–8.
28. Chang J, Kavanaugh A. Novel therapies for rheumatoid arthritis. Pathophysiology 2005; 12:217–25.
29. Feldmann M, Brennan FM, Maini RN. Role of cytokines in rheumatoid arthritis. Annu Rev Immunol 1996; 14:397–440.
30. van Schaardenburg D, Breedveld FC. Elderly-onset rheumatoid arthritis. Semin Arthritis Rheum 1994; 23:367–78.
31. van der Heijde DM, van Riel PL, van Leeuwen MA, van Hof MA, van Rijswijk MH, van de Putte LB. Older versus younger onset rheumatoid arthritis: results at onset and after 2 years of prospective follow up of early rheumatoid arthritis. J Rheumatol 1991; 18:1285–9.
32. Glennas A, Kvien TK, Andrup O, Karstensen B, Munthe E. Recent onset arthritis in the elderly: a 5-year longitudinal observational study. J Rheumatol 2000; 27:101–8.
33. Deal CL, Meenan RF, Goldenberg DL, Anderson JJ, Sack B, Pastan RS, *et al*. The clinical features of elderly-onset rheumatoid arthritis: a comparison with younger-onset disease of similar duration. Arthritis Rheum 1985; 28:987–94.
34. Ferraccioli GF, Cavalieri F, Mercadanti M, Conti G, Viviano P, Ambanelli U. Clinical features, scintiscan characteristics and X-ray progression of late onset rheumatoid arthritis. Clin Exp Rheumatol 1984; 2:157–61.
35. Kavanaugh AF. Rheumatoid arthritis in the elderly: is it a different disease? Am J Med 1997; 103:40S–8.

CHAPTER 16

Vesiculobullous Disorders in Elderly

• Surabhi Dayal • Priyadarshini Sahu • N Asokan

Key Points

- Geriatric patients are generally prone to bullous disorders of varying aetiology.
- Proper understanding of various blistering disorders facilitates prompt diagnosis and management.
- Patients should be evaluated carefully and treated properly, as this population usually has multiple co-morbidities.
- Multiple treatment modalities including conventional and biological therapies are available for managing these blistering disorders, but no standard therapy has yet been established.

Introduction

Among all the dermatologic patients, "Geriatric patients" constitute a special group because of its higher prevalence of dermatologic and systemic diseases. Concentrating on the dermatological conditions, blistering disorders constitute a significant cause of morbidity and mortality in this elderly population. With the advancing age of this population, the incidence of bullous disorders, especially bullous pemphigoid is expected to rise. So, it is critically important for clinicians to diagnose the condition correctly, as the management and prognosis differ greatly depending on the disease process. The classification of bullous disorders in elderly patients is given in Table 16.1. Owing to the relative rarity of these diseases, standard therapy is based on published evidence, expert opinion and consensus. In this chapter, authors have reviewed the important bullous

TABLE 16.1: Classification of bullous disorders in geriatric patients

Autoimmune causes

Intraepidermal: Pemphigus (pemphigus vulgaris, pemphigus foliaceus, IgA pemphigus)
- Subcorneal pustular dermatosis (SCPD)
- Transient acantholytic dermatosis (TAD)

Subepidermal:
- Bullous pemphigoid
- Mucous membrane pemphigoid
- Epidermolysis bullosa acquisita
- Dermatitis herpetiformis
- Linear IgA bullous dermatosis
- Bullous lupus
- Lichen planus pemphigoides
- Paraneoplastic pemphigus

Infectious
- Viral (herpes simplex, varicella zoster, others)
- Bullous tinea
- Bullous impetigo
- Blistering dactylitis

Allergic/drug hypersensitivity
- Acute allergic contact dermatitis
- Drug hypersensitivity:
  - Bullous erythema multiforme
  - Stevens-Johnson syndrome
  - Toxic epidermal necrolysis
  - Acute generalised exanthematous pustulosis
- Insect bite reactions
- Vasculitis

Pompholyx/dyshidrotic eczema

Metabolic: Porphyria/pseudoporphyria
- Bullous diabeticorum/diabetic bullae
- Bullous amyloidosis

Mechanical: Coma/pressure bullae
- Bullous lymphedema

disorders especially in geriatric patients, as well as key clinical features, diagnostic test and its management.

AUTOIMMUNE BLISTERING DISORDERS (ABD)

Etiopathogenesis

Elderly patients are particularly susceptible to autoimmune and metabolic bullous diseases. This may be secondary to loss of structure and function of adhesive molecules that normally maintain the integrity of cell-cell and cell-matrix adhesion. There is flattening of dermal papillae, which results in gradual loss of strength of dermo-epidermal adhesion increasing the risk of blister formation.[1] In addition, the incidence of immune dysregulation increases with age, resulting in a higher incidence of autoantibody production leading to several ABD.[2]

For making the diagnosis skin biopsies are frequently necessary. Direct immunofluorescence (DIF) or indirect immunofluorescence (IIF) may be required for making definite diagnosis.[3]

Histopathology

Biopsy of early, intact vesicle with adjacent skin is the ideal specimen

DIF: The ideal specimen is perilesional uninvolved, non-sun-exposed skin. For patients with diseases manifesting primarily with mucosal involvement, uninvolved lower labial mucosa is most suitable for DIF.

IIF: Blood, serum or blister fluid may be used. In IIF, patient serum is tested for the presence of circulating autoantibodies using various substrates such as monkey or guinea pig oesophagus and rodent bladder epithelium.

Newer serum tests, specifically enzyme-linked immunosorbent assay (ELISA) and electron microscopy may be useful adjuncts. Table 16.2 outlines the characteristic DIF and IIF findings in well-characterised immunobullous disorders.[3]

BULLOUS PEMPHIGOID (BP)

It is one of the most commonly encountered immunobullous diseases in elderly population.[4]

Etiology

Patients have bound and circulating IgG autoantibodies specially directed against BP230 (or BP antigen 1) and BP180 (BP antigen 2).

Epidemiology

A recent nationwide cohort study performed in Olmsted County, Minnesota over 6 decades presented an adjusted incidence of 2.4 per 100,000 person-years.[5] On comparing various studies, it has been shown that the incidence has increased within last 10 years.[6,7] Factors for increased incidence include growing elderly population, improved ability to diagnose BP, increased prevalence of neurological disorders, and increased use of medications.[4] It affects both sexes equally with no strong association with race or geographical location.

Clinical Features

The mean age of onset is 80 years.[8] BP initially presents as pruritic, urticarial plaques with notable absence of blisters lasting for a few weeks to months (called prodromal non-bullous stage) followed by the development of blisters (bullous stage). The classical bullous lesions are tense, containing clear fluid (Fig. 16.1). Rarely haemorrhagic exudates can also be observed. Nikolsky sign is negative and the blisters spontaneously rupture after several days, leaving erosions and crusts on the surface. Ruptured bulla most commonly heal spontaneously without scarring. Post-inflammatory hyperpigmentation (PIH) and hypopigmentation are commonly seen. It has asymmetrical distribution, commonly involving the upper limbs, abdomen, and trunk. Mucosal sites such as eyes, nose, oesophagus and anogenital areas can be affected, out of these oral mucosa is the most common site.[4]

TABLE 16.2: DIF and IIF in various autoimmune blistering disease

Bullous disorders	Antigens targeted	DIF findings	IIF findings	Substrate for IIF
Bullous pemphigoid	BP230 (BPAG1) BP180 (BPAG2-NC16a)	Linear BMZ C3, IgG	Linear IgG along blister roof	SSS
Cicatricial pemphigoid	BP180, BP230	Linear BMZ C3, IgG and IgA	Linear IgG along blister roof (in majority of cases)	SSS
Epidermolysis bullosa acquisita	Type VII collagen	Dense linear BMZ IgG, C3, IgA, IgM	Linear IgG along blister base	SSS
Bullous lupus	Type VII collagen	Variable pattern BMZ IgG ± IgA, IgM, C3	Linear IgG along blister base	SSS
Linear IgA bullous dermatosis	BP180	Linear BMZ IgA	Linear IgA along blister roof	SSS
Pemphigus vulgaris	Desmoglein 3, Desmoglein 1	Intercellular IgG and/or C3	Intercellular IgG	Monkey oesophagus
Pemphigus foliaceus	Desmoglein 1	Intercellular IgG and/ or C3	Intercellular IgG	Guinea pig oesophagus
Paraneoplastic pemphigus	Desmoglein 1, desmoglein 3, desmoplakins I/II, envoplakin, periplakin, BP230	Intercellular and/or BMZ (linear or granular) IgG/C3/ both	Intercellular IgG	Rodent bladder
IgA pemphigus	Desmocollin 1, others	Intercellular IgA	Intercellular IgA	Monkey oesophagus
Dermatitis herpetiformis	Epidermal transglutaminase	Papillary dermal granular/ fibrillar IgA	Negative	N.A.

SSS: Salt split skin; Human skin is incubated first in 1M NaCl to separate the epidermis from the dermis at lamina lucida. Staining may be localised to the blister roof (epidermal side) or blister base (dermal side) or both.

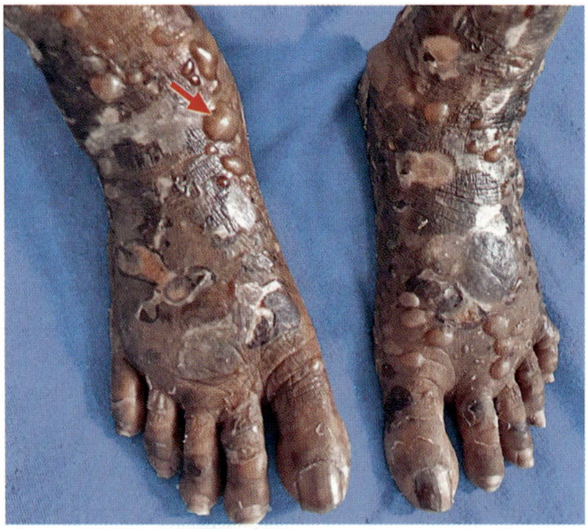

Fig. 16.1: Bullous pemphigoid: Multiple tense bullae (shown by red arrow) and crusting healing with post-inflammatory hypopigmentation

Other clinical variants of BP include dyshidrosiform pemphigoid, prurigo nodularis-like, ecthyma gangrenosum like, intertrigo like, papular, eczematous, lymphomatoid papulosis like, vegetating and erythrodermic pemphigoid. Lichen planus pemphigoid (LPP) is a rare disorder characterised by lesions of lichen planus occurring simultaneously with BP.[9]

Association

Blood eosinophilia may occur in association with BP but is not present in most patients. The risk factors include neurological disorders, psychiatric disorders, bedridden condition, and with use of drugs (such as furosemide, amoxicillin, ciprofloxacin, gliptin with metformin, spironolactone, neuroleptics and captopril).[10] There is no conclusive evidence for an association with malignancy or other autoimmune diseases.[2,11] However, recently few studies have shown weak association with gastric cancer and haematological malignancy.[9]

Diagnosis

The diagnosis is supported by classical histopathology which includes subepidermal bulla with a dermal inflammatory cell infiltrate partly composed of eosinophils. It can be confirmed with DIF and IIF (Table 16.2). ELISA kits can be used to measure serum levels of antibodies to both BP180 and BP230, out of which BP180 ELISA is more sensitive.[8]

Treatment

Management should aim to control symptoms with minimal adverse effects as elderly patients often have multiple comorbidities. When bullae are large or at troublesome site such as sole of foot, they may be drained with a sterile needle, but it is crucial not to de-roof the blister, as it functions as a natural dressing and prevents secondary bacterial infection.[8]

In elderly high potency topical corticosteroids such as clobetasol propionate 0.05% cream applied twice daily is considered as first line of treatment, especially in localised disease. Clobetasol cream has quicker clinical improvement with fewer complications. A practical pitfall of using topical corticosteroids is application over extensive area on regular basis and higher cost of obtaining topical corticosteroid is higher than oral steroids. Hence, systemic corticosteroids (i.e. prednisolone or methylprednisolone) are widely used worldwide as initial therapy in the treatment of BP.

Immunosuppressive agents (e.g. azathioprine, mycophenolate mofetil [MMF], methotrexate, dapsone or sulfonamides) can be used as an adjunct to systemic steroids for their steroid sparing effect. Anti-inflammatory antibiotics such as tetracycline, doxycycline, minocycline or lymecycline with nicotinamide and erythromycin have also been used. Intravenous immunoglobulin (IVIg), rituximab and omalizumab should be considered in recalcitrant cases.[8]

MUCOUS MEMBRANE PEMPHIGOID (MMP)/ CICATRICIAL PEMPHIGOID (CP)

MMP is a rare chronic subepithelial blistering disorder characterised by predominant involvement of the mucosae, with a tendency towards scarring of affected areas. Any mucous membrane lined by a malpighian epithelium can be involved.

Etiology

Autoantibodies usually IgG against BP180 (BPAG2), laminin-332, $\alpha6\beta4$ integrin or type VII collagen are found.

Epidemiology

MMP is a rare condition with limited epidemiological data available on its incidence. Female predominance without any racial or geographical predilections has been demonstrated. A high mortality rate is reported in patients with anti-laminin-332 MMP.

Clinical Features

It mostly affects elderly patients aged from 60 to 80 years. Its variants include: Classical form, single-site forms such as pure ocular or oral cicatricial pemphigoid, anti-laminin-332 form, and Brunsting-Perry form.[12]

In the classical form, tense blisters develop mainly on mucous membranes. Buccal mucosae are the most frequently affected (≈80–90%).[13] Erosions of buccal membranes, hard and soft palate, and desquamative gingivitis are frequently observed. Gingival lesions heal with scarring and atrophy. Other mucosal sites such as eyes, ear, nose, throat and genitalia may be involved. Cutaneous manifestations are seen in 25% of patients of MMP.[4] Blisters may arise from erythematous plaques and heal with milia and atrophic scars. Nevertheless, it is vital to check for other mucous membrane involvement during every patient assessment.

The diagnosis of anti-laminin-332 CP is ascertained by immunological investigation, as it is clinically indistinguishable from the classical form of MMP. In Brunsting-Perry pemphigoid, patients have recurrent head, neck and upper trunk vesiculobullous lesions, followed by subsequent ulceration and residual atrophic scarring. Mucosal involvement may be absent or minimal.[13]

Associations

A positive association exists between antibodies to anti-laminin 332 and an underlying malignancy.[14] Methyldopa, penicillamine, and clonidine have been reported to trigger MMP but the evidence is not strong.[4]

Diagnosis

Histopathology is similar to that of BP, with a subepidermal vesicle and mixed inflammatory infiltrate. The presence of plasma cells in the infiltrate is not uncommon in oral mucosa. DIF and IIF are gold standard for diagnosis (Table 16.2).

Treatment

No international consensus or guideline is available for the treatment of MMP. Generally, the treatment of MMP is guided by the areas of involvement and severity of mucous membrane involvement.

Local Agents

- Oral involvement: Regular use of antiseptic mouth washes is effective in preventing inflammation and recurrent infections. Topical anaesthetics are used to reduce pain. For inflamed areas, corticosteroids orabase or mouthwashes can be used. Topical tacrolimus has shown beneficial effect in few case studies of oral MMP.
- Ocular involvement: Regular use of preservative-free artificial tears for maintaining adequate moisture to prevent the ocular damage. Corticosteroid eye drops and topical cyclosporine may be used. Ophthalmology consultation and regular follow-up are vital to providing optimum care.

Systemic Agents

In mild-to-moderate MMP, dapsone is effective and may be considered as first line therapy. It is more effective for lesions of buccal mucosa as compared to ocular inflammation. Cyclophosphamide, IVIg, rituximab, etanercept and bortezomib has been used in patients with recalcitrant MMP.[4,15]

EPIDERMOLYSIS BULLOSA ACQUISITA (EBA)

EBA is an acquired subepidermal blistering disease.

Etiology

It is associated with IgG autoantibodies against type VII collagen.

Epidemiology

Limited epidemiological data are available for accurately assessing the true incidence of EBA. An incidence of 0.2–0.5 cases/million/year is reported in Central Europe, Singapore, and Kuwait.[16, 17]

Clinical Features

There are five main clinical presentations: Classical form, BP-like form, MMP-like form, Brunsting-Perry-like form, and linear IgA bullous dermatosis-like form.[9]

Classic EBA manifests as a non-inflammatory bullous disease with an acral distribution. Patients have skin fragility and develop tense vesicles and bulla (Fig. 16.2). Nail dystrophies, flexion of the fingers, milia and scarring alopecia are often seen in chronic EBA. An inflammatory phenotype of EBA also exists that mimics BP know as BP-like form. EBA

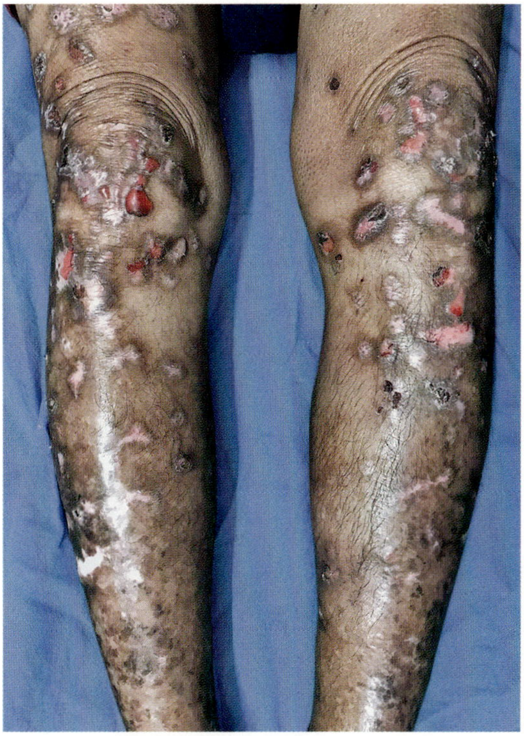

Fig. 16.2: Epidermolysis bullosa acquisita: Blisters arising on bilateral lower limb at trauma prone area and healing with atrophic scarring and pigmentary changes

may also present with an MMP phenotype with predominant and chronic mucous membrane involvement. Brunsting-Perry-like form is rare, presenting with discrete and isolated vesiculobullous lesions predominantly on the head and neck areas, which heal with atrophic scars. Patients with the linear IgA bullous dermatosis-like form develop tense vesicles arranged in an annular pattern along with involvement of mucous membranes.

Associations

A few studies showed its positive possible association with inflammatory bowel disease, i.e. Crohn's disease.[18] A few studies of EBA exacerbated by ultraviolet treatment or combined hormonal treatment have been reported.[19, 20]

Diagnosis

Histology reveals a subepidermal bulla with minimal inflammatory infiltrate in classic EBA but varying degree of inflammation with lymphocytes, neutrophils and eosinophils in the inflammatory type. DIF and IIF are given in Table 16.2.

Management

Managing EBA may be difficult, as it is often but invariably refractory to conventional therapy. Avoidance of trauma to prevent blister formation and prompt attention towards ulceration to reduce secondary bacterial infection is warranted.

Anti-inflammatory Agents and Corticosteroids

Dapsone has been used in EBA in conjunction with other treatments. It can be beneficial in EBA patients, especially in the presence of neutrophils in their dermal infiltrate. Colchicine has also been used either alone or with other immunosuppressants.

Immunosuppressive Agents

Cyclosporine has been tried with some good response. A recent study has shown its standalone utility without corticosteroids at a lower dose of 4 mg/kg/day. Nevertheless, the side-effect profile of cyclosporine limits its long-term use in the elderly patient.

Miscellaneous Drugs

Rituximab and IVIg have been shown to be effective in treating recalcitrant EBA.[9]

PEMPHIGUS

It is an autoimmune mucocutaneous blistering disease that has been reported in many countries. It has been classified into three major subtypes: (1) Pemphigus vulgaris (PV); (2) Pemphigus foliaceus (PF); and (3) Paraneoplastic pemphigus (PNP).

Epidemiology

The incidence is variable worldwide, ranging from 0.05 to 2.7 cases per 100,000 individuals per year. PV is more common in Europe, US and India, whereas PF is more common in Brazil and Africa.[9]

PEMPHIGUS VULGARIS (PV)

It is the most common form among the pemphigus family, accounting for approximately 70% of all cases of pemphigus.[21]

Etiology

Autoantibodies target desmosomal cadherin, especially desmoglein (dsg) 3 (130 kd) protein only, or both dsg 3 and dsg 1 (160 kd). Patients with autoantibodies to dsg 3 have been associated with only mucosal involvement, whereas autoantibodies to both dsg 1 and 3 have both cutaneous and mucosal involvement. Autoantibody titers to dsg 1 and 3 frequently correlate with disease activity.

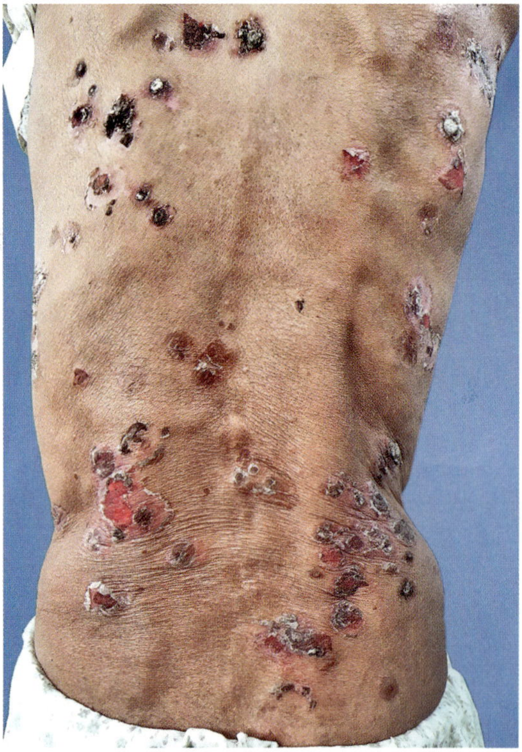

Fig. 16.3: Pemphigus vulgaris: Multiple erosions with crusting present on back of the patient

Clinical Features

In PV, flaccid blisters on the skin erupt and rupture easily, leaving painful denuded surfaces (Fig. 16.3). The disease usually begins in the oral cavity. The disorder may be localised or it may become generalised and involve 20 to 50% of the skin in severe disease. In severe disease, there can be involvement of ocular, nasal, pharyngeal, laryngeal, esophageal, vaginal, penile, and anal mucosa. Healing usually occurs without scarring, often with PIH.

Pemphigus vegetans is a variant of PV, which can affect both mucosal and cutaneous tissues. Patients with pemphigus vegetans present with a "cerebriform" tongue and vegetating lesions characteristically present in the intertriginous areas.

Diagnosis

Skin biopsies from early lesions demonstrate characteristic histology of acantholysis and suprabasal bulla. DIF and IIF aid in the diagnosis (Table 16.2). There are several serologic assays that can be used to demonstrate autoantibodies such as immunoblot assay and ELISA.

Management

Patients with limited disease, localised treatments for specific area of involvement can facilitate healing and prevent the use of systemic agents. Localised PV can be treated with topical and intralesional corticosteroids. Limited benefit has been reported with cyclosporine and topical tacrolimus. Systemic corticosteroids are often considered the mainstay of therapy for extensive, progressive, and severe PV. Adjuvant anti-inflammatory and immunosuppressive agents have been used to avoid prolonged use of corticosteroid and its side effects.

Drugs with anti-inflammatory effects include dapsone, minocycline, or tetracycline, in combination with nicotinamide. Immunosuppressive agents include azathioprine, methotrexate, cyclophosphamide, cyclosporine, and MMF. Pulse therapy (dexamethasone with intravenous cyclophosphamide), plasmapheresis, IVIg, and rituximab have been used in severe disease not responding to conventional therapy. The mortality in elderly pemphigus is secondary to prolonged immune suppression or a direct consequence of high dose long-term immunosuppressive therapy.[21]

PEMPHIGUS FOLIACEUS (PF)

PF is considered a less severe form of the disease and rare in the elderly.

Etiology

Autoantibodies IgG_4 subclass against dsg 1 is present.

Clinical Features

Patients develop recurrent crops of superficial blisters that erode easily forming crusted erosions. Mucous membrane is rarely involved. The cutaneous lesions are most commonly present on seborrhoeic sites, but rarely progress to erythroderma. Pemphigus erythematosus (also known as Senear-Usher syndrome) represents about 10% of all cases of PF, with features of lupus erythematosus.[22]

Associations

Other autoimmune diseases and thymoma.

Diagnosis

Histology of an early lesion demonstrates split directly beneath stratum corneum. DIF and IIF are help in making diagnosis (Table 16.2). Autoantibody titers to the keratinocyte cell surface antigen and dsg 1 correlate with disease activity.

Treatment

As PF is a more benign subtype of pemphigus, the treatment of PF is usually less challenging as compared with PV. Management options are similar to those used in PV including systemic corticosteroids, dapsone and other immunosuppressants. Patients with erythrodermic and refractory forms of PF often require high-dose systemic corticosteroids along with immunosuppressive agents for disease control. Opportunistic infections and malignancy are reported causes of mortality. Elderly patients must be monitored for side effects of prolonged immune suppression.[21]

PARANEOPLASTIC PEMPHIGUS (PNP)

It is also known as "paraneoplastic autoimmune multiorgan syndrome". It most commonly occurs in individuals aged between 45 and 70 years. According to study, overall survival rate is 49%, 41% and 38% at 1, 3 and 5 years.[24] The leading cause of death for these patients is sepsis, respiratory failure, and progression of underlying malignancy.[23]

Epidemiology

Actual incidence is unknown but it is much less common than other autoimmune blistering disorders. Approximately 300 total cases of PNP have been reported in the literature.[24]

Etiology

In PNP, autoantibodies to dsg1 and 3, and to members of the plakin family of molecules, including desmoplakin I and II, envoplakin, periplakin, plectin, BP antigen 230, and a 170-kDa protein has been identified.

Clinical Features

Florid oral mucosal lesions with stomatitis are usually the foremost and the most consistent findings of PNP. Erosions with crusting are typically seen on the vermilion of the lips and lateral aspects of the tongue; though it can occur on any of the other mucosal surfaces. Patients usually develop generalised polymorphous cutaneous eruptions by definition, which may resemble pemphigus, pemphigoid, erythema multiforme or lichenoid dermatitis. It is important to note that more than one morphology can appear at any given time throughout the disease progression. Gastrointestinal and respiratory tracts can be involved in PNP.[25]

Associations

PNP is almost invariably associated with malignancy such as lymphoproliferative disorders including Castleman's disease, non-Hodgkin lymphoma and chronic lymphocytic leukaemia.[2] Erythema multiforme like skin lesions have been identified as a poor prognostic factor with two-fold increase in the death rates.[23] In up to one-third of cases, the diagnosis of PNP antedates the discovery of the underlying malignancy.[4]

Diagnosis

The histologic findings are equally variable and may show suprabasilar acantholysis, basal vacuolization and dyskeratotic keratinocytes, or lichenoid dermatitis. DIF and IIF are unique to PNP given in Table 16.2.

Management

Outcomes are favourable mainly in patients with resectable benign tumours. The outcome is much poorer when associated with malignancy. It has been suggested that perioperative infusion of IVIg, may allow blockage of autoantibody release from the tumour during the operation.

Despite effective local resection and chemotherapy, some patients have persistent or progressive PNP. High dose corticosteroids are often used for immunosuppression in these cases. Adjuvants agents such as azathioprine, MMF and cyclosporine can be used in conjunction with systemic corticosteroids with inconstant and unpredictable results. A few case studies have shown promising outcomes with rituximab. Alemtuzumab has also been used in a patient with B cell chronic lymphocytic leukaemia.[4]

SUBCORNEAL PUSTULAR DERMATOSIS (SCPD)

SCPD is also known as Sneddon-Wilkinson disease. It is rare benign chronic relapsing blistering disorder. Women in their fourth to fifth decades are most commonly affected.

Etiology

It is still unknown.

Clinical Features

SCPD presents as crops of pustules in an annular or polycyclic pattern on normal or erythematous skin. The lesions are mostly distributed over the trunk and flexural surfaces and heal with PIH and without scarring.

Associations

IgA monoclonal gammopathy, pyoderma gangrenosum, inflammatory bowel disease, lymphoproliferative disorders and rheumatoid arthritis may be associated.

Diagnosis

On histology a subcorneal pustule mixed with superficial perivascular inflammatory cell infiltrate can be present in the underlying dermis. DIF and IIF are usually negative.

Management

The treatment includes systemic corticosteroids, dapsone (50–150 mg daily) and sulfapyridine. Acitretin and colchicine (1.5 mg daily) and other immunosuppressants have been used anecdotally for treatment of recalcitrant variety.[26]

IgA PEMPHIGUS

Some cases previously diagnosed as SCPD had demonstrated intercellular IgA and have been reclassified as IgA pemphigus. It is more common in elderly as compared to SCPD.

Etiology

Antibodies to desmocollin 1 (SPD type) and dsg 1 or 3 (IEN type) are demonstrated.

Clinical Features

The average age of onset is 45 years, reported cases in children and elderly. There are two distinct groups:

a. IgA confined to upper epidermis (subcorneal pustular dermatosis—SPD type)
b. IgA throughout the epidermis (intraepidermal neutrophilic IgA dermatosis—IEN type)

SPD type presents with similar annular, crusted vesicles and pustules in the axilla and groin. The IEN type may preferentially involve the trunk rather than intertriginous area.

Associations

It has increased frequency of association with IgA monoclonal gammopathy as compared to SCPD. IgA antibodies present in approximately 50% of cases.

Diagnosis

Histopathology shows subcorneal or intraepidermal spilt with neutrophils underlying the spilt. Early lesions show neutrophil exocytosis and neutrophils at the dermoepidermal junction. DIF shows:

- SPD type: Intercellular IgA deposition in upper dermis
- IEN type: Intercellular IgA in lower or throughout epidermis

IIF is unreliable and only 50% have detectable circulating IgA.

Treatment

Initially, dapsone 25 to 100 mg daily is used. If dapsone-intolerant: Start sulfapyridine 500 mg twice a day and increase slowly. A few case reports include colchicine or retinoids as effective treatment options.[26]

TRANSIENT ACANTHOLYTIC DERMATOSIS (TAD)/GROVER'S DISEASE

Etiology

Unknown but linked to heat and sweating.

Clinical Features

It presents with pruritic papules and vesicles with crusting on sun-exposed skin areas of chest and back. It usually affects middle to older aged adults. There are 3 variants: Transient eruptive, persistent pruritic and chronic asymptomatic.[22] Prolonged exposure to ultraviolet light and heat are known exacerbating factors.

Diagnosis

Histology demonstrates intraepidermal vesicles with focal acantholysis and dyskeratosis. Four histologic patterns can be seen: Darier-like, Hailey-Hailey-like, pemphigus vulgaris-like, and spongiotic. DIF is negative.

Treatment

It is generally self-limiting and heals without scarring. For localized lesions, high potency topical steroids can be used to control the disease. In case of extensive disease, systemic agents including systemic corticosteroids, retinoids, dapsone and psoralens with ultraviolet A (PUVA) can be used.[22]

LINEAR IgA BULLOUS DERMATOSIS (LIgABD)

LIgABD is an autoimmune subepidermal blistering disease with several clinical variants. In the adult form, the average age of onset is 60.

Etiology

The immunological targets are a group of BMZ antigens including 285 kDa, 97 kDa and 120 kDa proteins that are likely components of the extracellular domain of BP 180.

Association

LIgABD disease has been reported secondary to intake of drugs, especially with vancomycin. Other important drugs include captopril, penicillins, cephalosporins, and NSAIDs.[2]

Clinical Features

Patients usually present with pruritic, grouped, annular vesicles and bullae on trunk and extensors (Fig. 16.4) that are often excoriated. Oral and conjunctival involvement can occur. Atypical presentations include forms resembling erythema multiforme, TEN or morbilliform eruption. Drug-induced LIgABD appears within 7 to 14 days of starting the causative medication.

Diagnosis

Histologic findings include subepidermal bullae with neutrophils, but DIF and IIF are confirmatory (Table 16.2).

Management

Treatment involves withdrawal of the suspected inciting drug and improvement is typically evident within 3 weeks. Some patients may require conventional therapies including dapsone or systemic corticosteroids.[21]

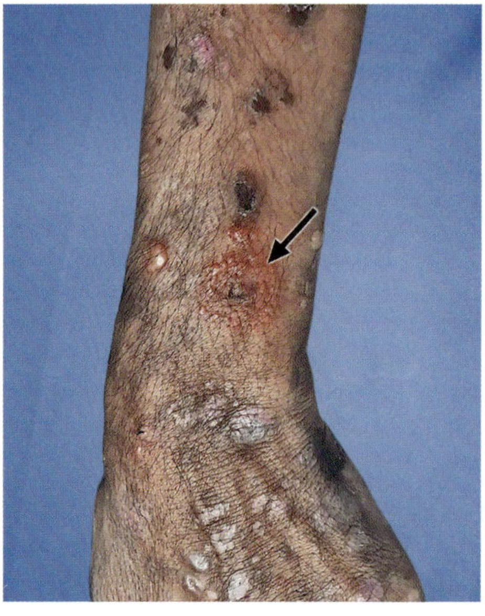

Fig. 16.4: Linear IgA disease: Arrangement of multiple vesicles around an erythematous plaque

DERMATITIS HERPETIFORMIS (DH)

It is rare chronic sub-epidermal autoimmune blistering disorder that rarely affects elderly. It has higher male predominance.

Etiology

Studies have revealed association between DH and certain HLA types such as HLADQ2 and to lesser extend HLADQ8. Gluten sensitive enteropathy has been reported in minority of patients.

Clinical Features

Patients present with grouped pruritic erythematous papules, vesicles or plaques. There is a symmetric distribution on the neck, elbows, buttocks, sacrum, knees, and extensor surfaces of the extremities.

Diagnosis

The histology demonstrates a sub-epidermal blister with an infiltrate consisting of neutrophils at the tips of the dermal papillae. DIF is characteristic (Table 16.2). Circulating IgA autoantibodies to endomysium, and more specifically to transglutaminase, have been reported to be present in the sera of DH patients.

Management

Two major treatment modalities:

- Dapsone is the treatment of choice. For cutaneous lesions, potent topical steroids can be used. If dapsone is contraindicated, sulphamethoxypyridazine, sulphapyridine or sulphasalazine can be used as an alternative agent.
- Another aspect is gluten-free diet. This can prevent relapse of the disease and allow discontinuation of systemic therapy.[9]

BULLOUS SYSTEMIC LUPUS ERYTHEMATOSUS (BSLE)

Etiology

Autoantibodies to type VII collagen (290 kDa protein) are found.

Clinical Features

It is characterized by herpetiform vesicles or more often large tense fluid filled to haemorrhagic bullae on sun-exposed area. Patients generally meet the criteria for SLE.

Diagnosis

Histopathology reveals subepidermal blister with neutrophils without interface changes. DIF and IIF are given in Table 16.2.

Treatment

Initially, patients are treated with dapsone (100 mg per day in an adult).[10] Combination of dapsone and prednisolone or azathioprine is the treatment of choice for recalcitrant disease. Methotrexate and rituximab have also been reported to be effective in few patients.[26,27]

NON-IMMUNE BLISTERING CONDITIONS

There are rare non-immune blistering conditions that can also present in geriatric patients. Few of these conditions relevant to geriatric age group are being discussed.

PORPHYRIA CUTANEA TARDA (PCT)

PCT is a metabolic photosensitive disease that can present with vesiculobullous lesions on sun-exposed area. It is reported to be autosomal dominant or acquired. Mean age of onset is about 45 years of age; but this disease is included in the differential for bullous diseases in all age groups including the elderly.

Epidemiology

Incidence varies but in most countries is around 1 in 10,000.[9]

Etiology

It results from the deficiency of UROD (uroporphyrinogen decarboxylase) leading to the accumulation of uroporphyrin. Uroporphyrin diffuses from plasma to the surrounding tissues, causing a photo-toxic reaction in sun-exposed skin leading to the formation of blisters.

Clinical Features

Patients presents with serous or haemorrhagic vesicles or tense bulla on light-exposed skin. Other cutaneous features such as scarring alopecia, hypertrichosis and sclerodermoid thickening may be associated. Healing occurs with milia formation, scarring and PIH. Alcohol, oestrogen and polychlorinated hydrocarbons are exacerbating factors.

Diagnosis

Patients have elevated porphyrin (uroporphyrins I and III) levels in a 24-hour urine specimen. A reddish pink colour of urine can also be seen with a Wood's lamp. Other porphyrin abnormalities include elevated plasma porphyrin, heptacarboxyl porphyrin, fecal heptacarboxyl porphyrin and isocoproporphyrin. On histology, a subepidermal blister with sparse inflammatory infiltrate and "festooning" of dermal papillae base are seen. On DIF deposition of IgG, IgM and C3 can be seen in the capillary walls and at the BMZ.

Management

Exacerbating factors should be avoided. Physical sunscreens should be used. In addition, patients can undergo bi-weekly phlebotomy. Definite treatment with venesection or low dose antimalarials is required in almost all patients.[9]

DIABETIC BULLAE/BULLOSIS DIABETICORUM

Etiology

Both insulin- and non-insulin dependent diabetic patients can develop such bullous lesions. Diabetic bullae are more frequently observed in older patients and have been associated with microangiopathy and neuropathy in diabetics.[22]

Clinical Features

The lesions often present as tense blisters on the upper and lower extremities. Lesions heal within several weeks without scarring and may become dark as they dry up.

Diagnosis

Histopathology shows subepidermal blister with a sparse perivascular infiltrate in early lesions. Later lesions show intraepidermal blisters with surrounding spongiosis, which likely represents healing. DIF and IIF are negative.

Treatment

Management is conservative. Spontaneous healing of blister occurs within 3 to 5 weeks.[21]

BULLOUS DISEASE OF THE COMATOSE/ COMA BULLAE (CB)

Etiology

It is due to tissue ischaemia caused by local pressure necrosis and systemic hypoxia. Various medical conditions especially with neurological conditions and drugs, i.e. barbiturate over dose are associated with CB.

Clinical Features

The lesions develop within 48–72 hours after loss of consciousness and arise at the site of pressure.

Diagnosis

Biopsy demonstrates presence of a subepidermal bulla or intraepidermal spongiotic vesicle with focal necrosis of all epidermal appendages. Eccrine sweat gland and duct necrosis is the most remarkable and significant change. DIF can be negative or sometimes demonstrate deposition of IgM and C3 in the dermal vessels.

Treatment

Management consists of supportive measures, such as elimination of causative agents, control of underlying medical conditions, postural changes to reduce pressure and prevention of infections. Healing occurs within a period of 2 to 4 weeks without scarring.[21]

FRICTION BLISTER

Etiology

It occurs in population involved in vigorous activity. Development is linked to magnitude of frictional force.

Clinical Features

Most commonly occurs on thick horny layer that is held tightly to underlying dermis. It includes site such as tips of toes, balls of feet and posterior heel.

Diagnosis

History and location are most important. Histopathology shows necrosis just below stratum granulosum or in the upper stratum spinosum.

Treatment

Larger lesions may be drained. Blister roof must be maintained intact in order to speed healing time.[21]

BULLOUS LYMPHEDEMA

Etiology

It is due to physical insult caused by poorly controlled oedema due to concurrent medical conditions (heart failure, renal failure, lymph node dissection) contributing to volume overload.

Clinical Features

It presents with tense bullae on lymph edematous skin.

Diagnosis

On histopathology, subepidermal split is seen. DIF and IIF are negative.

Treatment

Correction of underlying medical condition and optimizing volume status with low salt diet and diuretics are prime treatment modalities. Symptomatic management is done for the bullous lesions.[21]

ALLERGIC CONTACT DERMATITIS (ACD)

Etiology

In ACD, sensitization occurs when Langerhans cells present allergens to T-lymphocytes causing clonal expansion of sensitized lymphocytes. On subsequent exposure, cell-mediated, delayed type hypersensitivity develops.

Clinical Features

There are two types of presentations:

- Acute presentation has blisters that develop after 24–48 hours following exposure of allergen (Fig. 16.5).
- Chronic presentation manifests as hyperkeratosis, fissuring and lichenification.

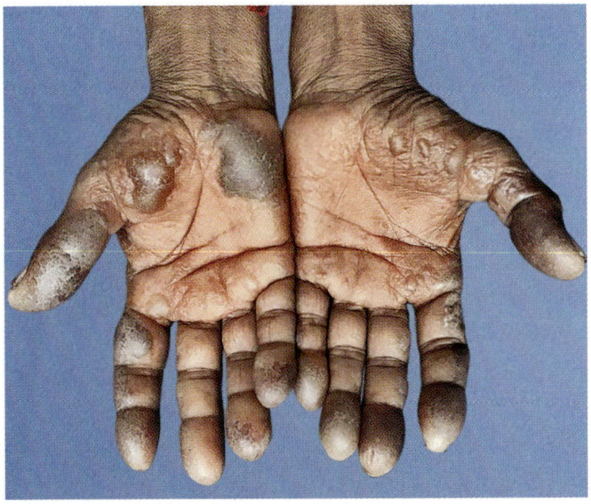

Fig. 16.5: Acute contact dermatitis: Multiple vesicle and bulla on bilateral palms with cement exposure

Diagnosis

Patch testing is the gold standard for identifying specific allergens. Biopsy shows spongiotic vesicles present at different horizontal and vertical levels of the epidermis. Superficial perivascular and interstitial infiltrate with eosinophils present in the dermis. DIF is negative.

Treatment

Avoidance of exposure to allergens is the first line of treatment. Potent or moderately potent topical steroids are usually effective in resolving the symptoms. Systemic steroids are indicated for widespread involvement with severe symptoms.

ARTHROPOD BITE

It can cause subepidermal blister characterized with urticarial papules or blisters. Sometimes, it appears in groups (e.g. breakfast, lunch and dinner sign). Histopathology shows, subepidermal split with spongiosis and a superficial and deep perivascular infiltrate with numerous eosinophils, which can be wedge shaped. Prevention is advised and lesions are treated with class I topical steroids.[21]

Prognosis of bullous disease in elderly:[4] Prognosis in elderly is generally worse than in younger individuals due to:

- Slow healing process especially in patients with nutritional deficiencies or systemic diseases.
- Extensive loss of fluids and electrolytes.
- Increased chances of secondary bacterial infections and sepsis.
- Prone to develop to ulcers due to increased local pressure in immobile and bedridden patients.
- Temperature regulation may be compromised following loss of large area of epidermis.

Presently, the commonest cause of death is secondary to therapeutic agents used.

CONCLUSION

This chapter discusses the major blistering diseases in the geriatric population. Recognition and proper management is quite essential as the population is ageing, and immune system evolves with senescence. For this population medication choices may be challenging due to comorbidities and susceptibility to adverse effects. In conclusion, as a dermatologist a proper understanding into the pathogenesis and various treatment modalities is essential for proper management of geriatric patients.

References

1. Farage MA, Miller KW, Berardesca E, Maibach HI. Clinical implications of aging skin: cutaneous disorders in the elderly. Am J Clin Dermatol. 2009; 10:73–86.
2. Miller RA. The aging immune system: primer and prospectus. Science. 1996; 273:70–4.
3. Parker SR, MacKelfresh J. Autoimmune blistering diseases in the elderly. Clin Dermatol. 2011; 29: 69–79.
4. Kim M, Borradori L, Murrell DF. Autoimmune Blistering Diseases in the Elderly: Clinical Presentations and Management. Drugs Aging. 2016; 33:711–23.
5. Brick KE, Weaver CH, Lohse CM, Pittelkow MR, Lehman JS, Camilleri MJ, *et al*. Incidence of bullous pemphigoid and mortality of patients with bullous pemphigoid in Olmsted County, Minnesota, 1960 through 2009. J Am AcadDermatol. 2014; 71:92–9.
6. Bernard P, Vaillant L, Labeille B, *et al*. Incidence and distribution of subepidermal autoimmune bullous skin diseases in three French regions: Bullous Diseases French Study Group. Arch Dermatol. 1995; 131:48–52.
7. Joly P, Baricault S, Sparsa A, *et al*. Incidence and mortality of bullous pemphigoid in France. J Invest Dermatol. 2012; 132:1998–2004.
8. Venning VA, Taghipour K, MohdMustapa MF, Highet AS, Kirtschig G. British association of Dermatologists' guidelines for the management of bullous pemphigoid 2012. Br J Dermatol. 2012; 167:1200–14.
9. Schmidt E and Groves R. Immunobullous diseases. In: Griffiths CEM, Barker J, Bleiker T, Chalmers R, Creamer D (editors). Rook's Textbook of Dermatology. 9th ed. UK: Wiley-Blackwell Publications; 2016. P. 50.01–52.
10. Bastuji-Garin S, Joly P, Lemordant P, Sparsa A, Bedane C, Delaporte E, *et al*. French Study Group for Bullous Diseases. Risk factors for bullous pemphigoid in the elderly: a prospective case-control study.J Invest Dermatol. 2011; 131:637–43.
11. Borradori L, Joly P. Toward a practical renaming of bullous pemphigoid and all its variants: cutaneous pemphigoid. JAMA Dermatol. 2014; 150:459.
12. Kurzhals G, Stolz W, Meurer M, *et al.* Acquired epidermolysis bullosa with the clinical feature of Brunsting-Perry cicatricialbullous pemphigoid. Arch Dermatol. 1991; 127:391–5.
13. Bernard P, Antonicelli F, Bedane C, *et al.* Prevalence andclinical significance of anti-laminin 332 autoantibodies detectedby a novel enzyme-linked immunosorbent assay in mucousmembrane pemphigoid. JAMA Dermatol. 2013; 149:533–40.
14. Caux F, Prost-Squarcioni C. Mucous membrane pemphigoid. In: Murrell DF, (editor). Blistering diseases. Sydney: Springer, Inc.; 2015. p. 363–73.
15. Saeed L, Schmidt TH, Gensler LS, Gross AJ, Fox LP, Scharschmidt TC, *et al.* successful treatment of mucous membrane pemphigoid with bortezomib. JAAD Case Rep. 2017; 4:81–83.
16. Nanda A, Dvorak R, Al-Saeed K, Al-Sabah H, Alsaleh QA. Spectrum of autoimmune bullous diseases in Kuwait. Int J Dermatol. 2004; 43:876–81.
17. Wong SN, Chua SH. Spectrum of subepidermal immunobullous disorders seen at the National Skin Centre, Singapore: a 2-year review.Br J Dermatol. 2002; 147:476–80.
18. Reddy H, Shipman AR, Wojnarowska F. Epidermolysis bullosa acquisita and inflammatory bowel disease: a review of the literature. ClinExpDermatol. 2013; 38:225–9.
19. Jappe U, Zillikens D, Bonnekoh B, Gollnick H. Epidermolysis bullosa acquisita with ultraviolet radiation sensitivity. Br J Dermatol. 2000; 142: 517–20.
20. Kubo A, Hashimoto K, Inoue C, *et al*. Epidermolysis bullosa acquisita exacerbated by systemic estrogen

and progesteronetreatment and pregnancy. J Am Acad Dermatol. 1997; 36:792–4.

21. Sami N, Yeh SW, Ahmed AR. Blistering diseases in the elderly: diagnosis and treatment.DermatolClin. 2004; 22:73–86.
22. Hurley MY, Mattox AR. Diagnosis and management of bullous disease. Clin Geriatr Med. 2013; 29: 329–59.
23. Leger S, Picard D, Ingen-Housz-Oro S, Arnault JP, Aubin F, Carsuzaa F,*et al*. Prognostic factors of paraneoplastic pemphigus. Arch Dermatol. 2012; 148:1165–72.
24. Zimmermann J, Bahmer F, Rose C, Zillikens D, Schmidt E. Clinical and immunopathological spectrum of paraneoplastic pemphigus. J Dtsch Dermatol Ges. 2010; 8:598–605.
25. Zhang J, Qiao QL, Chen XX, *et al*. Improved outcomes after complete resection of underlying tumors for patients with paraneoplastic pemphigus: a single-center experience of 22 cases. J Cancer Res Clin Oncol. 2011; 137:229–34.
26. Alsanafi S, Kovarik C, Mermelstein AL, Werth VP. Rituximab in the treatment of bullous systemic lupus erythematosus. J ClinRheumatol 2011; 17:142–4.
27. Malcangi G, Brandozzi G, Giangiacomi M, Zampetti M, Danieli MG. Bullous SLE: response to methotrexate and relationship with disease activity. Lupus 2003; 12:63–6.
28. Mutasim DF. Autoimmune bullous dermatoses in theelderly: diagnosis and management. Drugs Aging 2003; 20:663–81.

CHAPTER 17

Aesthetic Concerns in the Elderly

• Aarti Sarda • Varsha Vaidyanathan

"Youth is a gift of nature but age is a work of art."

Introduction

The world is ageing and India is no exception. Advances in the field of medicine, technology, infrastructure, economy and hygiene have increased the average life expectancy and changed the Indian demography. It is estimated that the geriatric population which currently is at 7.2% will grow to 20% by the year 2050.[1] This geriatric boom brings with it, its own set of health issues making geriatric health one of the top five challenges to be faced by the healthcare systems in the future.[2]

While it is logical to assume that the average elderly person will have more pressing health issues to grapple with, such as hypertension, diabetes, declining organ function or reduced mental acuity, it is important to realize that even at an advanced age, beauty, cosmesis, and grooming are vital to a sense of well-being and happiness.

Beauty is no longer the desire and domain of youth alone. The elderly are now just as motivated to look good and feel good as their younger counterparts, and it has been noted that an improvement in one's physical appearance brings with it a sense of psychological well-being, happiness, satisfaction and a better quality of life.[3]

In this chapter, we will discuss the aesthetic concerns unique to the ageing skin.

PHYSIOLOGY OF THE AGEING SKIN[4]

Epidermis

There is a generalized thinning of the epidermis with fewer melanocytes, Langerhans' cells, and stem cells. The ability of the skin to recover from DNA damage is adversely affected. There is a reduction in the production of lipid layer in the stratum corneum. Although the thickness of the stratum corneum remains the same, the individual corneocytes are larger. The skin is more permeable to chemical substances.

Dermis

In the aged skin, the dermis too is thinned out. Collagen content decreases and the collagen fibrils are disorganized. This, combined with increased collagenase results in poor wound healing. Elastic fibres decrease in number and size and are fragmented. The ground substance mucopolysaccharides, glycosaminoglycans and proteoglycans are reduced, leading to loose and lax skin.

There is vessel wall thinning with reduced vasculature especially in the dermal papillae.[5] Similar changes are seen in lymphatic vessels. The upshot of these changes is decreased lymphatic drainage, disruption of thermoregulation and compromised immune function because of decreased ability of endothelial cells to induce white cell adhesion. The ageing dermis is thus rigid, inelastic and unable to heal well after injury or stress.

Subcutaneous Tissue, Muscles and Bone

Accumulation of the age pigment, lipofuschin, in the facial muscles along with reduced neuromuscular control leads to formation of wrinkles. Subcutaneous fat is resorbed from certain facial regions like the forehead, preorbital, buccal, temporal and perioral regions combined with an increase in fat deposition in areas like the submental region, jowls, nasolabial folds and the lateral malar areas. This contributes to sagging and drooping of the skin giving rise to the 'aged look'. Sleeping in the same position leads to folding of the skin on one side of the face giving rise to 'sleep lines'. Due to bone resorption affecting the mandible, maxilla, and frontal bones, there is enhanced facial skin droopiness and obliteration of the demarcation of the contour between jaw and neck.

Hair[6]

Melanin is not produced during telogen which is a stage lengthened with advancing age leading to greying and eventual whitening of the hair. There is a slight decrease in the number of hair follicles due to atrophy and fibrosis. Remaining hairs may be smaller and grow more slowly. Hair is also dull, dry, rough and brittle. Balding results primarily from the androgen-dependent conversion of dark thick terminal hairs to lightly pigmented short fine vellous hairs. Women are affected less often and far less severely than men. In postmenopausal women, hair loss is also due to decreased estrogen levels. Hair is lost from other areas too such as lower legs, axilla and pubis. There may be mild facial hirsutism in women especially on the chin and upper lip. Males may develop bushier eyebrows and visible hairs develop around the external auditory meati.

Nails[6,7]

Nails are affected in the elderly due to impaired circulation, connective tissue changes, concomitant dermatological and systemic diseases and treatments taken for the same. The ageing nails have increased calcium and decreased iron. The nail plate keratinocytes are increased in size with increased number of 'pertinax bodies' which are remnants of keratinocyte nuclei. The nail bed dermis shows thickening of blood vessels and degeneration of elastic tissue. There is a decrease in the rate of linear nail growth. Senile nails may appear pale, dull and opaque with colour ranging from white or yellow to brown or grey. There is an increased transverse curvature to nails with a decreased longitudinal curvature. Altered turnover of the matrix cells may lead to longitudinal striations. Transverse ridges and pitting are also found frequently. In the elderly, the nail plate thickness may increase, decrease or remain unchanged.

COSMETIC SKIN CONCERNS IN THE ELDERLY

1. Wrinkles[8,9]

Wrinkles are the hallmark of ageing skin. They may be defined as creases or furrows in the skin surface. Deepening of the furrows occurs with advancing age. Wrinkles less than 1mm in width and depth are referred to as fine wrinkles whereas those greater than 1 mm are said to be coarse wrinkles. Histologically, there is epidermal thinning, decrease in chondroitin sulphate and deposition of abnormal elastic tissue in the papillary dermis.

Morphologically, wrinkles are of three types:

Crinkles: Refer to fine wrinkling which disappears on stretching the skin degeneration of the vertically-oriented elastic fibres which occurs with physiological ageing and also hastened by sun exposure leads to formation of crinkles.

Glyphic wrinkles: Sun induced photodamage of normal skin resulting in elastotic degeneration of leads to accentuated normal skin markings especially noticeable on the back and sides of neck.

Linear furrows: These are facial linear or curved lines present over forehead, lateral canthus of eyes (crow's feet), side of chin (marionette lines), frown lines and glabellar lines and laugh lines (corners of mouth).

Management[9–16]

Preventive strategies: Although wrinkles cannot be prevented per se, their appearance can be delayed by avoiding factors which contribute to skin ageing

- Regular use of moisturisers and sunscreens
- Avoidance of tobacco and alcohol
- Adequate sleep and exercise
- Avoidance of strong winds, pollution
- Balanced diet

Medical interventions: These are oral and topical medicaments including cosmeceuticals which have some modest improvement especially with fine wrinkles.

- Topical retinoids: Topical tretinoin, adapalene, tazarotene decrease the appearance of fine wrinkles and improve the overall texture of the skin
- Glycolic acid: Increases the collagen, elastin and glycosaminoglycan synthesis causing the dermis to 'plump up' with an improved appearance of wrinkles
- Vitamins C and E: Can be used both orally and topically. Act as antioxidants
- Oral retinoid: Isotretinoin increases the skin thickness and elasticity and improves wrinkles.
- Oral estrogen/hormone replacement therapy (HRT): In postmenopausal women, reverses the hormone-induced changes, increases elasticity and turgor of skin.

Surgical interventions

- Chemical peels: Cause exfoliation of the epidermis and rejuvenation of the dermis. Of use in fine wrinkles. Various peels can be used like glycolic acid, lactic acid, pyruvic acid, yellow peel, ferulic peel or a combination of the above.
- Microdermabrasion: For fine wrinkles. Increases collagen formation and causes epidermal rejuvenation.
- Dermabrasion: For fine wrinkles. Epidermal and dermal resurfacing causing new collagen synthesis.
- Microneedling
- Lasers: Er:YAG, Nd:YAG, CO_2, IPL can be used for treating fine as well as coarse wrinkles.
- Botulinum toxin: A potent neurotoxin that inhibits release of acetylcholine at the neuromuscular junction. Injection into a muscle causes localized muscle relaxation, smoothening of the overlying skin and disappearance of wrinkles. Particularly effective in both fine and coarse wrinkles.
- Fillers: Fillers containg collagen, hyaluronic acid or PMMA are used to fill up the grooves due to shallow or deep nasolabial folds and other facial wrinkles.
- Threads: Absorbable and non-absorbable threads are used in the dermis and subcutis to pull up and tighten lax skin.

2. Photoageing (Dermatoheliosis)[17,18]

Wrinkles do not occur in isolation in the aged skin. Invariably they are accompanied by some element of photoageing. The damage to the skin as a result of UV exposure is understood to be due to the effects of reactive oxygen species such as superoxide anion, peroxide and singlet oxygen.

The following changes are produced in the photoaged skin: Coarsening, deep wrinkling, furrowing, dryness, roughness, laxity, sagging, solar lentigenes, seborrhoeic keratoses, freckles, telangiectasias, purpura, pseudoscars and finally, a tendency to develop premalignant and malignant lesions.

TABLE 17.1: Glogau classification

Type I	Early photoageing	Minimal wrinkles, mild pigmentary changes	Requires little to no make-up	20s to 30s
Type II	Early to moderate photoageing	Wrinkles in motion, early senile lentigenes	Requires some make-up to hide it	30s to 40s
Type III	Advanced photo-ageing	Wrinkles at rest, dyschromia, telengiectasia	Always requires heavy make-up to hide	50s to 60s
Type IV	Severe photoageing	Wrinkles throughout, with no normal skin, yellow-gray colour, precancerous lesions	Cannot be covered with make-up	70s and older

There are 4 types of photoageing as per the Glogau classification (Table 17.1).[19]

a. **Cutis rhomboidalis nuchae:** This is an example of the textural and pigmentary changes that occur on the neck of chronically sun-exposed persons. Deep furrows are present in a criss-cross fashion, creating a rhomboidal or diamond-shaped pattern on thickened, leathery skin.
b. **Solar lentigenes:**[20] Also called liver spots, coffin spots and senile lentigo, they occur more often on sun-exposed areas of caucasian skin. Lesions are flat, brown and are more common on dorsa of hands. The lesions are usually multiple and have circumscribed, well-defined round borders. Histologically, rete ridges are elongated with increased numbers of benign melanocytes. Preventive strategies include use of adequate sun protection. Management involves electrocautery, radiofrequency, topical adapalene and tretinoin or use of lasers like QS Nd:YAG and ablative CO_2.
c. **Senile comedones:** These are seen in elderly people, especially in the periorbital areas. Most patients have had a high amount of sun exposure over the course of a lifetime. Elastotic degeneration of the dermis leads to dilatation of the pilosebaceous duct opening which is clogged by the inspissated keratinocytes. They appear as multiple, grouped, open or closed blackheads over the sundamaged skin around eyes and cheeks. Treatment involves topical retinoids and use of comedo extractor.
d. **Solar elastosis (actinic elastosis):** This is a degenerative change in the dermis caused by prolonged sun exposure. It is characterized clinically by thickening and yellowish discolouration and histologically by degeneration of elastic fibres of the upper and middle dermis which become curled and fibrillar to form thick, irregular masses. At a later stage, the elastotic degeneration becomes more diffuse, forming long, swollen bands of irregular texture, with finely granular elastin and dense microfibrillar masses.

   Favre-Racouchot disease: The combination of solar elastosis with senile comedones, especially in the periorbital area and temples of older individuals, is known as Favre-Racouchot disease. Dermatoheliosis is the necessary background.
e. **Solar purpura (Bateman's senile purpura):** Purpura frequently occurs on the severely sun-damaged skin on the dorsal forearms of the elderly. It occurs due to lack of support to the blood vessels. Lesions appear after minor trauma or apparently spontaneously. They are usually asymptomatic and vary in size from a few mm to several cm across. They are often arranged linearly, and may show a linear or geometric shape.

The appearance of the lesions is characteristic, with irregular red to dark purple patches that show little inflammatory reaction and do not have the sequential colour changes expected from a normal bruise. They may persist for several weeks. Treatment is usually not necessary or possible, however, patients must be investigated to look for underlying platelet disorders or use of concomitant antiplatelet medications.

f. **Stellate and discoid pseudoscars:** Stellate pseudoscars are white, irregular or 'star-shaped' atrophic scars. The term 'pseudoscar' is a misnomer since these are true scars resulting from the tearing of fragile photodamaged skin. They are common on light-exposed skin, particularly on the extensor aspects of the forearms, often in association with senile purpura. These are seen mostly in patients aged 70–90 years, and a much less common presenile form occasionally occurs before the age of 50 years. Brown pseudoscars may also develop over the shins of diabetic patients with no history of trauma.

3. Benign Neoplasms[21, 22]

With advancing age, there is an increased tendency for the development of certain benign neoplasms which can be a source of concern from the aesthetic viewpoint.

a. **Cherry angioma:** Also known as senile hemangiomata or Campbell de Morgan spots, cherry angiomas are produced by spherical and tubular dilatations of capillary loops in the dermal papillae. These bright red or purplish papules are particularly common on the trunk of middle-aged or elderly people. They disappear in extreme old age. They do not empty on pressure and may bleed on trauma. No treatment is indicated however larger lesions can be excised or treated with a vascular laser under local anaesthetic if they are unsightly.

b. **Skin tags (acrochordons):** They are very common in the elderly. They are soft, fleshy, pedunculated lesions with a connective tissue core and occur most commonly on the sides of the neck and in the axillae. Their size varies from a pin-head to pea-sized. These teardrop-shaped tags feel like small bags. Occasionally, as a result of twisting of the pedicle, one will become inflamed, tender, and even gangrenous. They may be associated with diabetes mellitus. Histologically, acrochordons are characterized by epidermis enclosing a dermal fibrovascular stalk. The bag-like papillomas generally show a flattened epidermis. Smaller lesions often demonstrate seborrhoeic keratosis-like acanthosis and horn cysts. Small lesions can be clipped off at the base with anaesthesia. Light electrodesiccation can also be effective. For larger lesions, anaesthesia and snip excision are preferred.

c. **Colloid milium:** Colloid milium is a degenerative change characterized clinically by the development of yellowish, translucent papules or plaques on light-exposed skin, and histologically by the presence of colloid in the dermal papillae. Sun exposure is implicated in older patients. Small dermal papules 1–2 mm in diameter, yellowish brown and sometimes translucent, develop slowly and more or less symmetrically in irregular groups in areas exposed to sunlight especially in the periorbital region, the dorsa of the hands, the back and sides of the neck and the ears. These milia can be manually extracted.

d. **Cutaneous horn:** This is a clinical diagnosis. Horny outgrowths can be caused by various epidermal changes, such as epidermal naevus, wart, molluscum contagiosum, keratoacanthoma, seborrhoeic keratosis, or marsupialized trichilemmal or epidermoid cyst. In most of these cases, the primary diagnosis is suggested by the appearance and clinical course. Clinical examination shows a hard, yellowish brown horn, which is curved with circumferential ridges. They are most common on the exposed areas especially on the upper part of the face. They are commonly single, but may be multiple. Tretment is excision.

e. **Seborrhoeic keratoses:** The precise etiology is unknown—genetics, sun exposure and infections have all been implicated. These are extremely common benign epidermal neoplasms seen in middle-aged and elderly individuals. They usually begin as well circumscribed dull, flat, brownish patches. As they grow, they become more papular and take on a waxy, verrucous, 'stuck on' appearance. Of particular cosmetic concern is the presence of dermatosis papulosa nigra which are small dark papules found on the face of individuals with Fitzpatrick skin type IV or greater. Histologically, they are identical to seborrhoeic keratosis. Symptomatic or cosmetically undesirable seborrhoeic keratoses can be treated with either cryotherapy, electrodessication, curettage or chemical cautery.

f. **Sebaceous hyperplasia:** This is merely a benign proliferation of the sebaceous gland. The sebaceous glands sometimes become prominent in middle-aged or elderly people especially on the forehead and temples and are of no clinical significance however they can be cosmetically unappealing. Treatment is rarely required but some physical treatments such as light cautery, cryotherapy, trichloroacetic acid, and carbon dioxide and pulsed dye laser may be offered.

4. Eczematous Dermatitis[23,24]

Certain eczematous conditions are problematic not just because of the associated symptoms but also the unsightly appearance.

a. **Stasis or gravitational eczema:** It is the eczema that can accompany chronic venous hypertension and is quite common in the elderly. There is scaling, erythema, pigmentation and fibrosis associated with pruritus. Secondary bacterial infection may lead to cellulitis and lymphangitis.

b. **Asteatotic eczema:** Asteatotic dermatitis (eczema craquele) is an eczematous eruption common in the elderly and is characterized by dry, cracked, and fissured patches on the limbs. It is essentially a type of xerosis which is common in winter. Sun, wind, and low humidity are predisposing factors.

5. Disorder of Pigmentation

a. **Idiopathic guttate hypomelanosis:** This is common especially in the elderly and is a source of anxiety especially in a country like India because it is mistaken for vitiligo or leprosy. The lesions usually occur in sun-exposed areas of the limbs.

b. **Melasma:** There is a significant reduction in the prevalence of melasma after the age of 50 possibly due to reduction in hormone levels as also decrease in melanocyte activity with advancing age.[25] Nevertheless, it still remains a source of cosmetic concern for many elderly women.

6. Disorders of Hair[6]

a. **Androgenetic alopecia:** This is a genetically determined non-scarring, patterned hair loss. It is the most common type of hair loss seen in the elderly and is more prevalent with increasing age. In men, it begins with a bitemporal recession of frontal hairline followed by thinning and balding on the vertex eventually leading to the presence of only a strip of hair on the back of the head Finasteride has been shown to be effective even in the older age group.[26]

b. **Senile alopecia:** This is a non-androgen mediated hair loss characterized by slowly progressive thinning of hair on the scalp and body of elderly persons.

c. **Greying and whitening of hair:** This most obvious and striking characteristic of advancing age is inevitable. It occurs due to a lack of melanin in the hair and for which there is no treatment per se.

7. Disorders of Nails[6]

a. **Brittle nails:** Increased fragility of the nail plate is manifested clinically by onychorrhexis and onychoschizia. This is quite common in the geriatric population. Treatment consists of soaking nails in lukewarm water for 25 minutes daily, use of urea-based moisturisers, and supplementation with iron and biotin.

b. **Onychogryphosis:** Frequently present in the elderly, this is characterized by the presence of a grossly thickened, discoloured, opaque nail plate which is curved to resemble a claw. Treatment involves removal of the nail plate either surgically or through nonsurgical methods like use of urea ointments.

CONCLUSION

Aesthetic concerns in the geriatric population are subjective—what may seem like a normal and natural part of the ageing process and merely a minor concern to one may be causing undue distress to another. It is up to the dermatologist to give a patient hearing to every elderly patient, find the cause of their apprehensions, not be dismissive of their desire to be attractive and offer them treatment options whenever possible.

References

1. Population Division, Department of Economic and Social Affairs, United Nations Secretariat. World Population Prospectus: 2002 Revision and World Urbanization Prospectus 2001 Revision. Available from: http://esa.un.org/unpp.
2. Singh Z. Ageing. The triumph of humanity—are we prepared to face the challenge? Indian J Public Health 2012; 56:189–95.
3. Hayakawa Y, Shoji I, Kumon H, Tokita M, Kamata M, Arao T. Feasibility and effectiveness of a cosmetic intervention program for institutionalized older women in Japan. Prev Med Rep. 2016 Jun 16;4:242–7.
4. Yaar, M. and Gilchrest, B. (2012). Ageing of Skin. In: L. Goldsmith, S. Katz, B. Gilchrest, A. Paller, D. Leffell and K. Wolff, (eds) Fitzpatrick's Dermatology in General Medicine, 8th ed. McGraw Hill, pp. 1213–26.
5. Bentov I, Reed MJ. The effect of ageing on the cutaneous microvasculature. Microvasc Res. 2015 Jul; 100:25–31.
6. Maddy AJ, Tosti A. Hair and nail diseases in the mature patient. Clin Dermatol. 2018 Mar–Apr; 36(2):159–66.
7. Singh G, Haneef NS, Uday. Nail changes and disorders among the elderly. Indian J Dermatol Venereol Leprol 2005; 71:386–92.
8. Burrows NP, Lowell CR. Disorders of Connective Tissue. In: Burns T, Breathnach S, Cox N, Griffiths C, eds. Rook's Textbook of Dermatology. 8th edn., Oxford: Wiley-Blackwell publication 2010:45.1–70.
9. Manrique JJ, Cataldo K, Vera-Kellett C, Harz-Fresno-I. Wrinkles. BMJ Clin Evid. 2014; 2014:1711.
10. Khunger N. Ageing Skin. In: Khunger N, Sachdev M (eds) Practical Manual of Cosmetic Dermatology and Surgery, 1st Ed, New Delhi: Mehta Publishers: 2010; 177–92.
11. FisJ Eur Acad Dermatol Venereol. 2010 Mar; 24(3):281–92. cher TC, Perosino E, Poli F, Viera MS, Dreno B. Chemical peels in aesthetic dermatology: an update 2009.
12. Fernandes M, Pinheiro NM, Crema VO, Mendonça AC. Effects of microdermabrasion on skin rejuvenation. J Cosmet Laser Ther. 2014 Jan; 16(1):26–31.
13. Ooe M, Seki T, Miura T, Takada A. Comparative evaluation of wrinkle treatments. Aesthetic Plast Surg. 2013 Apr; 37(2):424–33.
14. Small R. Botulinum toxin injection for facial wrinkles. Am Fam Physician. 2014 Aug 1; 90(3):168–75.
15. Ballin AC, Brandt FS, Cazzaniga A. Dermal fillers: an update. Am J Clin Dermatol. 2015 Aug; 16(4): 271–83.
16. De Masi EC, De Masi FD, De Masi RD. Suspension Threads. Facial Plast Surg. 2016 Dec; 32(6):662–663.
17. Poon F, Kang S, Chien AL. Mechanisms and treatments of photoageing. Photodermatol Photoimmunol Photomed. 2015 Mar; 31(2):65–74.
18. Bilaç C, Sahin MT, Öztürkcan S. Chronic actinic damage of facial skin. Clin Dermatol. 2014 Nov-Dec; 32(6):752–62.
19. Glogau RG. Aesthetic and Anatomic Analysis of the Ageing Skin. Semin Cutan Med Surg. 1996 Sep;15(3):134–8.

20. Ortonne JP, Pandya AG, Lui H, Hexsel D. Treatment of solar lentigines. J Am Acad Dermatol. 2006 May; 54(5 Suppl 2):S262–71.
21. Jindal R, Jain A, Roy S, Rawat SD, Bhardwaj N. Skin Disorders Among Geriatric Population at a Tertiary Care Center in Uttarakhand. J Clin Diagn Res. 2016 Mar; 10(3):WC06–8.
22. Thomas VD, Swanson NA, Lee KK. Benign Epithelial Tumors, Hamartomas and Hyperplasias. In: Wolff K, Goldsmith LA, Katz SI, Gilchrest BA, Paller AS, LEffell DJ, (eds). Fitzpatrick's Dermatology in General Medicine. 7th edn. McGraw Hill publication. 2008: 1054–67.
23. Darjani A, Mohtasham-Amiri Z, Amini KM, Golchai G, Sadre-Eshkevari S, Alizade N. Skin Disorders among Elder Patients in a Referral Center in Northern Iran. Dermatol Res Pract. 2013; 2013: 193–205.
24. Souissi A, Zeglaoui F, El Fekih N, Fazaa B, Zouari B, Kamoun MR. Skin diseases in the elderly: a multi-centre Tunisian study. Ann Dermatol Venereol. 2006 Mar; 133(3):231–4.
25. Handel AC, Miot LD, Miot HA. Melasma: a clinical and epidemiological review. An Bras Dermatol. 2014 Sep-Oct; 89(5):771–82.
26. Whiting DA, Olsen EA, Savin R, *et al.* Efficacy and tolerability of finasteride 1 mg in men aged 41 to 60 years with male pattern hair loss. Eur J Dermatol. 2003; 13(2):150–60.

CHAPTER 18

Pigmentary Disorders in Elderly

• *Vibhu Mendiratta*

Introduction

Chronological ageing modifies the pigmentary system of skin. The number of enzymatically active melanocytes depletes by 10–20% per decade. Skin looks thinner, paler, and clear (translucent) on ageing.[1] Photoageing contributes to skin pigmentation and habitually photo exposed areas bear twice the number of melanocytes and appear blotchy with specific pigmented dermatoses in elderly. Melanocytic naevi are rarely seen beyond 80 years. Elderly patients can develop both hyper and hypopigmentation. Some common hyperpigmented conditions include lentigines, blotchy pigmentation secondary to photoageing, drug induced pigmentation, notalgia paraesthetica, post-inflammatory pigmentation , oral and genital melanosis, etc. (Table 18.1) and pigmentation secondary to systemic diseases and exogenous agents (chemicals) (Table 18.2). Vitiligo, idiopathic guttate hypermelanosis, lichen sclerosus et atrophicus, mycosis fungoides, Hansen's disease constitute some hypopigmented disorders in the elderly (Table 18.3).

TABLE 18.1: Hyperpigmentation in elderly

- Lentigines: Simple lentigo, solar lentigo, PUVA lentigo
- Drug-induced pigmentation: Anti-malarials, amiodarone, minocycline, clofazimine, hydantoin, psychotropic drugs (trifluoperazine, imipramine)
- Acquired brachial cutaneous dyschromatosis
- Notalgia paresthetica
- Macular amyloidosis
- Smokers melanosis
- Genital melanosis
- Erythema ab igne
- Post-inflammatory (eczemas/photodermatitis/stasis dermatitis)

TABLE 18.2: Conditions associated with generalised pigmentation in elderly

- Endocrinopathies (Addison's disease, Cushing's syndrome, hyperthyroidism)
- Nutritional (Vit A, Pellagra, Vit B_{12}, Vit C, folic acid deficiency, vagabond disease)
- Hypermelanosis in other systemic disorders (chronic hepatic and renal failure, primary biliary cirrhosis, POEMS syndrome)
- Hypermelanosis in malignancy: Malignant melanoma, carcinoid syndrome
- Non-melanin pigmentation: Hemochromatosis, jaundice, carotenemia, tatto
- Metals: Silver (argyria), arsenic, bismuth, gold (chrysiasis)

TABLE 18.3: Hypopigmented disorders

- Vitiligo
- Idiopathic guttate hypomelanosis
- Mycosis fungoides
- Progressive macular hypomelanosis
- Lichen sclerosus et atrophicus
- Leprosy
- Post-inflammatory hypopigmentation

HYPERPIGMENTATION IN ELDERLY

Senile Lentigo

These are benign, multiple hyperpigmented macules, size (few mm >1 cm across), having a regular/irregular border, mottled appearance without scaling, infiltration or hyperkeratosis (Fig. 18.1). More than 90% of Caucasians develop lentigos. Hyperpigmentation of the basal layer with an increase in the dopa-positive epidermal melanocytes and elongation of rete ridges are the most important histopathological features.

Lentigo Maligna

Lentigo maligna is more common in type 1 skin but can occur in type 3 also. It occurs more commonly in men, outdoor workers, between 60–80 years and in association with solar damage). They have a large size: >6 mm and often several centimetres in diameter at diagnosis. Lentigo maligna has irregular shape, smooth surface with a variegate pigmentation—colours may include light brown or tan, dark brown, pink, red or white (Fig. 18.2). Thickening in the part of lentigo or any colour change such as blue/black or ulceration and bleeding are suggestive of development of melanoma. Confirmation of diagnosis is by dermatoscopy/confocal microscopy and excision biopsy.[2]

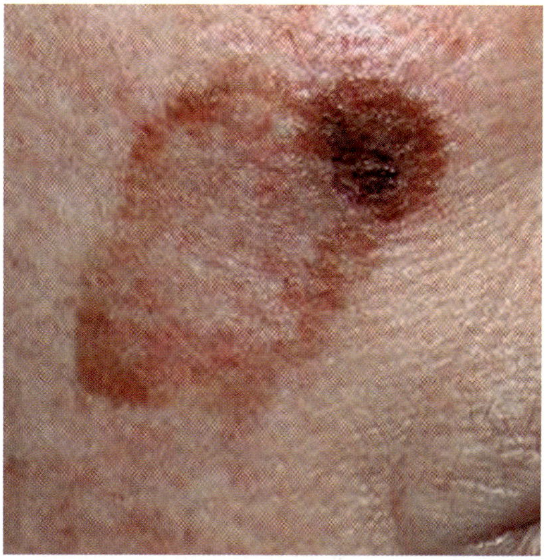

Fig. 18.2: Lentigo maligna

Notalgia Paraesthetica

Notalgia paresthetica (NP) is a sensory neuropathic syndrome affecting the skin over midback. It is classically described as an asymmetrical, small, hyperpigmented patch over infrascapular area (Fig. 18.3). It may present with episodic itching or pain on a small hyperpigmented patch over the mid back, usually an area of skin just past easy reach.[3]

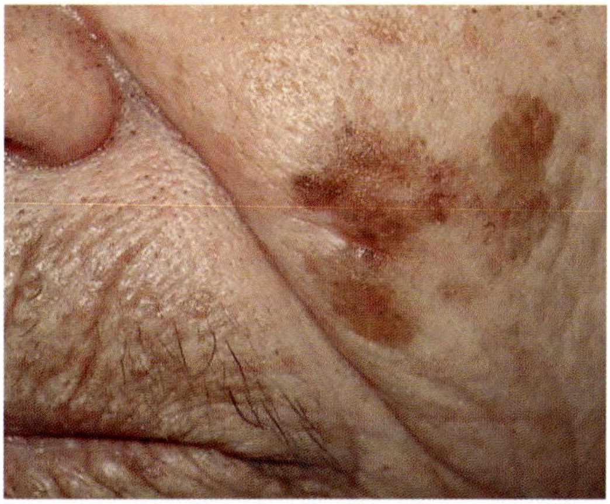

Fig. 18.1: Senile lentigo

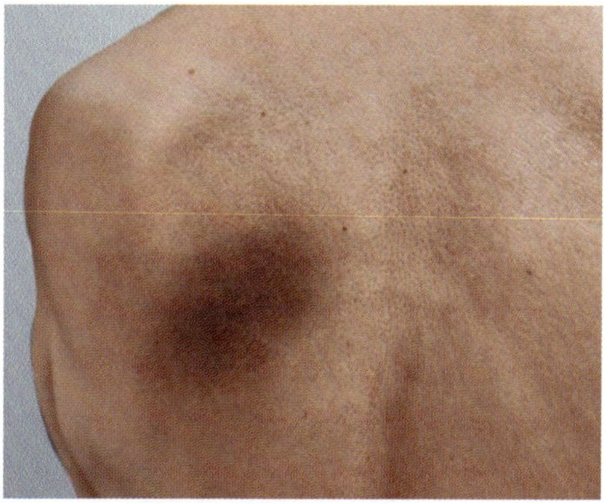

Fig. 18.3: Notalgia paraesthetica

Acquired Brachial Cutaneous Dyschromatosis

Acquired brachial cutaneous dyschromatosis (ABCD) is a newly described disorder of pigmentary change that occurs on the dorsal aspects of the forearms in postmenopausal women. It is characterized by asymptomatic, irregular, gray-brown patches with geographic borders, which were occasionally interspersed with hypopigmented, slightly atrophic macules. For treatment depigmenting agents, chemical peels, lasers have been used.

Brachioradial pruritus also belongs to the category of neuropathic itch and like NP is common in subjects >60 years. Symptoms include pricking/stabbing sensations along with burning and pruritus. Like NP it is associated with neural compression syndromes or spinal canal stenosis. Application of ice, local application of capsaicin cream provides partial relief.[3]

Smoker's Melanosis

Appears as a brown to black pigmentation of the oral tissue, i.e. the gums, cheeks or palate as well as in larynx to the naked eye. It is most often seen in the lower labial gingiva of tobacco users (Fig. 18.4).

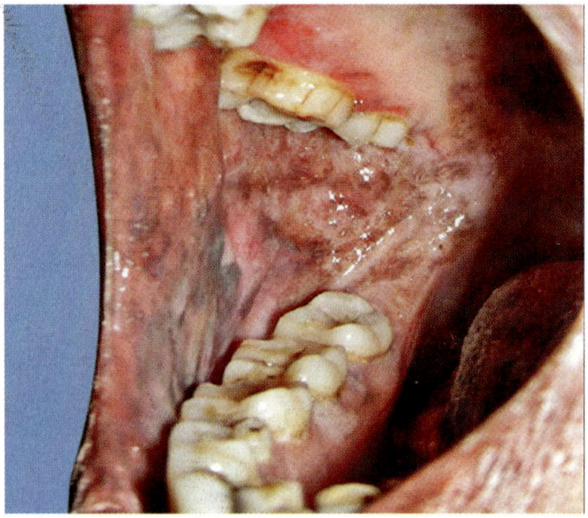

Fig. 18.4: Oral melanosis

Genital Melanosis

Asymptomatic hyperpigmented macules are present on penis, vulva, vagina (Fig. 18.5). No treatment is required. Q-switch laser is an effective treatment.

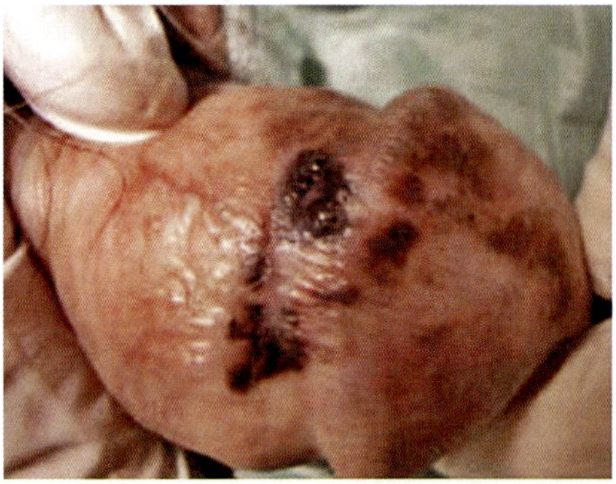

Fig. 18.5: Genital melanosis

Erythema Ab Igne (EAI)

It is a common pigmentary dermatosis in elderly who often use heaters to keep them warm during winters. EAI is characterized by localized areas of reticulated erythema and hyperpigmentation due to chronic and repeated exposure to infrared radiation (Fig. 18.6). Patients with erythema ab igne have a history of repeated exposures to heat at a lower level than that which causes a thermal burn. Its incidence has been rising as heating sources are being used to treat chronic pain. Use of an electric blankets also is known to promote EAI.

Treatment includes removal of offending heating device, topical tretinoin or 5-FU application or, Q-switch lasers.[4]

Drug-induced Pigmentation

Polypharmacy in elderly population predisposes them to develop drug-induced skin eruptions. Drug-induced pigmentation must be considered in subjects who receive multiple drugs. Pathogenesis of drug-induced pigmentation is variable according to the causative medication and may involve accumulation of melanin, sometimes following a nonspecific cutaneous inflammation and often worsened by sun exposure, an accumulation of the triggering drug itself, or synthesis of special pigments under the direct influence of the drug or deposits of iron following damage to the dermal vessels. Various drugs are implicated in inducing skin pigmentation namely nonsteroidal anti-inflammatory drugs, antimalarials, amiodarone, cytotoxic drugs, tetracyclines, heavy metals and psychotropic drugs. Clinical features are very variable according to the triggering molecule, with a large range of patterns. Histological findings are variable. Coloured particles are often concentrated within dermal macrophages which are sometimes localized in a distinctive fashion with respect to dermal structures such as vessels or adnexes. Treatment is limited to sun-avoidance and interruption of the offending drug. Laser therapy can help reduce the pigmentation. Drug induced pigmentation may last for a long time or may even become permanent in a small percentage of patients.

Post-inflammatory Pigmentation

History is suggestive of pre-existing inflammation. The pattern of pigmentation may provide clues to underlying condition. The lesions are ill-defined and may show areas with patchy hypopigmentation.[5]

Macular Amyloidosis

Primary localised cutaneous amyloidosis (PLCA) refers to amyloid deposition in the skin without any previous skin disease. Whereas deposition of amyloid with pre-existing cutaneous lesion (s), is called secondary localised cutaneous amyloidosis. Primary localised cutaneous amyloidosis can be of various types, i.e. lichenoid, papular or macular type. Rare varieties include nodular, bullous, poikilodermatous, vitiliginous or ichthyosiform amyloidosis. Macular amyloidosis is non-itchy, reticulate macular, brownish pigmentation in a rippled pattern

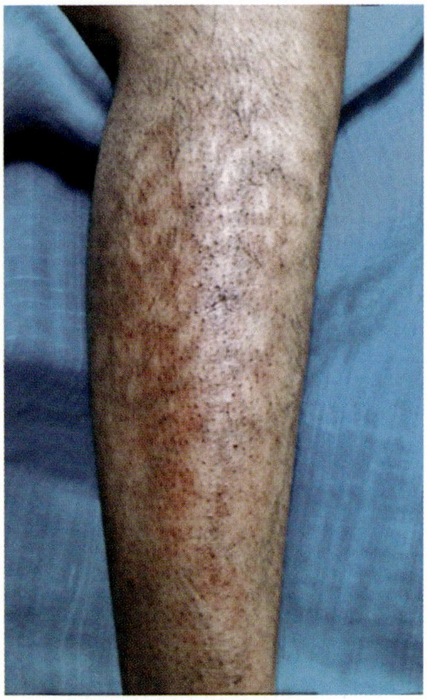

Fig. 18.6: Erythema ab igne

over interscapular area, shins, arms and the neck (Fig. 18.7). Frictional melanosis secondary to use of loofah any other rubbing or scrubbing device in elderly can cause hyperpigmentation poikiloderma like cutaneous amyloidosis was reported in a 62-year-old man. Diagnosis of this unique condition is a challenge and a skin biopsy is necessary in such instances topical treatment with corticosteroids with or without occlusion, 10% DMSO, retinoic acid derivatives is advocated, but is often unsatisfactory. Dermabrasion may be beneficial for lichen amyloidosis over the shins. Etretinate appears to be helpful in relieving the pruritus in PLCA, but the condition soon relapses after the drug is stopped.[6]

Should there be a mention of lichen planus pigmentosus?

HYPOPIGMENTATION IN ELDERLY

Vitiligo

Vitiligo causes psychological stress in elderly also and they also have cosmetic concerns,

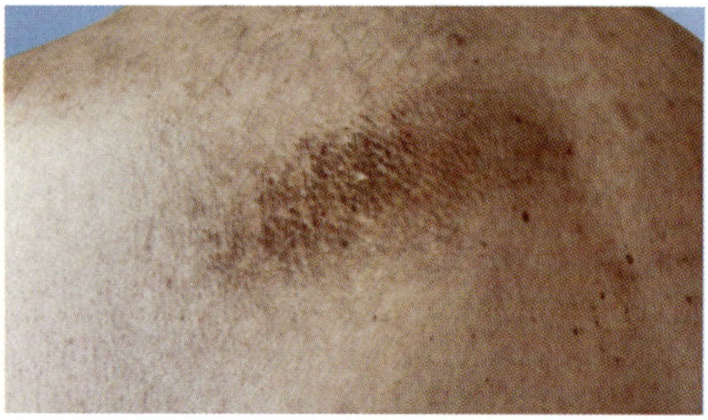

Fig. 18.7: Macular amyloidosis

thus treatment is actively sought for late onset vitiligo. Vitiligo is an autoimmune disorder characterized by localized and/or generalized depigmentation of the skin and/or mucous membranes, well circumscribed, ivory or chalky white macules which are flush to the skin surface. Although 20% cases begin before 20 years, a significant number of patients have a late onset vitiligo, that begins after 50 years. A study from India showed that majority of the patients were between 55 and 60 years of age, had a female preponderance. Vitiligo vulgaris was the commonest variant. Head and neck were common sites of onset (Fig. 18.8). The majority of patients had a stable course of disease. Acquired autoimmune disorders were noted in 21.4% cases suggesting an active search for thyroid disorders, diabetes and rheumatoid arthritis.[7,8] Vitiligo can occur over bald scalp and genitalia. Vitligo must be differentiated from chemical leukoderma in the elderly. First line therapy includes—topical calcineurin inhibitors (tacrolimus) and topical steroid. Narrow-band ultraviolet B (NB-UVB), targeted phototherpy (excimer lamp and lasers) are some other options. Nutritional rehabilitation is also helpful.

Idiopathic Guttate Hypomelanosis (IGH)

IGH is a common acquired leukoderma characterised by multiple, discrete round or oval, porcelain-white macules on sun-exposed areas, especially on the extensor surface of forearms and pretibial areas (Fig. 18.9). It usually affects individuals aged over 40 years.

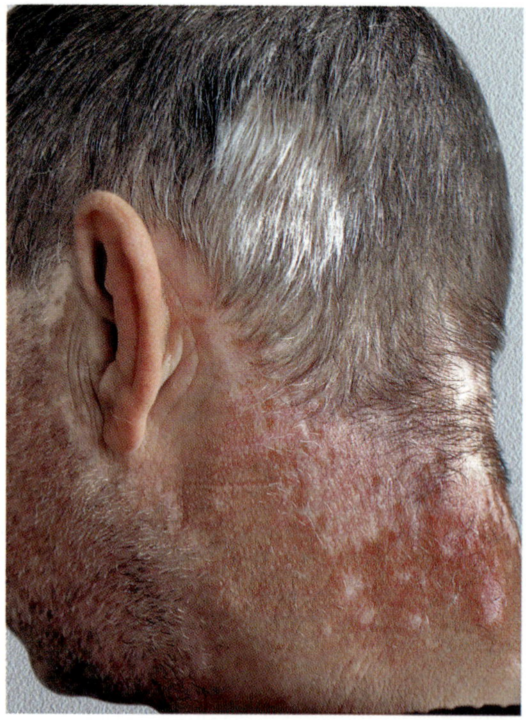

Fig. 18.8: Vitiligo

The spots increase with age. Aging, ultraviolet exposure, trauma, genetic factors, autoimmunity, and local inhibition of melanogenesis are some of the factors proposed in its pathogenesis. IGH has a benign course of progression. Numerous medical and surgical treatments including topical corticosteroids, topical retinoids, topical calcineurin inhibitors, phenol peeling, cryotherapy, superficial dermabrasion, skin grafting, and ablative and non-ablative lasers have been tried with mixed results. The condition needs to be differentially diagnosed from lichen sclerosus et atrophicus and guttate morphea.[9]

Mycosis Fungoides

Hypopigmented mycosis fungoidesis a subtype of mycosis fungoides. Most patients with hypopigmented mycosis fungoides are younger than patients typically diagnosed with classical mycosis fungoides. Adults more >30 years can present with hypopigmented

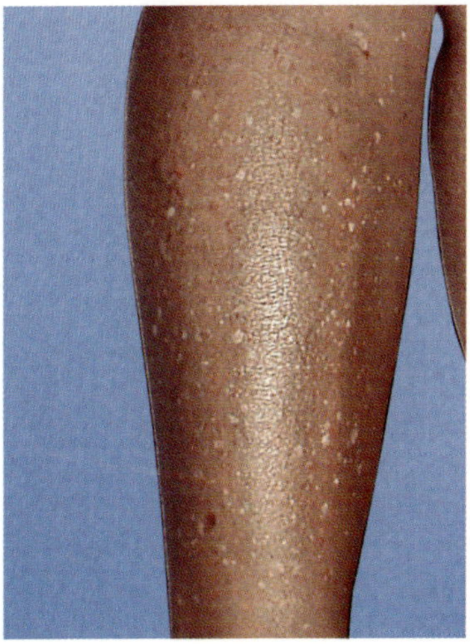

Fig. 18.9: Idiopathic guttate hypomelanosis

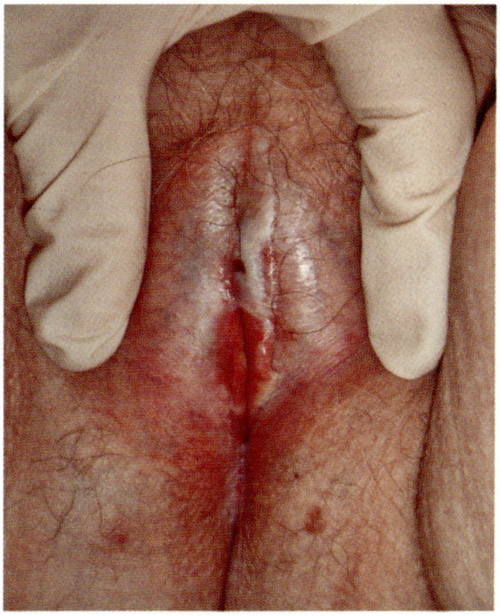

Fig. 18.10: Lichen sclerosus et atrophicus

patches which are diagnosed late after a couple of years. The prognosis for hypopigmented mycosis fungoides is much better than for classical mycosis fungoides: Hypopigmented mycosis fungoides is diagnosed when there are only patches of affected skin, and lesions usually will not progress beyond terminal stages, although they can persist for many years. Diagnosis should involve clinicopathologic correlation: Skin biopsy analysis often reveals intense epidermotropism, characterized by haloed, large, and atypical CD8+ lymphocytes with convoluted nuclei, in contrast to mild to moderate dermal lymphocytic infiltrate.[10]

Lichen Sclerosus et Atrophicus (LSEA)

Vulvar lichen sclerosus (VLS) is a chronic inflammatory dermatosis characterized by ivory-white plaques or patches with glistening surface commonly affecting the vulva and anus. Common symptoms are irritation, soreness, dyspareunia, dysuria, and urinary or fecal incontinence. Anogenital lichen sclerosus (LS) is characterized by porcelain-white atrophic plaques, which may become confluent extending around the vulval and perianal skin in a figure of eight configuration (Fig. 18.10). Thinning and shrinkage of the genital area make coitus, urination, and defecation painful. LS is not uncommon in India and present as an itchy vulvar dermatosis. There is often a delay in diagnosis of VLS due to its asymptomatic nature and lack of awareness. Regular follow-up is required as there is a risk of developing squamous cell carcinoma. Bullous LSEA has been reported in a female patient aged 55 years. Some of these lesions evolved with haemorrhagic blisters. The patient was treated with high-potency topical corticosteroid for two months, resulting in remission of bullous and haemorrhagic lesions.[11]

Penile lichen sclerosus, also known as balanitis xerotica obliterans, is a chronic inflammatory condition of the penis which can occur at all ages. The inflammation leads to the formation of white plaques most commonly on the foreskin or penis, and can lead to inability to retract the foreskin or blockage to the flow of urine (Fig. 18.11). Cancer may occur rarely. Penile lichen sclerosus is a progressive, sclerosing, inflammatory dermatosis of the glans penis and foreskin which is of uncertain aetiology. Recent studies have shown a link between lichen sclerosus and

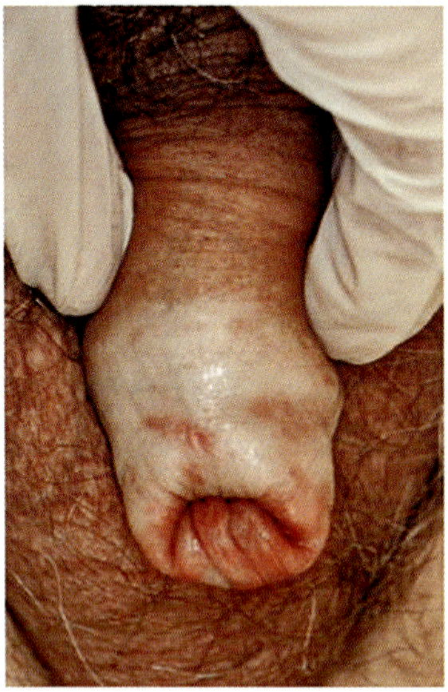

Fig. 18.11: Balanitis xerotica obliterans

squamous cell carcinoma of the penis. Meatoplasty was performed in one patient with a meatal stenosis. No coexistence of penile cancer was observed. Statistically significant improvements were observed in subjective and objective findings after treatment. In conclusion, BXO with phimosis in elderly patients should be considered as a cause of lower urinary tract symptoms.[12]

Hansen's Disease

Late onset leprosy occurring after 50 years is well known although there is lack of consolidated data on the same. Elderly patients can also present with late onset neuropathy, trophic ulcers and osteomyelitis. They are more likely to present with deformities and osteomyelitis. Cutaneous examination might show hypopigmented macules or atrophic patches in case of burned out disease.

References

1. Waller JM, Maibach HI. Age and skin structure and function, a quantitative approach (I): blood flow, pH, thickness, and ultrasound echogenicity. Skin Res Technol. 2005 Nov; 11(4):21–35
2. Flat pigmented macules on sun-damaged skin of the head/neck: Junctional nevus, atypical lentiginous nevus, or melanoma in situ? Clinics in Dermatology. 32, (1) Jan-Feb; 2014; 88–93.
3. Pereira MP, Lüling H, Dieckhöfer A, Steinke S, Zeidler C, Ständer S. Brachioradial Pruritus and Notalgia Paraesthetica: A Comparative Observational Study of Clinical Presentation and Morphological Pathologies. Acta Derm Venereol. 2018 Jan 12;98(1):82–8.
4. Huynh N, Sarma D, Huerter C. Erythema ab igne: a case report and review of the literature. Cutis. 2011 Dec;88(6):290–2.
5. Passeron T.Post-inflammatory hyperpigmentation. Ann Dermatol Venereol. 2016 Dec; 143 Suppl 2:S15–S19.
6. Heng JK, Ho SA, Tan KB. Poikiloderma-like cutaneous amyloidosis—a rare presentation of primary localized cutaneous amyloidosis.Dermatol Online J. 2016 Jan 15;22(1).
7. Dogra S, Parshad D, Handa S, Kanwar AJ. Late onset vitiligo: A study of 182 patients. Int J Dermatol 2005; 44:193–6.
8. Mason CP, Gawkrodger DJ. Vitiligo presentation in adults. Clin Exp Dermatol 2005; 30:344–5.
9. Koh WS1, Kim JE1, Ro YS1, Ko JY1. Comparative study of ablative fractional photothermolysis versus topical retinoid cream in the treatment of idiopathic guttate hypomelanosis.J Cosmet Laser Ther. 2018 Mar 16:1–5.
10. Rodney IJ, Kindred C, Angra K, Qutub ON, Villanueva AR, Halder RM. Hypopigmented mycosis fungoides: a retrospective clinicohistopathologic study. J Eur Acad Dermatol Venereol. 2017 May; 31(5):808–14.
11. Lima RS, Maquiné GÁ, Schettini AP, Santos M Bullous and hemorrhagic lichen sclerosus—case report. An Bras Dermatol. 2015 May-Jun; 90(3 Suppl 1):118–20.
12. Nemoto K, Ishidate T. [Balanitis xerotica obliterans with phimosis in elderly patients presenting with difficulty in urination]. Hinyokika Kiyo. 2013 Jun; 59(6):341–6.

CHAPTER 19

Cutaneous Tumours in Elderly

• *Meghana Madhukar Phiske*

Key Points
- Elderly
- Skin cancers
- Basal cell carcinoma
- Squamous cell carcinoma
- Melanoma

Introduction

In the last two decades there is a worldwide surge in incidence of cutaneous malignancy reaching an epidemic proportion, contributing to overall burden of cutaneous conditions in elderly, determining significant morbidity, mortality and health-related costs. Lifetime sun exposure, cumulative exposure to carcinogens, increasingly ageing population and age-related factors are contributory to high prevalence.[1] Factors like social isolation, skin changes and medical comorbidities, cause neglect of malignant tumours, leading to advanced stages.[2]

Epidemiology

White-skinned elderly population represents largest patient group at-risk for developing skin cancer. The National Institute on ageing classifies elderly into young-old (aged 65–75), old (aged 76–85) and oldest-old (older than 85 years). Prevalence is 2.1–8.3% obtained from geriatric units, as opposed to 9–12% reported in elderly attending dermatology clinics. Causes for disparity in prevalence are: (1) Selection bias, (2) different study designs, case-definitions and geographical origin of studies. Improved methods of screening/diagnosis, increased disease awareness and an ageing population also increase incidence.

Non-melanomatous skin cancer (NMSC) is commonest cancer, with basal cell carcinoma (BCC) representing largest portion (3 million cases annually). BCC incidence has increased by 10% in the last decade, being highest in white individuals of old and oldest old age, ranging from 13 to 12,100 per 100000 person/years, varying depending on skin phototype and geographical location.[1,2]

SKIN CANCERS IN ELDERLY

Cutaneous malignancies have epidermal, melanocytic or mesodermal origin. They comprise cutaneous melanoma and NMSC, encompassing heterogeneous clinical spectrum in terms of morbidity and mortality. NMSC (80% of all cutaneous tumours) category includes several types of tumours, but BCC (70%) and cutaneous squamous cell carcinoma (cSCC) (20%) are most important from an epidemiological and clinical perspective.[1]

Table 19.1 mentions benign and malignant tumours in elderly.[3]

TABLE 19.1: Benign and malignant tumours in elderly

Benign tumours	Malignant tumours
Seborrhoeic keratoses	Bowen's disease
Keratoacanthoma	Basal cell carcinoma
Epidermal cyst	Squamous cell carcinoma
Sebaceous hyperplasia	Melanoma
	Actinic keratosis

Table 19.2 mentions characteristic features of tumours.[3]

TABLE 19.2: Characteristic features of tumours

Tumour type	Characteristic features
Epidermal tumours	Scaling, hyperkeratosis and loss of surface lines May occasionally be pigmented
Melanocytic tumours	Brown to black in colour
Mesodermal tumours	Papulonodular in appearance and red or yellow colour

BENIGN TUMOURS IN ELDERLY

A. Benign Tumours of Epidermis (Epidermal Tumours)

1. Seborrhoeic Keratosis[3,4]

They are among the most common benign skin tumours, being confused with solar lentigo.

Clinical features

They develop after middle age and occur in both sexes, commonly seen on face, sparing palms/soles. They are multiple, sharply defined, brown to black, round to oval papules with uneven, hyperkeratotic and verrucous, dull surface with multiple plugged follicles (Fig. 19.1). They may be hundreds, appearing primarily on back, chest and face.

Diagnosis

Histology shows hyperkeratosis, acanthosis and papillomatosis, interwoven tracts of basoloid and squamoid cells with true horn or pseudohorn cysts. Lower border of tumour is in a straight line with that of adjoining normal skin. Dermal infiltrate may be mild, band-like or eczematous.[4]

Treatment

Treatment is required for cosmetically unacceptable, inflamed or atypical lesions and includes curettage, cryosurgery, electrodessication or laser ablation. In patients with numerous lesions, topical alpha hydroxy acid is effective.[3,4]

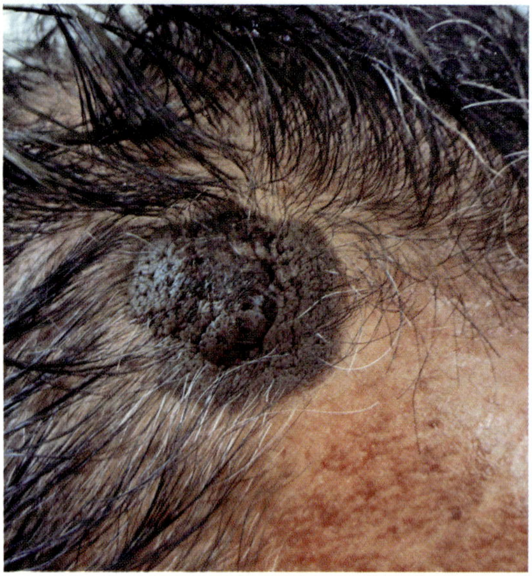

Fig. 19.1: Seborrhoeic keratoses

2. Keratoacanthoma (KA)

It is squamoproliferative benign tumour of hair bearing skin, rarely progressing into SCC.[4]

Epidemiology and etiopathogenesis

It occurs on sunexposed areas, common in light colored individuals, with peak incidence in sixth and seventh decade. In temperate regions 70% KA occurs on face while in subtropics they are seen on arms, dorsal aspects of hands and lower extremities. It develops due to interaction between genetic predisposition, ultraviolet radiation, chemical agents like tar, viral infections, trauma and immunosuppression.[4]

Clinical features

It presents as solitary, flesh coloured, dome shaped nodule with a central keratin plug (Fig. 19.2). Its evolution occurs in three stages: proliferating, mature and resolving. It appears suddenly, grows rapidly over 1–2 months; stabilizes for weeks and then regress, leaving large, scarred, depressed area over 4–6 months. Multiple eruptive lesions can occur. It can recur in 8%.[3,4]

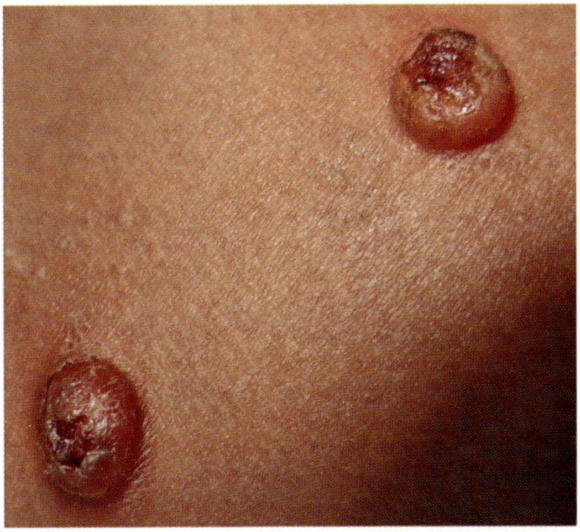

Fig. 19.2: Keratoacanthoma

Diagnosis

Histopathology shows a keratin filled invagination of epidermis. Below epidermis are epidermal strands protruding into dermis that is poorly demarcated from surrounding stroma consisting of mixed infiltrate. Epidermal strands show atypical cells with nuclear atypia and atypical mitoses and dyskeratotic cells. Fully developed lesions show epidermal extension on sides of keratin filled crater like a lip with irregular downward proliferation of epidermis. Keratinization is advanced giving epidermis glassy appearance. There are many horn pearls.[4]

Treatment[3,4]

Various treatment modalities for KA are mentioned in Table 19.3.

TABLE 19.3: Various treatment modalities for KA

Various treatment modalities for KA	Utility
Surgical excision	Used for solitary KA (treatment of choice) Used for accurate histologic examination Used for cosmetic reasons Used for multiple lesions not responding to other treatment modalities
Mohs surgery	Done for lesions over critical anatomic sites or for large lesions
Systemic therapy (retinoids, methotrexate, 5-FU, cyclophosamide)	Used for multiple lesions
ILS chemotherapy with 5-FU	Used for large, mutilating lesions or for lesions on nose and lips
Other treatment modalities Interferon α-2a, bleomycin, intralesional triamcinolone, topical imiquimod Cryosurgery, electrodessication radiotherapy, curettage, laser surgery	

3. Epidermal Cyst

They usually occur on head, neck and trunk, having smooth surface, with sloping borders. Boundaries are appreciated on palpation and lesion is always larger than clinically suspected. Treatment includes surgical excision with removal of tumour sac to reduce recurrence.[3]

4. Sebaceous Hyperplasia

It usually occurs on face presenting as multiple, 1 to 3 mm, yellowish, dome-shaped papules with small telangiectatic vessels over surface and central umbilication. Treatment includes cryosurgery and/or bichloracetic acid application.[3]

5. Other Benign Tumours

These include junctional, dermal, compound, halo and blue nevi. They are black to blue to light brown. Their number increases up to fourth decade and then begins to involute. Appearance of new nevi after 40 years requires follow-up or biopsy to rule out malignancy.[3]

B. Melanocytic Skin Tumours

These appear first from birth to adolescence and throughout their existence, they may change colour, shape and size, which are normal, being associated with ageing, irritation or pregnancy. Removal and histological evaluation is indicated if suspicious changes occur.[3]

C. Mesodermal Skin Tumours

Mesodermal tumours in elderly are mentioned in Table 19.4.[3]

Benign Mesodermal Tumours

1. **Angiomatous lesions:** These are red to blue and ooze blood on light pressure.
2. **Cherry angiomas:** These are common, appearing as bright-red papular lesions on trunk.
3. **Venous lakes:** These are common blue papular-nodular lesions occurring on face, especially lips.
4. **Angiokeratomas of Fordyce:** They are small, red to blue-black papular tumours seen on scrotum; first appearing in middle age, becoming multiple.
5. **Dermatofibromas:** They are common on legs and arms presenting as firm, brown to pink papules or nodules.
6. **Fibroepitheliomas:** They are papillomatous lesions occurring over neck, axillae, groin and inframammary regions.[3]

   Benign tumours can be removed by electrodessication and excision.

Malignant Mesodermal Tumours

1. **Kaposi's sarcoma:** It is uncommon elderly patients, seen in immunosuppression states (renal transplantation/AIDS). It is seen on lower legs, as blue papule or plaque. Therapy consists of local radiation or chemotherapy with vinblastine or cyclophosphamide.

TABLE 19.4: Mesodermal tumours in elderly

Benign lesions	Malignant lesions
Angiomatous	Kaposi's sarcoma
Cherry angioma	Angiosarcoma
Venous lake	
Angiokeratoma	
Dermatofibroma	
Fibroepithelioma	

2. **Angiosarcoma:** It is an aggressive, asymptomatic tumour presenting as reddish purple nodules usually on scalp with poor prognosis. Treatment includes wide excision, with grafting.[3]

D. Premalignant Tumours of Epidermis

1. Actinic Keratosis (AK)

It is a premalignant lesion occurring on sun damaged skin, being an early stage in the biological continuum of SCC.[4]

Epidemiology and etiopathogenesis[4]

It is a common tumour in Caucasian Australian population, mainly men, with mean prevalence of 20%. Intermittent and cumulative sunexposure is risk factor. UVB and UVA are responsible; leading to UV induced mutation in telomerase and tumour suppressor gene on chromosome 17p132. Suspectible individuals include:

1. Fair skin
2. History of sunburn
3. Presence of solar lentigenes, solar elastosis, freckles and red hair.
4. People residing at low latitude or high altitude
5. Advancing age
6. High fat diet

Clinical features

It occurs on face, bald scalp, sides of neck, dorsa of hands and presents as multiple, keratotic papules or red, scaly macules. It is easily felt than seen, due to its rough quality. Increase in size, bleeding, ulceration, induration suggests malignant transformation. 5 to 10% of AK evolve into SCC, with extremely low potential for metastasis.[4]

Diagnosis

Histopathology shows intraepidermal neoplasm characterized by atypical keratinocytes showing large nuclei with prominent nucleoli and pale cytoplasm, loss of polarity, mitotic activity and dyskeratoses involving variable depth of epidermis.[4]

Treatment[3,4]

Treatment modalities for AK are mentioned in Table 19.5.

TABLE 19.5: Treatment modalities for AK

Medical therapy	Surgical therapy
5% imiquimod	Cryotherapy (for solitary or multiple, hypertrophic and resistant lesions)
Intralesional interferon	Curettage
5-fluorouracil (for numerous poorly defined actinic keratoses on face, scalp and ears)	Shave excision
Systemic retinoids	Electrosurgery Excision (for resistant lesions) Dermabrasion Chemical destruction with trichloroacetic acid and salicyclic acid Laser surgery Photodynamic therapy with 5 aminolevulinic acid

2. Bowen's Disease (BD)

It is intraepidermal-epidermoid carcinoma *in situ*, occurring mainly in fair skinned individuals, in sixth to eight decades, on exposed and covered areas. 3% of BD can advance to invasive SCC.[4]

Epidemiology and etiopathogenesis[4]

It arises from outer root sheath of hair follicle or epidermal cells of acrotrichum.

Various other causes for BD are included in Table 19.6.

TABLE 19.6: Various other causes for BD

- Chronic sun exposure
- Arsenic exposure
- HPV
- Genetic factors
- Trauma
- Chronic irritation
- Chemical carcinogens
- Tobacco exposure
- X-ray radiation
- Thermal injury
- Therapeutic immunosuppression in organ transplant

Clinical features

Lesions are circumscribed, round to oval, pink to salmon red scaly patches or plaques, small to large which may become hyperkeratotic, crusted, fissured or ulcerated.[3, 4]

Diagnosis

Histopathology shows full thickness epidermal dysplasia with pagetoid cells, which are atypical large pale keratinocytes with abundant ground glass cytoplasm and loss of polarity, are distributed haphazardly throughout epidermis giving windblown appearance.[4]

Treatment

Various treatment modalities for BD are mentioned in Table 19.7.

TABLE 19.7: Various treatment modalities for BD

Medical therapy	Surgical therapy
5 FU	Simple excision
Imiquimod	Mohs surgery
PDT	Curettage
X ray radiation	Electrodessication
	Cryotherapy
	Lasers like Nd: YAG and CO_2

MALIGNANT TUMOURS IN ELDERLY

1. Basal Cell Carcinoma (BCC)

BCC are clinically slow-growing tumours, characterized by local tissue invasion and very low rate of metastatic invasion (<0, 05%). It can invade underlying structures, causing local tissue destruction, functional impairment and aesthetic mutilation.[1]

Etiology

Predisposing factors are genetic and environmental; others are included in Table 19.8.

TABLE 19.8: Risk factors for development of BCC
• Male sex
• Old age
• Ionizing radiation
• Immunosuppression
• Fair skin phototype (Fitzpatrick I or II)
• Chronic arsenic ingestion
• Family history

BCC arises from hair follicle stem cells or from progenitor cells in interfollicular epidermis. Genetic studies have identified germline mutations in hedgehog (Hh) signaling pathway, key component of which is receptor protein called smoothened (SMO), which constitutively stimulates cell proliferation, by activating nuclear transcription factors. This signaling pathway is kept in check by a transmembrane protein, patched (PTCH). BCC carcinogenesis is characterized by aberrant activation of Hh pathway, resulting from either genetic inactivation of PTCH or activating mutations in SMO.[1]

Clinical Features[1]

It has variable appearance, being small erythematous and/or crusted patch or nodule, scar-like or ulcerative, seen commonly in light-skinned males. 93% occur on head and neck, 60% above a line drawn from ear to corner of mouth and 7% on trunk.

Different clinical subtypes include:

1. **Noduloulcerative:** It is most common, less aggressive type, presenting as waxy or pearly nodule with central ulceration and telangiectatic vessels threading over translucent, rolled, sloping borders.
2. **Superficial:** It is less aggressive, presenting as multiple, superficial, sharply marginated plaques, with pearly, thread-like borders and central crust.
3. **Sclerodermiform:** It is more aggressive.
4. Pigmented
5. Ulcerated
6. **Rare type:** Inside BCC lesion, there can be squamous features without clear separation; this mixed morphology is called baso-squamous carcinoma, which is aggressive, has higher tendency for recurrence and metastases. Delayed diagnosis leads to extensive, giant tumours more than 10 cm, causing local tissue destruction, disfigurement and major surgical defects.

BCC are classified into low and high-risk tumours based on risk of recurrence, number of lesions, size, location and clinicopathological phenotype.

Diagnosis

Clinical suspicion, dermoscopy and biopsy aid in diagnosis.[1] Histopathology shows presence of nests of basoloid tumours with hyperchromatic nuclei and scanty cytoplasm, palisading of cells at periphery and retraction artifact.[4]

Treatment Modalities[1,2]

Various treatment modalities are mentioned in Table 19.9.

2. Cutaneous Squamous Cell Carcinoma (cSCC)

It develops from malignant transformation of keratinocytes of epidermis and its appendages. It is seen in advanced age, with more than 80% cases occurring in old patients.[1]

Etiology

Invasive cSCC represents 20% of NMSC, developing *de novo* on chronic sun-exposed skin or from precursor lesions. Its incidence increases with age and cumulative, chronic sun-exposure is main risk factor.

Other predisposing factors are mentioned in Table 19.10.

Epidemiology

There has been dramatic increase (50–200%) in incidence in past three decades, reflecting an increase of cumulative UV-exposure and an ageing population.[1]

TABLE 19.9: Various treatment modalities for BCC

Treatment	Treatment modality	Uses
1. Topical	Imiquimod	Used for superficial BCC in low-risk areas, providing local control and reduced chance of recurrence
	5-fluorouracil	Used for superficial BCC in low-risk areas, providing local control and reduced chance of recurrence
	Photodynamic therapy	—
2. Systemic	a. Vismodegib First oral, small-molecule of class of inhibitors of Hedgehog (Hh)-signalling to receive FDA-approval in 2012 for BCC treatment b. Retinoids c. New target therapy (SMO inhibitor)	Locally advanced BCC Unresectable BCC Metastatic BCC BCC not managed with surgery/radiotherapy Local recurrence after an initial operation Patients not suitable for surgery or radiation
3. Destructive (Physical treatments)	Electrodessication	For superficial BCC in low-risk areas
	Curettage	For superficial BCC in low-risk areas
	Cryotherapy	For superficial BCC in low-risk areas
	Lasers	
	Radiotherapy	
4. Surgical	a. Surgical excision with primary wound closure b. Multi-stage surgery with skin grafts/ flaps	For advanced lesions and nodular, sclerodermiform and infiltrating lesions in high-risk areas For larger lesions requiring complex defect repairs For larger lesions with adjuvant radiation therapy
	c. Complex surgical procedure and reconstruction	—
	d. Mohs micrographic surgery with histological excision-margin control	—

TABLE 19.10: Predisposing factors for cSCC[1,4]

- Exposure to ionizing radiation
- Toxic chemicals (arsenic acid, polycyclic hydrocarbons)
- Very long-lasting cutaneous inflammation associated with chronic wounds, ulcers, radiodermitis, old burn and scars
- Immune suppression (organ transplant recipients and during treatment of haematogical conditions)
- Premalignant lesions like tar/arsenical/thermal keratosis or lesions with full thickness dyspalsaia or carcinoma *in situ*

Clinical Features

It usually develops on head, neck, dorsal aspects of upper limb in 90% of cases. It can spread to locoregional lymph nodes (85% of cases) and to distant sites as metastatic disease (lungs, bone, liver, brain), risk of which ranges from 3 to 16.4% depending on intrinsic tumour prognostic factors.

Risk of metastases varies in low- vs. high-risk tumours in terms of clinical outcomes and prognosis. High-risk cSCC are aggressive with risk of local recurrence (10–47.2%), regional/

distant metastasis (11–47.3%) and lower survival (70%).[1]

1. **Keratotic invasive SCC:** It presents as raised, firm, pinkish papule or plaque with smooth, verrucous or papillated surface and indistinct margins.
2. **Nodular SCC:** It is similar to keratotic SCC but is more elevated.
3. **Arsenic-induced SCC:** It presents as keratotic growth or painful non-healing indurated ulcers.
4. **Thermal SCC:** Develops on a background of erythema ab igne.
5. **Radiation-induced SCC:** It presents as scaly plaque/ulcer on background of radiation induced skin changes.
6. SCC developing in scars presents as indurated non-healing ulcer.
7. SCC may develop *de novo* as an indurated keratotic nodule or plaque.
8. SCC of lip is seen as noduloulcerative indurated ulcer.

Diagnosis

Dysplastic epidermal keratinocytes show downward proliferation and invasion into dermis as long slender strands or large bulky masses. Tumour may be well, moderately or poorly differentiated which is predicted by degree of size variation and shape of dysplastic keratinocytes, nuclear atypia, loss of polarity, absence of intercellular bridges, degree of keratinization, atypical mitosis and demarcation of tumour from surrounding stroma. Degree of keratinization is greater in well-differentiated tumours, manifesting as horn pearls.[4]

Treatment

Treatment is based on several factors which include[3]

1. Cell type
2. Tumour size
3. Ease of defining margins clinically
4. Depth of invasion as indicated by biopsy.

Treatment options are mentioned in Table 19.11.[1]

Treatment modalities for various spectrum of SCC is mentioned in Table 19.12.[1]

3. Cutaneous Melanoma in Elderly

CM is most dangerous of all skin cancers[3] and elderly population is at highest risk of developing it.[1] Increased incidence (due to increasing age) and poorer prognosis may be explained by following factors:

1. Increased proportion of acral lesions
2. Decreased tumour surveillance by elderly
3. Increased tendency of elderly to delay medical care.

Etiology

Melanoma associated with chronic sun-damage is seen on head and neck areas, dorsal-distal aspects of extremities, along with clinical signs of chronic, cumulative sun exposure. This sub-group presents variable molecular profile, with KIT and NRAS gene

TABLE 19.11: Treatment options for cSCC[1]

Surgical	Destructive	Topical	Systemic
Simple standard excision	Electrodessication and curettage	Topical 5-FU	Chemotherapy
Flap surgery	Cryotherapy	Photodynamic therapy	Biologic response modifiers
Mohs surgery	Lasers		New target therapy (EGFR inhibitor)
	Radiotherapy		Immunotherapy

TABLE 19.12: Treatment modalities for various spectrum of SCC[1]

Spectrum of SCC	Treatment modalities
1. Primary invasive cSCC	Complete surgical excision with histopathological control of excision margins
2. SCC on lips, periorificial areas, nose, ears	Standard surgical excision and Mohs micrographic surgery (allows preserve normal tissue function and achieves adequate cosmetic results).
3. Multiple and recurrent cSCC on head and neck area	Extensive surgery and plastic reconstruction.
4. Inoperable cSCC or locally advanced tumours	Radiotherapy, either as an elective or as an adjuvant treatment option.
5. Inoperable tumour recurrences and in transit metastasis of cSCC	Radiotherapy, electrochemotherapy or chemotherapy, aiming at disease control or palliation.
6. Highly-selected cases	Electrochemotherapy a complex, inpatient based procedure, combining high-dose bleomycin and cisplatin with electrical-mediated cell membrane permeability with a good efficacy and safety profile.

mutations, with an initially more radial, intra-epidermal growth pattern.[1]

In light skinned individuals risk factors for developing melanoma are mentioned in Table 19.13.[4]

There is 2–3 times increased risk of melanoma in patients having another family member with melanoma. Mutations in genes CDKN2A/p16 on chromosome 9p21 and CDK4 on chromosome 12 have been noted in melanoma families. But melanoma in general population does not show mutations in these genes and DNA repair genes may play more important role. In acral melanoma there is no role of UV radiation.[4]

TABLE 19.13: Risk factors in light skinned individuals for developing melanoma

- High exposure to sunlight in the childhood and later in life
- Multiple sunburns
- Lighter skin colour
- Multiple nevi
- Dysplastic nevi
- Large nevi
- Immune deficiency
- Familial predisposition

Epidemiology

Highest rate of increase in incidence is reported in United States (40% of melanomas seen above 65 years, resulting in 60.2% of melanoma-related mortality) and Australia, mainly in elderly white-male population and in lower socio-economic areas. Prevalence of thick melanomas increases up to 20% by 80 years, especially in males.[1]

Clinical Features

Melanoma in elderly has distinct clinical and disease-course suggesting divergent biological and molecular profiles, as mentioned in Table 19.14.[1]

TABLE 19.14: Characteristics of melanoma in elderly[1]

- Higher proportion of tumours presenting in head-neck area
- Greater mean Breslow tumour thickness
- Higher frequency of adverse histologic markers (ulceration, high mitotic index)
- More advanced tumour stages at diagnosis than in younger patients
- 10% lower disease-specific survival rates compared to younger ones

Clinicopathological variants are classified in Table 19.15.

TABLE 19.15: Clinicopathological variants of melanoma

- Superficial spreading melanoma
- Nodular melanoma
- Lentigo maligna melanoma
- Acral lentiginous melanoma

Lentigo maligna and acral lentiginous melanoma occur more frequently in elderly, with worse prognosis depending on depth of invasion.[3] There is increased prevalence of melanoma associated with chronic sun damage and nodular melanoma. Superficial spreading melanoma is less frequent (~31.6%) in advancing age, involving intermittently sun-exposed areas, displaying distinct molecular profile associated with BRAF-mutations.[1]

Clinical Types of Melanoma in Elderly

1. **Lentigo maligna melanoma (LMM):** It is chronic sun-damage associated melanoma variant, accounting for 11.1–24.2%, with mean age of diagnosis being 65 years. It represents intraepidermal, *in situ* stage of disease presenting as large, irregular pigmented macule or patch on sun-exposed skin with slow, indolent radial expansion, often changing size, shape or contour. If left undiagnosed/un-treated, it progresses to frank, invasive tumour (50 %), switching to vertical growth phase, with risk of loco-regional (lymphatic) or systemic (haematogenous) dissemination (10% metastasize).[1,3]
2. **Nodular melanoma:** It represents 15–33.9% of diagnosed melanomas in old to very old patients (>85 years) having negative prognostic factor. It is aggressive, seen as rapidly growing nodular lesion with high risk of loco-regional and metastatic spread.[1]
3. **Acral lentiginous melanoma:** It is rare variant (1–2%), seen on glabrous palmo-plantar skin, not associated with chronic sun-damage.[1]

Diagnosis[1,5]

Biopsy remains confirmatory although various molecular and imaging techniques work as adjuncts to histopathology. Delay in diagnosis leads to advanced stages, with thick, ulcerated, rapidly growing, invasive lesions with poor outcome.

Various diagnostic tests for melanoma are included in Table 19.16.

TABLE 19.16: Various diagnostic tests for melanoma

Various diagnostic tests for melanoma	Utility
Dermoscopy	1. Used to diagnose melanoma with high accuracy (90–95%), differentiating melanoma subtypes and improving clinico-histological correlations. 2. Can improve diagnostic accuracy 3. Help direct optimal and adequate tissue sampling in very large lesions or those in cosmetically or functionally sensitive areas
Skin biopsy	It is used to confirm definitive diagnosis
Reflectance confocal microscopy (RCM)	Used to diagnose melanoma with high accuracy
Electrical impedance spectroscopy	—
Gene expression analysis	—
Optical coherence tomography	—

IMMUNOHISTOCHEMISTRY

It is important in confirming melanocytic origin of tumours that lack compelling morphologic indicators, like pigmentation, nesting and pagetoid scatter. For this antibodies used include Sox10 and S100, which are sensitive but less specific and Melan-A/MART1, HMB45 and tyrosinase, which are more specific for melanocytic differentiation.[5]

Treatment

1. Lentigo Maligna

Topical therapy: Imiquimod is TLR-7 agonist and it is an alternative option to surgery, giving 78% clinical and 76% histological clearance rate, leading to discrete risk of local recurrence (~3%).[1]

Surgical treatment: Complete surgical excision with 0.5 to 1.0 cm margins, results in 90% cure. If patient is not good candidate for surgery, conventional radiation and orthovoltage (90% cure rate) should be considered.[3]

Mohs micrographic surgery or staged excision with paraffin-embedded permanent sections is used for melanoma *in situ*, lentigo maligna on face, ears, or scalp for tissue-sparing excision and histologic assessment of peripheral margins.[5]

2. Localized/Primary Melanoma (Stages I–II)

It is treated surgically and old age is associated with variations in surgical management, with high-risk of local recurrence.[1]

3. High-risk Melanoma, Locoregional Disease (Stage III) and Metastatic Disease (Stage IV)

It includes combining surgery, intralesional/regional therapy, systemic therapies and radiotherapy, to improve survival. Adjuvant treatment is given after complete surgical resection to prevent disease progression. Adjuvant treatment includes high-or low-dose interferon-alpha regimens and immune checkpoint inhibitors. The inhibitors include two main groups of monoclonal antibodies, ipilimumab, targeting CTLA-4 (cytotoxic T-lymphocyte antigen-4), and PD-1 inhibitors, with nivolumab and pembrolizumab targeting programmed-death-1 antigen. Both types modulate activation of T cells by blocking inhibitory signals in priming or in effector phase of immune response, restoring an effective immune response against tumour cells.[1]

SENTINEL LYMPH NODE BIOPSY (SLNB)

SLNB status is important in melanoma-staging, being useful for identifying patients at high-risk of progression qualifying for completion lymph node dissection (CLND). It is convenient, minimally invasive procedure, done under general anaesthesia.

Deciding factors for performing SLNB include:

1. Pure chronological age
2. Performance status
3. Tumour location (head and neck primaries)
4. Surgeon's and patient's preference.

When SLNB is positive (micro- or macro-metastasis), an immediate or delayed CLND is performed.[1]

CONCLUSION

Incidence of skin cancers in elderly is rising, but it is underestimated, as all tumours are not recorded in cancer registries. Diagnosis depends on tumour's characteristics and morphology, aided by dermoscopy and biopsy. Treatment depends on character of lesion, its location and patient's general condition and includes curettage, cryosurgery, chemosurgery, excision and radiotherapy. Combination therapies including surgical excision with local radiation therapy are used whenever feasible. Vismodegib, is now approved for treatment of advanced, non-resectable BCC.[1,3,6]

References

1. Garcovich S, Colloca G, Sollena P, Andrea B, Balducci L, Cho WC, *et al*. Skin Cancer Epidemics in the Elderly as An Emerging Issue in Geriatric Oncology. Ageing Dis. 2017; 8:643–61.
2. Bisgaard E, Tarakji M, Lau F, Riker A. Neglected skin cancer in the elderly: a case of basosquamous cell carcinoma of the right shoulder. J Surg Case Rep. 2016; 2016: rjw134.
3. Beacham BE. Common skin tumours in the elderly. Am Fam Physician. 1992; 46:163–8.
4. Khandpur S, Ramam M. Skin tumours. S Sacchidanand (editor). IADVL textbook of Dermatology, 4th ed. Bhalani publishing house Mumbai India; 2015, pg 2075–153.
5. Swetter SM, Tsao H, Bichakjian CK, Lewandrowski CC, Elder DE, Jeffrey E. Gershenwald, *et al*. Guidelines of care for the management of primary cutaneous melanoma. Journal of the American Academy of Dermatology. 2019; 80:208–50.
6. Dhiwakar M, Khan NA, McClymont LG.Surgery for head and neck skin tumours in the elderly. Head Neck. 2007; 29:851–6.

CHAPTER 20

Vascular Reactions in Elderly

• *Vijay Zawar* • *Manoj Pawar*

Geriatric dermatology is quite unexplored but interesting and challenging branch of dermatology as the proportion of elderly/ aging people has gradually increased around the world. According to the United Nations' World Population Ageing Report, people aged 60 years or older are considered to be ageing people. The increasingly aged population worldwide means more people are living with chronic diseases, reduced autonomy, and taking various medications. Health professionals should take these into consideration when managing dermatological problems in elderly patients.[1]

Elderly and non-elderly patients may have differences in the clinical characteristics of several diseases as in elderly individuals there is a 20% reduction in dermal thickness, up to 50% loss of the mast cells in the dermis, and basal and cutaneous blood flow are decreased by approximately 60%. Also, various usages of medicines and the ageing process may interfere with pharmacokinetics and pharmacodynamics of the drugs, resulting in different responses to treatments.[2]

Multiple skin disorders present with ring-like or annular lesions, e.g. urticaria, tinea corporis, granuloma annular, erythema multiforme, etc. However, certain reactive inflammatory skin conditions do not necessarily lead to a specific underlying diagnosis and may pose diagnostic and therapeutic challenge.

Urticaria, urticarial vasculitis and erythema multiforme.

URTICARIA

Urticaria is a highly prevalent condition which ranges between 0.3 and 11.3% depending on the study population. It has been estimated that approximately 20% of the population will experience an episode of acute urticaria (AU) at some point in their lifetime.

Urticaria is a heterogeneous group of diseases that share a distinct skin reaction pattern, i.e. the sudden appearance of wheals and/or angioedema, associated with itching or, sometimes, a burning sensation, and of transient nature, with the skin returning to its normal appearance in usually 1 to 24 hours. Wheal is a cutaneous swelling of variable size, which is surrounded by a reflex erythema in most of the cases.

Magan et al have observed that the elderly patients with urticaria tend to have shorter disease duration, higher percentages of antithyroglobulin antibodies, and positive autologus serum skin test (ASST) in comparison with the non-elderly patients with urticaria.[3] Some authors have found the equal sex distribution of chronic idiopathic urticaria (CIU) in the elderly population and was found to be characterized by fewer wheals and angioedema, lower rates of concomitant physical urticaria, and lower ASST positivity.[4,5]

Classification urticaria can be classified on the basis of its duration, presence or absence of inducing factors (induced *vs* spontaneous) and presence or absence of angioedema. Acute urticaria (AU) is characterized by the occurrence of wheals or hives and/or angioedema for less than 6 weeks, whereas episodes lasting longer than 6 weeks are regarded as chronic urticaria (CU).

The classification of urticaria is presented in Table 20.1.

Etiology and Pathogenesis

The etiological factors especially in ageing patients of acute urticaria include:[6]

- Viral infections, e.g. prodrome of Hep B infection, infectious mononucleosis, Hep C.
- NSAIDs, penicillin, sulfa group of drugs, anticonvulsants, radio-contrast media, vitamins, supplements.
- Food allergies, e.g. nuts, shellfish, scombroid fish poisoning, food additives, beverages.
- Insect stings
- Immunisation, e.g. tetanus toxoid.
- Contact allergy

The IgE-mediated hypersensitivity reaction is mainly responsible for acute urticaria especially in patients treated with antibacterials or having occupational contact with antibacterials. Aspirin and NSAIDs interfere with the metabolism of arachidonic acid causing episodes of acute urticaria whereas the ACE inhibitors inhibit kininase II and resulting overproduction of bradykinin leads to vasodilatation and an increase in vascular permeability. This leads to extravasation of interstitial fluid leading angioedema.

In contrast, symptoms of chronic spontaneous urticaria appear spontaneously, i.e. without any identiable exogenous stimulus. Whereas, in some patients, nonspecific exogenous triggers such as exercise, environmental changes, and stress for the development of wheals in chronic spontaneous urticaria are present

Autoreactivity and Autoimmunity

Cutaneous mast cell degranulation induces hive formation. Also, there is infiltration with granulocytes (neutrophils, eosinophils, and basophils), CD41 with a mixture of TH1 and TH2 subtypes, monocytes, and very few number of B lymphocytes. In 30% of patients when their own serum is injected intra-

TABLE 20.1: Classification of urticaria subtypes (presenting with wheals and/or angioedema) based on the different eliciting stimuli

Types	Subtypes	Dentition or inciting agent/factor
Spontaneous urticaria	Acute urticaria	Wheals and/or angioedema <6 wk
	Chronic urticaria	Wheals and/or angioedema >6 wk
Urticarias induced by physical agents	Cold contact urticaria	Cold objects
	Delayed pressure urticaria	Vertical pressure (wheals arising with a 3–12 h latency)
	Heat contact urticaria	Localized heat
	Solar urticaria	UV and/or visible light
	Urticaria factitia/dermographic urticaria	Mechanical shearing forces (wheals arising after 1–5 min)
	Vibratory urticaria/angioedema	Vibratory forces, e.g. pneumatic hammer
Other urticaria	Aquagenic urticaria	Water
	Cholinergic urticaria	Increase of body core temperature due to physical exercises, spicy food
	Contact urticaria	Contact with urticariogenic substance physical
	Exercise-induced anaphylaxis/urticaria	exercise

dermally into their skin, it results in wheal and are reaction termed autoreactivity and led to considerations of autoimmune (i.e. immunoglobulin) mechanisms for the initiation of mast cell degranulation. Approximately 5 to 10% of patients have circulating IgG anti-IgE, which is functional and subsequently, 30 to 40% of patients were found to have IgG antibody to the a subunit of the IgE receptor resulting activation of cutaneous mast cells in a selective fashion.

The remaining 55 to 60% of patients lacking such autoimmunity are considered to have chronic idiopathic urticaria. In these patients antireceptor antibody binding to the a subunit of the IgE receptor causing activation of the classical complement pathway with release of C5a, and subsequent activation of basophils and mast cells may contributes to recruitment of granulocytes and monocytes by its chemotactic activity.[7]

Diagnostic Approach to Urticaria

The diagnosis of urticaria is usually based on clinical findings. Generally, the history is characteristic. Sudden onset of signs and symptoms, such as hives, angioedema, diffuse erythema, pruritus raise the suspicion of anaphylactic reaction.

The diagnostic measures are utilised to identify the type of urticaria and to identify the underlying causes. Thorough and proper clinical history is sufficient in most of the cases but sometimes a limited initial workup is needed. Investigations are necessary to confirm the diagnosis, identify unknown etiological agents, and to direct the prevention of new episodes.

AU is associated with a rapid recovery, and the identification of its provocating agent can be helpful to prevent recurrence especially when allergy is the culprit. Diagnostic workup is needed especially when type I allergy is suspected to be the underlying cause of acute spontaneous urticaria.

While evaluating a case of chronic spontaneous urticaria, the thorough and careful acquisition of patient history, physical examination, ruling out of systemic diseases and specific provocation and laboratory tests is needed to confirm the diagnosis as the etiology of it changes according to the subtype. The diagnostic work-up should be carried out on an individual basis in patients with long-standing, severe, or persistent urticaria. If physical urticaria is suspected, the diagnostic workup should include physical stimulation tests. Ice cube or cold water tests are used widely for cold urticaria, and exercise challenge tests are used for cholinergic and exercise-induced urticaria. Screening for thyroid autoimmunity may be considered. Oral provocation tests with aspirin are available since one-third of CSU patients have aspirin/NSAID hypersensitivity. Challenge tests with food additives may be necessary in CSU patients suspected to have food or food-additive allergy. The ASST is the only generally available test to screen for autoantibodies against either IgE. A skin biopsy may be needed to rule out other etiologies such as urticarial vasculitis and Schnitzler syndrome.

Treatment

As with all medications, the choice of antihistamine agent must be tailored to the needs of the individual. First-generation antihistamines should be avoided in treatment of urticaria in the elderly as age-related physiological changes can enhance or complicate the actions of anti-H1-receptor drugs, especially when these drugs are taken concurrently with other medications and/or in the presence of comorbid disease. Being lipophilic first generation antihistamines cross the blood–brain barrier easily, resulting adverse effects such as lack of coordination, alterations in memory, dyskinesia, anxiety, confusion, sedation, vertigo, somnolence or the activation of epileptogenic foci. Also due to their anticholinergic, antiserotonergic and antidopaminergic activity they can cause urine retention, arrhythmias, peripheral vasodilatation, postural hypotension, tachycardia, mydriasis in elderly patients.[8] Second-generation H1-receptor antagonists provide excellent, safe, and effective alternatives to first-generation antihistamines. Adjustments in dosages are necessary when some agents are used in patients with renal and/or hepatic disease; however, overall, the use of the newer non-sedating antihistamines is safe, effective, and gratifying in the elderly. Except ebastine, rest all newer antihistamines are eliminated through renal excretion, hence in patients of renal impairment ebastine is safest choice. Conversely, ebastine should be used judiciously in patients of hepatic impairment owing to its hepatic excretion, whereas rest second-generation antihistamines are safe in patients of hepatic insufficiency.[9]

Antihistamines remain the initial treatment of choice and approximately 50% of patients respond sufficiently to require no further treatment. If there is no response to standard doses then rapid increase to 4 tablets/day is recommended. Patients who do not respond to this regimen are unlikely to be benefitted from leukotriene antagonist, i.e. montelukast.

According to European Academy of Allergy and Clinical Immunology (EAACI) and the World Allergy Organization (WAO) in antihistamine-resistant cases the best treatment is omalizumab.[7]

Patients with antihistamine-resistant who fail to respond to omalizumab, the most effective of the remaining possibilities is cyclosporine. A typical dose for an adult is 200 mg/day with monitoring of blood pressure and renal function every 6 weeks.

Other agents considered in earlier guidelines include sulfasalazine, methotrexate, and HCQ.

Corticosteroids are effective for CSU, but it should be used in short courses for acute amelioration of severe urticaria/angioedema episodes and should not be used for long term owing to its side effects outweigh the efficacy.

A severe urticarial episode with or without angioedema can be treated with 40 mg/day for 3 days; then decrease by 5 mg each day for a total of 10 days.

The Prognosis of Urticaria

The prognosis of AU is excellent, with most cases resolving within days. In adults, longer disease duration is an important risk for poorer prognosis. If a patient continues to be exposed to a trigger, urticaria may become chronic.

The prognosis of CU is variable. Spontaneous remission occurs in 30 to 50% of patients within 1 year, and another 20% within 5 years. If angioedema is present, the prognosis is worsened.

URTICARIAL VASCULITIS

Urticarial vasculitis is a clinicopathologic disorder characterized by recurrent episodes of urticaria with or without angioedema and histopathological features of leukocytoclastic vasculitis. In most of the patients, this condition is idiopathic, but it can occur in the context of autoimmune disorders especially systemic lupus erythematosus (SLE), infections, drug reactions, or as a paraneoplastic syndrome. Besides cutaneous manifestations, it can potentially affect other organs, such as the joints, lungs, kidneys, and eyes and systemic manifestations are likely to be associated with a low complement level.

Epidemiology

The prevalence of urticarial vasculitis ranges from 2 to 20%. Urticarial vasculitis is more common in women than men, and has a peak incidence in the fourth decade of life.

Urticarial vasculitis has been divided into three groups based on complement levels:

1. Normocomplementemic Urticarial Vasculitis (NUV)

NUV is typically a self-limited, generally idiopathic, and benign form. Patients with NUV usually have either no associated systemic involvement or minimal involvement and thus have a better prognosis.

2. Hypocomplementemic Urticarial Vasculitis (HUV)

All patients with hypocomplementemic urticarial vasculitis have systemic involvement. It is characterized by overlapping features of SLE such as renal involvement, arthralgia/ arthritis, raised ESR, low serum complement, autoantibodies, and an interface dermatitis characterized by immunoreactant deposition at the dermal-epidermal junction in a pattern essentially equal to the lupus band test.[10]

3. HUV Syndrome (HUVS)

HUVS is a rare but potentially severe form of UV with multiorgan involvement. It is characterized clinically by persistent urticarial skin lesions, a variety of systemic manifestations, including severe angioedema, laryngeal oedema, ocular inflammation, arthritis, arthralgia, obstructive lung disease, recurrent abdominal pain, and glomerulonephritis and leukocytoclastic vasculitis.

Clinical Features

The cutaneous features include mostly painful, burning or sometimes pruritic skin lesions which last more than 24 hours, palpable purpura, and residual hyperpigmentation following resolution of the lesions. Almost 42% of the patients experience angioedema.

Systemic Features

Systemic involvement occurs in patients with decreased complements levels. The most common extracutaneous feature is musculoskeletal complaint characterised by arthralgia and/or arthritis which accounts for 50–75% of patients. The joint complaints are usually transient and migratory, which develop during the course of cutaneous disease, and typically affect the peripheral joints, i.e. joints of the hands, elbows, knees, ankles and feet.

Approximately 17–30% of the patients experience gastrointestinal symptoms such as abdominal pain, nausea, vomiting, and diarrhoea.

Renal involvement is almost exclusively seen in hypocomplementemic UV (HUV) than the normocomplementemic UV (NUV). Proteinuria or hematuria are the most common laboratory findings in the HUV group of patients with renal involvement.

Pulmonary involvement in the form of chronic obstructive pulmonary disease (COPD) is seen in 20–30% of the patients. The incidence of COPD occurs in late 30s to 40s.

Ophthalmologic complications occur in form of episcleritis, uveitis, or conjunctivitis occur in less than 10% of patients.

Other rare systemic findings include haemoptysis, pleural effusions, pericarditis, cardiac tamponade, angioedema, livedo reticularis, pseudotumour cerebri, dermatographism, Raynaud's phenomenon, myositis, lower cranial nerve palsies, and transverse myelitis.

Laboratory Findings

An elevated erythrocyte sedimentation rate (ESR) which occurs in almost 75% of patients and hypocomplementemia are the most common laboratory abnormalities in urticarial vasculitis. An elevated ESR is nonspecific, and it bears no relationship between disease severity or associated disorders. Hypocomplementemia with low serum complement level C1q, C3, C4 and C1q antibodiesis a sensitive marker for systemic disease. The role of anti-C1q antibodies are implicated in lung and kidney involvement in UV. Low-titer antinuclear antibodies without antidouble-stranded DNA distinguished it from SLE. Rheumatoid factor, false positive syphilis serologies, cryoglobulins, and elevated polyclonal immunoglobulin levels are occasionally present. If renal involvement is suspected, urinalysis with microscopy, protein quantification, 24-hour urine protein should be done. Renal biopsy is indicated if there is suspicion of a nephritic syndrome.

Histology

Lesional skin biopsy is the gold standard for the diagnosis of urticarial vasculitis remains. The histopathology of urticarial vasculitis is leukocytoclastic vasculitis of the capillaries and postcapillary venules, characterised by perivascular infiltrate of mostly neutrophils and less commonly, lymphocytes and eosinophils with fibrinoid necrosis and erythrocyte extravasation. Nuclear dust, i.e. fragmented neutrophils due to leukocytoclasis is frequently seen in the infiltrate. The fibrin thrombi as a result of deposition of fibrin within and around vessel wall may also occlude the vessel lumen. Direct immunofluorescence of HUVS lesions show immune complex and complement deposition in a granular pattern in or around blood vessels in the upper dermis and a striking deposition of immunoglobulins and complement along the dermoepidermal junction.

Pathophysiology

The pathogenesis of UV is immune complex mediated which gets deposited in the vessel walls. Through the classical pathway, complement pathway is activated, and anaphylotaxins, i.e. C3a and C5a are generated which induce mast-cell degranulation and *de novo* synthesis of chemokines and cytokines, resulting in increased vascular permeability, neutrophil chemotaxis, and further aggravation of immune complex deposition. Phagocytes consume neutrophils and later release lysosomal protolytic enzymes, leading to further tissue damage and oedema.

Differential Diagnosis

The most common differential is chronic urticaria which should be ruled out when patient presents with a possible UV case. Other disorders such as Muckle-Wells syndrome; Cogan's syndrome; Schnitzler syndrome; arthritis, hives, and angioedema (AHA); SLE; mixed cryoglobulinemias; and Sharp syndrome should be kept in mind while evaluating a case of UV.

Treatment

The treatment of urticarial vasculitis is dictated by the severity of disease. For the symptomatic control of pruritis antihistamines are useful for, and may be adequate for mild limited, cutaneous disease without systemic involvement. In cases of intermittent exacerbations of cutaneous or extra-cutaneous disease, short course of corticosteroids may be needed to control the symptoms. Dapsone has been used with success especially when combined with pentoxifylline. Dapsone acts through inhibition of neutrophil chemotaxis, and inhibition of the alternate pathway of complement activation. Hydroxychloroquine is effective in 50% of patients with urticarial vasculitis limited to cutaneous manifestations. It stabilises lysosomal membrane and thus inhibit lysosomal enzyme release and interleukin-1 release. Corticosteroid sparing immunosuppressive agents such as azathioprine, cyclophosphamide, cyclosporine, and mycophenolate mofetil are useful in treating patients with resistant disease. Cyclosporine has been found to be effective in treatment of hypocomplementemic urticarial vasculitis syndrome especially urticarial vasculitis patients with lung involvement. In recalcitrant cases of urticarial vasculitis, plasmapheresis may provide rapid, yet temporary result. Patients with hepatitis C infection and urticarial vasculitis should be treated with interferon alpha and ribavirin, which are effective in suppressing the hepatitis C infection and the consequent urticarial vasculitis episodes.[11]

ERYTHEMA MULTIFORME

EM was first described by the Austrian dermatologist Ferdinand von Hebra in 1860. EM was later divided into EM minor and EM major by Bernard Thomas in 1950. Erythema multiforme (EM) was previously considered as a part of spectrum of Stevens-Johnson syndrome and toxic epidermal necrolysis ranging from mild to severe adverse drug reaction. Nowadays, EM is classified into EM minor and EM major as part of one spectrum, which often follows infections (especially with herpes virus) and sometimes after drug exposure.[12]

EM is regarded as a cytotoxic dermatitis resulting from cell mediated hypersensitivity directed towards drugs or infection. Clinically it presents with macular, papular or urticarial lesions, as well as the acral iris or 'target lesions'. Lesions may involve the palms or trunk, as well as the mucosal membranes, which are associated with painful erosions.

Epidemiology

EM is rare under the age of 3 year and after 50 year, however, it can occur at any age including in neonates or young children. The disease usually occurs in patients in their 3rd and 4th decade of life.

Clinical Features

Erythema multiforme minor; papular or simplex form: Around 80% cases of EM fall into this group. Clinically, it manifests as macular, papular or urticarial lesions, as well as the classic iris or 'target lesions' which are mostly distributed on the acral sites although it may involve the palms or trunk, and less frequently oral or genital mucous membranes. Typical cases show target (or iris) lesions which consists of three zones: A central area of dusky erythema or purpura, a middle pale zone of oedema and an outer well-defined ring of erythema. Elevated atypical papular target lesions appear as round, oedematous, palpable and reminiscent of EM, but with only two zones and/or a poorly defined border. The lesions appear in successive crops for a few days and fade within few weeks leaving behind dusky discoloration.[13]

Localized vesiculobullous form: This is intermediate form in severity. It presents as erythematous macules or plaques, with a central bulla and ring of vesicles at margin, i.e. herpes iris of Bateman in acral distribution. Mucous membranes are often involved.

EM major: This is the most severe form of EM associated with extensive target lesions and mucous membrane involvement. There may be a prodromal systemic illness a week or two before the eruption appears but usually onset is sudden.

Triggering Factors

In almost 50% of cases, there is no known provoking factor. The most common association is with a preceding herpes simplex infection. Mycoplasma infection is mainly suspected when conjunctival and corneal involvement occurs. Other viral, bacterial and fungal (histoplasmosis) infections and vaccination have also been incriminated.

The commonly implicated drugs in EM are: Sulphonamides and cotrimoxazole, sulphones, penicillins, rifampicin, barbiturates, hydantoin derivatives, carbamazepine, phenothiazines, pyrazolone derivatives (phenylbutazone), phenolphthalein, chlorpropamide, and thiazide diuretics.

Topical medications or agents which can induce EM like eruptions are balsam of Peru, chloramphenicol, econazole, ethylenediamine, furazolidone, mafenide acetate cream used to treat burns, the muscle relaxant mephenesin, neomycin, nifuroxime, promethazine, scopolamine, sulphonamides, ophthalmic anticholinergic preparations (scopolamine hydrobromide and tropic amide drops), vitamin E, the antimycotic agent pyrrolnitrin, as well as proflavine, topical steroids, topical nitrogen mustard, sesquiterpene lactones in herbal medicine and phenylbutazone, nitroglycerin patch, tea tree oil and paraphenylenediamine, and nickel, formaldehyde, trichloroethylene, the insecticide methyl parathion, a glyphosate pesticide, epoxy compounds and cutting oil.

Etiopathogenesis

The etiology of EM is complex and poorly understood. In a patient of EM, immune complexes, autoantibodies against epithelial cells, desmosomal plaque proteins desmoplakin I and II have been demonstrated in skin and circulation which results finally in suprabasal acantholysis.

It has been speculated that peripheral blood mononuclear antigen presenting cells phagocytose herpes simplex virus (HSV) DNA and transport fragments to distant skin sites which activates SP1 viaHSV protein Pol. Also activation of interferon-α (IFN-α) upregulates SP1 target genes such as TGF-β which leads to localized inflammation, and recruitment of HSV specific CD4 Th1 cells that produce further IFN-α. Thus, an inflammatory cascade is initiated which increases sequestration of circulating leukocytes, monocytes and natural killer (NK) cells, and the recruitment of autoreactive T cells.

In drug-induced EM, drug hapten specific T cells play a major role.

Pathology

EM is a prototype example of interface dermatitis. On histology, there is necrotic keratinocytes in the epidermis, vacuolar liquefaction degeneration of the basal layer, epidermotopism of lymphocytes, subepidermal blister formation and pigmentary incontinence with papillary melanophages. Dermal inflammatory changes, with an interstitial and perivascular lymphohistiocytic infiltrate can be present in severe cases, sometimes with eosinophils if the etiology is drug. Subepidermal bullae and necrosis of the whole epidermis can occur in more severe bullous EM cases. Immunofluorescence study shows granular deposits of IgM and C3 around superficial blood vessels and focally at the dermal–epidermal junction have been described.

Treatment

In the limited papular and localized bullous forms, symptomatic treatment only is often sufficed. For severe cases, along with good nursing, prednisolone 30–60 mg/day, decreasing over a period of 1–4 weeks needed. In EM triggered by herpes simplex infections, antiviral therapy with aciclovir or valacyclovir does not show promising results once the eruption starts. In individuals with HSV-associated EM with frequent recurrences, prophylaxis for at least 6 months with oral aciclovir (10 mg/kg/day in divided doses), valacyclovir (500–1000 mg/day) or famciclovir (250 mg twice daily) should be considered. Ocular involvement requires early referral to an ophthalmologist.

To prevent relapses of recurrent EM, thalidomide has been found to be useful in a few cases. Other drugs used in EM are dapsone, azathioprine, mycophenolate mofetil and ciclosporin.

References

Urticaria

1. The uses of epidemiology in the study of the elderly. Report of a WHO Scientific Group on the Epidemiology of Ageing. World Health Organ Tech Rep Ser. 1984; 706:1–84.
2. Farage MA, Miller KW, Elsner P, *et al*. Functional and physiological characteristics of the ageing skin. Ageing Clin Exp Res 2008; 20:195–200.
3. Magen E, Mishal J, Schlesinger M. Clinical and laboratory features of chronic idiopathic urticaria in the elderly. Int J Dermatol. 2013; 52:1387–91.
4. Ban GY, Kim MY, Yoo HS, Nahm DH, Ye YM, Shin YS, *et al*. Clinical features of elderly chronic urticaria. Korean J Intern Med. 2014; 29:800–6.
5. Chuamanochan M, Kulthanan K, Tuchinda P, Chularojanamontri L, Nuchkull P. Clinical features of chronic urticaria in ageing population. Asian Pac J Allergy Immunol. 2016 Sep; 34(3):201–5.
6. Frigas E, Park MA. Acute urticaria and angioedema: diagnostic and treatment considerations. *Am J Clin Dermatol.* 2009; 10(4):239–50.
7. Kaplan AP. Chronic Spontaneous Urticaria: Pathogenesis and Treatment Considerations. Allergy Asthma Immunol Res. 2017 November; 9(6):477–482.
8. Kaliner MA. H1-antihistamines in the elderly. Clin Allergy Immunol. 2002; 17:465–81.
9. Dávila I, del Cuvillo A, Mullol J, Jáuregui I, Bartra J, Ferrer M, Montoro J, Sastre J, Valero A. Use of second generation H1 antihistamines in special situations. J Investig Allergol Clin Immunol. 2013; 23 Suppl 1:1–16.

Urticarial Vasculitis

10. Venzor J, Lee WL, Huston DP. Urticarial vasculitis. Clin Rev Allergy Immunol. 2002 Oct; 23(2):201–16.
11. Buck A, Christensen J, McCarty M. Hypocomplementemic urticarial vasculitis syndrome: a case report and literature review. J Clin Aesthet Dermatol. 2012 Jan; 5(1):36–46.

Erythema Multiforme

12. Yager JA. Erythema multiforme, Stevens-Johnson syndrome and toxic epidermal necrolysis: a comparative review. Vet Dermatol. 2014 Oct; 25(5):406–e64.
13. Sola CA, Beute TC. Erythema multiforme. J Spec Oper Med. 2014 Fall; 14(3):90–2. Review.

CHAPTER 21

Principles of Topical Drug Therapy in Elderly

• *N Asokan*

Key Points

- Topical therapy is valuable in treating skin diseases of elderly as many of them have systemic co-morbidities.
- The changes in structure and function of skin associated with ageing can alter the pharmacokinetics of several drugs.
- Factors affecting the efficacy of topical drugs include the concentration, type of vehicle, and the frequency and quantity of the drugs used.
- Daily skin care has to be attended to in all elderly persons, especially in those who present with skin diseases.
- Frequent emollient use is necessary in the regular care of skin of most elderly persons, especially those with ichthyosis/xerosis.
- Barrier creams are important to prevent pressure ulcers and moisture associated skin damage.
- Use of topical corticosteroids should be more careful among elderly persons, as they are more likely to manifest their adverse effects such as atrophy, striae and purpura.

Introduction

Among all medical disciplines, dermatology utilizes topical therapy the most. As the pathology of most skin diseases is in epidermis or dermis which can be reached by topical agents reasonably easily, skin diseases are best treated using a topical delivery system. Topical drugs can be supposed to be 'targeted' to reach the required areas, ensuring perhaps a greater efficacy compared to the rather circuitous and often unpredictable route by which a systemic drug can reach these areas. Being the organ with largest surface area, skin offers an attractive option for delivering drugs in several systemic diseases too. Topical administration of drugs for skin diseases saves the patient from various complications associated with systemic therapy. The need to have a healthy liver and kidney is not as significant in topical therapy as in systemic therapy. Often, though not always, topical therapy is cheaper. The 'autonomy' it provides to the patients is often welcomed by them. Patient can be an active participant in choosing when, how and what quantity of drugs has to be used.

Elderly skin offers certain challenges to topical therapy. There will be atrophy of almost all components of skin, perhaps most noticeable in dermis, in old age. Decreased production of collagen leads to decreased tensile strength. Decreased number of elastin fibres results in increased laxity of skin. Epidermis becomes thinner in many places.[1] Dermo-epidermal junction gets flatter.[2] Epidermal cell turnover rate is reduced and barrier function is impaired.[3] Permeability of skin to chemical substances is altered in ageing.[4] There will be decreased water holding capacity of stratum corneum.[5]

FACTORS AFFECTING TOPICAL THERAPY

Several factors affect the effectiveness of a topically administered drug.

Concentration

Each of the topical drugs has an optimum concentration, which maximizes its penetration into the skin. Any alteration is better avoided as it may result in decreased efficacy, increased irritancy and increased cost of therapy.

Vehicle

These substances, though not necessarily active pharmaceutically, can affect the efficacy and tolerability of topical drugs. Common types of vehicles are the following:

Ointments

Ointments are semisolid vehicles, almost exclusively in lipid phase. They usually have additional occlusive and emollient properties.

Creams

Creams are biphasic, having both aqueous and lipid phases. Emulsions are usually in liquid state and can be either oil in water type (aqueous cream or vanishing cream, which have a cooling effect) or water in oil type (oily creams which are mildly occlusive).

Gels

Gels are semisolid preparations having polymers such as carboxymethylcellulose. They dry up on the surface of skin, letting the active ingredient to penetrate into the deeper layers.

Powders

Powders are made up of fine solid particles and can reduce friction between adjoining skin surfaces (e.g. talcum powder) or can absorb moisture (e.g. starch powder).

Pastes

Pastes are mixtures of powders in liquids or semisolids (either in lipid or aqueous phase). Pastes in semisolid lipid phase (e.g. zinc oxide paste, Lassar's paste) usually have occlusive and protective properties. Those in liquids are called cooling pastes and have a drying effect on the skin.

Lotions

Lotions are either suspensions of insoluble particles in liquids (e.g. calamine lotion) or solutions (corticosteroid or antifungal lotions).

Paints

Paints may be based on alcohol (e.g. tinctures), water or both. They evaporate quickly leaving the active ingredient on the skin surface.

Collodion

These liquid preparations, leave a film at the site of application (skin or mucosa), allowing prolonged contact of the active medication, not much affected by external moisture.

Other topical delivery systems in dermatology include foams, sprays, micro sponges and liposomal preparations, all having their own advantages and disadvantages.

Frequency of Application

This depends on the agent used, and the type and stage of the disease being treated with it. Usually emollients are recommended to be applied several times a day. The older topical corticosteroids are recommended to be applied twice a day, at the beginning of therapy. As the dermatoses respond, the frequency can be reduced to once a day or even to once in a few days, to minimize the adverse effects. Most of the newer topical corticosteroids carry a recommendation of once a day application, at the beginning of treatment.

Quantity

It is difficult to define the optimum quantity of topical drugs to be used, but applying more than a thin layer is considered useless. An exception to this dictum may be some of the topical drugs which protect skin from external agents, such as barrier creams and sunscreens. For most topical agents, the fingertip unit method provides an approximate guideline about the quantity to be applied and prescribed.

COMMONLY PRESCRIBED TOPICAL AGENTS AMONG ELDERLY

Topical drugs, which have a special significance and relevance among elderly, are discussed briefly in the following section.

Cleansers

Frequent use of soaps with alkaline pH can irritate elderly skin more easily. It may be advisable to avoid soap and water as a means of regular cleansing among elderly.[6] Syndets made of surfactants with a neutral pH and skin protectants are more gentle to the skin and have been reported to reduce the incidence of pressure ulcers.[7] Soap free cleansers which contain agents such as cetyl alcohol and stearyl alcohol have emulsifying as well as emollient properties. These are useful in cleansing elderly skin, particularly if there is concomitant ichthyosis or xerosis.

Emollients and Humectants

Emollients are agents which soften and moisturize the surface of skin. The most commonly used emollients are mineral oils extracted from petroleum—liquid paraffin, white soft paraffin, petrolatum and vaseline. Mineral oils and greases are usually preferred to vegetable oils as the former are more stable and do not get rancid. Other useful emollients include vegetable butters (shea or cocoa), alcohols, fatty acids and esters, triglycerides and ceramides.[8] Frequent use of emollients is crucial for its success in relieving xerosis.[9]

Humectants are hygroscopic (having a high affinity to water) and attract water to stratum corneum from deeper layers of skin. Examples are glycerine, propylene glycol, alpha and beta hydroxy acids and urea.

Barrier Creams

These are helpful in preventing irritation of the skin from urine, faeces and excessive moisture. These are usually made of an emulsifying base, silicon-based agents such as dimethicone and zinc or titanium oxides.[6] Barrier creams are very useful in bed ridden patients to prevent development of pressure ulcers. They are also useful to protect skin constantly or repeatedly exposed to moisture, from developing moisture associated skin damage.

Astringents

Astringents precipitate proteins and exhibit antimicrobial and healing properties. Examples are Condy's solution (dilute potassium permanganate solution—1:5000–1:10000), Burrow's solution (aluminium acetate) and silver nitrate.

Healing Agents Used in Pressure Ulcers

There are reports that topical phenytoin, silver preparations and growth factors may be beneficial in the treatment of pressure ulcers.[10] But the results are inconclusive. Sucralfate can promote healing of skin and can be useful in treating pressure ulcers. Zinc oxide paste bandages have been used effectively in the treatment of chronic venous leg ulcers.[11]

Sunscreens

Physical sunscreens such as zinc oxide and titanium dioxide can block ultraviolet A (UVA), ultraviolet B (UVB) as well as visible light. Among chemical sunscreens, there agents that block mainly UVA (e.g. anthranilate), mainly UVB (e.g. PABA and its derivatives, cinnamates, salicylates) and both (e.g. benzophenones).

Anaesthetics

Eutectic mixture of local anaesthetics (EMLA) is a combination of lidocaine and prilocaine, 2.5% each, prepared in a cream base and useful for topical anaesthesia. Other agents useful for topical anaesthesia include tetracaine, liposome—encapsulated tetracaine and liposome—encapsulated lidocaine.[12]

Analgesics

These are used for treating neuropathic pain common among elderly. The approved agents include 5% lidocaine medicated plaster and 8% capsaicin patch.[13] Other agents tried include topical ketamine, alone or combined with other agents such as amitriptyline. Transdermal buprenorphine also has been reported for this condition.[14]

Anti-bacterials

Mupirocin, fucidic acid, bacitracin, polymyxin B, neomycin, framycetin, silver sulfadiazine, zinc sulfadiazine, clindamycin, erythromycin, metronidazole and retapamulin are some of the commonly used topical anti-bacterials. Their major features are summarized in Table 21.1.

In addition to these, antiseptics such as cetrimide, isopropyl alcohol, ethanol, formaldehyde, glutaraldehyde, hydrogen peroxide and iodine preparations are widely used for varying purposes—for cleansing, as disinfectants, as shampoos, for wound care and as dressings.

Anti-fungals

Commonly used topical antifungal drugs are imidazoles such as clotrimazole, ketoconazole, miconazole, sertoconazole, luliconazole; polyenes such as nystatin; allylamines such as naftifine, butenafine and terbinafine; hydroxypyridones such as ciclopirox olamine; thiocarbamates such as tolnaftate; morpholines such as amorolfine and other agents such as Whitfield's ointment, selenium sulfide and zinc pyrithione. Uses of these are summarized in Table 21.2.

TABLE 21.1: Common topical antibacterial drugs and their important features

Name of the drug	Group of bacteria against which the drug is mainly active	Comment
Bacitracin	Gram-positive	Commonly combined with neomycin and polymyxin B; high sensitization potential
Polymyxin B	Gram-negative	Commonly combined with neomycin and bacitracin
Neomycin	Gram-positive and Gram-negative	Commonly combined with bacitracin and polymyxin B; high sensitization potential
Fucidic acid	Gram-positive	Low sensitization potential
Mupirocin	Gram-positive	Useful to eradicate nasal carriage of *Staphylococcus aureus*
Framycetin	Gram-positive and Gram-negative	High sensitization potential
Retapamulin	Gram-positive, anaerobes	Efficacy comparable to fucidic acid
Silver sulphadiazine and zinc sulphadiazine	Gram-positive and Gram-negative	Low sensitization potential
Clindamycin	*Propionibacterium acnes*	Develop resistance quickly on mono-therapy
Erythromycin	*Propionibacterium acnes*	Develop resistance quickly on mono-therapy
Metronidazole	*Propionibacterium acnes*	Also useful in rosacea and decubitus ulcers

TABLE 21.2: Common topical antifungal drugs and their important features

Chemical group of the drug	Name of common drugs in the group	Type of fungi against which the drug is mainly active	Comment
Imidazole	Clotrimazole, miconazole, ketoconazole, sertoconazole, luliconazole	Candida, dermatophytes, malazzezia	Fungistatic, broad spectrum, various formulations
Polyene	Nystatin	Candida	Good for local action on mucosa, as it is poorly absorbed
Allylamines	Naftifine, butenafine, terbinafine	Dermatophytes	Fungicidal, fast response
Hydroxypyridone	Ciclopirox olamine	Dermatophytes, Candida, other moulds	Can be an option when more common agents fail
Thiocarbamate	Tolnaftate	Dermatophytes	Useful in intertriginous type of tinea pedis
Morpholine	Amorolfine	Dermatophytes, moulds	Effective in onychomycosis, as nail lacquer
Traditional agents	Whitfield's ointment (salicylic acid 3% and benzoic acid 6%)	Dermatophytes, malazzezia	May sometimes irritate skin
	Selenium sulfide	Malazzezia	Used as shampoo
	Zinc pyrithione	Malazzezia	Used as shampoo

Antiparasitic Drugs

Permethrin (5% for scabies and 1% for pediculosis), gammabenzene hexachloride (1%) and benzyl benzoate (12.5–25%) are some of the commonly used antiparasitic drugs used for treating scabies and pediculosis among elderly.

Corticosteroids

These drugs revolutionized treatment of inflammatory skin diseases in the latter half of 20th century. They are categorized based on potency. The most potent preparations are clobetasol propionate and halobetasol. The least potent is hydrocortisone. Between these two extremes there are various molecules of varying potency such as desonide, clobetasone butyrate, betamethasone valerate, fluocinolone acetonide, fluticasone propionate and mometasone furoate (listed somewhat in the order of increasing potency). In addition to the chemical structure, formulation also is an important factor affecting potency—ointments being more potent, whereas creams, gels and lotions being less potent. The most important limiting factors of the use of topical corticosteroids are their frequent adverse effects, such as atrophy, striae, purpura/ecchymosis, telangiectasia, acneform eruptions, rosacea, rebound phenomenon and sensitization. Adverse effects are more frequent and more severe with the use of more potent preparations.

Immunomodulators

Molecules belonging to the calcineurin inhibitor family such as tacrolimus and pimecrolimus are useful in the treatment of several inflammatory skin diseases such as atopic dermatitis. Unlike corticosteroids, they do not produce skin atrophy, though burning sensation is a common complaint of the patients who use them. Pimecrolimus has been reported as a useful second line treatment in several vulvar dermatoses.[15]

Retinoids

These agents which interact with retinoid receptors have a wide range of beneficial effects on skin such as normalization and regulation of keratinization, suppression of dysplasia and decrease in hyperpigmentation. The prototype molecule in this group is tretinoin (all-*trans*-retinoic acid) which constitutes an important component in the treatment of acne vulgaris and several other disorders of keratinization. Adapalene, commonly used in the treatment of acne vulgaris, is considered to be less irritant than tretinoin. Tazarotene is useful in the treatment of psoriasis. Bexarotene has a selective action on RXR receptors and is used in the topical treatment of cutaneous T cell lymphoma.

Vitamin D Analogues

These include tacalcitol, calcitriol and calcipotriol. Calcipotriol is a useful drug for treating psoriasis. It has also been tried in the treatment of several other diseases such as vitiligo, lichen planus and lichen amyloidosus.

Miscellaneous Agents

Imiquimod

Imiquimod 5% cream has been effectively used in the treatment of mycosis fungoides.[16]

5-fluorouracil

As a 5% cream, it has been used in the topical treatment of warts, actinic keratoses, Bowen's disease and basal cell carcinoma.

Tars

Tars, which are derived from distillation of organic substances, are of mainly three categories—wood tar (e.g. birch, pine), shale tars (e.g. ichthyol/ichthamol) and coal tar. Coal tar has anti-inflammatory and anti-proliferative properties and therefore is used in the treatment of several inflammatory skin diseases, particularly, psoriasis.

Dithranol

Anti-inflammatory and anti-proliferative effects of dithranol makes it useful in the treatment of psoriasis.

CONCLUSION

Topical therapy has an important position in the treatment of skin diseases. With the advancement in the knowledge on pathogenesis of skin diseases and developments in drug research, the armamentarium of topical drugs is expanding significantly. We can expect topical drugs with greater safety, efficacy and precision in future. In the treatment of elderly persons with several systemic co-morbidities, effective and safe topical therapy will always be an attractive option. In this era of evidence-based medicine we need more well-designed studies to establish the value of topical therapy further.

References

1. Tsugita T, Nishijima T, Kitahara T, Takema Y. Positional differences and aging changes in Japanese woman epidermal thickness and corneous thickness determined by OCT (optical coherence tomography). Skin Res Technol. 2013; 19:242–50.
2. Fenske NA, Lober CW. Structural and functional changes of normal aging skin. J Am Acad Dermatol. 1986; 15:571–85.
3. Cerimele D, Celleno L, Serri F. Physiological changes in ageing skin. Br JDermatol. 1990; 122 Suppl 35:13–20.
4. Konda S, Meier-Davis SR, Cayme B, Shudo J, Maibach HI. Age-related percutaneous penetration part 1: skin factors. Skin Therapy Lett. 2012; 17:1–5.
5. Raab WP. The skin surface and stratum corneum. Br J Dermatol. 1990; 122 Suppl 35:37–41.
6. Humbert P, Dréno B, Krutmann J, Luger TA, Triller R, Meaume S, et al. Recommendations for managing cutaneous disorders associated with advancing age. Clin Interv Aging. 2016; 11:141–8.
7. Thompson P, Langemo D, Anderson J, Hanson D, Hunter S. Skin care protocols forpressure ulcers and

incontinence in long-term care: a quasi-experimental study. Adv Skin Wound Care. 2005; 18:422–9.

8. Pons-Guiraud A. Dry skin in dermatology: a complex physiopathology. J Eur Acad Dermatol Venereol. 2007; 21 Suppl 2:1–4.

9. Shim JH, Park JH, Lee JH, Lee DY, Lee JH, Yang JM. Moisturizers are effective in the treatment of xerosis irrespectively from their particular formulation: results from a prospective, randomized, double-blind controlled trial. J Eur Acad Dermatol Venereol. 2016; 30:276–81.

10. Mao CL, Rivet AJ, Sidora T, Pasko MT. Update on pressure ulcer management and deep tissue injury. Ann Pharmacother. 2010; 44:325–32.

11. Parboteeah S, Brown A. Managing chronic venous leg ulcers with zinc oxide paste bandages. Br J Nurs. 2008; 17:S30,S32,S34–6.

12. Eidelman A, Weiss JM, Lau J, Carr DB. Topical anesthetics for dermal instrumentation: a systematic review of randomized, controlled trials. Ann Emerg Med. 2005; 46:343–51.

13. Sawynok J. Topical analgesics for neuropathic pain in the elderly: current and future prospects. Drugs Aging. 2014; 31:853–62.

14. Vadivelu N, Hines RL. Management of chronic pain in the elderly: focus on transdermal buprenorphine. Clin Interv Aging. 2008; 3:421–30.

15. Goldstein AT, Thaçi D, Luger T. Topical calcineurin inhibitors for the treatment of vulvar dermatoses. Eur J Obstet Gynecol Reprod Biol. 2009; 146:22–9.

16. Martínez-González MC, Verea-Hernando MM, Yebra-Pimentel MT, Del Pozo J,Mazaira M, Fonseca E. Imiquimod in mycosis fungoides. Eur J Dermatol. 2008; 18:148–52.

CHAPTER 22

Principles of Systemic Therapy in Elderly

• Rajesh Kumar • Manjeet Ramteke

Key Points

- Elderly populations are increasing gradually and progressively all around the world including India.
- Polypharmacy, drug interactions, nonadherence and adverse cutaneous drug reactions are common in elderly populations.
- It is imperative to know the prescribed drugs, its side-effects and drug interactions in elderly before prescribing a new drug.

Introduction

In India, according to 2011 population census, nearly 104 million people are above 60 years of age. The number will increase to 325 million by year 2050, constituting 20 percent of populations.[1] It is a real challenge to everyone including physicians, how to tackle it. Advancing age is characterized by many physiological changes which include changes in body composition and organ function. Inappropriate drug use or polypharmacy and self-medications are common in elderly.[2,3] With age, pharmacokinetic changes include a reduction in renal and hepatic clearance and an increase in volume of distribution of lipid soluble drugs (hence prolongation of elimination half-life), whereas pharmacodynamics changes involve altered (usually increased) sensitivity to several classes of drugs.[4] Thus knowledge of drug pharmacokinetic and pharmacodynamics are necessary in treating aged population. Concurrent age-related illnesses, availability of a drugs, cost-effectiveness and need should be taken into consideration before prescribing a particular medicine. There is a need of appropriate drug selection and proper adjustment of dosages in elderly. The emphasis of current chapter is on commonly used systemic dermatological agents in ageing population.

Pharmacokinetics

Pharmacokinetics, is the effect of body on the drug and it includes absorption of the drug, distribution of the drug to the various organs and tissues in the body, metabolism of the drug into other compounds, and hepatorenal excretion of the drug and its metabolites with subsequent elimination from the body.[4]

- *Absorption*: With ageing the common physiological changes includes, a slower rate of gastric emptying, a decrease in intestinal motility, a reduction in intestinal blood perfusion, and a diminished intestinal mucosal surface area.[5] However, there do not appear to be any significant changes in healthy elder patients in recent reports.[1] An age-dependent reduction of the extent or rate of absorption was shown for only a few drugs (indomethacin, prazosine, digoxin). Agents that delay propulsive gut motility (antimuscarinic drugs, antihistamines, tricyclic antidepressants, opioids) may retard intestinal absorption to a greater extent than aging does. The rate of absorption of topical agents may be either decreased or erratic due to thinning of the skin and its compromised barrier function.[2]

- *Distribution/ protein binding*: Once the drug is absorbed from the gastrointestinal (GI) tract, it gets distributed to various organs and tissues of the body. This drug distribution significantly differs in elder population as compared to adults. The total body weight of a person reduces in old age due to decrease skeletal muscle mass and increase in proportion of total body fat. Thus lipophilic drug like hydroxyzine will have a longer half life in older patients. The total body water content also declines and thus the volume of distribution of hydrophilic drugs therefore decreases, resulting in higher plasma concentrations.[3] There is general reduction in plasma albumin and an increase in α_1 acid glycoprotein leading to increase of free or unbound drug causing overdose.
- *Metabolism and bioavailability*: In aged population, there is overall reduction in size of liver and its functions, namely decrease blood and bile flow, decrease synthesis of proteins, lipids and glucose. There are two major pathways for metabolism of a drug, namely phase I reactions, which include oxidation, hydroxylation, reduction, and alkylation, and phase II metabolism includes glucuronidation, conjugation, and acetylation. The major enzymes involved in phase I reactions are cytochrome P450 (CYP), xanthine oxidase and alcohol dehydrogenase. About 80% of medications are processed by CYP, and the resulting metabolites often remain pharmacologically active.[4] The common dermatologic medications that can induce or inhibit CYP are diphenhidramine, cyclosporine, dapsone, erythromycin, fluconazole, itraconazole, griseofulvin and ketoconazole. Phase II or conjugation reactions usually are unchanged in old age, the activities of glutathione transferase and UDP glucuronyl transferase are not altered as it is extrahepatic. Examples of medications metabolized by phase II reactions include azathioprine (methyltransferase) and mycophenolate mofetil (glucuronidation).[5]
- *Excretion*: Physiological changes associated with old age are decrease in renal mass, decrease blood flow to kidneys and gradual reduction in the glomerular filtration rate (GFR). Consequently, there is a reduction in the filtration, active secretion, and tubular reabsorption of drugs. Common dermatological drugs that need dose adjustment in old age are acyclovir, famcyclovir, valacyclovir, hydroxyzine, cetirizine, azathioprine, cephalosporine, tertracycline, trimethoprim/sulphamethoxazole, choloroquin, colchicines, cyclosporine, fluconazole, terbinafine, methotrexate, andranitidne.[5,6]

Pharmacodynamics

Pharmacodynamics refers to the effect of drug on the body. Older people tend to have different response to some medications as opposed to young adults. The differences may include changes in the binding affinity for the drug, changes in the number or density of active receptors at the target organ, biochemical processes, homeostatic regulation, structural features, and physiological processes. Age-related changes at the receptor site may be responsible for an increase in sensitivity to medication, thus dose adjustment is required.[7] There are age related changes in the central nervous system leading to adverse drug reactions like dizziness, delirium, sedation. So, first generation antihistamines and anticholinergics drugs are best to be avoided in older patients.

Polypharmacy or Overuse

Polypharmacy (PP) or overuse is defined in many ways; however, 2 definitions are currently in use by many authors.[8] First, the administration of many drugs than clinically indicated and secondly, is defined as the use of four/five or more medications in the same individual.[9] The factors that contribute to polypharmacy are multiple disease states, time constraints on health professionals, multiple health care providers, use of non-prescription medications, patient-driven prescribing. PP in dermatology is not uncommon, it may increase from 5.6% in 1995 to 18.5% in 2009.[10]

Non-adherence

Medication non-adherence is described as when patients do not take the medicines, the way it is prescribed to them.[11] Like PP, this phenomenon is also not uncommon in elderly. To make it worse, patients are not reliably going to tell you about the medicines. Non-adherence not only leads to therapy failure and drug-resistance (anti-microbial), it may result in drug wastage and huge economic burdens on government. Non-adherence may be due to, miscommunication between health care providers, failure to understand the purpose of the medicines by older patients, and inability to take the medicines because of physiological changes in elderly like poor vision, arthritic changes in joints, and cognitive function.[12]

Self-medication

Self-medication is defined as self-administration of medicines without a prescription from a registered medical practitioner. The prevalence is somewhere between 20 and 60% even higher in villages.[13] In most of the cases, the medicines are suggested by relatives, friends or people who are not licensed to prescribe (quacks) and it happens because of sociocultural and behavioral factors.[13] The most common medicines used in this way are analgesics, anti-pyretic, anti-histamines, and in extreme cases topical and systemic corticosteroids.

Complimentary/Alternative Medicines

Medicines, other than the main stream medicines, are not uncommon to be in use in older populations. In our country, it could be either ayurvedic preparations or homeopathic medicines. It is a common belief that these medicines have no side effects and even cure the diseases from root. However, they may cause Stevens-Johnson syndrome, arsenic toxicity, pellagra like dermatitis, mercury poisoning and hypersensitivity reactions.[14,15] In our country, in one study it was found that 38% of the 120 samples of the ayurvedic preparations were adulterated with systemic corticosteroids.[16]

Adverse Drug Reactions

Adverse drug reactions (ADRs) are very common in elderly people because of age-related physiological changes.[17] The changes in pharmacokinetics and pharmacodynamics in older people results in altered handling of the drugs in the body. Older age is frequently accompanied by polypharmacy, comorbidity and frailty with decreased physiological reserves.[13,17] Polypharmacy has been identified as a major risk factor for adverse drug reaction.[18] The majority of ADRs in older people are type A reactions, i.e. they are attributable to a predictable known pharmacological effect of a drug which can be easily avoided and typically involved common prescribing medications.[18] ADRs can present as symptom or problem already prevalent in older people. Thus, it becomes difficult to identify the ADRs in elderly. The term 'geriatric syndrome' is used to capture those clinical conditions in older persons which are by their nature non-specific and do not fit into a single deficit diagnosis. Geriatric syndromes presenting acutely in older people (delirium, falls, dizziness, urinary incontinence) have been identified as particular targets for medication rationalization. These can be prevented by avoiding unsafe medications, recognizing when medications worsen activities associated with daily functioning, use of evidence-based medicine to determine first-line agents and tailored drug therapy to the individual, considering concomitant disease states and medications.[17]

Drug Interactions

Drug interactions are common in elderly as PP is common. One should know the drug interaction of commonly prescribed medications. Many antibiotics interact with warfarin.

Antifungals can interact with medications metabolized through CYP pathways. It is recommended to use online resources to confirm and alter the dose of prescribed medications.

Some of the commonly prescribed systemic drugs used in elderly for dermatology ailments patients are as follows.

ANTIHISTAMINES

Antihistamines are commonly used drug in various skin disorders in elderly.[17] The antihistamines are classified as first and second-generation antihistamine. First-generation antihistamines (i.e. brompheniramine, chlorpheniramine, clemastine, dexbrompheniramine, diphenhydramine), it crosses the blood–brain barrier and are associated with central nervous system adverse effects like drowsiness, fatigue, dizziness, impaired thinking and memory, agitation, and hallucinations; elderly may experience paradoxical excitation and agitation.[19] The H1 antihistamines are one of the causes of geriatric syndrome.

The side effects may increase in the risk of falls and falls related injuries leading to poor quality of life. There is a high risk of adverse reactions in elderly people due to the lack of receptor specificity and they frequently interact with other medications and so are best avoided. Thus, first generation H1 antihistamines are not recommended in elderly, if at all it should be given in lower doses.[20] The American Geriatrics Society (AGS) updated Beers list of potentially inappropriate medications in older adults includes five nonprescription first-generation H1 antihistamines (brompheniramine, chlorpheniramine, clemastine, dexbrompheniramine, and diphenhydramine) and seven prescription first-generation H1 antihistamines (carbinoxamine, cyproheptadine, dexchlorpheniramine, doxylamine, hydroxyzine, promethazine, and triprolidine).[21]

Second-generation antihistamines like fexofenadine, cetirizine, loratadine, levocetirizine, desloratadine, bilastine and ebastine can be used in elderly people and are safe and may cause less sedation as there is limited passage through blood–brain barrier.[21] Loratadine has more anti-cholinergic side-effects than the fexofenadine. However, the majority of second-generation antihistamines are metabolized by the cytochrome P450 enzyme system through the liver and excreted via kidneys, there dose should be lowered in patients of hepatorenal impairment. Concurrent use of second-generation antihistamines (particularly ebastine) with drugs (i.e. ketoconazole, macrolides, quinolones, and cimetidine) that inhibit microsomal enzymes of the liver could stimulate arrhythmias in older patients.

ANTIBACTERIAL AGENTS

Commonly prescribed antibiotics in elderly in dermatology practice are given below.

Drugs	Key points	Adverse effects
Erythromycin	Strong inhibitor of CYP3A4; may lead to increase in toxicity of coadministered drugs such as benzodiazepines, calcium channel blockers, cyclosporin, tacrolimus, and warfarin	
Ciprofloxacin	Inhibits the metabolism of theophylline by CYP1A2; may result in theophylline accumulation and toxicity	May increase risk of developing seizures
Cephalosporins	Cephalexin has renal clearance; many cephalosporins increase warfarin levels	
Dapsone	Metabolized by CYP3A3/3A4	
Macrolides	Increases warfarin levels (except for azithromycin); increases digoxin levels	
Metronidazole	Increases warfarin levels	May cause dysgeusia and aggravate anorexia in frail patients

ANTIFUNGAL AGENTS

The availability of various systemic antifungal agents has greatly improved the treatment of various dermatomycoses. These are broadly classified as allylamines (terbinafine), azoles (fluconazole, itraconazole, ketoconazole) and griseofulvin.[22]

Drugs	Key points	Adverse effects
Griseofulvin	• Weak to moderate CYP1A2/2C9/3A4 inducer leading to decrease in the levels of warfarin, itraconazole, calcium channel blockers, erectile dysfunction drugs, cyclosporine, dapsone and statins • Best absorbed with fatty meals	Headache, photosensitivity, disulfiram-like reaction with alcohol
Terbinafine	• Fungicidal • Renal clearance • CYP2D6 inhibitors	Dysgeusia, anorexia
Itraconazole	• Fungistatic • CYP3A4/3A5 inhibitor, hence many drug interactions.	Nausea, vomiting, stomach upset, diarrhoea
Fluconazole	• Renal clearance • CYP2C9 inhibitor • Increases warfarin levels	
Ketoconazole	• CYP3A4/3A5 inhibitor	

ANTIVIRAL AGENTS

The three major drugs which have efficacy against HSV1, HSV2 and varicella zoster virus are acyclovir, famciclovir and valacyclovir. They act by inhibiting viral DNA polymerase leading to DNA chain termination. All the three drugs have low protein binding, do not get metabolized in liver but are excreted majorly by kidney. As these drugs have no hepatic metabolism, they have minimal or no drug interaction. Special attention should be given to elderly patient while administering antiviral agents. The adverse effects encountered with the use of antiviral agents are neurotoxicity and nephrotoxicity commonly seen in elderly with or without renal dysfunction.[23] Overall, the dose of commonly used antivirals may be reduced in elderly keeping in mind the reduced renal reserve.

SYSTEMIC GLUCOCORTICOSTEROIDS

Systemic glucocorticoids (GCs) are frequently prescribed medication in the clinical practice. The effects of GCs are widespread and include alterations in carbohydrates (increased blood glucose levels), stimulation of amino acid release, maintenance of fluid and electrolyte balance, preservation of normal cardiovascular system function, immune system suppression, and decreased bone formation.[24] The potential adverse effects of GCs in older people are infections, metabolic complications like diabetes mellitus, psychiatric side effects like depression, mania delirium and psychosis, osteoporosis, heart failure, impairment of wound healing, dysarrhythmias, and myopathy. Older patients have compromised age-related changes in renal and heart, hence are susceptible to sodium and fluid retention, which may lead to hypertension and congestive heart failure. Potassium loss may cause general weakness. Systemic glucocorticoids use increases the risk of gastritis and peptic ulcers, and this risk further increases when it is combined with NSAIDs such as ibuprofen, aspirin, ornaproxen.

NON-STEROIDAL IMMUNOSUPPRESSIVE AND CYTOTOXIC AGENTS

Use of immunosuppressive other than GCs in dermatology is common especially in diseases which are immune mediated (psoriasis, pemphigus, bullous pemphigoids and SJS/TEN). The most commonly used agents are methotrexate, azathioprine, cyclosporine and cyclophosphamide.

METHOTREXATE

Methotrexate commonly used for patients with psoriasis and bullous pemphigoids in old age. The absorption of MTX is around 70% in elderly. Factors such as reduced liver and kidney mass can potentially affect MTX metabolism in elderly patients. Elderly patients are at increased risk for hepatotoxicity because of an increased tendency for elevated triglycerides, elevated liver function tests, and obesity that are often found in the aging population.[25] Myelosuppression is another rare side effect seen in the geriatric population associated with this medication. Therefore, the dose of methotrexate should be titrated keeping in mind the liver and kidney function tests.[26] Drug interactions are potentially fatal with trimethoprim, a commonly used antibiotic.

AZATHIOPRINE

Azathioprine a purine antimetabolite prodrug converted to 6-MP after intake; may inhibit synthesis of DNA, RNA, and proteins; interferes with cellular metabolism; may inhibit mitosis mainly use in immunobullous diseases, airborne contact dermatitis and photodermatoses. It is completely metabolized in liver by hypoxanthine-guanine phosphoribosyltransferase, xanthine oxidase and thiopurine methyltranferase.[27] It is excreted in urine, thus needs dose alteration in elderly patient. It decreases warfarin levels in elderly. Adverse effects in the beginning of therapy are nausea and vomiting which can be overcome by taking it along with food.

CYCLOSPORINE

Cyclosporine (CsA) is a potent immunosuppressant used in organ transplantation and autoimmune disorders, acts by inhibiting calcineurin leading to reduced activity of transcription factor and thus decreased production of IL2. As CsA is a lipophilic drug, and elderly have relatively more body fat than younger people, there is a decrease in volume of distribution. Cyclosporin is primarily eliminated via biotransformation by cytochrome P450 (CYP)3A in the gut wall and liver.[28] Pharmacokinetic interactions involving cyclosporine appear to be mediated primarily by modifications in its gastrointestinal absorption and by alterations in its metabolism associated with changes in cytochrome P-450 3A4 (CYP3A4) activity related to induction of, inhibition of, or competition for this isoenzyme. Patients taking cyclosporine were at risk for pharmacokinetic drug interactions when cyclosporine was used in combination with sertraline, losartan, valsartan, quinine, atorvastatin, simvastatin, pravastatin, fluvastatin, alendronate, digoxin, acyclovir and oxycodone.[27] As elderly patients eliminate CsA slower than younger patients and also had a larger proportion of the CsA within the T lymphocytes resulting in incidences of nephrotoxicity, neurotoxicity, and an increased risk of infection. Given the prevalence of cyclosporine-drug interactions and the expanding use of cyclosporine in the elderly, it is necessary to identify medications that alter cyclosporine pharmacokinetics in this population. CsA is better avoided in elderly, due to side effect (narrow therapeutic index) and vast drug interactions.

Prescribing in Elderly

Many factors affect the metabolism of a particular drug, when prescribed in elderly. Physiological changes include increased body weight, decreased body water and decreased physiological reserve may affect the metabolism of medication. Elderly population are prone to polypharmacy, increased risk of adverse reactions, non-adherence, and self-medications.[21,29]

Following points may guide in minimizing the ADRs, toxicity and drug–drug interactions.

- Avoid unnecessary medications. Ask a question, is it required?
- Evaluate the medications which is currently being taken (avoid polypharmacy).
- Consider the pharmacokinetics and pharmacodynamics of a particular drug.
- Ask for alternative medicines, if being taken.
- Ensure adherence, periodically reassess the list of medicines.
- Start with lowest possible effective dose and gradually increase the dose according to clinical response.

CONCLUSION

As the elderly population is rising, and there are lot of factors affect the drug metabolism in elderly, understanding age related physiological and pharmacological changes is must before prescribing a new drug.

References

1. PHD Research Bureau. Elderly in India- profile and Programme, 2016. http://phdcci.in/image/data/Research%20Bureau-2014/Economic% 20 Developments/Economic-2016/April/Elderly%20in%20India.pdf(accessed 11.03.2018)
2. Maher RL, Hanlon J, Hajjar ER. Clinical consequences of polypharmacy in elderly. Expert Opin Drug Saf. 2014 Jan;13(1):57–65.
3. Jerez-Roig J, Medeiros LF, Silva VA, Bezerra CL, Cavalcante LA, Piuvezam G, Souza DL. Prevalence of self-medication and associated factors in an elderly population: a systematic review. Drugs Aging. 2014 Dec;31(12):883–96.
4. Corsonello A, Pedone C, Incalzi RA. Age-related pharmacokinetic and pharmacodynamic changes and related risk of adverse drug reactions. Curr Med Chem. 2010;17(6):571–84.
5. McLean AJ, Le Couteur DG. Aging biology and geriatric clinical pharmacology. Pharmacol Rev. 2004 Jun; 56(2):163–84.
6. Schwartz JB. The current state of knowledge on age, sex, and their interactions on clinical pharmacology. ClinPharmacolTher. 2007 Jul; 82(1):87–96.
7. Waring RH, Harris RM, Mitchell SC. Drug metabolism in the elderly: A multifactorial problem? Maturitas. 2017 Jun; 100:27–32.
8. Maher RL, Hanlon J, Hajjar ER. Clinical consequences of polypharmacy in elderly. Expert Opin Drug Saf. 2014 Jan; 13(1):57–65.
9. Masnoon N, Shakib S, Kalisch-Ellett L, Caughey GE. What is polypharmacy? A systematic review of definitions. BMC Geriatr. 2017 Oct 10;17(1):230.
10. Gupta MA, Gupta AK, Fink NH. Polypharmacy in dermatology: analysis of a nationally representative sample of 46,273 dermatology patient visits in the United States from 1995 to 2009. Skinmed. 2013; 11(5):273–80.
11. Osterberg L, Blaschke T. Drug therapy—adherence to medication. N Engl J Med. 2005;353(5):487–97.
12. Advinha AM, Lopes MJ, de Oliveira-Martins S. Assessment of the elderly's functional ability to manage their medication: a systematic literature review. Int J Clin Pharm. 2017 Feb; 39(1):1–15.
13. Jerez-Roig J, Medeiros LF, Silva VA, Bezerra CL, Cavalcante LA, Piuvezam G, Souza DL. Prevalence of self-medication and associated factors in an elderly population: a systematic review. Drugs Aging. 2014 Dec; 31(12):883–96.
14. McAleer MA, Powell FC. Complementary and alternative medicine usage in rosacea. Br J Dermatol. 2008; 158(5):1139–41.
15. Niggemann B, Gruber C. Side-effects of complementary and alternative medicine. Allergy. 2003; 58(8):707–16.
16. Gupta SK, Kaleekal T, Joshi S. Misuse of corticosteroids in some of the drugs dispensed as preparations from alternative systems of medicine in India. Pharmacoepidemiol Drug Saf. 2000;9(7):599–602.
17. Endo JO, Wong JW, Norman RA, Chang AL. Geriatric dermatology: Part I. Geriatric pharmacology for the dermatologist. J Am Acad Dermatol. 2013 Apr; 68(4): 521.e1–10; quiz 531–2.
18. Young JWS, Shear NH. Cutaneous Drug Reactions in the Elderly. Drugs Aging. 2017 Sep;34(9): 655–672.

19. Kaliner MA. H1-antihistamines in the elderly. Clin Allergy Immunol. 2002; 17:465–81.
20. McCue JD. Safety of antihistamines in the treatment of allergic rhinitis in elderly patients. Arch Fam Med. 1996 Sep; 5(8):464–8.
21. By the American Geriatrics Society 2015 Beers Criteria Update Expert Panel. American Geriatrics Society 2015 Updated Beers Criteria for Potentially Inappropriate Medication Use in Older Adults. J Am Geriatr Soc. 2015 Nov; 63(11):2227–46.
22. Kaul S, Yadav S, Dogra S. Treatment of Dermatophytosis in Elderly, Children, and Pregnant Women. Indian Dermatol Online J. 2017 Sep–Oct; 8(5):310–318.
23. Sagawa N, Tsurutani Y, Nomura K, Okuyama T, Kondo M, Sata A, Miyao M, Mizuno Y. Acyclovir-induced neurotoxicity and acute kidney injury in an elderly diabetic patient treated with valacyclovir: report of a case. Nihon Ronen IgakkaiZasshi. 2014; 51:581–585.
24. Liu D, Ahmet A, Ward L, Krishnamoorthy P, Mandelcorn ED, Leigh R, Brown JP, Cohen A, Kim H. A practical guide to the monitoring and management of the complications of systemic corticosteroid therapy. Allergy Asthma ClinImmunol. 2013 Aug 15;9(1):30.
25. Bello AE, Perkins EL, Jay R, Efthimiou P. Recommendations for optimizing methotrexate treatment for patients with rheumatoid arthritis. Open Access Rheumatol. 2017 Mar 31; 9:67–79.
26. Menting SP, Dekker PM, Limpens J, Hooft L, Spuls PI. Methotrexate Dosing Regimen for Plaque-type Psoriasis: A Systematic Review of the Use of Test-dose, Start-dose, Dosing Scheme, Dose Adjustments, Maximum Dose and Folic Acid Supplementation. Acta Derm Venereol. 2016 Jan; 96(1): 23–8.
27. Meggitt SJ, Anstey AV, Mohd Mustapa MF, Reynolds NJ, Wakelin S. British Association of Dermatologists' guidelines for the safe and effective prescribing of azathioprine 2011. Br J Dermatol. 2011 Oct; 165(4):711–34.
28. Kovarik JM, Koelle EU. Cyclosporin pharmacokinetics in the elderly. Drugs Aging. 1999 Sep; 15(3):197–205.
29. Novaes PH, da Cruz DT, Lucchetti ALG, Leite ICG, Lucchetti G. The "iatrogenic triad": polypharmacy, drug–drug interactions, and potentially inappropriate medications in older adults. Int J Clin Pharm. 2017 Aug; 39(4):818–825.

CHAPTER 23

Dermatosurgery and Cosmetic Procedures in the Elderly

• *Sheilly Kapoor*

Key Points

- The rapid increase in the older adult demographic has given rise to a new field called geriatric aesthetics.
- The fastest-growing group to undergo cosmetic procedures is older patients.
- Recognizing health conditions of geriatric patients and responding correctly to their needs are the key components of geriatric aesthetics.
- A wide array of surgical procedures encompassing both the antiageing and cosmetic approaches as well as surgery for benign and malignant tumours is available to geriatric patients.
- In general, contrary to the assumption, cosmetic procedures can be performed safely even on very old patients, provided precautions are followed.

Introduction

Consideration of surgical and cosmetic concerns of the elderly is essential. It is important to appreciate that there can be a discrepancy between a person's chronological age and their perceived age. Gerontology literature has demonstrated that people who maintain a "middle-age" identity despite having an older chronological age are better adjusted and satisfied in life. Cosmetic surgery thus can be a mechanism to resolve the discord between an internal youthful state and an elderly physical appearance.[8]

A wide array of surgical procedures is available to geriatric patients. These interventions can enhance the appearance of patients and facilitate the removal of skin cancers. Enhanced appearance generally equates to an increased sense of well-being, stimulates endorphins and affects one's overall health.[2] The rapid increase in the older adult demographic has given rise to a new field called geriatric aesthetics. In the developing field of geriatric aesthetics, healthful grooming may be considered as important as healthful eating, as quality of life fades with lack of either.[1] Elderly patients are not just 'old adults' but undergo psychological, physiologic, and anatomic changes that affect all organ systems, including the skin. In addition, pre-existing medical conditions of geriatric patients such as diabetes, heart disease, hypertension, clotting disorders, renal insufficiency, and the general debility of old age must be considered comprehensively when selecting and performing cutaneous surgical procedures. If patients are treated holistically and comprehensively, their surgical experience can be enhanced and their health and appearance improved.[3]

Epidemiology

The increase in medical utilization seen in the elderly population is not limited to disease states, but equally in terms of aesthetic procedures. As aesthetic procedures become less invasive and more available to the general public, more elderly patients are undergoing cosmetic surgery.[8] According to statistics from the American Society for Aesthetic Plastic Surgery (ASAPS), the largest consumer group is still 35–50 years old, but the fastest-growing group to undergo cosmetic procedures is older patients. Older patients, as well as other age groups, tend to opt for more non-surgical cosmetic procedures than surgical procedures, although both the non-surgical and the surgical segments are increasing. According to the 1997 statistics, there were a total of 115,709 cosmetic procedures, both surgical and non-surgical, performed on patients older than 65, which was 5.5% of the total cosmetic procedures performed for all age groups. That increased in 2004 to 6.3% and in 2014 to 10.4% of all procedures for all age groups.[11] Overall, there is a 95% increase in total number of procedures since 2002 to 2014.[9]

The top five nonsurgical cosmetic procedures in 2005 were: Botulinum toxin injections (3,294,782), laser hair removal (1,566,909), hyaluronic acid fillers (1,194,222), microdermabrasion (1,023,931), chemical peels (556,172).[4]

It is also worth noting that elderly patients had more facial procedures performed than their younger counterparts, 62.9 percent to 12 percent, respectively.[7]

On the other hand, the progressive aging of the population has resulted in a rising skin cancer incidence. In an observational study on 247 successive patients older than 85 years of age who underwent dermatological surgery, the most common site of affection was head and neck (82.7%). The most frequent tumour was basal cell carcinoma (45.1%), followed by squamous cell carcinoma (38.7%) and melanoma (8.3%).[11]

Etiopathogenesis

As mentioned previously, there are multiple reasons for the increased demand for aesthetic dermatology procedures in the elderly population. There are multiple motivations that elderly patients have to seek a more youthful look. Elderly persons are living longer and healthier lives. Economic abundance, in particular among retiring baby boomers who have accumulated sufficient savings as they reach their retirement age. Many older adults are working longer and feel that they are better received in the workplace if they look younger and fresher. Many want to match their outward appearances to how they physically feel and want to look as young as they feel. Some pursue procedures because they feel it will allow them to compete in their job with younger employees in an era of ageism. Beauty and youth in many fields are a determinant of economic security as well as there are strong negative stereotypes with aging. A growing number seeking new potential mates and want to appear fresher and more sexually appealing. In women, many stipulate that signs of aging are perceived as a loss of femininity, sexual identity, social power, and social visibility. Males are equally seeing a dramatic increase in aesthetic procedures, with a 273% increase from 1997 to 2014. These procedures are mostly related to the face and body from the belief that it will enhance their job prospects or public image.[8]

From a societal standpoint, there has been a major influence in the last couple decades from the beauty industry. The push for antiaging products and social stigma against aging has led to a surge in aesthetic procedures. Cosmetic procedures are no longer viewed negatively as a sign of vanity. Society is more open today about self-improvement and multiple media sources, including the internet, provide a wealth of information about what is possible and available. Also, there is media-driven demand and hype promoted by some beauticians, medical practitioners, and the cosmeceutical and medical devices industries. In addition, there are improvements in techniques that have led to shorter recoveries and more options of treatments. Anesthesia is safer, and surgical techniques more refined. In a time of age-discrimination, maintaining self-confidence is important.[6]

There are three key components of geriatric aesthetics. It is very important for the treating clinician to recognise these before undertaking any procedure.[2]

1. ***Recognizing health conditions:*** It is valuable to recognize the characteristics of common

skin conditions including but not limited to—skin tags, senile purpura, milia, comedones, skin fragility (tears), bruising (trauma), wrinkles, lentigines, seborrheic keratosis, actinic keratosis, basal cell carcinoma, squamous cell carcinoma, melanoma, yellowing of the skin, general loss and thinning of hair to superfluous hair found facially and on ears, eczema, seborrheic dermatitis, reduced immune efficiency as well as influence of medications and supplements (vitamins, aspirin, statins, blood thinners for heart).

In addition, understanding the correlation of visible anomalies to other coexisting conditions including diabetes (feet, skin fragility), heart (medications), lungs (COPD-lying flat), psoriatic arthritis, eczema (beyond dry skin), cancers, hearing loss, vision loss, dementia, etc. is also important.

Additional issues of relevance when dealing with elderly include loss of mobility and dexterity, client positioning for breathing and back or hip pain. The duration of a procedure in elderly may be limited by exhaustion, pain or other factors. The skill of simple communication is the key.

2. ***Respond correctly:*** The second key in geriatric aesthetics is knowing how to respond to elderly patients with these needs. A specialised medical degree is not needed to handle these issues. All what is required is to be compassionate about particular patients needs and careful not to exacerbate existing conditions.
3. ***Refer for care:*** And finally, if recognized, consider referral for further care. Awareness about the special products that can make their lives easier may be helpful.

Dermatosurgical and Cosmetic Procedures

Local anesthesia: It is important to improve patient comfort during all procedures. Most dermato surgeries are performed in an outpatient setting and as daycare surgeries, under local anesthesia. The dermatologist's procedure room should be equipped to deal with any emergencies arising from administration of local anesthesia. This is even more relevant while dealing with elderly patients. Different methods of administration of local anesthesia include topical anesthesia, field block, ring block, local infiltration and nerve block. The dermatologist should be aware of the onset, dose, duration of action, side effects and drug interactions of various local anesthetic agents such as lignocaine, prilocaine and bupivacaine. Skin testing prior to administration of local anesthetic is recommended.[9]

As the popularity of cosmetic dermatology is increasing in the middle and upper classes, the aging face has become an attraction for cosmetic dermatologists. A wide variety of procedural treatments can be offered to geriatric patients as are outlined below.[10]

1. Anti-ageing and Cosmetic Approaches

a. ***Facial rejuvenation:*** First and foremost, a good skin care regimen and daily sun protection are essential to achieve healthier appearing skin.

   Microdermabrasion, chemical peels and/or laser treatment are helpful for sun spots, superficial wrinkles and skin discoloration. These procedures help remove outer layers of aged, discolored and irregular skin to reveal fresh skin which is usually smoother, less wrinkled and more even in colour. Mild treatments are recommended when treating **elderly** patients with thin skin to reduce the risk of abrasions.

   For persistent frown lines, forehead wrinkles or crow's feet, botulinum toxin treatment is well-established therapy. It is also used to improve neck lines and control excessive sweating. Seniors can receive botulinum toxin injections safely provided they are healthy and do not suffer from any neurologic issues.

   Cosmetic fillers restore volume, immediately smoothing out fine lines and wrinkles, creating a younger and natural appearance.

They can also be used to plump up lips and fill in scars. Different types of available fillers can be chosen depending on the indication.

Nonsurgical thread lift and radiofrequency are other useful antiaging tools for collagen remodeling and skin tightening. High intensity focused ultrasound uses ultrasonic waves to tighten and lift tissues.

Caution should be taken for elderly patients on blood thinners who desire to undergo botulinum toxin injections, soft tissue fillers and thread lift. Also in older patients, the interval between injection sessions must be shorter to retain the benefits of treatment.

b. ***Laser treatment:*** Laser and light-based technologies have revolutionized the therapeutic and cosmetic practice of dermatologic surgery. There is a wide spectrum of indications that can be undertaken by laser therapy.[13]

Laser resurfacing and skin rejuvenation: Laser resurfacing is a cosmetic solution for skin with significant sun damage, wrinkles, acne scars, freckles and age spots. This technique removes the top layers of skin as it gently smoothes and precisely contours the skin surface. Non-ablative lasers and light-based devices bypass the top skin layers to stimulate collagen production and tighten underlying skin without patient downtime. High energy, pulsed, and scanned CO_2 laser is generally considered the gold standard against which all other facial rejuvenation systems are compared. Erbium:YAG produces similar results.

Vascular lesions: Lasers have been used successfully to treat a variety of vascular lesions including **facial** telangiectasia, pyogenic **granulomas, Kaposi sarcoma and** poikiloderma **of Civatte. The pulsed dye laser is considered the laser of choice for most** vascular **lesions because of its** superior **clinical** efficacy **and low risk profile.**

Pigmented lesions and tattoos: Superficially located **pigment** is best treated with shorter wavelength lasers whilst removal of deeper **pigment** requires longer wavelength lasers that penetrate to greater tissue depths. Prior to any laser treatment of pigmented lesions, any **lesion** with atypical features should be biopsied to rule out malignancy. The QS laser systems can selectively destroy **pigment** without causing much damage to the surrounding skin. QS Nd:YAG is a suitable device for pigmented lesions.

Laser hair removal: Since the laser light attacks the melanin pigment, the procedure would not be effective on grey hair. This could be an issue in elderly subjects. Though laser treatments are less painful and much quicker than electrolysis but electrolysis can be a viable option for light coloured hair. Suitable devices include long-pulsed ruby and alexandrite lasers, diode (810 nm), millisecond Nd:YAG and non-laser intense pulsed light.

Keloids and hypertrophic scars: Vaporising lasers (CO_2 and erbium:YAG) and more recently PDL have been useful as an alternative to conventional surgery. This may require multiple treatment sessions or the simultaneous use of intralesional injections to gain good results.

Other uses: The CO_2 laser can be used to remove a variety of skin lesions including viral warts, seborrhoeic keratoses and skin cancers by vaporization or in cutting mode.

c. ***Hair restoration:*** The **older** patient is often the ideal candidate for **hair transplantation**. By this age the pattern of baldness has become more clearly defined and although androgenetic alopecia is progressive, the progress is more predictable. Because of their more predictable pattern of baldness and their more realistic expectations the surgeon and the patient are much more likely to have a positive experience.[12]

d. ***Scar improvement:*** High-tech lasers, dermabrasion, punch grafts and chemical peels are some of the more common treatments undertaken by dermatologic surgeons for scar (post-traumatic, surgical, acne) improvement.

Dermabrasion: Dermabrasion is a resurfacing procedure where the skin is mechanically smoothed to achieve a rejuvenated appearance. It is used to treat scarring, remove tattoos and minimize age spots, wrinkles and certain types of skin growths.

e. *Vein treatments:* Treatment options that minimize or remove the varicose or spider veins, most typically on the face or legs: Laser surgery or pulsed light therapy, sclerotherapy (injection of a solution to collapse the vein) and ambulatory phlebectomy (vein is removed via a series of tiny incisions along the path of the enlarged vein).

f. *Liposuction using local anesthesia:* The concept of using local anesthesia, often referred to as tumescent liposuction, allows the physician to perform the procedures in the office with increased safety and superior cosmetic results.

2. Benign and Malignant Tumours

Skin of the elderly is more prone to develop many types of tumours, both benign and malignant.[5]

Benign tumours: Notable benign tumours are cherry angioma, leukoplakia, seborrhoeic keratosis, actinic keratosis, and keratoacanthoma.

Cherry angiomas are bright red/purple popular lesions approximately 1–3 mm in diameter found mainly on the trunks of many elderly individuals. The lesions consist of endothelial lined dilated capillaries. Treatment with electrocoagulation or laser coagulation is usually for cosmetic reasons only.

Leukoplakia, premalignant white patches on mucosal surfaces that cannot be rubbed off. These can progress to an invasive carcinoma, hence draining lymph nodes must be assessed. Topical application of 5-FU can be done for localized areas electrocauterization and cryosurgery has also been used for limited patches, however, surgical excision is the best option for extensive patches.

Seborrheic keratoses have been covered in chapter on aesthetic concerns in elderly.

Actinic keratosis: Are present in light skinned individuals in the form of reddish-brown papules or small plaques most commonly over the sun exposed sites. These are premalignant lesions. Sun protection is fundamental to their prevention. Topical treatment includes application of 5-FU cream. They can also be removed by cryosurgery and curettage.

Keratoacanthoma: Seen as a dome shaped, asymptomatic nodule with a keratin filled central crater, variable sized (1 few cm), present most commonly over face. There is spontaneous regression in 1–2 years, however, excisional biopsy is advised to rule out squamous cell carcinoma.

Malignant tumours

Basal cell carcinoma: Is a common tumor in elderly. Noduloulcerative type is the most common. Low risk BCC includes those on the trunk, smaller than 1 cm, no history of radiation or organ transplant. Tumours >2 cm diameter, long duration, and histopathologically infiltrative, morphoea form are high risk in nature. Management depends on the risk factors, age, type of tumour. Mohs surgery and radiotherapy are specialized techniques and the choice between the above two depends on several variables.

Squamous cell carcinoma: A multifactorial malignant tumor seen secondary to sun exposure, human papillomavirus infections, burns and recipients of organ transplant. It appears as erosiocrusted plaque or as a noduloulcerative lesion. Topical agents like imiquimod 5% cream, 5-FU cream and cryotherapy are used for localized tumours. Large lesions are excised.

Malignant melanoma: The incidence is increasing in the elderly due to better longevity, increased exposure to UV light, immunosuppressants, lentigo maligna initially appears as a dark brown, variably pigmented macule over face commonly. Superficial spreading type is the most common type of melanoma.

Punch biopsy can be done in a lesion located over cosmetically important area. Details are covered in the chapter on skin tumors.

Since cosmetic surgery is elective, it should only be undertaken if the patient is at minimum risk. Older patients need more time and may need special assistance. Healing time may be longer and results may not be longer lasting. The elderly have sensory loss and benefit from extra attention, follow-up telephone calls, and therapeutic touch. The contribution and supervision of the family doctor who is familiar with the senior's medical history is crucial. Written handouts and instructions printed in large type are excellent. Dermatologic care should be kept as simple as possible with surgical closures designed to require minimal attention.[3]

Complications

Physiological age is far more important than chronological age when it comes to surgery.[6] An extensive review of information from May 2008 to May 2013 from the Cosmet Assure database illustrated that rate of postoperative complications among the elderly (65–79 years) was 1.94 percent and among octogenarian patients (>80 years) it was 2.2 percent, both statistically insignificant from the complication rate among younger patients, which was 1.84 percent. The similar complication rate occurred despite the greater-than-average presence of health-related indicators among the elderly in comparison to younger patients, including a higher body mass index (25.4 percent compared to 24.2 percent), and a higher incidence of diabetes (5.7 percent to 1.6 percent).[14]

CONCLUSION

In the evolving field of geriatric aesthetics, dermatologic surgeons can provide excellent care to elders provided they have a clear understanding of gerontologic issues and treat the patient holistically and comprehensively to enhance their health and appearance.

References

1. Geriatric Aesthetics. By Alison O'Neil, *Aging Well* Vol. 2 No. 3 P. 10 http://www.todaysgeriatricmedicine.com/archive/063009p10.shtml. Accessed March 16, 2018.
2. Elderly Esthetics: How is It different? http://www.skininc.com/treatments/wellness/alternativetherapies/-388211422 html. July 26, 2016.
3. Effectively Manage Older Patients with Skin Diseases; Q and A with Robert Norman. *Practical Dermatology.* 1st September, 2011 | 39.
4. Goh CL.The Need for Evidence-Based Aesthetic Dermatology Practice. *J Cutan Aesthet Surg*. 2009 Jul-Dec; 2(2): 65–71.
5. Norman RA. Geriatric dermatology. *Dermatologic Therapy.* Vol. 16, 2003, 260–268.
6. The American Society for Aesthetic Plastic Surgery, Inc. Commentary on: Safety of Cosmetic Procedures in Elderly and Octogenarian Patients; *Aesthetic Surgery Journal* 2015, Vol 35(7) 874–877.
7. American Society of Plastic Surgeons Study Reports Cosmetic Procedures Just as safe for Elderly as Young. https://www.plasticsurgery.org/news/press-releases 12th October, 2014.
8. Winocour J , Gupta V, Higdon K, et al. Elderly Face No Added Risk From Cosmetic Surgery. Textbook of Aging Skin. Springer-Verlag Berlin Heidelberg 2015.Farage MA et al. (eds.) DOI 10.1007/978-3-642-27814-3_148-1
9. Mysore V, Nischal KC. Guidelines for administration of local anesthesia for dermatosurgery and cosmetic dermatology procedures. Indian J Dermatol Venereol Leprol 2009;75, Suppl S2:68–75.
10. Common Dermatological Procedures https://www.urmc.rochester.edu/encyclopedia/content.aspx
11. Paradela S, Pitafernandez S, Pena C, et al. Complications of ambulatory major dermatological surgery in patients older than 85 years. *Journal of the European Academy of Dermatology and Venereology* 24(10):1207–13. March 2010.
12. Cohen IS. Hair Transplantation surgery in the Geriatric Patient. *J Geriatr Dermatol* 1995; 3(7): 239–246.
13. Lasers in dermatology | DermNet New Zealand https://www.dermnetnz.org/topics/
14. Yeslev M, Gupta V, Winocour J, et al. Safety of Cosmetic Procedures in Elderly and Octogenarian Patients. *Aesthetic Surgery Journal* 2015, Vol 35(7) 864–873.

CHAPTER 24

Nail Disorders in Elderly

• *Chander Grover* • *Richa Chaudhary*

Introduction

Nail disorders constitute up to 10% of the dermatologic disorders in an outpatient setup. These affect the geriatric population to a more significant extent.[1] Nail changes seen with growing age can be both physiological (senile or degenerative changes); or pathological (related to a specific pathology). Few of these conditions may only be a cosmetic concern, whereas others may be ominous clues to underlying systemic involvement. This chapter aims to discuss the gamut of nail changes seen exclusively or more commonly in the geriatric population. Both the senile morphological changes as well as the pathological conditions will be discussed as outlined in Table 24.1.

TABLE 24.1: Nail disorders in the geriatric age group

Senile nail changes	Pathological nail changes
• Biochemical changes • Histological changes • Nail growth changes • Nail colour changes • Contour changes • Surface texture changes • Nail plate thickness • Nail flexibility/strength	• Nail plate changes—chromonychia, fragilitym, etc. • Nail fold changes—paronychia, onychophosis, etc. • Nail bed changes—subungual corn, hematoma, etc. • Others—nail cosmetics side effects, nail tumours

Although, dermatoses (like psoriasis and lichen planus) affect elderly nails with an almost similar presentation as the general population; what is significantly different in this age group is the nail changes due to mechanical factors like altered gait, cumulative or repetitive trauma, ill-fitting shoes or lack of adequate care and grooming of the nails. This chapter summarises most of these disorders.

SENILE CHANGES IN NAILS

As a person ages, the nails also age. This is reflected grossly in changes affecting colour, surface, growth, contour, curvature, or texture of nails; and subtly as histological changes or changes in the biochemical composition. Such changes are mostly a result of impaired peripheral circulation (atherosclerosis, diabetes or neuropathy induced); years of UV exposure; cumulative or repetitive trauma; faulty biomechanics of the foot; prolonged or frequent wetting of nails (especially agricultural workers and homemakers); infections affecting nails; or systemic disease.[2,3] At least one of these changes can be seen in up to 98% of the elderly, though majority of them are not even aware of these. The changes seen as a part of ageing (Table 24.1) are detailed below:

- **Alterations in biochemical composition:** With ageing, there is a relative loss of inorganic material; leading to increase in the carbon content of nail keratins.[4] By corollary, total nitrogen decreases while sulphur content remains stable. Calcium content of ageing nails is higher while iron content decreases.[2] As nail lipids are under hormonal control, they are seen to decrease after menopause.[5]

- **Alterations in histology:** The nail plate keratinocytes show an increase in size as well as number of pertinax bodies (remnant of keratinocyte nuclei within the nail plate). Also, there is thickening of subungual blood vessels with loss of vascular elastic tissue.[6]
- **Alterations in nail growth rate:** The normal growth rate of finger nails (3.0 mm/month) or toenails (1.0 mm/month) is seen to be inversely proportional to age.[6] On an average, it decreases by 0.5% per year between 25 and 100 years of age.[7] In the female population, this slowing becomes significant by the sixth decade while in males, it is noticeable by the sixth to eighth decade.[8,9]
- **Alterations in nail colour:** Classic signs of ageing include dull, pale, lustreless and opaque nails reported in 70–90 % of elderly (Fig. 24.1).[6,10] Significant colour changes due to ageing range from white or yellow to brown or grey (Fig. 24.2). With advancing age, the visibility of the lunula also decreases; maximum visibility being still sustained in the thumb nails. A lunula is reportedly seen only in 50–78% elderly.[10,11]
- **Alterations in contour:** Ageing is associated with an increase in transverse curvature and decrease in longitudinal curvature of the nail plate (Fig. 24.2). Thus, conditions like platyonychia (21–65%) (Fig. 24.3), koilonychia (28–36%), dystrophic nails (5–13.5%) and pincer nails (5–13%) (Fig. 24.4) have been reported in senile nails.[12]
- **Alterations in surface texture:** Senile nails lose their smoothness and become noticeably friable. Longitudinal striations is the commonest surface pattern seen; superficial striations being called onychorrhexis (ageing being the commonest cause); while deep ones are called longitudinal ridging

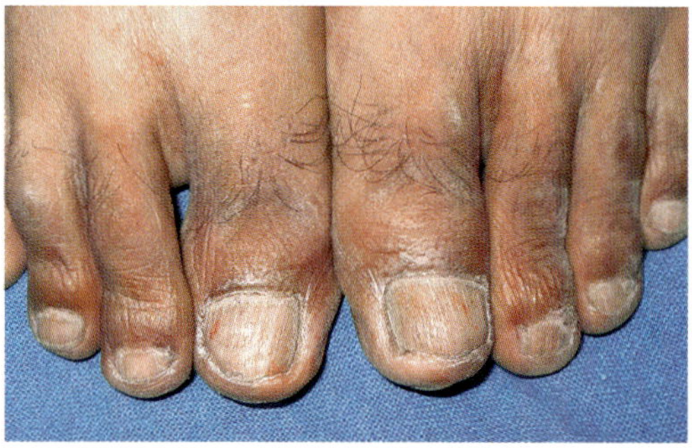

Fig. 24.1: Senile nails seen as dull, pale, lustreless and opaque appearing nails. Note the marked xerosis

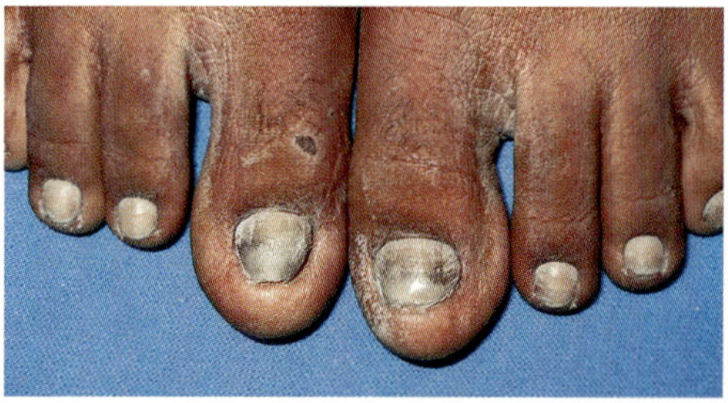

Fig. 24.2: Thickened nails in a 70-year-old man with significant colour changes in the form of whitish to yellow appearance with areas of darkening. Potassium hydroxide mounts were negative

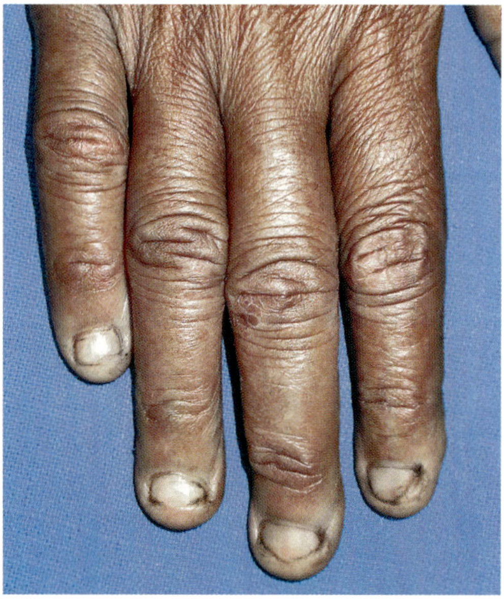

Fig. 24.3: Platynychia in an old lady. Thinned out nails giving a flat appearance

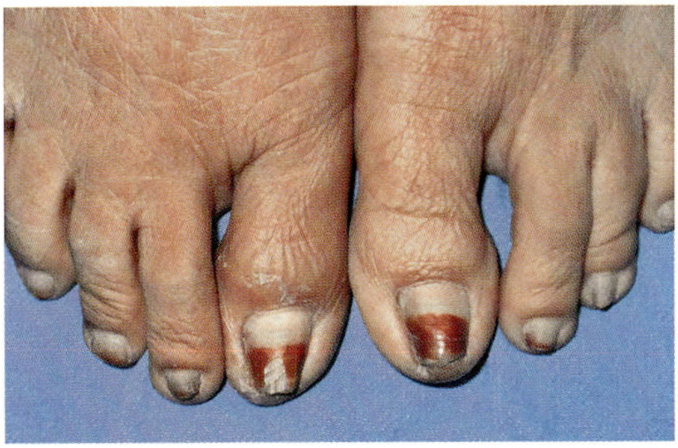

Fig. 24.4: Multiple pincer nails in a 68-year-old lady. These are seen as thickened nails with excessive curvature

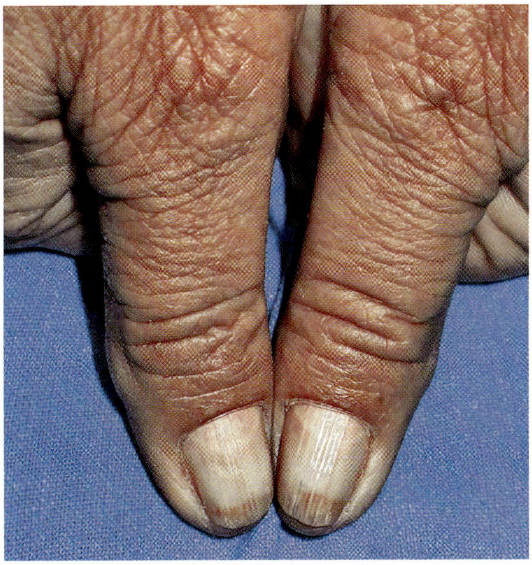

Fig. 24.5: Onychorrhexis in an old lady showing longitudinal ridging, beading and distal nicks

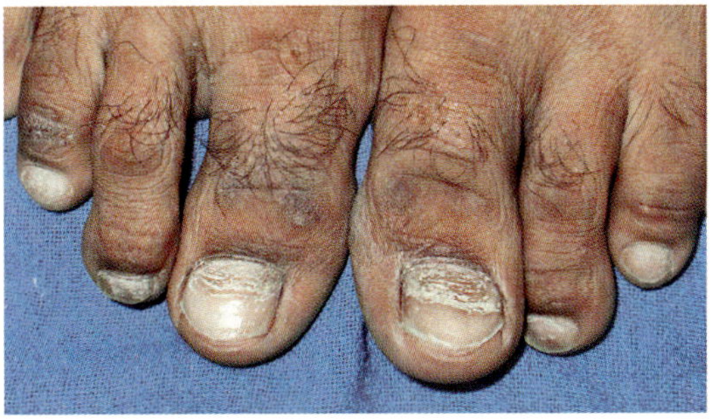

Fig. 24.6: Onychoschizia (lamellar splitting) involving great toenails

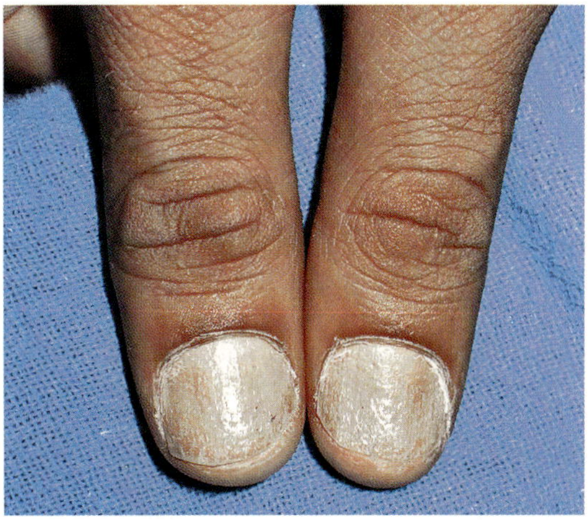

Fig. 24.7: Trachyonychia or sand paper appearance involving thumb nails

or beading (Figs 24.1 and 24.5). These are a result of altered epithelialisation, keratinization and nail matrix turnover.[6,7] Other surface changes like Beau's lines (transverse ridges), lamellar splitting (onychoschizia) (Fig. 24.6), pitting, roughening (trachyonychia) (Fig. 24.7), and fissuring are also frequently seen in ageing nails.[10–12]

- **Alterations in nail thickness:** Average nail plate thickness varies between sexes as well as between finger and toenails. Toenails are thicker (1.65 mm in males, 1.38 mm in females) than finger nails (0.6 mm in males, 0.5 mm in females). Also, thumbnail and great toenail are the thickest.[6,7,13] With ageing, nails may become thicker, thinner or may remain unchanged. Nail thickening can be seen in the form of onychauxis, pachyonychia, onychogryphosis or hemionychogryphosis.
- **Alterations in nail flexibility and strength:** Nail plate strength and flexibility depends on its water content, average being 18% (10–30%). Loss of moisture is an inevitable effect of ageing. Lifelong exposure to dehydrating chemicals is equally contributory. Brittle nails (seen in 20% of population) are even more frequent in the elderly. Toenails are more commonly affected, and may be accompanied by splitting, layering, peeling and easy breakability.[9,11,12]

NAIL DISORDERS IN ELDERLY

Although, disorders affecting the nails in the elderly are similar to the general population; essential differences exist with respect to morphology, frequency and presentation. A single disease process can affect nail components singly or multiple components may be involved. Below is an attempt to classify and summarise the disease processes involving geriatric nails as per the involvement of individual nail components (Table 24.2).

TABLE 24.2: Pathological nail changes encountered in the geriatric population

1. Nail plate changes
- a. Chromonychia
  - Leuconychia/pseudoleuconychia
  - Terry's nails
  - Half and half nails
  - Muehrcke's lines
  - Neapolitan nail
  - Melanonychia
- b. Brittle nails/fragilatus unguium
  - Onychoschizia
  - Onychorrhexis
- c. Infections
  - Onychomycosis
  - Scabies
  - Warts
- d. Onychauxis/pachonychia
- e. Onychogryphosis/Ram's horn nail
  - Hemionychogryphosis

2. Nail fold changes
- a. Paronychia
- b. Clubbing
- c. Onychophosis
- d. Onychocryptosis

3. Nail bed changes
- a. Subungual corn/onychoclavus
- b. Subungual hematoma
- c. Splinter hemorrhages
- d. Onycholysis
- e. Subungual hyperkeratosis

4. Other changes
- a. Ragged cuticle
- b. Adverse effects of nail cosmetics
- c. Nail tumours: Subungual exostosis, myxoid pseudocyst, Bowen's disease, subungual melanoma

A. Disorders of the Nail Plate

1. Chromonychia: Nail plate colour changes in the elderly are seen primarily due to changes in nail plate; however, few are just a reflection of the underlying nail bed involvement. Senile nails mostly appear as dull, pale and lustreless with various colour patterns:

a. *Leuconychia*: **True leuconychia** is reported in 22–58% of elderly.[11,12] It occurs as a result of nail matrix involvement leading to persistence of parakeratotic cells within the nail plate; and may be total or subtotal (transverse, punctate or longitudinal) as per the extent of the matrix disease process.[6] Although **leukonychia totalis** (hereditary) generally has an earlier age of onset; transverse leuconychia (leuconychia striata, or Mees' lines) can arise later, in the geriatric population, presenting as whitish discolouration running parallel to lunula and sometimes resolving spontaneously. The causation is attributable to systemic diseases like cirrhosis or heavy metal poisoning or vigorous trauma during manicures.[14] **Leuconychia punctata** appears after matrix injury as white spots while **longitudinal leuconychia** is associated with Darier's disease.[15] **Apparent leuconychia** is due to changes in the nail bed and fades or disappears on digital pressure.[11] In this setting, **leuconychia totalis** may be a classic sign of hypoalbuminemia seen with nephrotic syndrome, liver failure or as a side effect of sulphonamides. **Pseudoleuconychia** appears due to exogenous causes like nail enamel application (keratin granulation) or onychomycosis.

b. *Terry's nails:*[11,16] This is a special type of apparent leukonychia, where a proximal whitened nail is seen along with a short band of 0.5–3.0 mm width of normal pink colour distally. A decreased nail bed vascularity and increase in connective tissue is the suggested etiology. It is seen in up to 13% elderly other than in those with liver disease, diabetes mellitus, or congestive heart failure. Up to 80% patients with liver diseases are reported to have Terry's nails.[17]

c. *Half and half nails:* These nails are dull white proximally, with a distal 20–60% red-brown nail plate. These are commonly seen in uremic patients.[18]

d. *Muehrcke's lines:* These are paired narrow horizontal white bands parallel to lunula associated with conditions like hypoalbuminemia, nephrotic syndrome, glomerulonephritis, malnutrition, acrodermatitis enteropathica or chemotherapy.[19,20]

e. *Neapolitan nail:* It is the commonest form of chromonychia seen in old age, affecting about 10.5% of those aged 60 and above and 20% population older than 70 years.[12,21] Three distinct bands appear similar to those of Neapolitan ice cream, viz. proximal white band with absent lunula, middle pink band and opaque distal discolouration.[22] An association with osteoporosis and nail bed collagen abnormalities has been suggested.[21]

f. *Melanonychia:*[23,24] It is a brown or black discolouration of the nail in the form of longitudinal pigmented bands seen in up to 8% of the geriatric population.[11,12] The incidence of benign racial melanonychia is higher in darker population and increases with ageing. These bands arise more frequently in trauma prone digits. The proposed pathogenesis for these bands could be melanocyte activation (physiological, dermatological, iatrogenic or syndromic); melanocyte hyperplasia (nevus or melanoma); or invasion by a melanin producing pathogen (e.g. proteus sp., dermatophytes). The treatment hence depends on the underlying pathology.

2. *Brittle nails (fragilitas unguium):* Nail plate fragility is known to increase with age as well as with repeated cycles of hydration and dehydration, leading to brittle nails. These affect around 20% of general population; with prevalence increasing up to 60% in old age.[11,12] Morphological presentations of nail fragility can vary from onychoschizia to onychorrhexis of varying severity.

- *Onychoschizia* (Fig. 24.6): It refers to splitting of the nail plate due to loss of adhesion between nail plate corneocytes. The breakage involving lateral edges leads to transverse splitting, while that involving distal free edge leads to lamellar splitting. Onychoschizia is reported to affect 15–24% of the geriatric population.[12] Causation is attributable to factors altering the nail plate hydration like excessive domestic wet work, trauma, fungal proteolytic enzymes, cosmetics or dehydrating chemicals (nail enamel solvents and hardeners).[13] The first three fingers of the dominant hand are commonly affected.[25]
- *Onychorrhexis* (Fig. 24.8): Brittleness manifested as longitudinal ridging (deep splits) or onychorrhexis (superficial splits) is the commonest age related nail change affecting 85% of geriatric patients. Conversely, ageing is the commonest cause of onychorrhexis. Longitudinal ridging and splitting leads to triangular fragmentation of free nail edge producing V-shaped nicks. Abnormal keratinization due to nail matrix involvement could also be contributory.

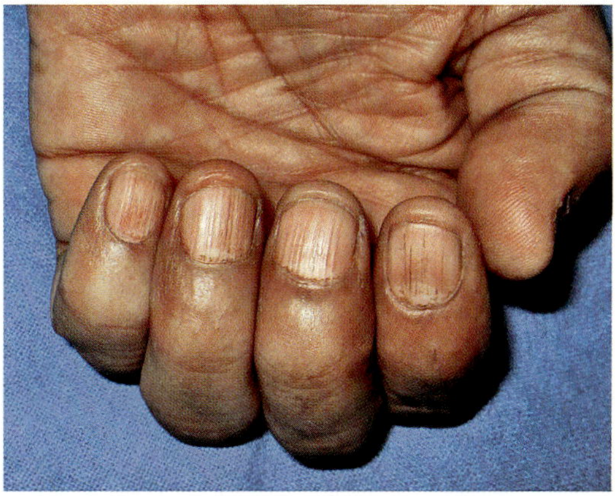

Fig. 24.8: Nail fragility in a 65-year-old man. Note the longitudinal ridging with beading (sausage bead appearance) in the middle finger; whereas the index finger shows more of superficial splits (made more visible by the brown external pigment)

Other contributory factors include abnormal vascularization and oxygenation (anaemia); metabolic diseases; endocrinopathies; or disorders of keratinization.[13]

Management of brittle nails depends on identifying causative and contributory factors. A differentiation based on predominant morphology suggests that onychoschizia mostly suggests role of exogenous factors, while onychorrhexis suggests endogenous factors affecting matrix keratinization. Preventive measures aimed at identifying and avoiding causative and exacerbating factors are important. Daily soaking in lukewarm water followed by application of phospholipid rich emollients under occlusion helps in maintaining nail plate hydration.[3,26] Mechanical nail plate protection with enamels and hardeners can be a double-edged sword as they themselves can cause dehydration; hence, should be used with caution.[27] Oral biotin, PABA, iron, thiamine, cystine, pantothenic acid, choline, and silicone have only a limited role.[28,29]

3. Infections: Bacterial, fungal or parasitic infections involving nails in the elderly primarily or secondarily (spread from surrounding structures) is commonly seen. The salient nail unit infections in the elderly include:

a. *Onychomycosis:* It is the commonest nail infection even in the geriatric population; caused by dermatophytes, yeast or non-dermatophyte molds.[30] It affects 10–20% of the general population and is characterised by changes like loss of lustre, distal onycholysis, subungual hyperkeratosis, brittleness or discolouration (Fig. 24.9).[30,31] An increased risk for onychomycosis is attributable to old age, smoking, immunocompromised status and genetic predisposition. Onychomycosis is more frequently seen in the geriatric population as compared to the general population, with up to 33%, cases involving finger nails and toenails simultaneously.[32] Influence of sexual predilection on the prevalence is controversial.[10,33] In up to 90% cases, dermatophytes are causative; commonly *Trichophyton rubrum and T. mentagrophytes* being involved. Yeasts such as *Candida* and nondermatophyte molds such as *Scopulariopsis brevicaulis, Hendersonula toruloidea* and *Scytalidium hyalinum* are responsible for the remaining cases; though, these are more frequent among elderly.[3,30] Potassium hydroxide mount, fungal culture, or histopathology with PAS stain are helpful in diagnosis and identification of the underlying pathogen. Treatment has to be tailored as per the individual and the pathogen. Factors like severity, number of nails involved, pathogen, comorbidities (and medications), potential side effects and cost have to be considered before choosing the treatment option, viz. topical or oral antifungals, mechanical (nail avulsion) or chemical removal, laser therapy or a combination of these.[34] Topical antifungals (ciclopirox, amorolfine) are preferred in elderly with limited nail involvement.[33] Terbinafine (continuous or pulse) is the most effective agent against dermatophytes and is preferred in the geriatric age group owing to fungicidal effect, high mycological clearance and low potential for drug

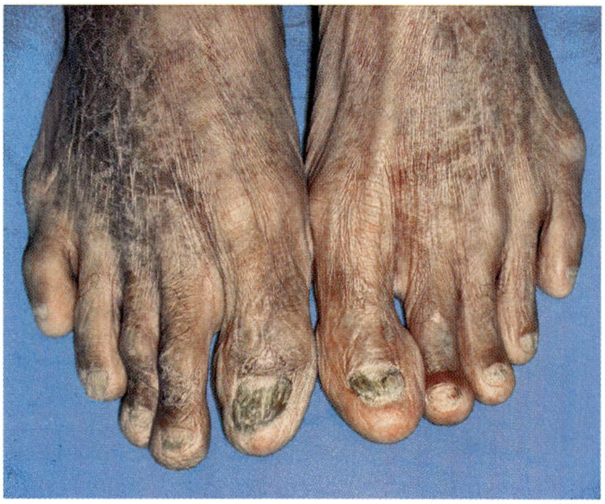

Fig. 24.9: Onychomycosis in an elderly male. Note the extensive involvement, yellowish discoloration and almost total destruction

interactions.[31,35] Owing to their fungistatic effect, azoles (fluconazole, itraconazole, ketoconazole) are less effective. Surgical intervention can be considered in recalcitrant cases involving a limited number of nails.[3,35]

b. *Sarcoptes scabiei infestation*: Scabies shows infrequent nail involvement; however, when involved, it is frequently a cause of epidemics in old-age homes or nursing homes. The mite resides in the subungual debris, leading to chronic infestation (Fig. 24.10).[11,36] Antiscabetic treatment, especially in the debilitated elderly, should be combined with cutting of nails and thorough brushing of nail tips with the scabicidal agent.[3,11]

c. *Periungual warts:* Involvement of nail folds or hyponychium by human papillomavirus (HPV) leads to periungual warts (Fig. 24.11). These are common amongst nail biters. Though, commoner in young adults, they can be seen in elderly patients on immunosuppressive therapy.[3,6]

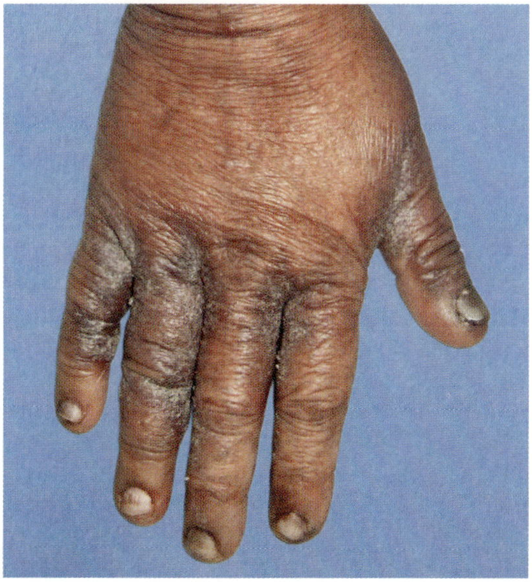

Fig. 24.10: Scabies in a 60-year-old male. There is extensive involvement with nail changes. The thumb nail shows subungual hyperkeratosis which was teeming with scabies mites

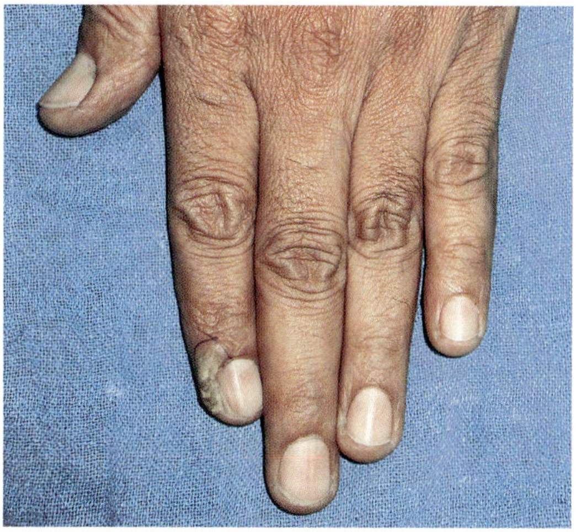

Fig. 24.11: Periungual wart

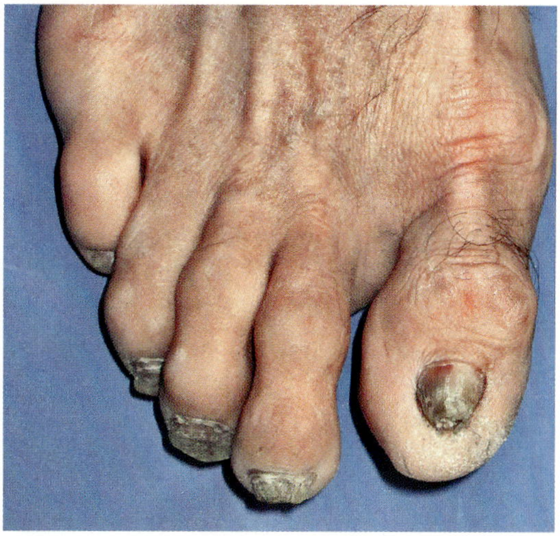

Fig. 24.12: Lustreless, narrow nails with a shrunken nail bed in a patient with lepromatous leprosy with extensive distal sensory loss

d. *Other infections:* Dry, lustreless, narrow shrunken nails with longitudinal ridging and subungual hyperkeratosis can be seen with leprosy (Fig. 24.12).[37] Treatment with clofazimine reflects as nail pigmentation.[38] Syphilis reportedly lead to dull, brittle nails with very large pits (elkonyxis) associated with nail shedding, Beau's line (secondary syphilis), paronychia and amber coloured nails (tertiary syphilis).[39,40]

4. Onychauxis/pachonychia: Onychauxis refers to localised thickening or overgrowth of nail plate without any deformity (Fig. 24.13). Pachyonychia is more diffuse thickening of the whole nail plate (Fig. 24.14). Clinically, it presents as an opaque, discoloured nail plate, which may be complicated with subungual hyperkeratosis, distal onycholysis, subungual haemorrhage or onychomycosis.[3,6,11] Advancing age along with faulty biomechanics (attributable in turn to incompatible foot-shoe ratio, overlapping or underlapping toes, contracted toes due to shortened flexors (Fig. 24.15) etc.) are the major contributing factors. This is the commonest pattern of nail thickening seen with ageing nails and involves toe-nails more frequently.[10,12] Periodic nail debridement (partial or total) is the initial step in management followed by chemical or surgical nail avulsion as per the case. In a few complicated cases, chemical or surgical matricectomy might also be required.[3,11,41]

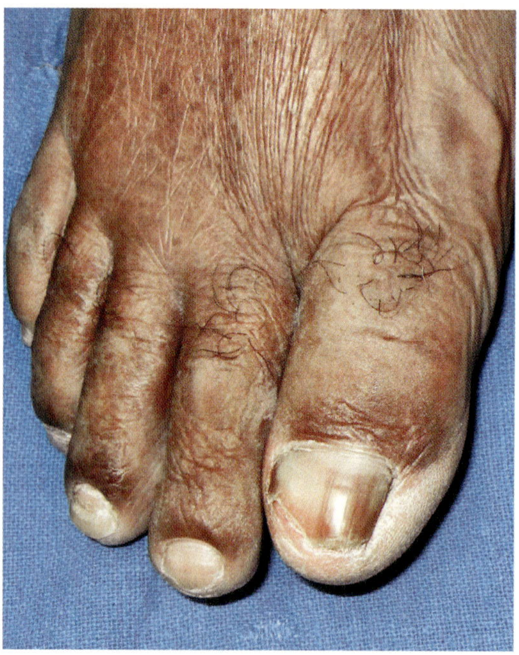

Fig. 24.13: Onychauxis or partial thickening of the nail plate in an elderly male. There is medial thickening of great toenail with discolouration

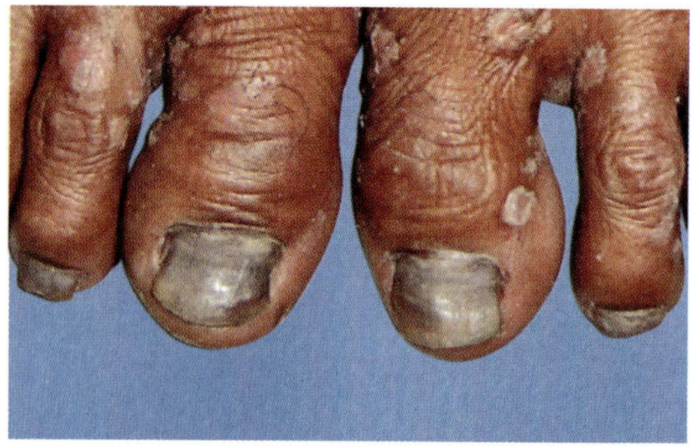

Fig. 24.14: Pachyonychia or almost complete thickening of the nail plate in an elderly male with cutaneous and nail psoriasis. Note the extensive discolouration

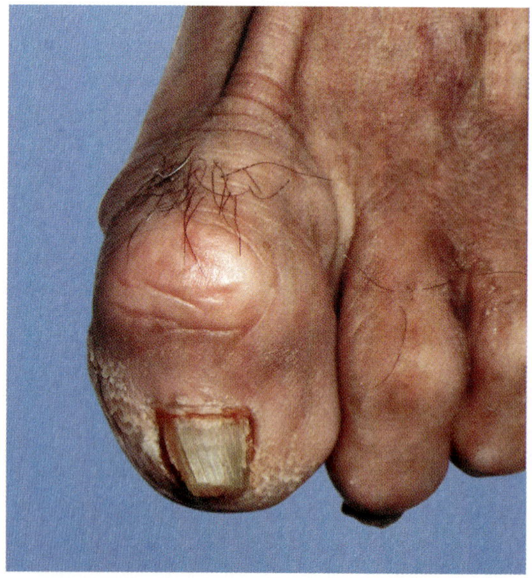

Fig. 24.15: Neuropathy in an elderly diabetic leading to flexion deformity of the toes (hammer toes). This has led to shortening of the flexor tendons and secondary nail changes in the form of pachyonychia, discolouration and extensive xerosis

5. Onychogryphosis (Ram's horn nail/oyster-like nail):[3,6] Thickening and excessive curvature of nail (akin to a claw or a horn) is termed onychogryphosis (Fig. 24.16). Here, the nail plate initially grows upwards, then laterally due to pressure from footwear or due to matrix activity. The toenails are commonly

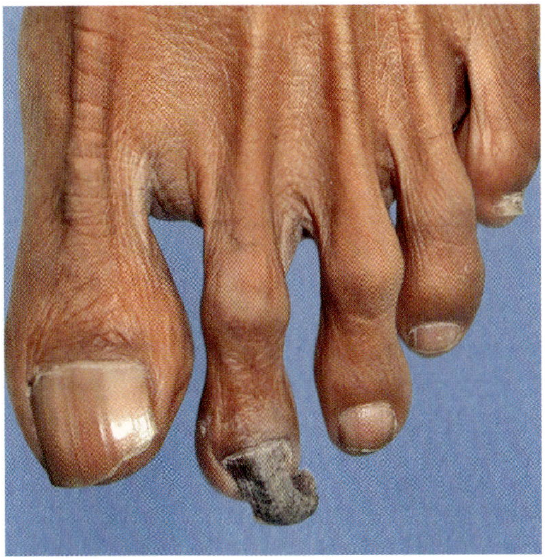

Fig. 24.16: Onychogryphosis (Ram's horn) affecting the second toenail in this elderly lady

involved; with the great toenail being the most frequently affected. Affected nails appear dirty, uneven, discoloured, and heaped up with multiple transverse striations. This condition is frequently seen in the elderly primarily due to self-neglect (infrequent cutting of nails), repetitive trauma, nailbed hypertrophy, and hallux valgus deformity. The congenital variant usually affects the fifth toenail and mostly remains asymptomatic.[42] Cases with altered peripheral circulation (diabetes mellitus, peripheral vascular disease, etc.) may develop gangrene also.[25] Management requires nail plate clipping with splitter or filing with an electric drill; subsequent regular nail cutting; and due care in those with a compromised blood supply. Surgical or chemical nail avulsion with or without nail matrix destruction (phenol or carbon dioxide laser) may be considered in those with good vascular supply.

Hemionychogryphosis[3,25] refers to a condition in which congenital malalignment of great toes leads to lateral nail plate growth, without upward growth, mimicking onychogryphosis. Regular foot care and periodic nail trimming is all that is required in these cases.

B. Diseases of the Nail Fold

1. Paronychia: Paronychia is an acute or chronic inflammation/infection of the nail folds (Fig. 24.17). It involves up to 10% of the geriatric population.[10–12] **Acute paronychia** is usually a trauma-induced bacterial infection of a solitary nail caused by *Staphylococcus aureus* or *Pseudomonas* species, manifesting as tender erythematous nailfold with/without abscess formation.[43,44] Management involves warm saline soaks with topical or systemic antibiotics and abscess drainage if required.[41,42] **Chronic paronychia** clinically presents as a red, tender boggy swelling of nail folds, loss of cuticle, patent proximal nail groove and secondary nail plate changes (transverse ridges). Though, there are multiple etiological factors involved, among the infective causes, *Candida* or gram negative bacteria (*Proteus* sp., *Klebsiella sp.*) are the pathogens implicated in the formation of chronic hypertrophic nail folds. Prolonged treatment with adequate protective measures are required. Patients are advised to keep the nail folds and surroundings dry and apply topical antifungals or antiseptics with a combination of steroids.[3,41,42]

2. Clubbing (hippocratic nails/watch glass nails): Clubbing is defined as an increase in both the transverse and longitudinal curvature of nail leading to decreased Lovibond's angle

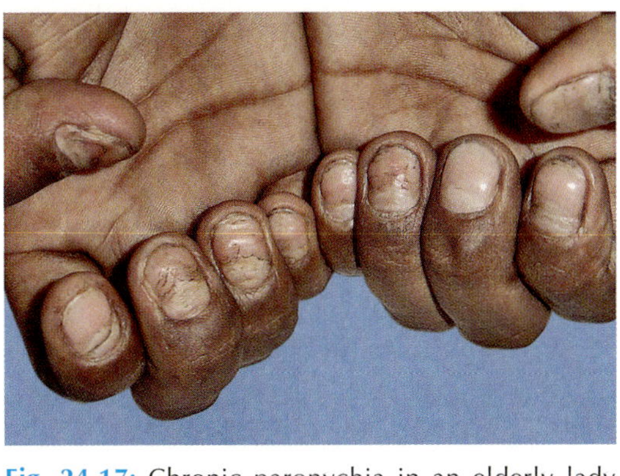

Fig. 24.17: Chronic paronychia in an elderly lady involved in repeated wet work. Note the secondary changes in the nailplate structure

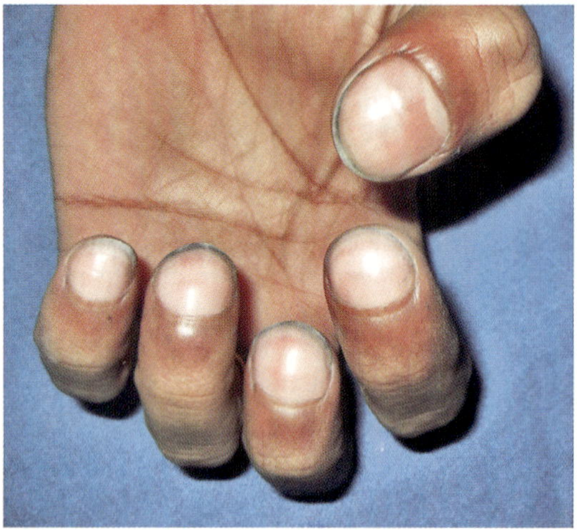

Fig. 24.18: Clubbing in an elderly smoker with severe chronic obstructive pulmonary disease

(<160°) (Fig. 24.18). It is reported to be present in 5–24.5% of elderly in various studies.[10,11,12] Clubbing serves as a clue towards systemic disease and warrants a thorough workup to find the etiology. Bilateral clubbing is the most common type and is associated with cardiopulmonary diseases in 4/5th of cases. Gastrointestinal disease, liver disease, kidney disease, endocarditis, congestive heart failure, cirrhosis of liver, etc. can cause bilateral clubbing. Lymphadenitis, Pancoast tumour of the lungs and erythromelalgia are known to cause unilateral clubbing. Local vascular tumours like aneurysm, arteriovenous fistula or peripheral shunt can cause unidigital clubbing.[45]

3. Onychophosis (callus in the nail sulcus):[3,6,46] This condition involves localised or diffuse growth of hyperkeratotic tissue (callus), in the sulcus between the nail plate and the proximal or lateral nail fold (Fig. 24.19). This may also extend subungually. It is a common finding in the elderly.[47] First and fifth toes are commonly involved. Factors like continuous rubbing and shearing force on the toes due to tight footwear; repeated minor trauma; nail fold deformity or hypertrophy; onychocryptosis; or xerosis may be the involved in

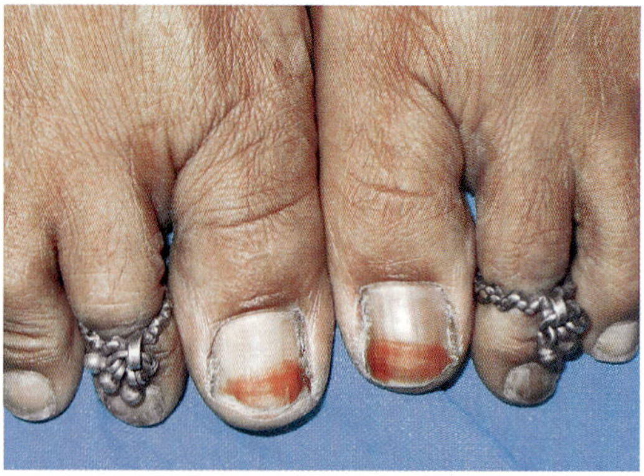

Fig. 24.19: Onychophosis involving the lateral nail folds in an old lady

the causation. Application of keratolytics (20% urea, 12% lactic acid, 6–20% salicylic acid) will help in debridement. A change of footwear will prevent recurrence. Nail wedge resection may be required in severe cases.

4. Onychocryptosis (ingrown toenail): This condition clinically manifests as inflammation of lateral nail fold due to impinging of the nail plate (Fig. 24.20). It occurs when the nail plate penetrates the lateral nail fold resulting in inflammation, swelling, redness, hypergranulation and secondary infection of the lateral nail fold. Three major types are known: Over curvature of the nail plate (pincer nail), subcutaneous ingrown toenail and hyper-

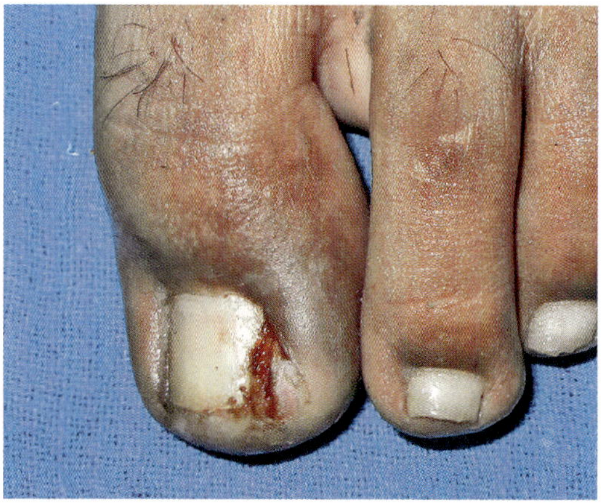

Fig. 24.20: Lateral ingrown toenail in a 60-year-old man

trophy of the lateral nail fold.[11] An improper cutting of nails (leaving a spike or spicule of the nail, or cutting the corners too far down) is the most common cause; even though, long toes, prominent nail folds, tight ill-fitted shoes, high heeled shoes, hyperhidrosis, or bony abnormalities can also be contributory.[3,6,11] In grown nail starts with a mild pressure on the lateral nail fold, associated with discomfort, progressing to pain, walking difficulty and disability. For management, the causative factors must be corrected. Properly fitting footwear is important, cutting of the nails straight across, and removal of any offending spicule is advisable.[48] Conservative management includes warm soaks, placing a wisp of cotton beneath the lateral free edge of the nail, sterile taping, topical and systemic antibiotics, etc.[11,13] Partial nail plate avulsion with lateral matricectomy (phenol, cryotherapy, CO_2 laser) can achieve cure.[49] Surgical decompression of the surrounding skin without matricectomy has also been reported to be successful.[50]

C. Diseases of Nail Bed

1. Subungual corn/onychoclavus/subungual heloma:[3,6] It is a hyperkeratotic process presenting as a tender hyperkeratotic area under the distal nail plate, commonly involving the great toenail (Fig. 24.21). It is very commonly confused with subungual melanocytic lesions, subungual exostosis, foreign body or epidermoid cyst. Repeated trauma or persistent pressure on toes (tight shoes, flexed digits, rotated toes) are the underlying cause and should be addressed properly while managing this condition. Enucleation of the excess tissue and correction of underlying bone abnormality are recommended. In elderly, velcrostraps/moulded shoes, protective pads or orthostatic inserts may be considered.

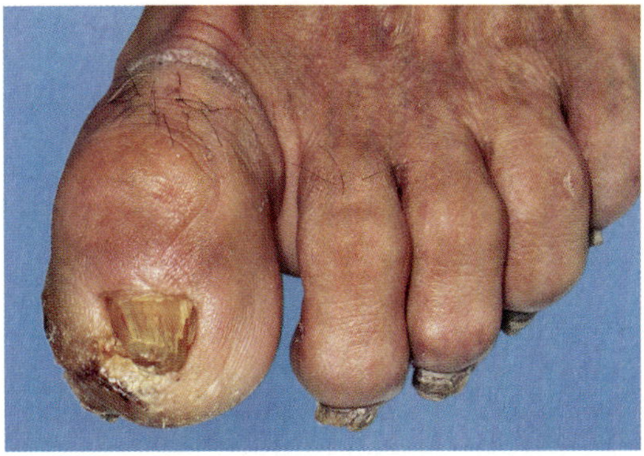

Fig. 24.21: Subungual corn (heloma) in an elderly diabetic. Note the thickening and discoloration of most of the nails and the flexion deformity of the toes due to diabetic neuropathy

2. Subungual hematoma: It is commonly seen in elderly population after a traumatic nail bed injury (Fig. 24.22).[3,11] Less commonly, it can be associated with diabetes mellitus, amyloidosis, or anticoagulant therapy. As a natural course, it progresses from an initial painful, red subungual discolouration to a bluish, less tender globule, carried forward with time.[51] This feature helps to distinguish it from melanocytic lesions of the nail bed. A suspicion of concomitant neoplasm should always be considered as blood may just be masking it. For management, large hematomas, which are acute and tender, may require drilling a hole through the nail plate to relieve the pressure; other lesions need to be managed with careful observation as the mainstay of management.[3,6,11]

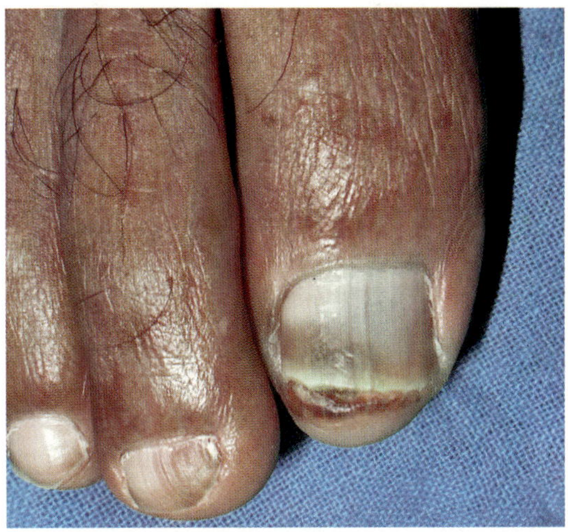

Fig. 24.22: Subungual hematoma in an elderly male. This was due to a poorly fitting shoe with a tight toebox

3. Splinter haemorrhages: These present as a linear subungual discolouration; with the location providing clue towards the etiology involved. Trauma-induced haemorrhages are distally located and brown to black in colour; while reddish proximal haemorrhage is induced by systemic diseases (cholesterol emboli, infective endocarditis, connective tissue disease), etc. In geriatric population, trauma associated splinter haemorrhages are more frequent and require assurance only as they resolve spontaneously.[3,6,11]

4. Onycholysis: It is defined as painless distal separation of nailplate from nailbed, reported in 48–68% elderly (Fig. 24.23).[11,12] Commonly it begins from the distal end and extends proximally. It may be idiopathic, trauma related, due to prolonged use of nail cosmetics or associated with dermatological (psoriasis, onychomycosis, hyperhidrosis) or systemic diseases (amyloidosis, diabetes mellitus, anaemia).[3,6]

5. Subungual hyperkeratosis: An excessive proliferation of nailbed and hyponychium leads to an accumulation of yellow soft keratin beneath the nail plate. In geriatric population it affects 60–90% cases.[11,12] This is not a disease *per se*, but is commonly seen in association with diseases of skin (psoriasis, eczema) and nail (onychauxis, onychogryphosis, onychomycosis, subungual warts).

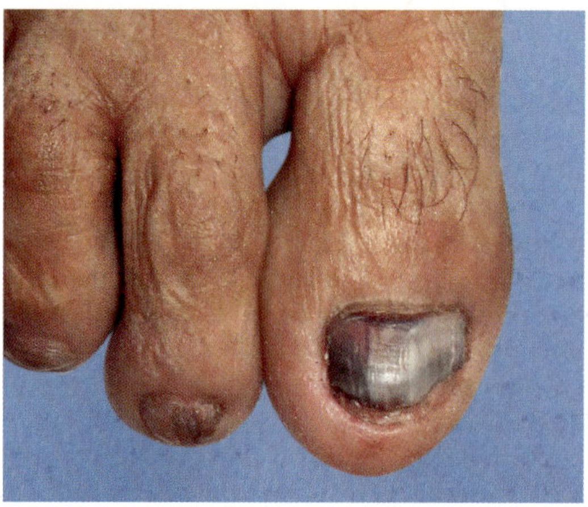

Fig. 24.23: Onycholysis involving the great toenail. There is brownish to blackish discolouration as well

D. Other Nail Disorders

1. Ragged cuticle: Cuticle has an important function of protecting the delicate nailbed; however, it can become hard, dry, and cracked due to repeated trauma (habitual, manicure, or household work) or in association with connective tissue diseases. Ragged cuticle is observed in 52–88% of elderly.[11,12] Patients are advised to keep the cuticle soft and apply moisturizer after every handwash.

2. Adverse effects of nail cosmetics: Prolonged use of nail cosmetics may lead to nail changes like staining, friability, thinning, keratin granulation, onycholysis, paronychia or contact dermatitis in the elderly. Various components of cosmetic agents like nail polish, nail polish remover, nail hardeners; acrylic or gel nails, nail adhesives, etc. produce variable manifestations in different individuals.[11,52] Nails may be affected by hair cosmetics as well.[52]

3. Nail tumours: Neoplastic conditions of nail apparatus are expectedly more frequent in the geriatric population. Benign (myxoidpseudocyst, subungual exostosis), as well as malignant tumors (Bowen's disease, melanoma) have recorded the highest incidence in elderly. Salient tumours are listed below.

- *Subungual exostosis:* It is benign overgrowth of bone and cartilage underneath the nailbed, manifesting as a tender, firm nodule which slowly grows upward from the nailbed, usually involving the medial side of great toe. Chronic irritation to the bone in patients with dystrophic nails, onychaux is or repeated trauma, is the presumed etiology. In these cases, a possibility of pyogenic granuloma, glomus tumour, or amelanotic melanoma should be thoroughly ruled out. Surgical removal of the overgrowth is planned only after an X-ray confirms its bony origin.[3,11,53]

- *Myxoid pseudocyst/ mucus cyst/ ganglion cyst/ synovial cyst:* It is a pseudocyst lacking a true capsule, and arising from degenerative connective tissue near the nail base. It presents as an asymptomatic smooth, shiny, semi-translucent nodule, which may release jelly like material (mucin) on manipulation (Fig. 24.24). Treatment options include intralesional steroids, sclerosant, cryotherapy or surgical excision. Recurrence is common.[2,11]
- *Bowen's disease:* Bowen's disease of nailbed and periungual area originates from the nail fold epithelium, and commonly affects the fingernails (Fig. 24.25). Trauma, arsenic, X-ray exposure, chronic paronychia and HPV infection[16,34,35] have a role in the pathogenesis. It clinically presents as an ulcerated hyperkeratotic tissue, either subungually or periungually; with onycholysis, paronychia or nail dystrophy. Only a few cases show local invasion while distant metastasis is rare. Moh's micrographic surgery is the treatment of choice.[13,53,54]
- *Subungual melanoma*: Malignant melanoma is associated with poor 5-year survival; when it involves the nail apparatus, diagnosis is further delayed leading to poorer prognosis as compared to cutaneous melanoma. Nail apparatus melanoma (NAM) is reportedly commoner in Japanese and African Americans; more frequent between 5–7th decade with no gender predisposition. NAM classically presents with longitudinal melanonychia (LM); although diffuse involvement may also be seen (Fig. 24.26). It is not uncommon for LM to

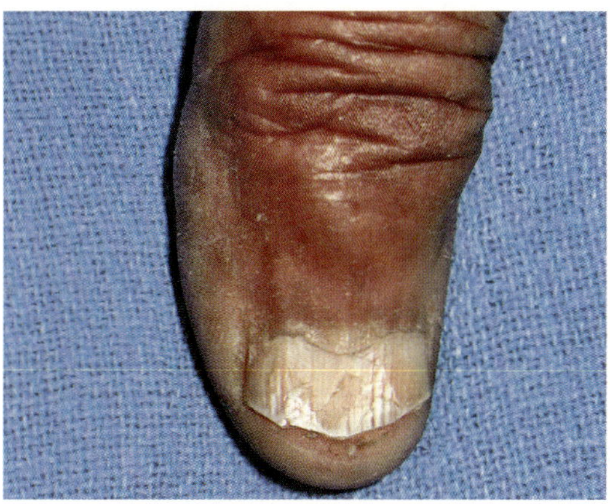

Fig. 24.24: Myxoid cyst presenting as a soft, globoid swelling just distal to the distal interphalangeal joint. The cyst has produced secondary pressure changes on the nail plate in the form of flattening with central depression

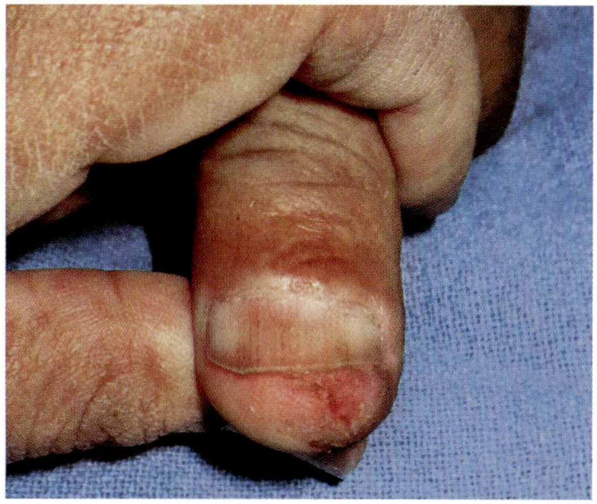

Fig. 24.25: Periungual Bowen's disease presenting as an ill-defined plaque involving the distal digital tip with erosions

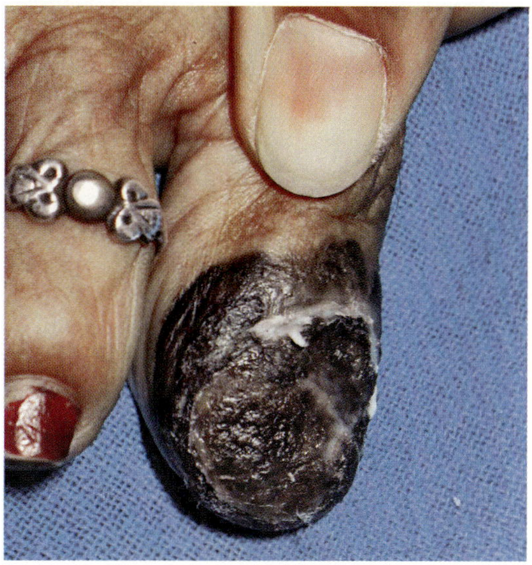

Fig. 24.26: Advanced melanoma of the nail unit in a 65-year-old lady

TABLE 24.3: Signs and symptoms suggestive of nail apparatus melanoma (ABCDEF rule)

A	Age, Afro-Americans, native Americans and Asians): fifth and seventh decades;
B	Nail Band: colour from brown to black, ≥3 mm wide, irregular borders
C	Change: rapid increase in size of band and/or change in nail morphology;
D	Digit involved: thumb > hallux > index finger, Dominant hand; only one Digit;
E	Extension: Hutchinson´s sign;
F	Family: personal or familial history of nevi dysplastic syndrome and melanoma.

go unnoticed or ignored by patients as well as physicians. Levit et al produced an aide-memoire (ABCDEF rule) to help distinguish alarming from non-alarming melanonychia (Table 24.3).[55] A high index of suspicion is the key to early diagnosis with histological confirmation. Treatment is as per the staging of melanoma.[53,54]

CONCLUSION

To conclude, nail abnormalities are quite commonly detected in the geriatric patient. As most of these abnormalities are just senile changes, and not pathologies, one needs to be aware of the spectrum of age-related changes in the nail. An astute clinician should be able to differentiate them deftly. Age-related nail changes can significantly affect the functionality of an individual (be it the toenail or the finger nail). Additionally, most of these can be significantly managed by advising the elderly regarding proper nail care, thus preventing secondary consequences. Among the pathologies affecting the aged nail, the etiological factors remain almost the same as the general population; however, the morphological presentations and the epidemiological factors vary. Apart from the dermatoses affecting nails (like psoriasis or lichen planus), a significant number of infections (fungal or otherwise) involve elderly nails. The role of altered pedal biomechanics in the elderly should always be kept in mind. Similarly, tumors, especially the pre-malignant or malignant variety, should always be kept at as possibility while dealing with elderly nail disorders. One needs to be very careful while managing these conditions as co-morbidities and co-medications in the elderly age group need to be taken into consideration before deciding on any form of therapy.

References

1. Raja Babu KK. Nail and its disorders. In: Valia RG, Valia AR, editors. IADVL Textbook and Atlas of Dermatology. 2nd ed. Mumbai: Bhalani Publishing House; 2001. p. 763–98.
2. Baran R, Dawber RP.The nail in childhood and old age. In: Baran R, Dawber RPR, editors. Diseases of the nails and their management. 4th ed. Oxford: Blackwell Science; 2012. p. 183–211.
3. Cohen PR, Scher RK. Geriatric nail disorders: diagnosis and treatment. J Am AcadDermatol 1992; 26:521–31.
4. Dittmar M, Dindorf W, Banerjee A: Organic elemental composition in fingernail plates varies between sexes and changes with increasing age in healthy humans. Gerontology 54:100, 2008.
5. Brosche T, Dressler S, Platt D: Age-associated changes in integral cholesterol and cholesterol sulfate concentrations in human scalp hair and finger nail clippings. Aging 13:131, 2001.
6. Cohen PR, Scher RK. Aging. In: Hordinsky MK, Sawaya ME, Scher RK, editors. Atlas of hair and nails. Philadelphia: Churchill Livingstone; 2000. p. 213–25.
7. Cohen PR, Scher RK. Nail changes in the elderly. J Geriatric Dermatol 1993; 1:45–53.
8. N Orentreich, N Sharp. Keratin replacement as an ageing parameter. J SocCosmChem 1967; 18:571-585.
9. Lewis BL, Montgomery H. The senile nail. J Invest Dermatol. 1955; 24:11–8.
10. Rao S, Banerjee S, Ghosh SK, Gangopadhyay DN, Jana S, Mridha K. Study of nail changes and nail disorders in the elderly. Indian journal of dermatology. 2011 Sep; 56(5):603.
11. Singh G, Haneef NS, Uday A. Nail changes and disorders among the elderly. Indian J Dermatol Veneveol Leprol. 2005; 71:386–92.

12. Snigdha J, Reddy BN, Prasad GK. A Study on the Pattern of Nail Changes and Nail Disorders in Geriatric Patients in a Tertiary Care Hospital in a Rural Setting. Sch. J. App. Med. Sci., 2016; 4(12C): 4394–4400.
13. Abdullah L, Abbas O. Common nail changes and disorders in older people. Canadian Family Physician. 2011 Feb 1;57(2):173–81.
14. Miles DW, Rubens RD (1995)."Images in clinical medicine.Transverse leukonychia". N. Engl. J. Med. 333 (2): 100. PMID 7777013.doi:10.1056/NEJM199507133330205.
15. Tüzün, Yalçýn; Karakuþ, Özge (2009). "Leukonychia" (PDF). Journal of Turkish Academy of Leukonychia: 1–3. Retrieved April 2, 2017.
16. Examination Medicine. Nicolas J Tally. MacLennan and Petty Pty Ltd. 2003.
17. Terry R. White nails in hepatic cirrhosis. Lancet. 1954; 266:757–9.
18. Singh G, Singh SJ, Chakrabarty N, Siddharaju KS, Prakash JC. Cutaneous manifestations of chronic renal failure. Indian J Dermatol Venereol Leprol 1989; 55:167–9.
19. Holzberg M. Nail signs of systemic disease. In: Hordinsky MK, Sawaya ME, Scher RK, editors. Atlas of hair and nails. Philadelphia: Churchill Livingstone; 2000. p. 59–70.
20. Baran R, Tosti A. Nails. In: Freedberg IM, Eisen AZ, Wolff K, Austen KF, Goldsmith LA, Katz SI, editors. Fitzpatrick's dermatology in general medicine. 6th ed. New York: McGraw Hill; 2003. p. 656–71.
21. Horan MA, Puxty JA, Fox RA. The white nails of old age (Neapolitan nails). J Am GeriatrSoc 1982; 30(12):734–7.
22. Cohen PR, Scher RK. The nail in older individuals. In: Scher RK, Daniel CR III, editors. Nails: Therapy, diagnosis, surgery. Philadelphia: WB Saunders; 1997. p.127–50.
23. Metzner MJ, Billington AR, Payne WG. Melanonychia. Eplasty. 2015; 15:ic48.
24. Julie Jefferson and Phoebe Rich, "Melanonychia," Dermatology Research and Practice, vol. 2012, Article ID 952186, 8 pages, 2012. doi:10.1155/2012/952186.
25. Baran R, Dawber RPR. Physical signs. In: Baran R, Dawber RP, editors. Diseases of the nails and their management. 2nd ed. Oxford: Blackwell Science; 1994. p. 35–80.
26. Drake LA, Dinehart SM, Farmer ER, Goltz RW, Graham GF, Hordinsky MK, et al. Guidelines of care for nail disorders. J Am AcadDermatol 1996; 34:529–33.
27. Van de Kerkhof PC, Pasch MC, Scher RK, Kerscher M, Gieler U, Haneke E, et al. Brittle nail syndrome: a pathogenesis-based approach with a proposed grading.
28. Hochman LG, Scher RK, Meyerson MS. Brittle nails: response to daily biotin supplementation. Cutis 1993; 51(4):303–5.
29. Scheinfeld N, Dahdah MJ, Scher R. Vitamins and minerals: their role in nail health and disease. J Drugs Dermatol 2007; 6(8):782–7.
30. Gupta AK, Ricci MJ.Diagnosing onychomycosis. Dermatol Clin 2006; 24(3):365–9.
31. Loo DS.Cutaneous fungal infections in the elderly. Dermatol Clin 2004; 22:33–50.
32. Demirseren DD, Kilinc F, Emre S, Ahmet M, Ankara DK. Nail Changes And Diseases In Geriatric Age Group: Assessment Of 249 Patients Admitted To Dermatology Outpatient Clinic. Turkish Journal of Geriatrics-Turk GeriatriDergisi. 2014 Jan 1; 17(2):119–24.
33. Weinberg JW, Vafaie J, Scheinfeld NS. Skin infections in the elderly. Dermatol Clin. 2004; 22:51–61
34. Gupta AK, Tu LQ. Therapies for onychomycosis: a review. Dermatol Clin 2006; 24(3):375–9.
35. Drake LA, Dinehart SM, Farmer ER, Goltz RW, Graham GF, Hordinsky MK, et al. Guidelines of care for superficial mycotic infections of the skin: onychomycosis. J Am AcadDermatol 1996; 34:116–21.
36. Witkowski JA, Parish LC. Scabies. Subungual areas harbor mites. JAMA 1984; 252(10):1318–9.
37. Jopling WH, McDougall AC. The disease. In: Handbook of leprosy. 5th ed. New Delhi: CBS Publishers and Distributors; 1996. p. 10–53.
38. Sharma VK. Leprosy: Classification and clinical features. In: Valia RG, Valia AR, editors. IADVL Textbook and atlas of dermatology. 2nd ed. Mumbai: Bhalani Publishing House; 2001. p. 1578–603.
39. King A, Nicol C, Rodin P. Venereal diseases. 4th ed. London: Balliere Tindall; 1980. p.15–43.

40. Misra RS, Kumar J. Syphilis: clinical features and natural course. In: Sharma VK, Bhargava R, Kar HK, Usman N, Sethuraman G, editors. Sexually transmitted diseases and AIDS. New Delhi: Viva Books Pvt Ltd; 2003. p.165–82.
41. Bartolomei FJ. Onychauxis. Surgical and nonsurgical treatment. Clin Pediatr Med Surg 1995; 12(2):215–20.
42. Sequeira JH (1923). "Case of Congenital Onychogryphosis". Proc. R. Soc. Med. 16:92.
43. Rich P. Nail disorders: diagnosis and treatment of infectious, inflammatory and neoplastic nail conditions. Med Clin North Am 1998; 82:1171–83.
44. Rigopoulos D, Larios G, Gregoriou S, Alevizos A. Acute and chronic paronychia. Am Fam Physician 2008; 77(3):339–46.
45. Meyerson MS, Scher RK. Nail signs of systemic disease. In: Callen JP, Jorizzo JL, Greer KE, Penneys NS, Piette WW, Zone JJ, editors. Dermatological signs of internal disease. 2nd ed. Philadelphia: WB Saunders Co; 1999. p. 368–75.
46. Neale D, Disorders of the nails. Common Foot Disorders, Diagnosis and Management, A General Clinical Guide. Edinburgh: Churchill Livingstone 1981; 103–114.
47. James, William; Berger, Timothy; Elston, Dirk (2005). Andrews' Diseases of the Skin: Clinical Dermatology. (10th ed.). Saunders. ISBN 0-7216-2921-0.
48. Dawber R, Bristow I, Turner W. Nail Disorders. In: Text atlas of podiatric dermatology. London: Martin Dunitz Ltd; 2001. p. 105–31.
49. Heidelbaugh JJ, Lee H. Management of the ingrown toenail. Am Fam Physician 2009;79(4):303–8.
50. Noël B. Surgical treatment of ingrown toenail without matricectomy. Dermatol Surg 2008; 34(1): 79–83. Epub 2007 Dec 5.
51. Huang YH, Ohara K. Medical pearl: subungual hematoma: a simple and quick method for diagnosis. J Am Acad Dermatol 2006; 54(5):877–8.
52. Dawber RPR, Baran R, De Berker D. Disorders of nails. In: Champion RH, Burton JL, Burns DA, Breathnach SM, editors. Rook/ Wikinson/ Ebling Texbook of dermatology. 6th ed. Oxford: Blackwell Science; 1998. p. 2815–68.
53. Salasche SJ, Garland LD. Tumors of the nail. Dermatol Clin 1985; 3:521–30.
54. Baran R, Richert B. Common nailtumors. Dermatologic clinics. 2006 Jul 31; 24(3):297–311.
55. Levit EK, Kagen MH, Scher RK, Grossman M, Altman E. The ABC rule for clinical detection of subungual melanoma. J Am AcadDermatol. 2000; 42:269–274.

CHAPTER 25

Scalp and Hair Disorders in Elderly

• *Vibhu Mendiratta*

Introduction

Hair is an important cosmetic asset. Hair diseases are common in the elderly and can have physical and psychological consequences. Some commonly encountered problems include androgenetic alopecia, telogen effluvium, scaly scalp, drug-induced alopecia, diffuse alopecia due to nutritional deficiencies, and anagen efflucium. Diffuse or patchy alopecia which presents suddenly, scalp nodules and erosio-ulcerative lesions mandate a thorough work up for any neoplastic association.

Pathophysiology

Ageing of appendages is a complex phenomenon due to interplay of genetic, hormonal, immunological and environmental factors. Ageing of hair is mediated by free radical generation leading to reduced number of keratinocytes, fibroblasts, and vascular network around hair bulb and glands, that results in slow hair growth. Ageing affects number of hair follicles, growth rate and diameter. Hair loss may occur due to: (1) Injury to the hair follicle (as in the cicatricial alopecias), (2) disruption of the hair cycle (as in telogen effluvium or alopecia areata) or (3) physical alteration of the pilosebaceous unit (as with aging). Conditions presenting with hair loss or scalp problems in elderly are given in Table 25.1.

TABLE 25.1: Scalp/hair disorders affecting the elderly population

- Scaly scalp
- Folliculitis
- Neurodermatitis
- Scalp dysaesthesia
- Senescent alopecia
- Androgenetic alopecia
- Telogen effluvium
- Anagen effluvium
- Alopecia areata
- Alopecia neoplastica
- Frontal fibrosing alopecia
- Erosive pustular dermatitis

SCALY SCALP

Dandruff (loose, greyish white scaling) is common in elderly (men > women). Inability to regularly wash the scalp and seborrhoea as in parkinsonism, post-stroke neuropathies, epilepsy, congestive heart failure, obesity, and chronic alcoholism predisposes to dandruff.[1] Seborrheic dermatitis appears as erythematous plaques with yellowish-white scales over scalp, face, retroauricular area, eyebrows, and nasal alae. Areas like chest, anus, and groin, can also be involved. Indians usually show white, minimally scaly patches over the eyebrows. Infection with Gram-positive bacteria is common due to repeated scratching. Scalp psoriasis should be suspected in recurrent, adherent scaling of scalp with underlying erythema. Frequent shampooing with ketoconazole/selenium sulphide/tar/ shampoos is helpful. Thick, adherent scales are treated with salicylic acid shampoos and lotions.

NEURODERMATITIS CIRCUMSCRIPTA OF SCALP

Neurodermatitis circumscripta (lichen simplex chronicus) is characterized by lichenified plaques as a result of constant scratching/ rubbing. The desire to scratch is secondary to a psychological urge. Commonly affected sites include nape of neck, ankles, anogenital region and scalp. Itch scratch cycle is paroxysmal and patient scratches until it bleeds which may even lead to sleep disturbance. Discrete, lichenified plaques of alopecia are noticed. Effective management depends on correction of associated psychological factors. Intralesional steroids, doxepin and psychotherapy are used in the treatment.[2]

SCALP NODULE

Nodular lesions such as pilar cysts, dermoid cysts are frequently seen over scalp. Warty dyskeratoma is a rare tumour that presents mainly as an isolated papule or nodule with a central keratotic plug on the scalp, face or neck in the middle-aged or elderly people. Multiple lesions are rare.[3] Folliculosebaceous cystic hamartoma (FSCH) is an uncommon, rarely reported non-neoplastic lesion which arises from the hair follicle. It is a rare cutaneous hamartoma composed mainly of follicular, sebaceous and mesenchymal elements. Clinicians always suggest cyst-like cutaneous lesion, soft tissue neoplasm, sebaceous gland hyperplasia or melanocytic nevus. It always presents as a painless, slowly growing single firm papule or nodule with a predilection for the central face, vulva, the nipple, the scrotum, the ear or scalp.[4] Differential diagnosis of scalp nodules in elderly must include metastases from adenocarcinoma lung, bronchus, pancreas. Skin biopsy is conclusive.

SCALP DYSAESTHESIA

It is characterized by localized pruritus, burning sensations or even pain over scalp. The pain and pruritus may be related to the chronic tension placed on the occipitofrontalis muscle and scalp aponeurosis secondary to the underlying cervical spine disease.[5] Single patch of alopecia on the vertex with pruritus and pain has to be considered as scalp dysesthesia. Trichoscopy can be helpful in establishing the diagnosis—broom hairs, block hairs and short hairs with trichorrhexis nodosa covering the alopecia patch, uniform in length, are considered characteristic for scalp dysesthesia.

ALOPECIA AREATA

Alopecia areata (AA) is characterized by round to oval patches of non-scarring hair loss with occult onset and spontaneous remission, although a remittent and fluctuating course is not uncommon. Progress of hair loss to involve the entire scalp (alopecia totalis, AT) or even the whole body (alopecia universalis, AU) can be seen in 5–10% of the patients. Association with nail changes, especially nail pitting, as well as history of atopy, vitiligo, autoimmune thyroiditis and other autoimmune diseases have been reported. A study by Wu MC et al reported that late-onset alopecia areata in the elderly represents a distinct subgroup with marked female predominance and milder disease activity with advancing age. The association with personal or family history of atopy is absent while the link to cancers needs to be further confirmed.[6,7]

DIFFUSE ALOPECIA

The most common cause of hair loss in aging men and women is ***androgenic alopecia***, or common balding. Individuals may start losing hair any time after puberty, but it is common for different balding patterns to clinically manifest first after 40 years. In late 60s, 80% of men have some substantial balding or thinning. Postmenopausal women are also affected, but hair thinning rather than balding is more noticeable.[8,9] Nutritional deficiencies (iron deficiency), thyroid and autoimmune connective tissue diseases and drugs (antithyroid, beta blockers, antidepressants and anticoagulents) also contribute to hair loss. **Effective control of diabetes with correction of nutritional deficiencies can improve hair loss.**

CONTACT DERMATITIS OF SCALP

Contact dermatitis over scalp is uncommon due to thick skin, which is rich in pilosebaceous units. Patients with scalp contact dermatitis often do not have evident skin lesions on the scalp, but instead present with acute or chronic scalp itch or hair loss. Typical eczematous lesions may be seen at the hairlines, on the ears, at the retroauricular region, and the neck. Patients may attribute their symptoms to a new shampoo or hair dye, various cosmetic products, keratin treatments, or other hair treatments. Eliciting a careful history is important since the scalp is exposed to many substances. Contact dermatitis can be to hair brushes, combs, metallic hair rollers, hair clasps and pins, hair dyes, shampoos, conditioners, hair gels or oils, as well as leave-on hair products. Common allergens identified include balsam of Peru, fragrance mix, carba mix, PG, ammonium persulfate (APS), preservatives, PPD, and minoxidil.

ANDROGENETIC ALOPECIA

Androgenetic alopecia (AGA) is the most common type of hair loss in men. It is characterized by visible loss of hair over areas of the scalp due to progressive miniaturization of hair follicles. One of the studies conducted on AGA in elderly population concluded that the majority of the variation in hair loss among elderly men can be attributed to genetic factors.

TINEA CAPITIS

Scalp ringworm is not rare in elderly. Only 3–5% of tinea capitis occur in adults over 20 years of age. Any pruritic, scaly or erosion crusted plaque on scalp should arouse clinical suspicion.[10] The adult hair seems to be relatively resistant to tinea capitis due to fungistatic properties of long chain fatty acids of sebum. An increase in tinea capitis among adults, particularly menopausal women has been reported by some authors. Adult men are involved only rarely. Factors causing tinea capitis at this age include hormonal changes (involution of sebaceous glands following decreased blood oestrogen levels), use of hair care products and services of hair salons.

ANAGEN EFFLUVIUM

AE is more common and severe with combination chemotherapy than with the use of a single drug, and the severity is generally dose dependent. While hair loss from anticancer therapy has traditionally been categorized as dystrophic anagen effluvium however both shedding patterns, i.e. dystrophic anagen effluvium and telogen effluvium can be seen. Accordingly, the hair may fall out very quickly in clumps or gradually depending on the mitotic activity of the hair follicle at the moment of the insult. Hair shedding usually begins 1 to 3 weeks after this incident. Normally, up to 90% of scalp hairs are in the anagen phase, and as such, hair loss is usually copious and results in alopecia that is quite obvious. The severity of hair loss after chemotherapy or radiation depends on timing and dose of chemo or radiotherapy on hair follicle melanocytes and inner root sheath epithelium. Radiation-induced alopecia may be reversible or permanent. Radiation-induced temporary hair loss may be observed following neuroradiologically guided embolization procedures. Regrowth after radiation therapy depends on type, depth, and dose-fractionation. Permanent follicular destruction is commonly seen, most likely due to irreversible damage to hair follicle stem cells. Permanent alopecia occurs with >30 Gy of deep X-rays or >50 Gy of soft X-rays. Persistent radiation-induced inflammatory changes that progressively damage the stem cells may lead to scarring alopecia even after cessation of radiation therapy. Many heavy metals are capable of disrupting the formation of hair shaft by binding with the sulphydryl group of the keratins in the hair. Thallium, mercury, bismuth, copper, and cadmium are the most common metals responsible for this kind of hair loss.

Diffuse, reversible alopecia was reported in 50% of patients receiving treatment with tyrosine kinase inhibitors such as sorafenib and sunitinib as well as monoclonal antibodies targeting the EGFR-like cetuximab can induce a constellation of cutaneous symptoms known by the acronym PRIDE (papulopustules and/or paronychia, regulatory abnormalities of hair growth, itching and dryness due to EGFR inhibitors). Some anticancer drugs are more frequently associated with hair loss, it is seen in 80% cases with antimicrotubule agents (e.g. paclitaxel), 60–100% for topoisomerase inhibitors (e.g. doxorubicin), >60% for alkylators (e.g. cyclophosphamide), and 10–50% for antimetabolites (e.g. 5-fluorouracil plus leucovorin).

TELOGEN EFFLUVIUM

Telogen effluvium is a form of nonscarring alopecia characterized by diffuse, often acute hair shedding. Telogen effluvium can occur in elderly. Acute telogen effluvium is described as an acute onset scalp hair loss occurring 2–3 months after a triggering event, which could be unidentifiable in up to 33% cases. Chronic telogen effluvium presents as telogen effluvium lasting more than 6 months, without any widening of central part or follicular miniaturization.

ALOPECIA NEOPLASTICA

The overall incidence of cutaneous metastasis from visceral carcinomas ranges from 0.7% to 9%. The presence of cutaneous metastasis is usually an indicator of a widespread disease and of poor prognosis. Alopecia neoplastica is characterized by single or multiple areas of cicatricial alopecia, which is the result of the neoplastic process involving the hair follicle and the surrounding skin (Fig. 25.1). Alopecia neoplastica has been associated with metastatic tumours like breast carcinomas, gastric carcinoma, desmoplastic and placental site trophoblastic tumour.

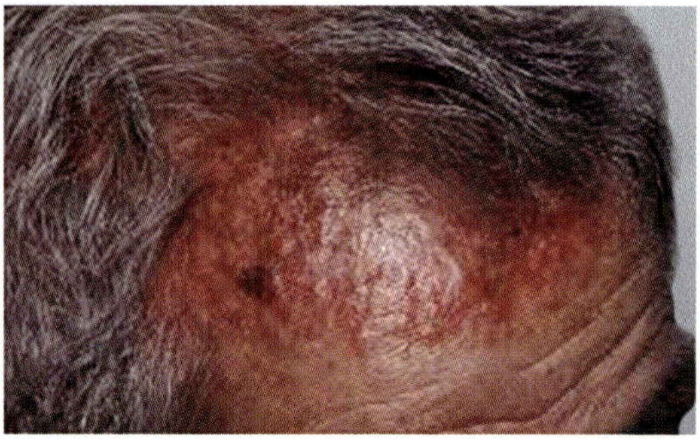

Fig. 25.1: Alopecia neoplastica

SCARRING ALOPECIA

Frontal Fibrosing Alopecia

Progressive frontal fibrosing alopecia is a clinically distinct variant of lichen planopilaris that affects middle aged to elderly women and frequently involves the eyebrows (Fig. 25.2). The basis for this lichenoid tissue reaction targeting frontal scalp follicles and eyebrows

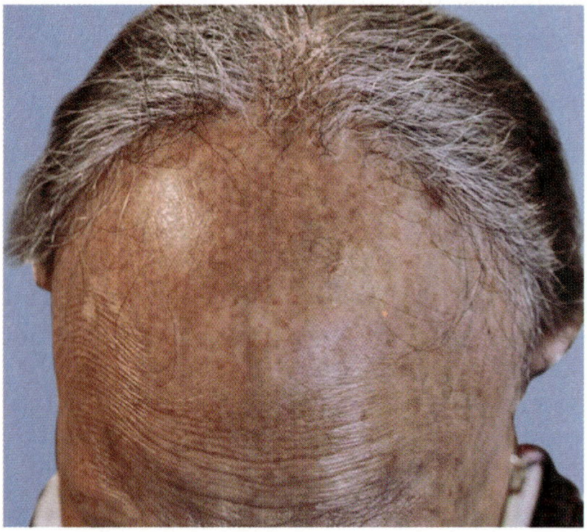

Fig. 25.2: Frontal fibrosing alopecia

is unknown. Treatment is not very successful. Antimalarials, retinoids and oral steroids have been used in the past.[12]

Erosive Pustular Dermatosis

Erosive pustular dermatosis of the scalp (EPDS) is a rare entity characterized by pustular, erosive and crusted lesions of the scalp with progressive scarring alopecia (Fig. 25.3). Several precipitating factors such as trauma, skin grafting, prolonged exposure to UV light, co-existence of auto-immune diseases have been reported to provoke it. Laboratory data, bacteriological and mycological investigations and histopathology are generally not diagnostic. A 45-year-old Caucasian man with 1-year-old pustular, erosive and crusted lesions on his bald scalp was seen. Laboratory data, including auto-immunity, bacteriological and mycological investigations were negative. Histopathology showed a diffuse polymorphous infiltrate involving the dermis. A diagnosis of EPDS was made. The patient was treated with topical and systemic antibiotics and steroids as well as oral nimesulide with no or partial response. Consequently, isotretinoin (0.75 mg/kg/day) was started obtaining complete resolution in a few months. EPDS represents a distinct disease with a history of relapsing and unsatisfactory response to common treatments. Systemic retinoids may be considered as a potentially resolutive choice.

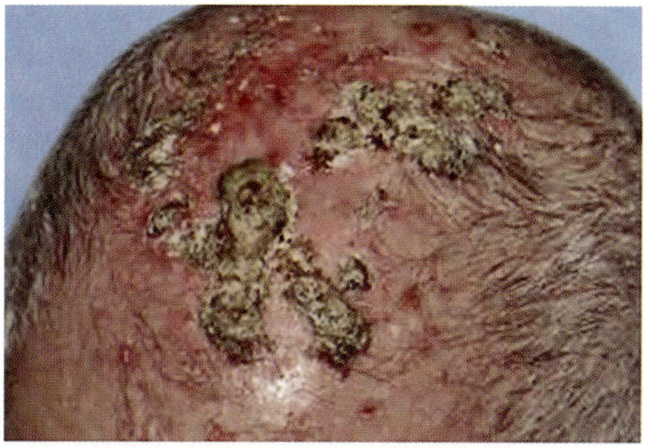

Fig. 25.3: Erosive pustular dermatosis

References

1. Prevalence and determinants of seborrhoeic dermatitis in a middle aged and elderly population: the Rotterdam Study. Sanders MGH, Pardo LM, Franco OH, Ginger RS, Nijsten T . Br J Dermatol. 2018 Jan; 178(1):148–153.
2. A case of neurodermatitis circumscipta of scalp presenting as patchy alopecia. Ambika H, Vinod CS, Sushmita J. Int J Trichology. 2013 Apr; 5(2):94–6.
3. Multiple warty dyskeratomas: case report. Ugras N, Adim SB, Kilicoglu M, Baskan EB Iran J Public Health. 2014 Aug; 43(8):1145–7.
4. Neuro-folliculo-sebaceous cystic hamartoma is a unique entity. Samaka RM, Alrahabi N. Pol J Pathol. 2015 Mar; 66(1):77–9.
5. Scalp dysesthesia related to cervical spine disease. Thornsberry LA[1], English JC 3rd. JAMA Dermatol. 2013 Feb; 149(2):200–3.
6. Late-onset alopecia areata: a retrospective study of 73 patients from Taiwan. Wu MC, Yang CC, Tsai RY, Chen WC. J Eur Acad Dermatol Venereol. 2013 Apr; 27(4):468–72.
7. Late-onset alopecia areata: descriptive analysis of 30 cases. Lazzarini R, Oliari CB, Erthal AL. An Bras Dermatol. 2016 Nov-Dec; 91(6):844–845.
8. Hair loss in elderly women. Chen W, Yang CC, Todorova A, Al Khuzaei S, Chiu HC, Worret WI, Ring J.Eur J Dermatol. 2010 Mar-Apr; 20(2):145–51.
9. Progressive hair loss. Power DV, Disse M, Hordinsky M. J Fam Pract. 2017 Aug; 66(8):521–523
10. Tinea capitis in the elderly. A report on two cases caused by *Trichophyton tonsurans*. Moberg S. Dermatologica. 1984; 169(1):36–40.
11. Alopecia neoplastica. Chansky P, Micheletti RG. BMJ Case Rep. 2017 Apr 11;2017.
12. Frontal fibrosing alopecia among men: A clinicopathologic study of 7 cases. Tolkachjov SN, Chaudhry HM, Camilleri MJ, Torgerson RR. J Am Acad Dermatol. 2017 Oct; 77(4):683–690.
13. Tardio NB, Daly TJ. Erosive pustular dermatosis and associated alopecia successfully treated with topical tacrolimus. J Am Acad Dermatol. 2011; 65(3):93–94.

CHAPTER 26

Cutaneous Manifestations of Internal Malignancy

• Nirmala Devi Palanivel • Selvam Arumugam • Sulochana Paul

Key Points

1. Cutaneous manifestations may be specific due to malignant deposits or non-specific due to paraneoplastic manifestations or secondary to immunosuppression due to the disease or treatment.
2. Geriatric age group is involved in 60% of malignancy and it is 7-fold higher in men and 4-fold in women.
3. Skin is the eighteenth most common site of metastases and in 0.5 to 1% it is the presenting manifestation. Usually they are common in primary breast, ovary, lung and GIT.
4. Paraneoplastic manifestations though rare are characteristic and helpful in detection of primary.
5. Knowledge about cutaneous manifestations helps in early recognition of malignancy and better outcome but high index of suspicion is necessary.

Introduction

Internal malignancies are associated with various skin changes which may be specific infiltrates (neoplastic) or non-specific (paraneoplastic or secondary). Specific infiltrates show malignant cells in histopathological examination and can be due to contiguous spread or noncontiguous spread. Non-specific lesions can be due to infections, non-infective conditions including paraneoplastic diseases (PND) or due to chemo- or radiotherapy. Skin is an infrequent site (18th most common) of metastases of internal malignancy.[1] It usually occurs in later stages of malignancy or may be the presenting symptoms and signs of the underlying malignancy. Nine percentage of patients with internal cancer had skin metastases and is the presenting feature in 0.5 to 1% of such patients.[2] The most common sources of cutaneous metastases are carcinoma of breast (69%) followed by carcinoma of lung (24%), colon (19%), stomach, upper aerodigestive tract, uterus and kidney. Paraneoplastic dermatosis may be a clue to the diagnosis of neoplasm and determines the prognosis. Secondary skin changes to malignancy has been reported in 27% of patients.[2]

Advancing age is a high risk factor for cancers with more than 65-year-old persons accounting for 60% of newly diagnosed malignancy and 70% of all cancer deaths.[3] It is 7-fold more in men and 4-fold more in women. Age adjusted cancer incidence rate is 2151/100000 population for over 65 when compared to 208/100000 for those under 65. Similarly, mortality rate of 10 to 68 Vs 67 per 1 lakh population between them has been established. Studies suggest that progressive decrease in DNA mismatch repair process in hematopoietic stem cells (HSC) of older individuals occur. Common malignancies in males (50% of all cancers) involve prostate and colon while in females (48% of all cancers), they involve breast, lung and stomach.[4]

CURTH'S POSTULATES

Curth's postulates describe 5 criteria that need to be fulfilled to establish an association between a skin disease and an internal malignancy.[5]

1. Concurrent onset of cutaneous disease and the internal malignancy or at the time of onset of the cutaneous disease, the internal malignancy is recognizable.
2. Parallel course of the skin disease and internal malignancy.
3. A specific type or site of malignancy is associated with certain specific skin disease.
4. A sound statistical evidence that the malignancy is more frequent in patients with the specific skin disease than in age and sex matched controls.
5. A genetic link existing between a syndrome with skin manifestations and an internal malignancy.

It is difficult to apply all the above criteria for all paraneoplastic conditions as many of the patients have not been detected of their primary at the time of presentation.

MAJOR TYPES OF CUTANEOUS MANIFESTATIONS

They can be classified fairly under four headings based on the specificity and nature of the manifestations and their relation to malignancies.

1. Paraneoplastic syndromes that occur due to circulating factors (proven or presumed) produced by the underlying malignancies.
2. Genetically determined syndromes with cutaneous component(s) (genodermatoses) with predisposition to certain malignancies.
3. Cutaneous metastases.
4. Secondary or reactive changes related to the malignancy or its treatment.

I. PARANEOPLASTIC DERMATOSES

Paraneoplastic diseases (PND) may be defined as hormonal, neurological or hematological disturbances and as clinical and biochemical imbalances associated with the presence of malignancies without direct association with primary tumor invasion or metastasis.[6]

Changes may occur in epidermis, dermis or subcutaneous tissue. Studies regarding exact incidence of paraneoplastic dermatoses are lacking though various studies exist regarding individual dermatoses and few reviews. Common manifestations in geriatric age group are discussed here though some are common in young and middle age group malignancies. They are classified according to the clinical features (Table 26.1).

A. Papulosquamous disorders
   - Tripe palms
   - Malignant acanthosis nigricans
   - Leser-Trélat sign
   - Bazex syndrome
   - Acquired ichthyosis
   - Pityriasis rotunda

TABLE 26.1: Characteristic paraneoplastic cutaneous manifestations in various common malignancies

Malignancy	Paraneoplastic manifestations/syndromes
Adenocarcinoma	Malignant acanthosis nigricans
Gastric and lung carcinoma	Tripe palms (associated with hypertrophic pulmonary osteoarthropathy in lungs)
Adenocarcinoma and lymphoproliferative disorders	Leser Trèlat sign
Esophageal carcinoma	Palmoplantar keratoderma (Howel-Evans syndrome)
Squamous cell carcinoma of upper aerodigestive tract	Bazex syndrome (Acrokeratosis paraneoplastica)
Hodgkin's disease	Acquired ichthyosis
Lung, esophageal and breast carcinoma	Erythema gyratum repens
Lymphoma	Paraneoplastic pemphigus
Hepatocellular carcinoma	Pityriasis rotunda
Alpha cell tumour of the pancreas	Necrolytic migratory erythema

B. Erythematous disorders
- Necrolytic migratory erythema
- Multicentric reticulohistiocytosis
- Erythema gyratum repens

C. Proliferative and inflammatory process
- Pyoderma gangrenosum
- Primary systemic amyloidosis
- Sweet's syndrome
- Scleromyxedema
- Dermatomyositis

D. Bullous disorders
- Paraneoplastic pemphigus
- Cicatricial pemphigoid
- Bullous pemphigoid
- Dermatitis herpetiformis
- Epidermolysis bullosa acquisita
- Porphyria cutanea tarda

E. Miscellaneous
- Exfoliative dermatitis
- Paraneoplastic pruritus and urticaria
- Acquired hypertrichosis lanuginosa
- Lichen planus
- Granuloma annulare
- Insect bite-like reactions
- Cutis verticis gyrata

A. Papulosquamous Disorders

Tripe Palms

It refers to wrinkled or ridged or rugose thick velvety appearance of palmar skin, and occasionally soles and caused by hypertrophy of epidermis (Fig. 26.1). It is also called pachydermatoglyphia or acanthosis palmaris and has the appearance similar to that of bovine foregut mucosa. In 1977, Clarke first coined the term. More than 90% patients with tripe palms (TP) have associated internal malignancy.[7] It manifests as paraneoplastic manifestation in 30–40%. It is most commonly seen with adenocarcinoma of gastrointestinal tract (associated with acanthosis nigricans) or squamous cell carcinoma of the lung (tripe palms occur alone in 53%). Other tumours associated with tripe palms include tumour of genitourinary tract and carcinoma breast.

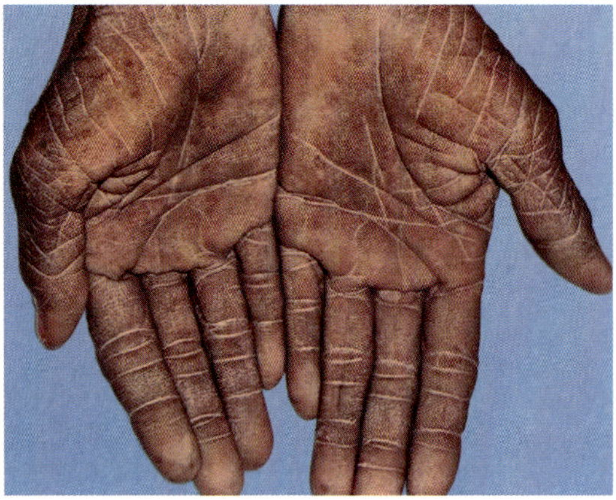

Fig. 26.1: Tripe palms in carcinoma stomach 3 months before diagnosis of primary

Malignant Acanthosis Nigricans

It appears as velvety, hyperpigmented, papillomatous, dirty looking skin. It is more frequently seen on the neck, axilla, groin, and dorsal aspect of hand surfaces. It has rapid onset, progression and severe. It may also involve the mucous membranes. Pathogenesis is due to production of transforming growth factor alpha, insulin like growth factor-1 or MSH alpha and cytokines by tumour cells. Histopathologically it is characterised by hyperkeratosis, irregular acanthosis and finger-like projections of dermal papillae. Paraneoplastic acanthosis nigricans is rare and most commonly associated with carcinoma of GIT (70–90%) especially gastric carcinoma.[5,7] Other malignant conditions are carcinoma ovary, uterus, liver, intestine, pancreas and breast.

Leser-Trélat Sign

It describes sudden appearance or rapid increase in size of multiple seborrhoeic keratoses. Clinically presents as a sudden onset of waxy, verrucous papules with stuck on appearance, frequently associated with itching, primarily on trunk and extremities. It is usually seen in adenocarcinoma of GIT especially colon (67%), tumours of female reproductive system and lymphoproliferative disorders (33%).[8] Individual reports of three PN dermatoses (tripe palms, acanthosis nigricans and sign of Leser-Trélat) coexisting in cases of CA ovary and gastric adenocarcinoma also reported.[9,10]

Bazex Syndrome

It is also known as acrokeratosis paraneoplastica. Bazex syndrome begins with acral violaceous erythema on the ears, nose, hands and feet. Early lesions may show small vesicles. As the lesions progress, they become hyperkeratotic and psoriasiform especially on the hands and feet. Paronychia and nail dystrophy are common. Later the eruption may generalise and the lesions on the face may appear dermatitis or lupus like. Skin biopsy will show hyperkeratosis, acanthosis and scattered parakeratosis. Eosinophilic and vacuolar degeneration of spinous cell layer may be present. This syndrome is more common in men and is associated with squamous cell carcinoma of the upper aerodigestive tract (60%).[7]

An another variant of Bazex syndrome inherited as an autosomal dominant disease is characterised by acral follicular atrophoderma, early development of multiple facial basal cell carcinoma and in some hypohidrosis.

Acquired Ichthyosis

It is characterised by small white to brown scales and they are mainly found over the extensor aspects of extremities and trunk (Figs 26.2 and 26.3). It is usually associated with drugs, systemic diseases, nutritional deficiencies, infection and malignancy. Histopathologically it is characterised by hyperkeratosis, parakeratosis and hypogranulosis. Dermis is normal. The most common malignancy is Hodgkin's disease (70%) and other lymphoproliferative disorders. Non-lymphoproliferative disorders associated with acquired ichthyosis are carcinoma ovary, leiomyosarcoma, transitional cell carcinoma, hepatocellular carcinoma and breast.

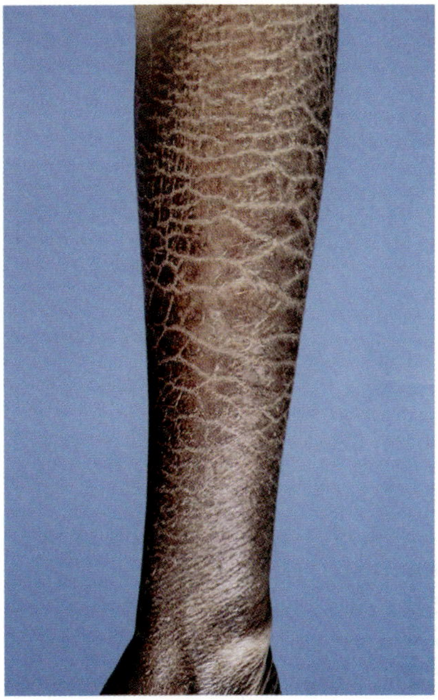

Fig. 26.2: Acquired ichthyosis following carcinoma colon after 1 year

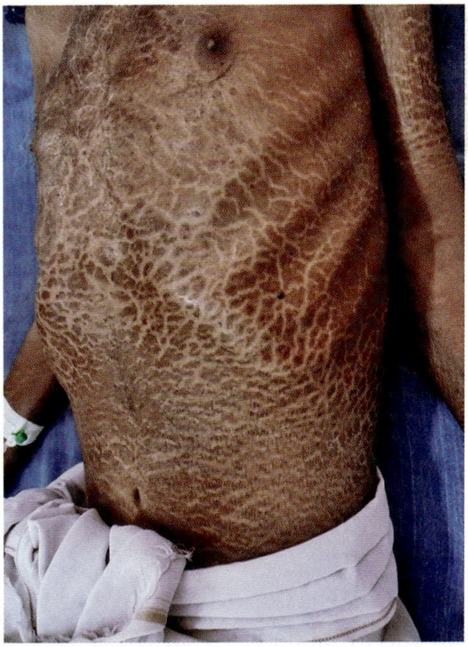

Fig. 26.3: Acquired ichthyosis following thymoma after 3 months of diagnosis

Pityriasis Rotunda

It describes the fixed, scaly, sharply defined, circular hyperpigmented patches on trunk, buttocks, and thighs. Scales are similar to ichthyosiform scaling with no inflammatory changes. It is usually associated with systemic illness particularly tuberculosis and malnutrition. It may be acquired cutaneous marker of malignancy. Sixteen percentage of patients are reported with hepatocelluar carcinoma.[7]

B. Erythematous Disorders

Necrolytic Migratory Erythema

Patches of intense erythema with irregular outline that coalesce to form polycyclic configuration occur in perioral region, intertriginous skin and acral extremities. It is associated with alpha cell tumour of the pancreas (glucagonoma syndrome).

Erythema Gyratum Repens

It is characterised by serpiginous, polycyclic and pruriginous erythema which may have fine scale and move up to 1 cm/day, producing concentric figures. Hands and feet are often spared. Tumour-induced antibodies can cross react with basement membrane of skin. Histopathologic features are of hyperkeratosis, focal parakeratosis, spongiosis and mononuclear lymphohistiocytic infiltrate around superficial vascular plexus. It is most commonly associated with carcinoma breast followed by lung and bladder cancer.

Multicentric Reticulohistiocytosis

Multicentric reticulohistiocytosis is a rare disease that mainly affects skin and joints in which papulonodular skin lesions affect the face, fingers or other extremities. Severe symmetrical polyarthritis is frequently reported in 45% of cases. It is also called lipoid dermatoarthritis and reticulocytoma cutis. Papules are seen around the nail fold which is called 'coral bead sign'. In histopathology epidermis will be thinned out and diffuse infiltration of multinucleate giant cells with ground glass cytoplasm and oncocytic macrophages occur predominantly in upper dermis. In immunohistochemistry, these cells show cytoplasmic staining with KP-1(CD68) and membranous staining with leucocyte common antigen (CD45) and CD3 also. Approximately 25% of cases are reported with internal malignancy such as carcinoma of breast, lung, colon, pancreas, stomach and ovary.[7]

C. Proliferative and Inflammatory Disorders

Pyoderma Gangrenosum (PG)

It manifests with superficial and bullous forms with surrounding erythema and rapid progression to deep purulent ulcerations with violaceous borders and healing leaves cribriform scars. Pretibial leg is the most common site involved.

Bullous pyoderma gangrenosum is associated with acute myeloid leukaemia, CML and ALL. Classical PG is associated with inflammatory bowel disease or rheumatoid arthritis. Other conditions associated with PG are monoclonal gammopathy, solid tumours (carcinoid, colon, bladder, prostate and breast) and non-Hodgkin's lymphoma.

Primary Systemic Amyloidosis

The cause of this disease is plasma cell dyscrasia and associated AL deposition of amyloid. The most common associated skin lesions are spontaneous ecchymoses that are seen most frequently on the skin areas like eyelids, neck, groin, axilla, umbilicus or oral mucosa following strenuous manoeuvres. The haemorrhagic lesions may occur on areas of clinically normal skin or in skin having waxy small papules, plaques, nodules or tumours. The bleeding is due to infiltration of blood vessel walls with amyloid protein with subsequent weakening of the vessels. Other less common skin lesions include alopecia, nail dystrophies, scleroderma like lesions, macroglossia, cutis verticis gyrata, bullous lesions and dyspigmentation. It is seen in patients with paraproteinemia and myeloma.[7]

Sweet's Syndrome

Sweet's syndrome occurs most commonly in women of 30 to 60 years age. It is characterised by acute onset of erythematous tender papules, plaques or nodules over face and extremities which are chronic, widespread and recurrent in nature. It is associated with fever, malaise and leukocytosis. The surface of the plaques often shows papulovesicles and pustules. It is frequently seen in haematological malignancy, most commonly AML.

Scleromyxedema

It is a rare systemic disease of mucin production and fibrosis. Characteristic features are the appearance of skin coloured firm waxy papules and nodules that coalesce into large plaques over head and neck, upper trunk, and extremities.

Approximately 80% of patients have a benign IgG gammopathy usually lambda type. Other conditions associated with scleromyxedema are lymphoma and Waldenstrom's macroglobulinaemia.

Dermatomyositis

Dermatomyositis (DM) is an autoimmune disorder affecting predominantly the skin and skeletal muscles. It is characterised by purplish erythema and slight oedema of the upper eyelids (heliotrope rash), thin papules or plaques with purplish hue on the dorsal knuckles of fingers, elbow and the knees, and poikiloderma on the V of the chest and upper trunk. Symmetric and progressive muscle weakness may be overt, subclinical, or absent.

Twenty to thirty percentage of patients with DM of old age onset may have associated malignancies like solid tumour malignancy involving ovary, lung, colon, stomach and male genitourinary system (mainly prostate) and rarely breast and uterus usually preceding or concomitant with the malignancy. They usually have therapeutically resistant musculocutaneous disease.[11]

D. Blistering Disorders

Paraneoplastic Pemphigus

It is an autoimmune mucocutaneous disease, characterised by severe mucosal erosions and blisters and erosions over the trunk and proximal extremities associated with underlying malignancy. Patients develop targetoid papules and plaques resembling erythema multiforme, vesicles and bullae which is similar to pemphigoid or pemphigus vulgaris, itchy purplish flat papules and plaques resembling lichen planus or graft-versus-host disease.[7] The tumours associated with PNP are non-Hodgkin's lymphoma, Castleman's tumour, thymoma and CLL.

Criteria to diagnose paraneoplastic pemphigus:

- Major criteria:
  - Polymorphic cutaneous eruption
  - Concurrent internal neoplasia
  - Serum antibodies with specific immunoprecipitative pattern
- Minor criteria:
  - Histologic evidence of acantholysis
  - Direct immunofluorescence showing intercellular and basement membrane staining
  - Indirect immunofluorescence showing staining with rat bladder epithelium.

Cicatricial Pemphigoid

It is a rare clinical variant that predominantly affects mucous membranes. Skin lesions often heal with scarring. It is usually associated with increased incidence of malignancy especially adenocarcinoma. About 30% of patients with antilaminin 332 presented with internal malignancy that is solid cancer.[7]

Bullous Pemphigoid

Bullous pemphigoid is reported with malignancies of breast, lung, thyroid, larynx and stomach.

Other Blistering Disorders

Dermatitis Herpetiformis

Dermatitis herpetiformis is associated with lymphoma and non-Hodgkin's lymphoma.

Epidermolysis Bullosa Acquisita

It is linked with myeloma and lymphoma.

Porphyria Cutanea Tarda

It is most commonly seen with hepatocellular carcinoma. Case reports are also present with myeloma and visceral carcinoma.

E. Miscellaneous Dermatological Disorders

Lichen Planus

Lichen planus may be associated with neoplasia. There will be increased risk in males especially of squamous cell carcinoma. All cases of oral squamous cell carcinoma should be looked for histopathological evidence of lichen planus.

Exfoliative Dermatitis

Erythroderma following malignancy mainly results from cutaneous T cell lymphoma followed by Hodgkin's disease.[12] Other neoplasms associated are non-Hodgkin's lymphoma, leukaemias and myelodysplasia. It is a severe pruritic condition and rubbing and scratching may produce secondary lichenification.

Paraneoplastic Pruritus and Urticaria

Generalised pruritus is a non-specific sign of internal malignancy. So, in any case of generalised pruritus we have to consider internal malignancy once the benign disease is ruled out. It is due to production of mediators such as histamine and serotonin by certain tumours.

Acquired Hypertrichosis Lanuginosa

It is an acquired excessive growth of silky non-pigmented lanugo hairs on face, neck, ears and trunk (Fig. 26.4). It is frequently associated with painful glossitis and angular cheilitis. Women are most commonly affected more when compared to males. Colorectal cancer is the most frequent association followed by lung and breast cancer.

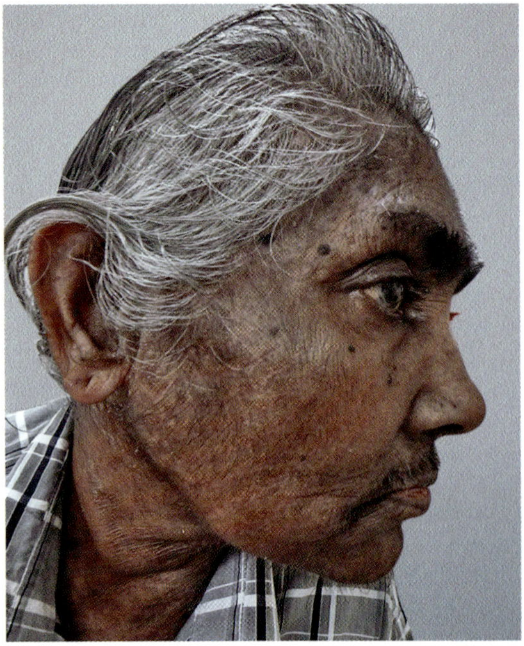

Fig. 26.4: Hypertrichosis lanuginosa following breast carcinoma at the time of diagnosis

Granuloma Annulare

Granuloma annulare is usually reported with lymphomas and other haematological malignancy such as lymphoma and uncommonly with solid tumours. Subcutaneous pattern of garanuloma annulare is the most common pattern with internal malignancy.[7]

Insect Bite-like Reactions

Insect bite-like reactions are reported in haematological malignancy such as chronic lymphocytic leukaemia.

Cutis Verticis Gyrata

Hypertrophy and folding of the scalp skin producing gyrate or cerebriform appearance is called cutis verticis gyrata (Fig. 26.5). It can

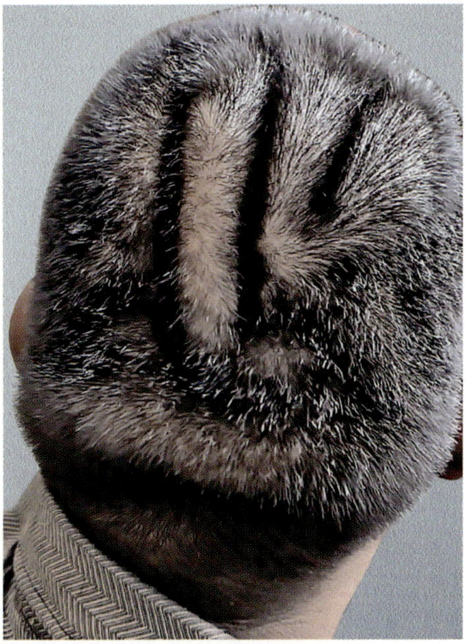

Fig. 26.5: Cutis verticis gyrata (4 months before diagnosis of primary)

be divided into primary or secondary. Primary may be sporadic in nature but familial cases are also reported. It is more common in men and typically develops after puberty. Cutis verticis gyrata may be secondary to internal malignancy. One case of carcinoma of fallopian tube has been reported with cutis verticis gyrata.[13]

II. GENODERMATOSES WITH MALIGNANCIES

Genodermatoses with predisposition to develop malignancies include:

- Cowden's syndrome
- Muir-Torre syndrome
- Gorlin's syndrome
- Gardner syndrome
- Neurofibromatosis type 1
- Tuberous sclerosis
- Birt-Hogg-Dube syndrome
- Peutz-Jegher's syndrome
- Howel-Evans syndrome
- Multiple endocrine neoplasia type 1 and 2A and B syndrome

Cowden's Syndrome

It is also known as PTEN multiple hamartoma syndrome which includes seven types. It is characterised by malignant and non-malignant tumours on skin, mucous membrane, breast, thyroid, and GIT which is inherited as autosomal dominant trait and the gene is located in chromosome 10q23.31.

Trichilemmomas, multiple oral papillomas, acral keratoses, palmoplantar keratoses, dermal fibromas, multiple skin tags and café au lait macules (CALM). Sclerotic fibromas and lipomas are also described. Facial trichilemmomas are considered as pathognomonic finding in Cowden's disease. Patients will develop mucocutaneous hamartomas during second and third decades of life.

Associated malignancies: Benign and malignant neoplasms of the breast and thyroid are the components of noncutaneous features. Breast carcinoma is most commonly reported in Cowden's disease. Follicular and papillary carcinoma of thyroid affects 3–10% of patients with Cowden's disease. Endometrial cancer reported in 5–10% of patients.[7]

Muir-Torre Syndrome (MTS)

The diagnostic criteria of MTS include sebaceous neoplasms like sebaceous adenoma, sebaceomas, sebaceous carcinoma in association with at least one internal malignancy of colon or genitourinary tract.

It is associated with hereditary nonpolyposis colorectal cancer (HNPCC) and other visceral malignancy and the genes involved are MLH1, MSH2 and MSH6 located in 2p21-p16 and 3p22.2. Fifty percentage of individuals with MTS are associated with colorectal cancer.

Gorlin's Syndrome

It comprises multiple basal cell carcinomas, mandibular odontogenic cyst, skeletal anomalies with palmoplantar pits. They will develop medulloblastoma and ovarian tumours. It is caused by mutation in PTCH 1 and PTCH 2 located in chromosomes 9q22 and 1p32 respectively.

Gardner Syndrome (GS)

Gardner syndrome is autosomal dominant disorder and is also known as familial polyposis of the colon. It has components of epidermoid cysts, desmoid tumours, fibromas, congenital hypertrophy of retinal pigment epithelium, osteomas, gastrointestinal adenomatous polyposis. GS is due to mutations in adenomatous polyposis coli gene (APC gene) in chromosome 5q22.2. Colorectal cancer is the most commonly reported carcinoma in GS and all patients with polyps will develop malignant degeneration. Other malignancies include carcinoma of ampulla of Vater, papillary carcinoma of thyroid and hepatocellular carcinoma.

Neurofibromatosis Type 1 (NF-1)

It is one of the most common genodermatoses with autosomal dominant inheritance and characterised by café au lait macules, neurofibromas, axillary or inguinal freckling, Lisch nodules, optic gliomas and skeletal defects and the genetic loci is located in chromosome 17q11.2 (neurofibromin-1 gene).

Tumours associated with NF-1 are optic gliomas, CNS tumours like malignant peripheral nerve sheath tumour, phaeochromocytoma, rhabdomyosarcoma, parathyroid adenoma and carcinoids.

Tuberous Sclerosis (TS)

TS is a multisystem hamartomatous disorder affecting skin, central nervous system, kidneys, and other organ system which consists of angiokeratomas, epilepsy and learning difficulties. It is also associated with astrocytomas and polycystic kidney disease and they are the most serious internal manifestations. Seventy percent (70%) of patients exhibit neurological manifestations. Multiple cortical tubers and calcifications are seen in tuberous sclerosis. Retinal hamartomas are seen in almost half of patients. Multiple bilateral angiolipomas present with benign course and are usually asymptomatic. The genes involved are TSC 1 and TSC 2 genes located in chromosomes 9q34.13 and 16q13.3 respectively.

Other features associated with TS are renal cell carcinoma, liver hamartomas and gastrointestinal polyps. Lymphangioleiomyomatosis occurs in female patients of tuberous sclerosis. Cardiac rhabdomyomas can be detected prenatally and usually self resolve by the age of 3 years.

Birt-Hogg-Dube Syndrome

BHD occurs in second and third decades of life characterised by triad of fibrofolliculomas, trichodiscomas, acrochordans, lung cyst, renal neoplasm and spontaneous pneumothorax and is caused by mutation in folliculin (FLCN) gene located in chromosome 17p11.2. Renal tumours may be unilateral or bilateral and seen in 41% of patients with BHD. Pavlovich and colleagues have demonstrated the association of BHD with renal cell carcinoma. They identified BHD to be most commonly associated with chromophobe/oncocytic hybrid that was seen in 50% of BHD patients followed by chromophobe in 34%, clear cell in 9%, oncocytoma in 5% and papillary in 2%.

Peutz-Jegher's Syndrome (PJS)

PJS is a rare genodermatosis characterised by mucocutaneous lentigines especially over the lips and benign gastrointestinal polyps and is produced by mutations in STK11 (serine/threonine protein kinase 11) mutation located in 19p13.3. Patients are at increased risk of developing gastrointestinal tumours, most commonly in the small intestine followed by stomach and colon. Patients have 70–93% increased risk of malignancy.

Howel-Evans Syndrome

This syndrome is composed of autosomal dominantly inherited focal palmoplantar keratoderma with the development of oesophageal carcinoma and is also associated with oral leukoplakia. The gene responsible is RHBDF2 (Rhomboid family member 2) located in 17q25.

Multiple Endocrine Neoplasia (MEN) Syndrome

MEN type1

MEN type 1 which has autosomal dominant inheritance is also called Werner syndrome and the gene MEN 1 is located in chromosome 11q13.1. Individuals with MEN 1 are associated with increased risk of malignancy involving parathyroid, pancreas and pituitary gland (3Ps). Other tumours include adrenocortical, thyroid and visceral malignancy and thymic neoplasm. Nonendocrine tumours are facial angiofibromas, collagenoma, meningioma, leiomyoma and lipomas.

MEN type 2A and 2B

They are linked with thyroid, parathyroid, adrenal medulla and medullary thyroid carcinoma. Pathology is due to RET protooncogene mutation located in chromosome 10q11.21 (for both 2A and 2B) with autosomal dominant inheritance. Other tumours include cervical neuroblastoma, pituitary adenoma and cerebellar hemangioblastoma. Additionally MEN 2B is characterised by mucosal neuromas, marfanoid and skeletal abnormalities.

III. CUTANEOUS METASTASES

Skin metastases usually occurs in late stages of internal malignancy (Fig. 26.6). The occurrence of cutaneous metastases from the onset of symptoms of internal malignancy varied from 2 months to 5 years.[1] Shortest duration of 2 months occurred with haematological dyscrasias. Incidence of cutaneous metastases range from 0.7 to 4.4% among cancer patients. Cutaneous metastasis is the first presentation in 0.7–10% of all metastases among internal malignancy. Overall in malignancies, the cutaneous deposits most

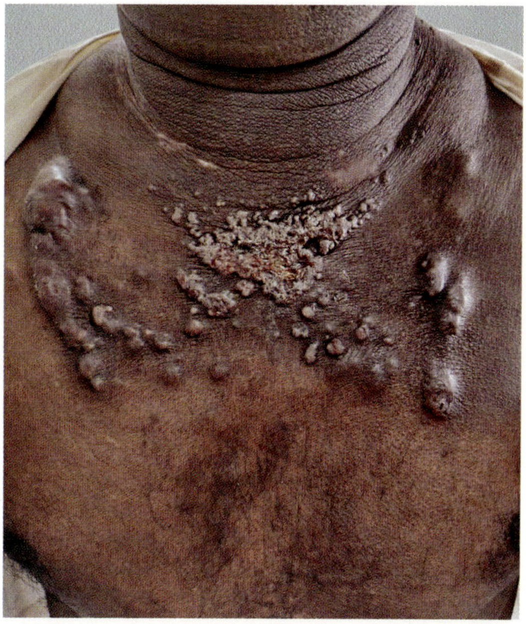

Fig. 26.6: Cutaneous metastases following anaplastic thyroid carcinoma after 3 years

commonly occur due to metastatic melanoma (45% chance).

Site of cutaneous metastases mainly depends upon the mode of spread of tumour whether through lymphatics or hematogenous spread. Spread may be in contiguous or noncontiguous sites. In males, contiguous cutaneous metastases occur most commonly due to CA lung and colon. In females, it commonly results from CA breast (Figs 26.7 and 26.8), colon and ovary.[14] Non-Hodgkin's lymphoma is the most common neoplasm to produce noncontiguous metastases. Common sites of secondary cutaneous deposits in order of occurrence are anterior chest, abdominal wall, lower limb, neck, back, upper limb, face, umbilicus, pelvis and scalp. Renal cell carcinoma has high rate of metastasis to the scalp[15] followed by thyroid. Clinically, it is usually present as skin coloured nodules at multiple sites. Rarely, it can present in a dermatomal pattern particularly adenocarcinoma (personal experience). Other cutaneous lesions are papules, plaques and ulcers.

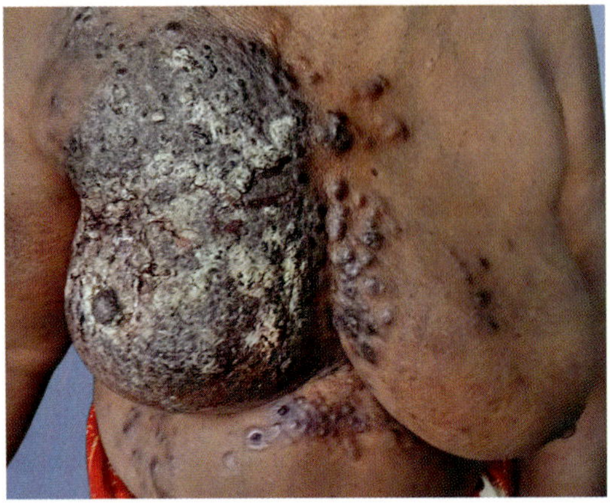

Fig. 26.7: Secondary cutaneous metastases at the time of diagnosis of breast carcinoma

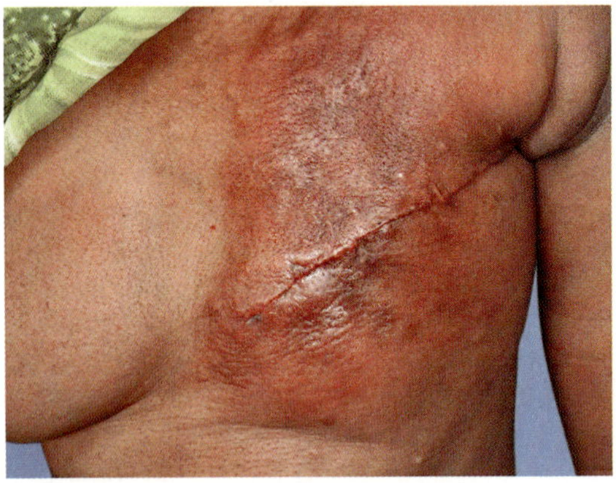

Fig. 26.8: Carcinoma erysipeloides in CA breast following 6 months of surgery

Cutaneous metastasis is a poor prognostic indicator. Patients have short life-expectancy after diagnosing cutaneous metastases which ranges from 2 months to 2 years.

IV. SKIN CHANGES RELATED TO THERAPY

A. Skin Changes Related to Chemotherapy

Cutaneous adverse events are the most commonly associated side effect with chemotherapy (Tables 26.2 and 26.3), next only to haematological toxicity.[16–20] Cytotoxic chemotherapeutic drugs act on tumour by interfering with DNA replication process that affects normal healthy tissues containing rapidly dividing cells such as hair, nails, skin and mucosae, e.g. alkylating agents, platinum compounds, antimetabolites.

Newer chemotherapeutic agents are introduced to improve the clinical outcome such as targeted therapies which contains small molecular drugs like epidermal growth factor receptor (EGFR) antagonists and multikinase (MK) inhibitors.[21–23] Other one is monoclonal antibodies (MAB) like rituximab, bevacizumab, trastuzumab, etc. They mainly act through signal transduction pathways. Compared to older drugs, newer targeted therapies are most commonly associated with cutaneous adverse events and are estimated to be 90%. They range from mild reactions like xerosis, alopecia, rash, pruritus, mucositis, hand–foot syndrome, dyspigmentation, acneiform eruption, nail and hair changes to severe fatal reactions like Stevens-Johnson syndrome, toxic epidermal necrolysis, urticarial vasculitis. These adverse effects are common with both cytotoxic drugs and targeted therapies. They occur commonly during initial 3–4 weeks of therapy.

Mucositis is the most severe and common side effect with EGFR inhibitors, antimetabolites (methotrexate) and alkylating agents and it occurs in 5–20% of all patients. Alopecia is the most distressing manifestation following cancer chemotherapy that occurs in 65% of patients. 5-fluorouracil and methotrexate are mostly responsible for telogen effluvium, whereas alkylating agents, topoisomerase inhibitors and taxanes are responsible for anagen effluvium. Other cytotoxic drugs associated are commonly with hand–foot syndrome, dyspigmentation, phototoxicity, nail changes, acral erythrodysesthesia and extravasation injury.

TABLE 26.2: Side effect profile of common chemotherapeutic drugs

Alkylating agents	Mechanism of action	Common side effects
Alkylating agents Mechlorethamine Cyclophosphamide Chlorambucil Melphalan Bendamustine Busulfan Dacarbazine	Forms the highly reactive carbonium ion intermediates. Covalently link to sites of phosphates, amines, sulfhydryl, and hydroxyl groups and cause alkylation of reactive amines, abnormal base pairing and DNA strand breakage. Alkylation also damages RNA and proteins.	Extravasation injury, alopecia (anagen effluvium), oral mucositis, hyperpigmentation of palms, soles, nails, photosensitivity Urticated plaques, morbilliform drug eruption and drug rash with eosinophilia and systemic symptoms (DRESS) (chlorambucil) Infusion reactions, papulopruritic eruption (bendamustine) Topical vesicant (mechlorethamine)
Antimetabolites	**Mechanism of action**	**Common side effects**
Methotrexate Pemetrexate	DNA synthesis inhibition—'S' phase specific Inhibits DHFR → impairs thymidylate synthesis → impairs pyrimidine synthesis Inhibits AICAR transformylase → impairs purine synthesis 6-thioguanine nucleotides (6-TGNs) (active metabolite), which are incorporated into nucleic acids, ultimately disrupting both the salvage and *de novo* pathways of DNA, RNA, and protein synthesis	Mucositis, alopecia, hyperpigmentation, radiation recall, toxic epidermal necrolysis, cutaneous rash, stomatitis, oral erosion, alopecia, acral pigmentation AGEP (pemetrexed)
Purine antagonist 6-TG, 6-MP	Inhibits thymidylate synthase → failure of DNA synthesis Prodrug of 5-FU	Alopecia, herpes zoster, verruca vulgaris, rarely malignant neoplasms, allergic contact dermatitis, azathioprine hypersensitivity syndrome
Pyrimidine antagonist 5-FU Capecitabine Gemcitabine Cytarabine	Inhibits DNA polymerase Inhibits DNA polymerase and thus blocks DNA synthesis.	Mucositis, hand–foot syndrome, photosensitivity, supravenous pigmentation, acral pigmentation (Fig. 26.9), diffuse or nail restricted hyperpigmentation Nail changes—onycholysis, pyogenic granuloma-like lesions, onychomadesis, subungual hyperkeratosis, and paronychia Mucosa—stomatitis, pyogenic granuloma, hyperpigmentation. Others—neutrophilic eccrine hidradenitis and eccrine syringosquamous metaplasia (cytarabine)
Platinum compounds	**Mechanism of action**	**Common side effects**
Cisplatin Carboplatin Oxaliplatin	Inter- and intra-strand crosslinking → abnormal base pairing → DNA damage → inhibits cell proliferation.	Patchy or localised hyperpigmentation, hypersensitivity reaction, maculopapular eruptions, oral hyperpigmentation, melanonychia, exfoliative dermatitis.

(contd.)

TABLE 26.2: Side effect profile of common chemotherapeutic drugs (*contd.*)

Microtubule damaging agents	Mechanism of action	Common side effects
Taxanes 1. Docetaxel 2. Paclitaxel	Bind to microtubular protein and inhibit polymerisation and assembly → mitotic spindle arrest and metaphase arrest	Alopecia (Fig. 26.10), hand and foot syndrome, hypersensitivity reactions, extravasation injury, mucositis, maculopapular eruption, photolichenoid reaction, hyperpigmentation PATEO (periarticular thenar erythema with onycholysis)(with non-albumin bound paclitaxel) Nail changes—paronychia, onycholysis, subungual haemorrhage and pyogenic granuloma Scleroderma-like changes (paclitaxel)
Vinca alkaloids	**Mechanism of action**	**Common side effects**
1. Vincristine 2. Vinblastine 3. Vinorelbine	Inhibit the microtubule polymerisation causing microtubule destabilisation	Vesicant—extravasation injury followed by ulceration Alopecia, xerosis, HFS, photosensitivity, Beau's lines, peripheral neuropathy
Topoisomerase inhibitors	**Mechanism of action**	**Common side effects**
Topotecan and irinotecan	Topoisomerase 1 inhibitor Stabilise DNA single strand breaks and inhibits strand resealing	Diffuse pigmentation, mucosal and nailbed pigmentation
Etoposide	Topoisomerase 2 inhibitor	Erythema multiforme, exanthema, hypersensitivity, SJS, urticaria, and alopecia
Antibiotics	**Mechanism of action**	**Common side effects**
Doxorubicin Daunorubicin	Directly binds with DNA and inhibits its synthesis.	HFS, mucositis, diffuse follicular rash, UV light recall, intertrigo like eruption, melanotic macules Cutaneous pigmentation, mucosal pigmentation and nail pigmentation Angioedema with generalised urticaria, alopecia, stomatitis, extravasation injury and infusion reactions, HFS
Bleomycin	Effect on cell cycle of G2 and M phase produces superoxide ions interfere with DNA strand chain scission inhibits repair mechanism	Pigmentation, alopecia, anaphylaxis, hypersensitivity reactions, mucositis, HFS, nailbed changes, and flagellate erythema

TABLE 26.3: Side effect profile of targeted chemotherapeutic drugs

Targeted drugs	Mechanism of action	Common side effects
Tyrosine protein kinase inhibitors Imatinib Nilotinib	Target BCR–ABL fusion protein and c-Kit oncogene	Xerosis, alopecia, dyspigmentation, generalised morbilliform eruption, folliculitis
Epidermal growth factor receptor inhibitors: Gefitinib, erlotinib, cetuximab	Inhibition causes arrest of growth and migration of keratinocytes	Acneiform eruption Hand and foot syndrome (Fig. 26.11) Xerosis Paronychia, periungual abscess
Angiogenesis inhibitor: Sunitinib Bevacizumab	Monoclonal antibody that blocks VEGF ihibitor	Mucositis, xerosis, hypersensitivity.
Proteasome inhibitor: Bortezomib	Inhibits nuclear factor kappa B signalling Induces cell death	Maculopapular rash, vasculitis EMF-like reaction Drug-induced lupus
Unarmed monoclonal antibodies Trastuzumab	Chimeric HER2 monoclonal antibody	Infusion reaction Morbilliform rash Infusion related urticarial reaction Flagellate erythema
Rituximab	Chimeric monoclonal antibody that targets CD20 antigen on B cells Complement dependant cell toxicity Antibody mediated cell cytotoxicity Direct antiproliferative effect	Urticaria Infusion related urticarial reaction

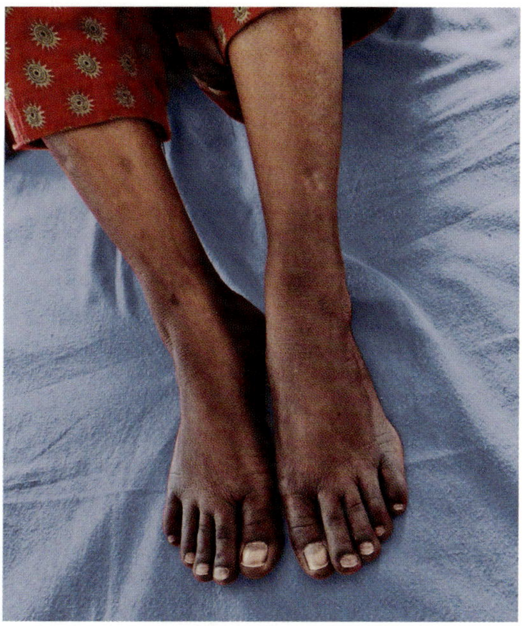

Fig. 26.9: Diffuse hyperpigmentation of feet following 3rd pulse of capecitabine

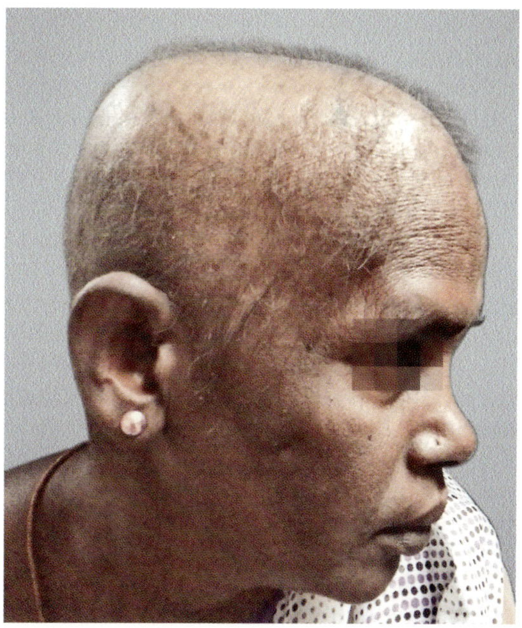

Fig. 26.10: Anagen effluvium following 1st pulse of docetaxel

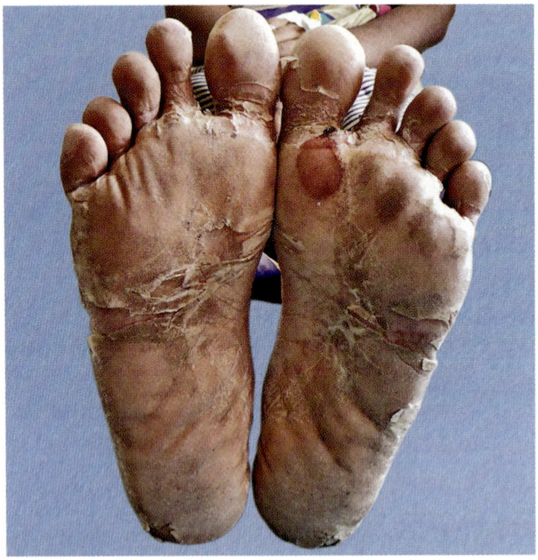

Fig. 26.11: HFS following 10 days of sunitinib

B. Radiotherapy-induced Cutaneous Side Effects

Radiotherapy (RT) can be used as the only therapeutic intervention for non-resectable locally advanced tumours, for patients in whom a non-surgical approach is preferred and for inoperable cases. Radiotherapy involves the use of high energy ionising radiations like photons (X-rays and γ-rays) and particle radiations like electrons, protons, neutrons, carbon ions, etc. Photons are produced by linear accelerators (LINAC) or gamma emitters (e.g. Cobalt-60 source).[24]

The radiation used for therapy not only damages the tumour cells but also affect the surrounding normal cells. The mechanism of cell damage is either by direct ionisation of the atoms in the target cells or indirectly by the production of highly reactive free radicals like H_2O^+ and OH^- ions. The early side effects that are observed during or shortly after RT within 3 months from the commencement of therapy are categorised as 'acute reactions' and those occurring after are categorised as 'late reactions'.[26] Acute reactions usually occur in tissues with high proliferative activity like epidermis, oral mucosa and epithelium of oesophagus and intestine.[24]

Even with the most modern RT techniques, up to 90% of the patients will experience a dose-dependent skin reactions at the exposed area. The severity of the reaction is related to the type of radiation, the dose per fraction, total dose delivered, use of bolus or other beam modifying devices, size of treatment field, site treated, use of concurrent chemotherapy or other agents and individual susceptibility.[26] The visible skin effects depend on the magnitude of the dose as well as the depth of penetration of the radiation. Unlike the skin lesions caused by chemical or thermal damage, the lesions caused by radiation exposures do not appear for hours to days following exposure, and burns and other skin effects tend to appear in cycles. While exposed to subsequent doses of radiation, the manifestations will have cumulative effect. The skin lesions pass through prodromal stage, latent stage, manifest illness stage, third wave of erythema and late effects.[27]

The severity of the skin reaction ranges from mild erythema (red rash) and dry desquamation (itchy, peeling skin) (Fig. 26.12) to more severe moist desquamation (open

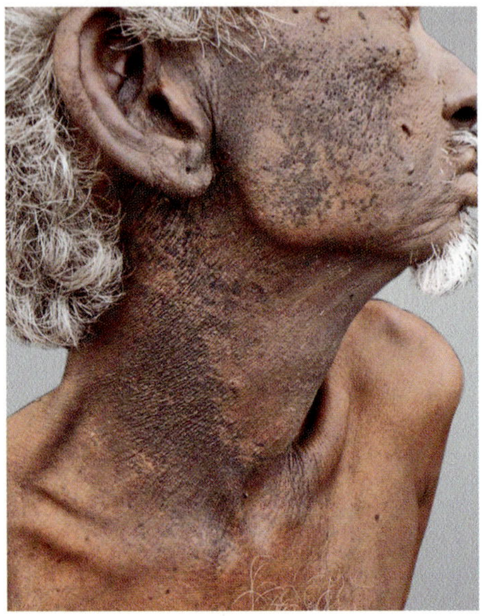

Fig. 26.12: Erythema, intense hyperpigmentation, hair loss and dry desquamation following 7 weeks of RT

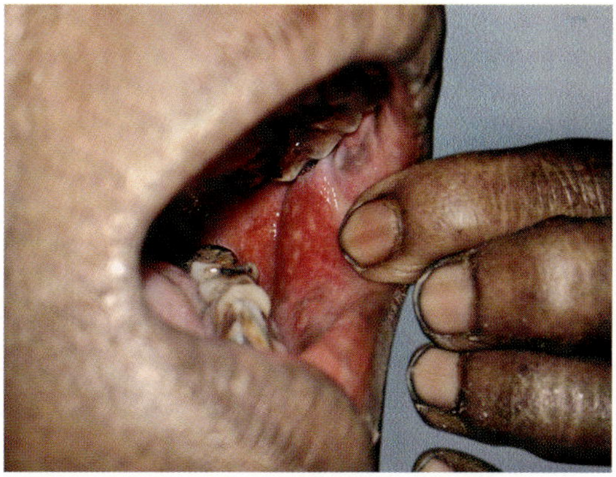

Fig. 26.13: Mucositis following 3 weeks of RT

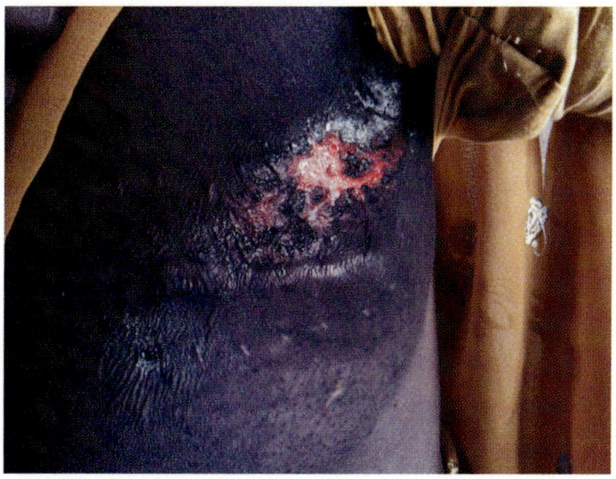

Fig. 26.14: Intense erythema and ulceration following 5 weeks of RT

wound) and ulceration.[26] The skin lesions such as early transient erythema occurs due to inflammation of the skin caused by activation of a proteolytic enzyme that increases the permeability of the capillaries. Dry desquamation occurs due to atypical keratinisation of the skin caused by the reduction in the number of clonogenic cells within the basal layer of the epidermis. Hair loss is caused by the depletion of matrix cells in the hair follicles. Moist desquamation occurs due to loss of the epidermis caused by sterilisation of a high proportion of clonogenic cells within the basal layer of the epidermis as well as due to infections.[27] Grading of RT injuries is done according to radiation therapy oncology group's (RTOG) acute radiation morbidity scoring criteria.[25] According to this, Grade I changes include faint erythema, epilation, dry desquamation and mucosal injection. Grade II changes include tender or bright erythema, patchy moist desquamation in skin folds and patchy mucositis (Fig. 26.13). Grade III reactions include confluent moist desquamation other than skin folds, pitting edema and confluent mucositis. Grade IV reactions include ulceration (Fig. 26.14), hemorrhage and necrosis.

CONCLUSION

Recognition of various cutaneous manifestations associated with internal malignancy and the knowledge of syndromes with predisposition to develop malignancies will help in early detection, and recognition with appropriate follow up, will lead to early intervention and better prognosis. Prospective well planned studies on this topic in India is the need of the hour. Since geriatric age group are at higher risk of developing malignancies regular periodical health screening which include dermatologists too among others is recommended.

References

1. Ayyamperumal A, Tharini GK, Ravindran V, Parveen B. Cutaneous manifestations of internal malignancy Indian Journal of dermatology. 2012; 57(4): 260–64.
2. Vora RV, Kota RS, Diwan NG, Jivani NB, Gandhi SS. Skin: A mirror of internal malignancy. Indian Journal of Medical and Pediatric Oncology. 2016; 37(4):214–22.
3. Nathan A, Berger P. Savvides, Siran M Koroukian, et al. Cancer in the elderly. Trans Am clin climatol Assoc. 2006; 117:147–56
4. Hansen J. Common Cancers in the elderly. Drugs Aging. 1998. (Dec); 13(6):467–78.
5. Karthik R, Mohan N, Ravikumar PT, Saramma Mathew Fenn. Cutaneous manifestations of internal malignancy. International Journal of Contemporary Medical Research 2017; vol 3 Issue 4:

6. Josenilson Antônio da Silva, Kleyton de Carvalho Mesquita, Ana Carolina de Souza Machado Igreja et al. An Bras Dermatol. 2013 Jan-Feb; 88(1):9–22.
7. Emtestam L and Sartorius K. Cutaneous markers of internal malignancy, ch. 147. In: Christopher Griffiths, Jonathan Barker, Tanya Bleiker, Robert Chamers, Daniel Creamer, editors. Rook's Textbook of Dermatology, 9th ed. United Kingdom: Blackwell Publishing Ltd; 2016; 4:147.1–147.27.
8. Thiers BH, Sahn RE, Callen JP. Dermatogical manifestations of internal cancer. Cancer Journal for Clinicians 1986; Vol 36(3):130–148.
9. Keberia MM, Belinson J, Kim R, Mekhali TM. Oral acanthosis nigricans, tripe palms and sign of Leser Trèlat, a hint to the diagnosis of early stage ovarian cancer: a case report and review of the literature. Gynecol Oncol. 2006 May; 101(2):353–5.
10. Pentenero M, Carrozzo M, Pagano M, Gandolfo S. Oral acanthosis nigricans, tripe palms and sign of leser trèlat in a patient with gastric adenocarcinoma. Int J Dermatol. 2004 Jul; 43(7):530–2.
11. Callen JP: Dermatomyositis. Lancet. 2000; 355(9197):53–7.
12. Yuste Chaves M, Unamunoperez P. Cutaneous manifestations of systemic malignancies. Actasderma 2013; 104:543–53.
13. Georgescu S R, Sârbu M , Mitran Cl. Cutis verticis gyrata in a patient with multiple basal cell carcinomas; case presentation and review of the literature: J Mind Med Sci. 2016; 3(1):80–87.
14. Rajagopal R, Arora PN, Ramasastry CV, Kar PK. Skin changes in malignancy. Indian Journal of Dermatology, Venereology, leprosy. 2004; 70:221–5.
15. Lim C , Chan R, Regan W. Renal cell carcinoma with cutaneous metastasis. Australas J Dematol. 2005; 46:158–60.
16. Rebecca M. Law; David TS. Chapter e99: Dermatologic Drug Reactions and Common Skin conditions. In: Pharmacotherapy: A Pathophysiologic Approach. LawDiPiro JT, L. Talbert R, Gary C. Yee, et al. editors. Philadelphia: McGraw Hill, 10th ed. Vol. 1:5567.
17. Donati A, Castro LGM. Cutaneous adverse reactions to chemotherapy with taxanes: the dermatologist's point of view. An Bras Dermatol. 2011 Aug; 86(4): 755–8.
18. Hammond-Thelin LA. Cutaneous reactions related to systemic immunomodulators and targeted therapeutics. Dermatol Clin. 2008 Jan; 26(1): 121–59.
19. Trüeb RM. Chemotherapy-induced alopecia. Semin Cutan Med Surg. 2009 Mar; 28(1):11–4.
20. Biswal SG, Mehta RD. Cutaneous adverse reactions of chemotherapy in cancer patients: A clinico-epidemiological study. Indian Journal of Dermatology. 2018 Jan 1; 63(1):41.
21. Lee JJ, Kroshinsky D, Hoang MP. Cutaneous Reactions to Targeted Therapy. Am J Dermatopathol. 2017 Feb; 39(2):67–82.
22. Hammond-Thelin LA. Cutaneous reactions related to systemic immunomodulators and targeted therapeutics. Dermatol Clin. 2008 Jan; 26(1): 121–59.
23. Ng CY, Chen C-B, Wu M-Y, Wu J, Yang C-H, Hui RC-Y, et al. Anticancer Drugs-induced Severe Adverse Cutaneous Drug Reactions: An Updated Review on the Risks Associated with Anticancer Targeted Therapy and Immunotherapies. Cancer management and Research. 2018. Volume 10: p1259-73 Available from: https://www.hindawi.com/journals/jir/2018/5376476/
24. Xavier Geets. Introduction to Radiotherapy. In: Marianne Kinggaard Federspiel, Peter Hogg, eds. *PET/CT Radiotherapy Planning*.Vienna: EANM, 2012:7–18.
25. Radiation Therapy Oncology Group—Acute Radiation Morbidity Scoring Criteria—Accessed online at http://www.rtog.org/ResearchAssociates/AdverseEventReporting/AcuteRadiationMorbidityScoringCriteria.aspxon 14.10.2014.
26. Salvo N, Barnes E, J. van Draanen, E. Stacey, G. Mitera, D. Breen, A. Giotis, G. Czarnota, J. Pang, C. De Angelis. In: Prophylaxis and management of acute radiation-induced skin reactions: a systematic review of the literature. Curr Oncol. 2010 August; 17(4):94–112.
27. Cutaneous Radiation Injury- Accessed online at http://www.bt.cdc.gov/radiation/criphysicianfactsheet.asp on 14.10.2014.

CHAPTER 27

Nursing Care for Elderly

• *Sunil Kumar Gupta*

Key Points

- Nursing care of geriatric patient needs multi-disciplinary approach.
- As skin is the largest body organ so its integrity is very important for geriatric health.
- A good quality of syndet based body wash with long acting emollient cream should be used in elderly patients.
- Oral hygiene must be maintained and high protein diet should be recommended in elderly.
- Psychotherapy is one of the important things to develop positive thoughts in elderly.

Introduction

Ageing is associated with structural and functional changes of the skin. The ageing process affects the whole body systems. Skin ageing is evidenced by impaired healing process, xerosis, exfoliation and pruritus[1]. Ageing is a complex process leading to biologic attrition at the cellular level that is manifested in many ways. Senescence and apoptosis play a role in the ageing processes of all cells by cumulative DNA damage from external and internal insults.[2–5]

GERIATRIC MODELS OF NURSING CARE

In the last three decades, various geriatric care models emerged; these include the geriatric consultation service, the ACE (acute care for the elderly) unit, the NICHE (nurses improving care for health system elders) initiative, the geriatric resource nurse (GRN) model and the HELP (hospital elder life program). These models target the prevention of complications that occur more commonly in older adults by employing evidence-based, ageing-sensitive interventions, promoting interdisciplinary communication and emphasizing discharge planning in hospital settings.[6] The most frequently implemented model is NICHE which focus on improving outcomes by positively influencing the geriatric nursing practice environment. Only NICHE aligns its approach to nurse involvement in hospital decision-making regarding care of older adults. NICHE is evidence-based program. The core components of a system-wide, acute care program designed to meet the needs of older adults are grouped into eight categories (guiding principles, leadership, organizational structures, the physical environment, patient- and family-centered approaches, ageing sensitive practices, geriatric staff competence, and interdisciplinary resources and processes.[7]

GERIATRIC SKIN

The term 'skin integrity' refers to the skin being a sound and complete structure in unimpaired condition. Conversely, impaired skin integrity is defined as an "altered epidermis and/or dermis, destruction of skin layers (dermis), and disruption of skin surface (epidermis)".[8] Geriatric skin undergoes numerous degenerative changes, which are

TABLE 27.1: Intrinsic changes that occur in ageing skin[9]

Intrinsic skin change	Effect on skin
Reduction in skin cell turnover. Skin gradually becomes more fragile as the epidermis thins and there is a reduction in integrity between epidermis and dermis	Papery appearance. Less effective barrier more prone to mechanical injury and damage from moisture, friction, and trauma
Reduction in key stratum corneum metabolites, including components of natural moisturising factor and the lipid lamellae	Decreased stratum corneum hydration and reduced integrity
Blood vessels become more fragile. Blood supply to the skin is reduced	Skin becomes more prone to bruising and damage
Collagen fibres that provide structural support stiffen elastic fibres thicken	Creases and wrinkles form. More prone to tearing and shearing
Production of sebum decreases	Skin becomes more dry. Vulnerable to splitting, cracking, and infection. Sensitivity to irritants increases
Sweat glands become smaller and secrete less sweat	Skin becomes more dry less effective temperature control
Localised overproduction of melanin	Blotchiness and uneven pigmentation
Reduction in subcutaneous fat	Less protection and insulation
Reduction in sensory receptors	Less sensitivity, so more risk of inadvertent damage

affected by both the intrinsic and the extrinsic factors (Table 27.1).[9] Intrinsic skin ageing is due to 'programmed cell death'. Extrinsic factors are basically environmental such as ultraviolet rays, pollution and drugs that accelerate the ageing in a cumulative basis.

SKIN CARE OF THE ELDERLY

Xerosis, fissures, and pruritus are common in older people. However, these conditions often go untreated. Xerosis brings with it an increased risk of eczema en craquele, dry discoid eczema and generalised pruritus. Xerotic skin also promotes secondary bacterial infection on it resulting into non-healing ulcers. It is estimated that xerosis affects 59–85% of older people.[10] So, management of xerosis with maintenance of skin hygiene are core elements during care of geriatric patients.

There are numerous skin cleansing and emolliating products available, although few have been developed specifically for older people.

Cleansers

The purpose of skin cleansing is to remove dirt, soil, and bacteria from the skin; but cleaning of skin in elderly leads to weakening of skin barrier function. Soap-based products are more damaging to the skin than syndets. Soaps and detergents can increase pH of the stratum corneum, which enhances protease activity and inhibits lipid lamellae synthesis. This results into defective skin barrier function. This potential skin barrier disruption is particular issues for older people, who are already having dry and fragile skin. So, there is need of milder cleansing formulations that interact minimally with the stratum corneum structure, but function effectively as cleansers. Skin cleansing products containing syndets or amphoteric surfactants compared with standard soap and water washing improved skin dryness and demonstrated skin-protecting effects.

Drying

After cleansing with water and a cleansing agent, drying of the skin is essential. It is generally achieved by towel drying using either a rubbing or patting action. Towel drying incurs the risk of direct mechanical damage to the stratum corneum; however, if the skin is not dried thoroughly, there is a risk of over-hydration and maceration.

Emollients

Aged skin is particularly prone to dryness, which can lead to the erosion of skin that allows irritants and allergens into the skin and precipitate or aggravate dermatitis. The use of certain 'complex' emollients can reduce the severity of eczema, and delay relapse of the condition. A good quality emollients should have ingredients, such as humectants, physiological lipids, and antipruritic agents. Humectants, including urea, attract and trap water in the stratum corneum. This can off-set the reduced levels of natural moisturising factor (NMF) and other natural moisturising agents in dry and older skin. Likewise, natural lipids, for example, ceramides, cholesterol, and free fatty acids, which are found in the stratum corneum, return the defective inter-cellular lipid matrix. Lauromacrogols are added to some products for their local anaesthetic and antipruritic action.

The ideal washing and emolliating intervention is one that removes oils and dirt from the skin whilst avoiding dryness or irritation to the skin, and which maintains or promotes skin integrity and comfort. Other measures like drinking plenty of liquids avoid smoking and sun tanning and use of broad spectrum sunscreens, keep the skin of elderly healthy.

HAIRS AND NAIL CARE

Graying of hairs is one of the clearest signs of ageing. Mostly in geriatric age group hair become white due to less melanin in hair follicles. Elderly people sometimes use hair dye to color their hairs. This practice often leads to severe contact dermatitis. So, they must be advised to use paraphenylenediamine (PPD) free hair colour and a do patch test before applying.

Complete or partial hair loss from scalp is also one of the important features in old age. Many men are nearly bald by the age of 60. Women can develop a similar type of baldness as they age. Hair become less dense and the scalp may become visible. With these changes on scalp of an aged person, he is more prone to develop sunlight damage like polymorphic light eruption. A broad brim hat or a hair wig should be advised that work aesthetically and prevent solar damage.

Nails also change with age. They grow more slowly and may become dull and brittle. They may also become yellow and opaque. Nails, particularly toenails, may become hard and thick. Ingrown toenails may be more common. The tips of the fingernails may break. Lengthwise ridges may develop in the fingernails and toenails. Brittle nails are easily infected by dermatophytes that can worsen the condition if generalized to involve the body. Application of moisturizer on nail with avoidance of trauma is important measures during nursing care of elderly people.

DENTAL CARE AND ORAL HYGIENE

Oral health is not separate from general health. Oral and dental care is difficult in geriatrics. Poor oral health can be a detrimental factor to nutritional status and health. Oral cavity disorders can lead to poor eating habits in the elderly. Loose painful teeth or ill-fitting dentures may result in a reduced desire or ability to eat. A compromised nutritional status, in turn can further undermine the integrity of the whole integumentary system in old age. The oral mucosa becomes increasingly thin, smooth with age and that it acquires satin like edematous appearance with loss of elasticity and stippling. The tongue in particular is reported to show marked clinical changes and to become smoother with loss of filiform papillae. With age, there is a tendency for development of sublingual varices and an increasing susceptibility to various pathological conditions such as *Candidal* infections and a decreased rate of wound healing.[11] Salivary gland secretion is reduced which precipitate xerostomia. This results in rampant caries, loss of denture retention and traumatic lesions and infections of the oral mucosa. Meticulous oral hygiene supplemented by mouthwashes with chlorhexidine and daily use of artificial salivary substitutes is important means to reduce complications to denture wearing in people with xerostomia.[12] The elderly person should be helped to develop the ability to brush effectively and thoroughly. Those who have diminished manual dexterity may benefit from the use of traditional mechanical toothbrushes, rotary electric toothbrushes, or manual brushes that have been adapted or customized for each person. A therapeutic rinse contains chlorhexidine, sodium benzoate, sanguinaria, a fluoride, or other remineralizing agents, can prevent oral disease and should be recommended to the elderly when appropriate.[13]

Nutrition

Nutritional care is a basic human right, as stated in Article 25 of universal declaration of human rights.[14] Nevertheless; under nourishment is known to be a frequent and serious health care problem among elderly hospitalised patients.

Adequate nutrition is a vital factor in promoting the health and well-being of the aged. In a study, 45% of elderly hospitalised patients in one large Norwegian university hospital were at nutritional risk.[15] Undernourishment in elderly patients increases the risk of disease-related complications, morbidity, and mortality. It lengthens hospital stay and expands health care costs. With ageing, appetite and food intake decreases which leads to decreased calorie requirement. This results into thin built in geriatric population. Approximately 8000 kJ (1900 kcal) is the required calorie requirement in 80 years old. An active elderly subject requires a protein intake of 0.97 g/kg of body weight per day. However, patients suffering from tissues necrosis or inflammation as in erythroderma, toxic epidermal necrolysis or pemphigus show an increase in protein turnover and requirements. Among the vitamins, most nutrients are recommended in the same amounts for elderly as for younger people. However, certain groups of elderly, such as those homebound, with no access to sunlight, may have insufficient vitamin D and develop osteomalacia. The other important nutrients required by the older individuals are ascorbic acid, iron, and potassium.[16]

GENITOURINARY CARE

Neurogenic bladder, impotence, balanoposthitis (candidal), urinary tract infections, and prostate hyperplasia and prostatic cancer, are common genitourinary problem in the elderly. Patients with neurogenic bladder present with symptoms such as incontinence and urinary retention. Urinary incontinence may lead to maceration and dermatitis in genitocrural area that can be managed by adult nappies and by application of barrier creams. Drugs like anticholinergic agents in the form of oxybutynin, flavoxate, and propantheline are effective bladder relaxants, and phenoxybenzamine, prazosin, and terazosin are commonly used as sphincter relaxants. Urinary tract infection is also very common in elderly. Lower urinary tract infections can be treated with almost any antibacterial agent. Upper urinary tract infections require full genitourinary evaluation and appropriate antibiotics should be used according to the urine culture sensitivity studies. Benign prostate hyperplasia is one of the most common genitourinary problems in elderly male causing hesitation and frequency of urine. Alpha-adrenergic antagonists and anti-androgenic agents have been found to relieve the symptoms of prostatic enlargement. Prostate cancer is the second most common malignancy in men. Diethylstilbestrol (stilboestrol), an oral estrogen, remains a commonly used agent to achieve castrate levels of androgens in advanced prostatic carcinoma. Agonist analogues, such as goserelin and leuprorelin, of gonadotrophin-releasing hormone (GnRH) [luteinising hormone releasing hormone (LHRH); or gonadorelin] achieve the same results as diethylstilbestrol but without the cardiovascular side effects. Antiandrogens are also being used in combination with GnRH agonists to produce complete androgen blockage, with mixed results.[17]

PSYCHOLOGICAL THERAPY IN ELDERLY

With advancing age, the psychomotor capacity is also decreased. The retirement from job and loss of the close family members or friends lead to development of negative feelings of loneliness and isolation. The loneliness in the elderly causes lack of confidence, lack of meaning in life, lack of social support, social inactivity, and sadness. It should also be noted that persons staying in the home environment more frequently suffered from numerous diseases and declared worse health conditions than care receivers in other comparable groups. All these feelings have enormous implications on health aspects and may lead to the development of depressive disorders frequently in association with the presence of general medical illnesses. Psychological counselling and behavioural therapy should be instituted in such cases to raise self confidence.

NURSING CARE IN HOSPITAL

The old people who suffer from chronic diseases are often dependent on others functionally and need long time caring.[18] Diseases like erythroderma, pemphigus and pemphigoid with other systemic disorders like stroke, diabetes and movement problems increase the risk of old people's transfer to nursing home by 50%.[19] Studies have shown that some older people have been transferred to nursing home voluntarily and some by obligation.[20] Another research reported that most family caregivers experience fatigue and increasing responsibility during the caring of older people at home.[21] Other studies have also indicated that some family caregivers encountered unsuitable care condition, lack of systems offering health services, and lack of formal support.[22] Findings showed that taking care of an old person at home requires a relatively full time presence of one family member, and this leads to persistent concern for caregivers. Health care providers are recommended to become familiar with challenges of family caregivers in taking care of an old person with chronic disease at home, and to organise their supportive and consultation actions according to family situations in order to improve the life quality of the old people and family caregivers.

CONCLUSION

Care of geriatric patients does not differ from pediatric care. This needs multispecialty approach from time to time and includes involvement of dermatologists to psychologists, physicians, urologists, dentists and dietician. Proper care of skin and appendages are as important as genitourinary and dental care. Geriatric patients need a healthy environment to prevent development of negativity in the last phase of life.

References

1. Gardiner, et al. Maintaining skin health in older people. Nurs Times. 2012; 108(49):16–20.
2. Fisher G, Kang S, Varani J, et al. Mechanisms of photoageing and chronological skin ageing. Arch Dermatol. 2002; 38:1462–70.
3. Yaar M. Mechanisms of ageing. Arch Dermatol. 2002; 138:1429–31.
4. Campisi J. The role of cellular senescence in skin ageing. J Invest Dermatol Symp Proc. 1998; 3:1–5.
5. Jenkins G. Molecular mechanisms of skin ageing. Mech Ageing and Develop. 2002; 123:801–10.
6. Steele JS. Current evidence regarding models of acute care for hospitalized geriatric patients. Geriatric Nursing 2010; 31:331–47.

7. Boltz M, Capezuti E, Zwicker D and Fulmer T (eds) (2012) Evidence-Based Geriatric Nursing Protocols for Best Practice, 4th edn. Springer Publishing Company, New York, NY.
8. North American Nursing Diagnosis Association. Nursing diagnosis for impaired skin integrity . // nandanursingdiagnosis.blogspot.co.uk/2011/08/ nursingdiagnosis- for-impaired-skin.html (accessed 26 February 2014).
9. Cowdell F. Older people, personal hygiene and skin care. MEDSURG Nursing 2011; 20(5):235–240. [MEDLINE: 22165782]
10. Beauregard S, Gilchrest BA. A survey of skin problems and skin care regimens in the elderly. Archives of Dermatology 1987; 123(12):1638–43. [MEDLINE: 3688904]
11. Papas AS, Niessen LC, Chauncey HH. Geriatric Dentistry—Ageing and Oral Health. St. Louis: Mosby Yearbook; 1991.
12. Vissink A, Spijkervet FK, Amerongen VA. Ageing and saliva: A review of the literature. Spec Care Dentist 1996; 16(3):95–103.
13. Persson RE, Truelove EL, LeResche L, Robinovitch MR. Therapeutic effects of daily or weekly chlor-hexidine rinsing on oral health of a geriatric population. Oral Surg Oral Med Oral Pathol. 1991; 72(2):184–91.
14. United Nations (UN). Declaration of Human Rights, Article 25. 1948. http://www.ohchr.org/EN/UDHR/Pages/Language.aspx?LangID=eng.Accessed 30 Nov 2016.
15. Eide HK, SaltyteBenth J, Sortland K, Halvorsen K, Almendingen K. Prevalence of nutritional risk in the non-demented hospitalised elderly: a cross-sectional study from Norway using stratified sampling. Journal of Nutritional Science. 2015; 4 e18: 1–9. doi:10.1017/jns.2015.8. In press.
16. Soini H, Routasalo P, Lauri S, Ainamo A. Oral and nutritional status in frail elderly. Spec Care Dentist 2003; 23:209–15.
17. Atala A, Amin M. Current concepts in the treatment of genitourinary tract disorders in the older individual. Drugs Ageing 1991 May; 1(3):176–93.
18. Sam Aram EA, Amin Aghai M. Social policies for the elderly in Japan and Sweden, and the proper role model for Iranian elderly. Iranian Journal of Ageing 2007; 1:88–100.
19. Pour-Reza A, Khabiri-Nemati R. Economics of health and ageing. Iranian Journal of Ageing 2007; 1:80–87.
20. Salarvand SH, Abedi HA. The causes and motives from the perspective of elderly nursing home residents in finding housing. FEYZ Journal of Kashan University of Medical Sciences. 2008; 12:55–61. [In Persian]
21. Babai M. Social problems of family caregivers of disabled elderly in the city of Karaj. Iranian Journal of Ageing, 2007; 2:177–81.
22. Mohammadi F, Dabbaghi F, Nikravesh M. Facilitator and barriers factors in family caregiving process of Iranian frail elderly: A qualitative study. Iran Journal of Nursing. 2008; 21:55–65. [In Persian]

CHAPTER 28

Drug Interactions and Polypharmacy in Geriatric Dermatology

• Yogesh S Marfatia • Reema R Baxi

Key Points

- Global population of elderly people is ever increasing.
- There is altered pharmacokinetics and pharmacodynamics of drugs in the elderly.
- Age-related decline in the functioning of liver and kidney takes place in the elderly.
- There is a trend to use herbal medicines, tonics and non-allopathic medications in India, which adds to problem of potential interactions.
- Prescriber has a crucial role to play in protecting patients from undesirable effects of drug interactions.

Introduction

According to the World Health Organization (WHO), the global population of elderly people aged 60 years or more was 600 million in 2000 and it is expected to rise to around 2 billion by 2050.[1]

With the rise in the elderly population, geriatric dermatology is a speciality that needs emphasis. Geriatric population offers altered physiologic status with altered pharmacokinetics and pharmacodynamics. Because of associated comorbidities, elderly population is on many medications. There is an increasing trend to use herbal medicines, tonics and non-allopathic medicines and all these add to the problem of potential drug interactions. As a result of drug interactions, there can be an increase or decrease in the efficacy of drugs as well as an increase in undesirable effects. Awareness on part of the prescriber and patient is a key to prevent drug interactions. Drug prescription in the elderly is an issue under addressed.

AGE-RELATED CHANGES AFFECTING PHARMACOKINETICS AND PHARMACODYNAMICS OF DRUGS

There are age-related changes in the physiologic status of the elderly leading to an alteration in the pharmacokinetics and pharmacodynamics of drugs.

1. **Absorption of drugs:** The absorption may be decreased due to gastrointestinal (GI) mucosal atrophy and associated atrophic gastritis or decreased blood flow to intestines. There might be an increase in the GI transit time.
2. **Distribution of drugs:** The volume of distribution tends to change with ageing.[2] Various factors responsible are:
   - Decrease in the muscle mass and total body water[2,3]
   - Increase in the adipose tissue fraction—lipophilic medications like hydroxyzine have an increased half-life in elderly.[2]
   - Decrease in the end-organ blood flow.
   - Plasma protein binding—albumin levels are decreased in malnourished elderly, so the chances of drug toxicity are more. For corticosteroids, endogenous carrier protein is cortisol binding globulin (CBG) whose levels are decreased by hypothyroidism, obesity and renal disease,

therefore leading to an increase in free fraction of corticosteroid. CBG levels are increased by estrogen therapy and hyperthyroidism which decrease the free fraction of steroid molecule available.

3. **Metabolism:** Diminution in the hepatic function leads to slow biotransformation of drugs, resulting in an altered first-pass effect of orally given drugs. There are two major phases of drug metabolic pathways in the liver.[2,4] These are discussed in Table 28.1.
4. **Excretion:** Renal function decreases as a function of both age-related decline and exogenous factors. Normally, there is a 30% decline in glomerular filtration rate (GFR) between 30 and 80 years of age.[5] Exogenous factors can contribute to renal insufficiency, including medications such as the chronic use of nonsteroidal anti-inflammatory drugs (NSAIDs) and chronic comorbid conditions, such as diabetes or hypertension.[5,6] There is an increase in the half-life elimination for drugs that are eliminated primarily unchanged in the urine.

Drug Interactions

Alteration in the effects of a drug by reaction with another drug or drugs, with foods or beverages, with herbs, or with a preexisting medical condition is known as drug interaction.[6,7] Drug interactions may be classified as drug-drug interactions, drug-food interactions, drug-medical condition interactions, or drug-herb interactions.[4,6,7] Drug interactions can be pharmacokinetic or pharmacodynamic.[4–7] A drug interaction occurs when two drugs are simultaneously present in the body and one drug alters the serum/tissue levels and mechanism of action of the other. Common pharmacokinetic drug interactions are listed in Table 28.2.

TABLE 28.1: Hepatic phase I and phase II metabolic pathways

Phase I reactions	Phase II reactions
• It includes oxidation, hydroxylation, reduction, and alkylation.	• It includes glucuronidation, conjugation, and acetylation.
• The most widely known phase I examples are the CYP450 pathway (80% cases), xanthine oxidase, and alcohol dehydrogenase.	• Phase II substrates consist of either active metabolites from phase I metabolism or the original drug itself.
• A decrease in some phase I pathways can occur with ageing, due to decrease in hepatic blood flow or volume.	• It does not seem to be affected by normal ageing, and it also occurs extrahepatically.
• *Example:* Cyclosporine and statins are substrates for CYP450.	• *Examples:* Azathioprine and mycophenolate mofetil.

TABLE 28.2: Cytochrome p450 enzyme inducers and inhibitors[2,17]

Induction	Inhibition
Drugs: Phenytoin, rifampicin, barbiturates, carbamazepine, griseofulvin[6]	Drugs: Allopurinol, azoles, erythromycin, metronidazole, sulfonamides, trimethoprim, ketoconazole[6]
Diet	Diet: Grapefruit juice
Age: Enzyme induction decreases with age.	Pesticides
Hormones	Carbon monoxide
Genetic factors	Genetic factors

Pharmacokinetic Drug Interactions

Pharmacokinetic drug interactions can be at the level of absorption, distribution, metabolism or excretion.

Absorption: The interaction can be due to alteration in gastric pH, motility or interaction with ions leading to chelation of drugs. Calcium, magnesium and iron supplements with tetracyclines lead to formation of chelated complexes and decreased absorption. Azole antifungals like itraconazole and fluconazole require acidic environment for their absorption, therefore administration of H_2 blockers or proton pump inhibitors with azole antifungals leads to impaired absorption.[5]

Hydroxyzine is known to have anticholinergic effects leading to decreased gastric motility and thereby reducing rate of intestinal absorption.[6]

Distribution: Majority of the drugs bind to albumin and serum albumin levels should always be estimated before starting a patient on methotrexate. Salicylates and sulphonamides compete with methotrexate (MTX) for plasma protein binding and lead to displacement of MTX from plasma proteins leading to an increase in the free fraction of MTX and increased chances of hepatotoxicity and myelosuppression.[7] Sulphonamides displace sulfonylureas from plasma protein binding sites leading to increased chances of hypoglycaemia.[4,8]

Metabolism: Alcoholism alters the metabolism of several drugs like metronidazole leading to increased chances of disulfiram-like reaction. Drugs causing cytochrome (CYP) enzyme induction and inhibition have a potential consequence leading to drug-drug interactions. Cytochrome P450A (CYP450A) is the most important enzyme responsible for metabolism of dermatologic drugs.[4,8] Ageing leads to significant reduction in liver volume and reduction in activity of some but not all CYPs. Oxidative metabolism is induced by substituting protein for carbohydrate in diet. Some dietary constituents such as caffeine and cruciferous vegetables can induce oxidative metabolism and grapefruit juice inhibits it.

Genetic polymorphism plays a role in the expression of various isoenzymes of CYP450.[9] Poor or slow metabolisers possess the homozygous autosomal recessive allele (usually mutant alleles), whilst the extensive or rapid metabolisers have the heterozygous or homozygous dominant allele. Factors responsible for induction and inhibition of cytochrome enzymes have been listed in Table 28.2.

Excretion: Levels of acyclovir are increased with probenecid due to inhibition of tubular secretion of acyclovir.[5,10]

Pharmacodynamic Interactions

Pharmacodynamic interactions are interactions where the effects of one drug are changed by the effect of another drug.[4,11] Interactions can be additive or synergistic when two drugs have the same pharmacological effect, antagonistic when two drugs have opposite actions.[5]

Table 28.3 describes the interactions of drugs used for dermatologic diseases with their consequences. Table 28.4 describes the interaction of drugs used for non-dermatologic diseases that are commonly prescribed in the elderly.

Drug-Food and Drug-Herb Interactions

Drug-food or drug-herb interactions occur when a food, beverage, or herb taken along with a drug interacts with a drug to either increase or decrease its effect.[11] Flavonoids in grape fruit juice are known to be potent inhibitor of several CYP enzymes, namely CYP3A4 and CYP1A2. Thus, the plasma concentrations of several drugs that are substances for these enzymes, including cyclosporine, and protease inhibitors such as saquinavir and buspirone are increased. Cruciferous vegetables[11] (such as broccoli, cabbage, and Brussels' sprouts) are known to increase CYP1A2 activity, whereas apiaceous

TABLE 28.3: Commonly prescribed dermatologic medications in the elderly with their drug-drug interactions and consequences[18]

Drug used in dermatology	Interacting drug and mechanism of action	Consequence
Antihistaminics	CYP3A4 inhibitors: Macrolides: Erythromycin >> clarithromycin/azithromycin Azole antifungals: Ketoconazole >> itraconazole, fluconazole	Increased risk of torsades de pointes[6] (mainly with terfenadine, which is now discontinued)
	CNS antidepressants	Additive sedative effect
Corticosteroids (CS)	Azole antifungals and macrolides: Potent CYP3A4 inhibitors	Increased serum levels and toxicity of various CS
	Anticonvulsants: Phenytoin and phenobarbital are CYP3A4 inducers	Decreased level of CS and increased level of anti-epileptics
	Anti-tubercular therapy Rifampicin is a CYP3A4 inducer	Rifampicin decreases level of CS
	Proton pump inhibitors	1. Prolonged use leads to rebound acid hypersecretion 2. Risk of hip, wrist and spine fractures due to decreased calcium levels 3. Infections like pneumonia, *C. difficile* diarrhoea 4. Mg levels fall that leads to tetany, arrhythmias and convulsions 5. Vitamin B_{12} deficiency
	Diuretics and salbutamol	Increased risk of hypokalaemia
Steroid sparing agents		
Azathioprine	ACE inhibitors, cotrimoxazole	Severe myelosuppression
	Anticoagulants: Warfarin	Decreased anticoagulant effect
	Allopurinol	Increased toxicity of azathioprine
Methotrexate (MTX)	Trimethoprim: Both synergistically act to suppress dihydrofolate reductase	Severe myelosuppression
	Systemic retinoids: Potentiates hepatotoxicity	Additive hepatotoxicity
	Probenecid, aspirin	Increased MTX toxicity due to decreased excretion of MTX
Cyclosporine (CyA)	Macrolides, ketoconazole, norfloxacin, CYP3A4 inhibitors	Increased levels of CyA
	Anticonvulsants (phenytoin), anti-tubercular drugs: CYP3A4 induction	Decreased levels of CyA
	Aminoglycosides, NSAIDs (indomethacin, naproxen)	Potentiates nephrotoxicity of CyA
Antibiotics		
Tetracyclines	Systemic retinoids: Acitretin, isotretinoin	Increased risk of pseudotumor cerebri
	Anticoagulants (warfarin): Tetracyclines lead to changes in gut flora	Increased serum levels of warfarin due to increased enterohepatic circulation.

(*contd.*)

TABLE 28.3: Commonly prescribed dermatologic medications in the elderly with their drug-drug interactions and consequences[18] (*contd.*)

Drug used in dermatology	Interacting drug and mechanism of action	Consequence
Antifungals Azole antifungals	Statins: Atorvastatin	Fatal rhabdomyolysis can occur.
Ketoconazole, itraconazole	Proton pump inhibitors	Decreased absorption of itraconazole.
	Anticonvulsants: Phenytoin is CYP inducer.	Decreased effect of itraconazole due to increased metabolism.
	Warfarin, oral contraceptive pills	Decreased metabolism of ketoconazole due to CYP3A4 inhibition.
	Erythromycin: CYP3A4 inhibitor	Increased toxicity of ketoconazole.
Griseofulvin	Warfarin and digoxin: Griseofulvin is a weak/moderate CYP1A2/2C9/3A4 inducer	Decreased levels of warfarin and digoxin
Allylamines: Terbinafine	Tricyclic antidepressants (TCA), selective serotonin reuptake inhibitors (SSRI): Allylamines are CYP2D6 inhibitors	Monitoring serum levels of TCA and SSRI required with terbinafine
Acyclovir	Probenecid	Increased bioavailability of acyclovir and decreased renal clearance due to decreased tubular secretion

TABLE 28.4: Drugs prescribed for non-dermatologic diseases having interaction with drugs used for dermatologic diseases in the elderly[18]

Medication prescribed	Drug interaction	Potential consequence
Omeprazole	Ketoconazole	↑ Gastric pH leads to ↓ ketoconazole absorption
	Cyclosporine	↑ Cyclosporine concentration; possible CYP450 inhibition
	Iron salts	↓ Iron absorption; iron requires acidic environment for absorption.
ACE inhibitors	Potassium chloride	ACE inhibitors ↑ serum potassium
Atorvastatin, simvastatin	Erythromycin: CYP3A4 inhibition	↑ Atorvastatin concentration
Warfarin	Macrolides, quinolones	Increased risk of bleeding, due to altered warfarin metabolism.
NSAIDs (naproxen)	Alendronate	Increased incidence of gastric ulceration; mechanism is unknown.

vegetables (such as carrots and celery) are known to decrease enzymatic activity.[11,12.] St. John's wort (*Hypericum perforatum*) is an over-the-counter dietary supplement that has been implicated as substrate of several CYP450 enzymes.[12,13] Patients with dermatological diseases are tempted to switch over to herbal medicines and alternative medicines due to the chronicity of diseases. There is a dearth of Indian data and an increasing trend to use Chinese and herbal medicines as well as drugs from indigenous systems of medicine.

Alcohol and Smoking

Concomitant alcohol intake along with ingestion of antihistaminics may cause CNS depression. An abuse reaction or disulfiram like reaction occurs when an alcoholic patient takes cyclosporine, ketoconazole, metronidazole or griseofulvin and is characterised by nausea, vomiting, flushing, dizziness and tachycardia. Smoking also leads to induction of CYP450 enzymes.[14]

Polypharmacy

Polypharmacy is inadvertent prescription of unnecessary or redundant medications. It can be defined as unintentionally prescribing too many medications (more than four), taking medications with duplicate mechanisms of action or inadvertently adding medications that interact with others.[2] The types of polypharmacy have been listed in Table 28.5.

Medication reconciliation is the process of creating a list of all medications a patient is taking. This is particularly useful in geriatric patients who are on multiple medications. Various methods have been designed like medication appropriateness index (MAI) which assesses the appropriateness of medications with respect to indication, effectiveness, dosage, drug-drug interactions, duration, duplication and cost.[15]

TABLE 28.5: Examples of polypharmacy[2]

Type of polypharmacy	Examples
Numerous medications	Patient having multiple medical conditions.
Duplicate mechanism of action	Urticaria patients simultaneously taking hydroxyzine and cetrizine Cetrizine is a metabolite of hydroxyzine so this combination is redundant Dose of cetrizine can be maximised and H2 antagonist can be added.
Drug-drug interaction	Digoxin for atrial fibrillation and doxycycline for acne vulgaris/rosacea leads to digoxin toxicity Cholinesterase inhibitor for Alzheimer's disease and diphenhydramine for pruritus—dementia can be exacerbated.
Prescribing cascade	Medication side effects are misinterpreted as either normal aging or a new medical condition, which leads to additional medications to treat the iatrogenic condition.

CONCLUSION

Geriatric dermatology as a subject should be introduced in residency curriculum. Since geriatric population have altered pharmacokinetics and pharmacodynamics, the chances of drug interactions are more. The impact of food-drug interactions, herb-drug interactions should not be underestimated. Clinical trials should not exclude the elderly population so as to have adequate data regarding efficacy and safety of drugs in the elderly. It is desirable that the product insert includes details of drug prescribing in elderly. There are various ready to use software programs and mobile applications or personal digital assistant (PDA) which can be useful for knowing about drug interactions. This PDA drug interaction software derives information from familiar handbooks, textbooks, and internet sources that need to be updated regularly. There are many software programs like Micromedex, iFacts and Lexi-interact.[16]

References

1. Buckinx F, Rolland Y, Reginster J, Ricour C, Petermans J, Bruyère O.Burden of frailty in the elderly population: perspectives for a public health challenge. Archives of Public Health 2015; 73(1):19.
2. Endo J, Wong J, Norman R, Chang A. Geriatric dermatology. Journal of the AmericanAcademy of Dermatology 2013; 68(4):521–692.
3. Norman RA. Geriatric dermatology. Dermatologic therapy 2003; 16(3):260–8.

4. Coondoo A, Chattopadhyay C. Drug interactions in dermatology: What the dermatologist should know. Indian Journal of Dermatology 2013; 58:249–54.
5. Flammiger A, Maybach H. Drug dosage in the elderly: dermatologicdrugs. Drugs and Aging 2006; 23(3):203–15.
6. Wolverton SE. Drug interactions. In: Wolff K, Goldsmith LA, Katz SI, Gilchrest BA, Paller AS, Leffell D. Fitzpatricks's Dermatology in General Medicine, 7th edition. New York: McGraw Hill; 2008. p. 2238.
7. Shapiro LE, Shear NE. Drug interactions. In: Wolverton SE. Comprehensive Dermatologic Drug Therapy, 2nd edition New Delhi: Saunders Elsevier; 2007. p. 949–76.
8. Roos TC, Merk HF. Important drug interactions in dermatology. Drugs 2000; 59(2):181–192.
9. Rothenbacher D, Klenk J, Denkinger M, Karakas M, Nikolaus T, Peter R et al. Prevalence and determinants of chronic kidney disease in community-dwelling elderly by various estimating equations. BMC Public Health 2012; 12:343.
10. Pantuck EJ, Pantuck CB, Garland WA, Min B, Wattenberg L, Anderson, et al. Stimulatory effects of brussels sprouts and cabbage on human drug metabolism. Clinical Pharmacology and Therapeutics 1979; 25(1):88–95.
11. Cyriac MJ. Drug interactions of some commonly used drugs in dermatology. Indian Journal of Dermatol Venereol Leprol 2004; 70:54–6.
12. Sorensen. Herb-drug, food-drug, nutrient-drug, and drug-drug interactions: Mechanisms Involved and Their Medical Implications. The journal of alternative and complementary medicine 2004; 8(3):293–308
13. O'Mahony MS, Woodhouse KW. Age, environmental factors and drug metabolism. Pharmacology and Therapeutics 1994; 61(1):279–87.
14. Fraser A. Pharmacokinetic Interactions between Alcohol and Other Drugs. Clinical Pharmacokinetics 1997; 33(2):79–90.
15. Somers A, Mallet L, van der Cammen T, Robays H, Petrovic M. Applicability of an adapted medication appropriateness index for detection of drug-related problems in geriatric inpatients. The American Journal of Geriatric Pharmacotherapy 2012; 10(2): 101–109.
16. Roblek T, Vaupolic T, Mrhar A, Lainscak M. Drug-drug interaction software in clinical practice: a systematic review. European Journal of Clinical Pharmacology 2015.
17. Gonzalez FJ. The molecular biology of cytochromes P450s. Pharmacology and Therapeutics 1990; 45(1):1–38.
18. Kinirons, O'Mahony. Drug metabolism and ageing. British Journal of Clinical Pharmacology 2004; 57(5):540–44.

CHAPTER 29

Psychocutaneous Disorders in Elderly

• Usha Naraindas Khemani • Megha Valjibhai Kakani

Key Points

- The skin and nervous system have a common embryological origin; this supports the connection between skin changes and psychological phenomenon.
- As people age, the skin related disorders increase. Ageing could be intrinsic ageing (natural changes) and extrinsic ageing (external factors like diabetes mellitus, hypertension, smoking, which reduce the body's ability to heal.
- Skin is a part of NICE (neuro-immuno-cutaneous-endocrine) system, stress can induce or exacerbate many dermatological conditions.
- The primordial relationship between the skin and mind and the interaction of neuroendocrine and immune systems due to various factors results in disturbance in equilibrium of neuro-immuno-cutaneous system resulting in various pyshocutaneous disorders.
- As advances in medical care have expanded the elderly demographics, there is a need to evaluate various pyschocutaneous disorders in growing geriatric population.
- Pyschocutaneous diseases in old patients can have psychological implications and severe impact on quality of life.
- Geriatric pyschodermatosis is a challenging job for a doctor in terms of diagnosis, management and follow-up.
- A different and more sensible approach is necessary when dealing with elderly patients is that we should always treat the patient and not the disease.
- Stress can worsen many skin conditions and leads to psychiatric comorbidity.
- Psychiatric comorbidity is common in many dermatological conditions. Antipsychotics, antidepressants, mood stabilizers and anxiolytics may be needed for the management.
- Unless we manage the underlying psychological issues, response to the therapy will be less.
- Psychotherapies like habit reversal supportive therapy, relaxation procedures and cognitive behaviour therapy are highly useful in stress-related dermatology cases.
- Patients with dermatological illness suffer high rates of psychiatric comorbidity particularly those with chronic dermatoses.
- The treatment of these disorders requires an effective liaison between a dermatologist, psychiatrist and psychologist.

Introduction

Skin is a window to ageing changes, a biological reality.

The skin is an important organ of communication throughout the lifespan.

The skin is not only the largest organ of the body but also a strong part of the immune system that protects us from the external environment. It bears the brunt of ageing from both the external and internal environments, resulting in pathological processes that can ultimately affect the health and quality of life of older patients. A large proportion of patients with skin disorders are associated with various degrees of psychic disturbances which may be the cause and/or effect. Disfiguring dermatological conditions often run a chronic course, resulting in profound psychological morbidity, leading to secondary psychiatric disorders (SPsDs). These patients need to be addressed with a special approach assisting their psychological need, pharmacotherapy for their psychiatric morbidity, and skin disease; hence, a complete holistic treatment approach to the patient.[1]

The relationship between skin and psyche is getting increasing attention and several theories postulate psychophysiological mechanisms underlying various dermatological disorders. Since both skin and brain originated from the same ectoderm, skin diseases can affect mind and vice versa.

Interface between Geriatrics, Psychiatry and Dermatology

Human embryogenesis involves the development of both the progenitors of nervous system as well as the skin from the ectoderm primary germ cell layer. Neural crest cells pigmentize the skin via melanocytes while simultaneously shaping the connections of the central and peripheral nervous systems via ganglia. Similarly, the epidermis of the skin as well as the epithelia of the pineal and pituitary glands share a common progenitor in the form of surface ectodermal cells. Both neuroendocrine and immune systems interact in a complex pattern with a disturbance in equilibrium of either component of the neuro-immuno-cutaneous system (NICS) resulting in a plethora of dermatological manifestations. Therefore, it is not surprising to unearth psychological problems in over 30% of patients presenting with a primarily dermatological complaint.[2] Geriatric age group presents the most important psychodermatological disorders of the elderly—an age group already at increased susceptibility to both psychiatric as well as dermatological ailments owing to a variety of factors including immunocompromise, lifestyle, chronic diseases such as diabetes mellitus and rheumatoid arthritis, polypharmacy, as well as financial and social adjustment among others.

Geriatric patients have special needs related to issues such as concurrent comorbidities, social isolation, and logistical limitations including difficulty with transportation or even basic activities of daily living

The objective here is to enhance the interaction between the fields of primary care, geriatrics, dermatology, and psychiatry (Table 29.1) such that the diagnosis, referral and ultimately management of the needy are superlative—a synergy that is at present lacking.

TABLE 29.1: Koo and Lee classification of geriatric psychodermatological disorders[15]

Classification	Age of presentation in years
Psychophysiologic disorders	
Psoriasis	20–30 and 50–60 +
Atopic dermatitis	<5 and 50–70
Hyperhidrosis	25
Urticaria	All age groups
Herpes simplex virus infection	14–49
Seborrhoeic dermatitis	2 weeks–12 months and 30–40+
Apthosis	<30
Rosacea	>30
Pruritus	All age groups
Psychiatric disorders with dermatological symptoms	
Dermatitis artefacta	18–60
Delusion of parasitosis	50+
Trichotillomania	9–13
Obsessive compulsive disorder	Juvenile: 10, and Adult: 21
Phobic states	20
Neurotic excoriation	30–45
Psychogenic pruritus	64
Dermatologic disorders with psychiatric symptoms	
Alopecia areata	<30
Vitiligo	20–30+
Generalized psoriasis	20–30 and 50–60+
Chronic eczema	20
Rhinophyma	30–50
Miscellaneous	
Glossodynia	55–60
Vulvodynia	25
Chronic itching in scalp	30–50+
Psychogenic purpura syndrome	14, 40
Pseudopsychodermatologic disease	21, 68

Note: Mean age of presesntation does not exclude incidence in geriatric population

(*Courtesy:* Geriatric Psychodermatology, Mohammad Jafferany, MD)

Epidemiology

The famous old saying OLD IS GOLD does not apply to human skin as elderly people are recognized by their wrinkled and dull skin. India has acquired the label of an ageing nation with 7.7% of its population more than 60 years.

Geriatric population is increasing worldwide. Elderly patients are afflicted with many dermatological concerns, not only because of normal ageing process but the additional stressors acquired from environmental causes.

Psychocutaneous diseases can present as primary psychiatric diseases such delusions of parasitosis or as secondary psychiatric disorders such as anxiety and depression. Geriatric psychodermatology is already complicated by pre-existing age-related decline in cognition, decreased physical capabilities, activities of daily living, and disabilities among others. Multiple morbidities along with their medications and treatment plans as well as complex social and financial relationships add numerous variables to this already challenging field. The elderly patient may use the skin as a heliograph for elevated psychological distress. It is, therefore, imperative that clinicians understand, diagnose and treat this impending deluge of humanity in an integrative and holistic manner. There is a crosspollination of psychiatric and dermatological referrals.

Pathogenesis

The complex inter-relationship between mind and skin has been investigated at both molecular and cellular levels and it has been recorded that patients with depression suffer more from physical illness and patients with chronic illness suffer more often from major depressive illness, suggesting that the state of mind has a marked bearing not only on how an illness is perceived but also on its severity and content.[4,5]

Stress and Psychoneuroimmunology

The neuroimmuno-cutaneous-endocrine model proposed by O'Sullivan et al explains the mind and body relationship. It forms the basis of many inflammatory cutaneous dermatoses that are triggered or exacerbated by psychological factors. These organs share a complex language of neuropeptides, cytokines, glucocorticoids, and other effector molecules (Fig. 29.1).[6–9] Stressors activate two major neural pathways—hypothalamo-pituitary-adrenal (HPA) axis and sympathetic nervous system. The activation of these two neurochemical pathways and release of hormones and transmitters have profound downstream effects on immune function. As a result, the body produces in-numerable hormones, cytokines and other neuro-hormonal chemical mediators which trigger and maintain the skin disease without much response to therapy. Hypothalamic pituitary axis (HPA) responds to psychological stress with upregulation of stress hormones (corticotrophin-releasing hormone, adrenocorticotrophin releasing hormone, cortisol, and prolactin), sympathetic nervous system activation leading to elevated catecholamine levels, and the release of neuropeptides and neuromediators (substance P and calcitonin gene-related peptide).

Flowchart 29.1 describing interplay of various factors leading to skin disorders originating from psychological stress.

These bind to receptors on cutaneous blood vessels, including vasodilatation, increased vessel permeability, chemotaxis, exocytosis and activation of neutrophils. These peptides in conjunction with with keratinocyte-derived CRH and nerve growth factor NGF act on mast cells resulting in the degranulation of these cells, secretion of TNF-α, histamine, tryptamine leading to cutaneous inflammation. It is observed that stress will increase the production and release of proinflammatory cytokines and nitric acid from macrophages and this leads to selective redistribution of immune cells from one organ to another. Stressors also activate intracellular transcription factors that play a central role in mediating

Flowchart 29.1: Flowchart describing interplay of various factors leading to skin disorders originating from psychological stress

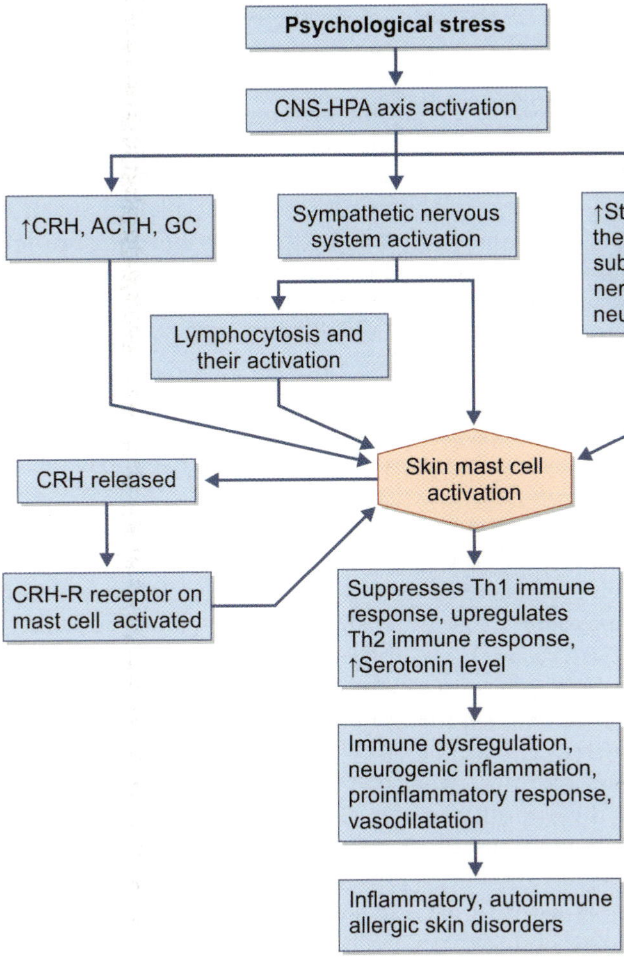

Source: Yadav S et al. Psychodermatology: A comprehensive review. Indian J Dermatol Venereol Leprol 2013; 79:176–92.

the physiological effects of proinflammatory cytokines. Stress has a significant role in the initiation and maintenance of cutaneous inflammatory response. Skin mast cells are an important target of key stress hormones and mediators, and their activation leads to immune dysregulation and various skin disorders. Arc et al suggested that skin is exquisitely well innervated and has its own neuroendocrine system, equivalent of the HPA axis, local stress response system, which is tightly linked to systemic neuroendocrine axis.[9]

The term of alexithymia, introduced by Nemiah and Sifneos,[10] is characterised by reduced symbolic thinking, a poor fantasy life, and a limited ability to identify and verbally express emotions, which results in altered physiologic and immune body responses.[11] Various studies have reported a high incidence of alexithymia in alopecia areata (58%),[12] psoriasis (35%),[13] chronic urticaria (50%),[14] and vitiligo (35.5%).[15]

The doctor–patient relationship is the keystone of the entire medical practice. The number of individuals 65 years of age and older is constantly increasing as well as the life expectancy in many countries. As people age, their chances of developing skin-related disorders increase. Geriatric patients have special physical, emotional, social and psychological needs.

Difficult Geriatric Patients

Difficult geriatric patients can also be challenging. Difficult patients can take up the doctor's time and physical and emotional energy.

These patients are more likely have mental disorders when compared with non-difficult patients. Also that difficult patients had lower satisfaction rates, more functional impairment and used the health care system more often. Patients that are labelled as difficult by clinician are angry, anxious, depressed, feeling guilty, frustrated, helpless, hostile, self-loathed, uncooperative, ungrateful and unpleasant.

Managing difficult patients can be a challenge for many doctors. When dealing with these types of patients, it can be helpful to utilize certain strategies such as empathizing with the patient, listening carefully, and involving the patient and their family in medical decisions and all aspects of the treatment process. Verbalizing the problem as well as conveying a positive attitude by focusing on solutions as opposed to disagreements can also be effective technique showing empathy can motivate the patient to pursue treatment, listen carefully and read the patient's state of mind. The patient should be involved along with his family, verbalize the difficulty and staying positive and to focus on finding solutions.

DIFFERENT TYPES OF PYSCHOCUTANEOUS DISORDER IN ELDERLY

Pychodermatologic disorders can be classified under 3 broad categories: Psychophysiologic disorders, primary psychiatric disorders (PPsDs) and secondary psychiatric disorders (SPsDs).

Psychophysiologic Skin Disorders

Psychophysiological disorders are those in which the course of a given skin disease is affected by the psychological state of a patient. These disorders are often precipitated or exacerbated by emotional stress and/or anxiety in a significant number of cases and include skin disorders like alopecia areata, atopic eczema, psoriasis and urticaria, mucocutaneous herpes simplex infection, hyperhidrosis, and chronic telogen effluvium (Table 29.2). All these conditions are not uniformly affected by stress. There are persons who are non-stress responders, where mental stress does not play any role. The role of stress in lichen planus, vitiligo, psychogenic purpura, rosacea, acne and seborrhoeic dermatitis is unclear.

Skin and mind are interrelated. Stress can precipitate or aggravate skin disease (stress responders). The relation between stress and certain skin disorders is well established. Stressors are events or factors that disturb one's mental balance. Reaction to stress depends on the genetic make up of the individual and how one perceives the event. The perception depends on external factors such as life events, natural environment and individual factors such as attitude, temperament and previous experiences. Stress activates hypothalamohypophyseal-adrenal axis and sympathetic nervous system to

TABLE 29.2: Percentage of patients reporting exacerbation with stress

Disease	% of patients
Psoriasis	54–60
Acne	50
Alopecia areata	60
Rosacea	58
Urticaria	16
Pompholyx	17
Vitiligo vulgaris	47

Source: Yadav S, et al. Psychodermatology: A comprehensive review. Indian J Dermatol Venereol Leprol 2013; 79:176–92.

liberate glucocorticoids and catecholamines, respectively. Both inhibit Th1 response suppresses cell-mediated immunity and promotes Th2 response. This activates mast cells, eosinophils and B cells causing inflammation. Stress disturbs epidermal permeability barrier. It also liberates histamine, vasoactive neuropeptides and causes variation in skin temperature, blood flow and sweat response which contribute to itch–scratch cycle.

While dealing with these patients, dermatologists should always try to ascertain the extent of role played by psychosocial and occupational stress in a given case to prevent the vicious cycle of stress-disease exacerbation and, finally, deterioration of the primary disease. These patients generally have a good insight into their diseases, but most are unable to decipher the role of psychological factors on their skin disease. Non-pharmacological as well as pharmacologic therapy such as with benzodiazepines (BDZ) and selective serotonin reuptake inhibitors (SSRIs) are helpful. In non-responders, a psychiatric referral is required psoriasis.

Aetiology of psoriasis is multifactorial involving genetic and environmental disorders. Among the latter, stress has an important role in the onset and exacerbation of psoriasis. In normal individuals, stress activates hypothalamo-pituitary-adrenal (HPA) axis and sympathetic-adrenal medullary (SAM) axis, but in psoriasis, stress reduces hypothalamo-pituitary-adrenal (HPA) response and upregulates sympathetic-adrenal-medullary (SAM) response. Hence, stress reduces cortisol levels, increases the levels of epinephrine and norepinephrine both of which stimulate the release of mast cells, affect skin barrier function and upregulate pro-inflammatory cytokines. The proportion of patients, who are stress responders, ranges from 37 to 78%. The incubation period between stress and exacerbation varies from 2 days to 1 month. 44% of patients with psoriasis, a chronic erythematosquamous, inflammatory and proliferative dermatitis with obscure aetiology and unpredictable evolution, report a stressful event before the disease onset, and 80% of them correlate the relapse episodes with stress. Stress responders tend to self-report greater disease severity compared to non-stress responders. Apart from increasing the severity of psoriasis, it also affects outcome of treatment. Early onset psoriasis (onset before the age of 40 years) is triggered more readily by stress than late onset psoriasis attributable to the fact that younger psoriatics have greater difficulties in assertion and expression of anger which adversely affects their ability to cope with stress. Stress-induced psoriatics have better long-term prognosis, especially if they have high levels of insight.[16–18] On the other hand, psoriasis chronic character, long-term treatment and its disfigurating lesions may be the cause of depression and suicidal ideation.[19,20] Psychological interventions along with standard skin care may improve the course of the disease.

Alopecia areata is a T cell-mediated autoimmune disease characterised by localised patches of hair loss on the scalp, sometimes involving other areas such as beard, moustache and eyebrows. The hair regrow after varying periods of time. Progressive cases of alopecia totalis and universalis have an unfavourable prognosis. Various precipitating factors, such as febrile illnesses, drugs and trauma have been reported stressors, can also act as potential trigger. Stressful life events such as personal, family and job-related problems have been reported in the preceeding 3 months of onset of the disease.[21]

Hair Disorders in the Elderly

As life expectancy is growing along with longer professional and social activity, the aesthetic appearance is gaining increasing importance. The quality of hair seems to be significant to the self-esteem, self-confidence and often to the mental attitude of elderly individuals. Hair changes and hair loss can lead to psychological problems and influence the quality of life. The most common hair-related problems in the elderly patients are hair greying and hair loss.

Several intrinsic and extrinsic factors may lead to premature hair greying. The intrinsic factors include medical conditions such as stress, thyroid insufficiency, Werner syndrome, Williams syndrome or pernicious anaemia. Extrinsic factors include smoking, ultraviolet radiation, toxins and nutritional deficiencies.[22–24] The most frequent cause of hair loss in the elderly population is androgenetic alopecia (AGA). Androgenetic alopecia is an androgen-related condition, which develops in genetically predisposed individuals. Androgenetic alopecia has a significant impact on the quality of life. However, for many men, loss of hair is associated with a significant psychological distress.[25,26] There is a correlation between the severity of balding and the impact of disease on the quality of life. Women and men with long-lasting androgenetic alopecia develop some coping mechanisms, such as avoiding negative emotions from their surroundings by reducing their outdoor activities or by wearing hats or wigs to prevent discomfort. The goal of current treatment in androgenetic alopecia is rather to decelerate ongoing hair loss than to achieve full hair regrowth. Taken into consideration that the disease has a significant impact on the quality of life and that the treatment results may be disappointing, dermatologists should devote sufficient time to consultation at the first visit to discuss the planned treatment timetable, the therapeutic options and patient's expectations. Psychological counselling may be required in certain patients in parallel to pharmacological management of hair loss.

Also most psychologically distressing type of hair loss in the elderly population is chemotherapy-induced alopecia. Hair loss can be associated with serious psychological consequences, particularly anxiety, depression and an impairment in the quality of life. The patient's expectations and the therapeutic options should be discussed in detail. It is important not to underestimate the psychological importance of hair appearance, also in elderly patients who may have other coexisting medical conditions, seem into the physician more—serious.[26–28] Corticotrophin- releasing hormone, the key stress hormone, is present in the hair follicle. Stress affects local CRH expression and HPA activity causing hair loss.

Atopic Dermatitis

Atopic eczema is a common endogenous dermatitis characterized by pruritus, recurrent eczema and an atopic diathesis. It starts in the second or third month of age and continues into adulthood. Various factors, such as genetics, infections, weather, food, tobacco, aeroallergens such a house dust mite and stress, have been implicated. There is typically itch–scratch cycle stressors cause itching and scratching initially relieves it. With time, constant scratching causes structural inflammatory changes causing more itching more scratching leading to a vicious cycle. Stressful life events have been reported preceding the onset of disease at a rate of 70%.

Several studies have shown association of stress with onset of flares and worsening of atopic dermatitis. In children, stress and family environment are predictors of symptom severity.

In atopic dermatitis, a blunted HPA axis responsiveness with a concurrent over a activity of the sympathetic adrenomedullary system may increase susceptibility to inflammation causing stress-related worsening of eczema. The reduced endogeneous cortisol production under stress would impair anti-inflammatory effect of this hormone. Patients with atopic dermatitis thus have a hyperacute response to stress with T cell and mast cell activation, HPA dysregulation, neurogenic inflammatory mediator expression and release and disruption of normal epidermal barrier function. Psychotherapeutic interventions such as stress management, habit reversal and relaxation training can reduce itching and scratching causing improvement.[30–32]

Sweating (hyperhidrosis) to emotional stimuli can occur in the context of psychosomatic disorders such as atopic dermatitis and can cause psychiatric symptoms such as social phobia, anxiety and depression or there may be a delusional theme without any clinical objective skin signs in patients with dismorphophobia.[33,34]

Urticaria is characterised by localised or generalised wheals with or without angioedema. In nearly 70% of cases, an underlying cause cannot be determined. Psychological factors play a role in about 50% of patients. Several studies have reported that urticarial patients frequently have stressful life events before the onset of disease. The effect of stress is mediated by CRH which is known to cause degranulation of mast cells. This hormone is elevated during stress and in depression and correlates with the severity of urticaria.[35]

Stress intervention in the reactivation of latent herpes infection is well documented, numerous studies revealing a reverse correlation between stress levels and CD4+/helper/inducer lymphocytes involved in antivirus defense mechanism. Another incriminated mechanism in reactivation of herpes infection seems to be the stress released catecholamines, cytokines and glucocorticoids which lead to the cell-mediated immune response alteration.[36]

Lichen planus: Various triggers like drugs, stress and infections have precipitated this condition. Pychosocial stressors have also been implicated in oral lichen planus.

Vitiligo is a common depigmentary condition affecting the melanocytes. It has been found that vitiligo patients experience more number of stressful events than controls suggesting that psychological distress may contribute to the onset of disease.[37]

Psychogenic purpura, also called autoerythrocyte sensitisation syndrome, is a spontaneous recurrent painful ecchymosis most commonly in woman who is always preceded by severe stress and emotional trauma. Psychiatric comorbidity such as depression may be present.

Rosacea and Acne

It is a chronic skin condition characterised by facial erythema with telangiectasias, papules and pustules occurring predominantly over the central parts of face such as forehead, nose and cheeks, affects women between 30 and 50 years of age. The exact cause is unknown but various triggers, like stress, have been implicated. Studies have shown increased sympathetic nerve activity in the facial skin in response to trigger events. Neurovascular interactions with release of proinflammatory and vasodilatory neuropeptide mediators are key to the pathogensis of certain types of rosacea.

Also emotional stress has a significant impact on acne. Stress leads to increased secretion of adrenal androgens causing sebaceous hyperplasia and comedones. Stress also releases neuropeptides from peripheral nerves causing proliferation and differentiation of sebaceous gland with increased sebum secretion. In acne excoriee, during stressful periods, patients pick at their acne causing hyperpigmented crusted skin lesions, usually there is associated psychiatry comorbidity such as depression, anxiety, dysmorphophobia or OCD.[38,39]

Primary Psychiatric Disorders (PPsDs) with Dermatological Symptoms

Primary abnormality of psyche or mind of a person can lead to dermatological diseases. Primary psychiatric disorders can lead to self-inflicted secondary dermatological diseases. The dermatologist plays an important role in these disorders, initially to suspect and establish the diagnosis and later to provide appropriate management. These patients often

TABLE 29.3: List of primary psychiatric disorders

Disorder of dermatologic beliefs	Delusion of parasitosis
Disorder of body awareness	Body dysmorphic disorder, anorexia nervosa
Impulse control disorder	Trichotillomania, neurotic excoriations, acne, excoriee, neurodermatitis, onychotillomania, prurigo nodularis
Factitious skin diseases	Dermatitis artefacta, dermatitis simulate, dermatitis passivata
Psychogenic pruritus	
Cutaneous phobias	Mole phobia, venereophobia, wart phobia and steroid phobia
Atypical pain disorder	Glossodynia, vulvodynia, scrotodynia, anodynia

Source: Yadav S, et al. Psychodermatology: A comprehensive review. Indian J Dermatol Venereol Leprol 2013; 79:176–92.

have an underlying psychological functional problem such as delusion, obsessive compulsive disorder (OCD), anxiety, depression, impulse control disorder, and personality disorder, which is essential to be identified and managed accordingly (Table 29.3). In addition, the supportive skin therapy must be given.

The underlying psychological problem needs to be managed essentially before dermatological management for a successful result of the skin problem.

Delusion of Parasitosis

Delusion of parasitosis (DP), also known as Ekbom's syndrome, is a rare disorder and exact prevalence is unknown. In this, the patients have delusional belief that their bodies are infested with parasites. *Diagnostic and Statistical Manual of Mental Disorders,* Fourth Edition (Text Revision) (DSM-IV-TR) defines it as a delusional disorder of somatic type. Hebbar et al. found it to be the most common subtype of delusional disorders.[40] Among 4234 psychiatry outpatients, 1% and 0.5% had delusional disorders and delusional parasitosis, respectively. The underlying psychiatric problem is a "monosymptomatic hypochondriacal psychosis".

Characteristic profile: Usually seen in a middle aged/elderly females presenting in anxious, ruminative, and overwhelmed state after having visited several doctors without satisfaction. The patients explain about visual and tactile hallucinations of the parasites crawling, burrowing, and biting all over their body. Manipulations of the skin in an attempt to remove the assumed parasites are common acts that lead to excoriation, erosions, cuts and burns. Most of the times, they often present with an evidence of parasite infection in the form of clothing lint, skin crust, or debris, which are misinterpreted as parasite parts, larva, ova, or the entire organism. Morgellons disease is largely considered a manifestation of DP by both the dermatologists and psychiatrists. Firstly actual infestation must be ruled. Also they may apply various lotions, antimicrobial ointments, chemicals, sometimes burn the area also.

Differential diagnosis: Psychiatric disorders such as schizophrenia, psychotic depression, psychosis episode in a maniac patient, formication without delusion, organic causes such as withdrawal from cocaine, amphetamines or alcohol, vitamin B_{12} deficiency, multiple sclerosis, syphilis, and cerebrovascular disease.

The attendants/family of the patient should be counselled regarding the patient's illness. Antipsychotic medication can be started by the dermatologist in consultation with psychiatrist before referral. Pimozide works well.[40]

Disorder of Body Image

Body dysmorphic disorder (BDD), also known as dysmorphophobia or dermatological non-disease, is a disorder characterised by distortion of psychological body image. The patient is preoccupied and distressed with an uncorrectable imagined defect in appearance or an excessive concern over a trivial defect. BDD is defined in DSMIV and classified as a somatoform disorder. The newly published DSM-V classifies body dysmorphic disorder (BDD) in the obsessive-compulsive and related disorders (OCRDs) category. BDD has been included in this category due to similarities with OCD, including repetitive behaviours, although BDD is characterised by poorer insight than OCD. The preoccupation causes social, occupational, family, personal and other areas dysfunction and makes them seek corrective procedures in the imagined disfigurement. There is an underlying co-morbid mental disorder including mood disorders such as depression, OCD, social phobia, and/or avoidant personality disorder. In some patients, the belief is of delusional intensity, then it is classified under psychotic disorders. It has a prevalence varying from 0.75 to 12%.[41–43] Usually seen in females in their 30's, however, later decades of life arguably represent a time when appearance concerns become more legitimate. Women present with complaints related to mainly face, breast, hair, nose, and stomach, while men presented with concern related to hair, nose, ear, genitals, and body build. As appearance is believed to be very important, people with BDD perceive themselves as unattractive and they evaluate themselves negatively and have low self-esteem. Changes in physical appearance due to ageing skin can make some patients, especially women, feel unattractive and this may trigger symptoms of BDD as they initiate a quest for the fountain of youth through repeated cosmetic procedures.[44,45] Male patients often show complaints related to scalp (hair thinning), nose, ears, body allure and genitals (scrotal redness, urethral discharge or venerophobia). These negative beliefs about their appearance often lead them to anxiety, shame and sadness, which in turn lead to maladaptive coping strategies, such as excessive mirror gazing and/or avoidance behaviours. Suicidal ideation and suicide attempts are common in BDD patients, with studies showing a rate of attempted suicide to 30%.[46,47] There are two types of patient with BDD: Those with insight and those without. Often, those without insight are also diagnosed with delusional disorder, somatic type. Management of BDD is extremely difficult, every attempt to explain the trivial nature of skin complaints is futile. In case of poor insight, it is difficult to intervene. The difficulty is to shift the focus from the primary dermatological illness to the one that requires psychiatric treatment. In patients with insight, it is relatively easy to address as they are open to discussion, compliant to medications and behavioural interventions.

Body dysmorphic disorder in the elderly is not frequent. Patients over 65 years of age may present with body dysmorphic symptoms or concerns but these could be due to an adjustment disorder caused by the ageing process. Gupta and Gupta (2013) refer to cutaneous body image (CBI) to describe an individual's mental perception of the appearance of his or her integumentary system.[48] CBI dissatisfaction can contribute to significant morbidity in dermatologic disorders and is often the primary consideration in deciding whether to proceed with some cosmetic procedures. Assessment of CBI has important clinical implications because it can significantly affect the patient's quality of life. CBI dissatisfaction can increase the overall morbidity in dermatologic disease and has been associated with intentional self-injury, such as self-induced dermatoses and suicide. Poor CBI has been shows to be an important factor in adherence to treatment in chronic disorders. Normal intrinsic ageing is often viewed as a medical and social problem that needs to be addressed by health care professionals. Even in later life, the patient may be highly invested in his or her CBI. Finally, we should remember to assess the risk of self-harm and suicide in patients with BDD, body image, or cutaneous body image symptoms or concerns.

Somatoform Disorders

In these patients, no objectifiable symptoms can be found, but they complain a number of symptoms that cannot be explained. The dermatological symptoms usually consist of pruritus (itching), pain, dysaesthesias, formication, feeling of disfiguration, or non-objectifiable hair loss (Table 29.4).

Somatization Disorders

These include the occurrence of a pattern of recurrent, multiple clinically significant somatic complaints leading to medical treatment. Usually seen features are: Pain symptoms, gastrointestinal, sexual, and pseudoneurological symptoms. In dermatology, environmental physical complaint, the so-called

TABLE 29.4: Overview of somatoform disorders in dermatology[49]

Somatization disorder	Environmental syndrome	Ecosyndrome, multiple chemical sensitivity syndrome, sick-building syndrome
	Special forms	Food allergies, sperm allergy, detergent allergy, light allergy electrosmog, amalgam-related complaint syndrome
Hypochondriacal disorder	Hypochondriacal disorder in the actual sense	Infections (bacteria, fungi, viruses, parasites) Neoplasia, other nosophobias
	Body dysmorphic disorder	Whole body: Dorian Gray syndrome. Regional: Head, breast, genitals
	Special form	Botulinophilia
Somatoform autonomic function disorder	Erythrophobia Goose bumps Hyperhidrosis Special form: Undifferentiated somatoform idiopathic anaphylaxia	
Persistent somatoform pain disorder	Cutaneous dysathesias	Glossesodynia-orofacial pain syndrome Trichodynia Vulvodynia, phallodynia, anodynia
Other somatoform disorders	Sensory complaints	Itching A. Localised somatoform itching B. Generalized somatoform itching (pruritus sine material) C. Paraesthesias D. Burning stabbing

Source: Primary Psychiatric disorders—cutaneous manifestations. Ravindra Munoli Handbook of Psychodermatology by Abdul Latheef EN 2016

ecosyndrome, is in the foreground of the somatization disorders, whereby multiple fluctuating complaints attributed to various intolerances. In the ecosyndrome, patients have different subjective presentations of disease in various organ systems coupled with conviction of being sick because of environmental toxins.

Persistent Somatoform Pain Disorder

Cutaneous Sensory Syndrome: Chronic Cutaneous Dysaesthesias

Atypical pain disorder/burn syndrome: Underlying psychiatric disorder—comorbid affective disorder, personality vulnerability, anxiety, depression.

Cutaneous sensory disorder or chronic cutaneous dysaesthesia, also known as hallucinatory dysaesthesia is a disorder consisting of 2 parts. The first part is the patient has disagreeable cutaneous sensations, e.g. itching, burning, stinging and the second part is the sensation lacks a neurologic, psychiatric, or medical explanation for the dysaesthesia, glossonydia, vulvodynia, scrotodynia, anodynia.

Pain/Burning/Dysaesthesias in Skin or Mucous Membranes with no Identifiable Pathology

This sensation can affect any body region but tends to develop in areas with greater density of epidermal innervation, most commonly involving the face, scalp, or perineum. Often the associated body parts with cutaneous sensory disorder are termed as vulvodynia, scrotodynia, glossodynia or burning mouth syndrome or stomatodynia. Most of the time, there are no apparent dermatologic or medical conditions that explain symptoms and all work-up appears negative.

Epidemiology: Chronic cutaneous dysaesthesia affects all genders and ages but predominantly affects females with an increased prevalence with age and during perimenopause. Geriatric population is particularly prone.[50–52]

Classification: Chronic cutaneous dysaesthesias are typically referred either by affected anatomy or known pathogenesis.

Head

- Glossodynia
- Stomatodynia or burning mouth syndrome
- Scalp dysaesthesia
- Trichodynia

Urogenital

- Vulvodynia
- Orchiodynia
- Urodynia
- Urethral syndrome
- Phallodynia
- Prostatodynia
- Coccygodynia
- Perineal pain syndrome
- Anodynia
- Proctodynia known pathogenesis
- Erythromelalgia
- Trigeminal neuralgia
- Postherpetic neuralgia
- Proctalgia fugax

Pathophysiology: Various neurologic and clinical factors are involved in the pathogenesis of cutaneous sensory syndrome. A better understanding of the pathophysiology of sensation will allow us to better understand therapeutic options for chronic cutaneous dysaesthesia. There are two main types of nociceptive afferents—the Aδ fibres and C fibres. The Aδ fibres transmit signals for fast, well-localised sharp pain and temperature. The C fibres transmit signals for slow, diffuse, aching pain, temperature, pressure, and itch. These fibres activate nociceptors in skin. Current research shows that nociceptors are activated via TRP (transient receptor potential) and purinergic receptors, which allow Na^+ and Ca^{2+} through the membrane of free nerve endings. The TRP channels can be directly modulated by H^+, capsaicin, noxious temperature or force, and the purinergic receptors can be directly modulated by ATP. TRP channels are further potentiated at GPCR (G-protein coupled receptors) by bradykinin, histamine, prostaglandin, and serotonin. Once the nociceptors are activated, the peripheral nervous system utilises substance P and calcitonin gene-related peptide to transduce the signal from primary afferent to the anterolateral system. Centrally, the sensation of pain is inhibited by enkephalinergic interneurons and by glutamate, norepinephrine, and serotonin neurotransmitters. Anxiety and depression are commonly seen in cutaneous sensory syndrome. Emotional and psychological trauma suffered in life causes grave psychological consequences for an individual and leads to—dissociation and conversion of emotional symptoms into cutaneous somatic symptoms. The dissociation process plays a central role in the development of medically unexplained symptoms and somatization.

Psychiatric factors noted in chronic sensory syndrome are related to somatization phenomenon. Somatization appears to be an important factor in cutaneous sensory syndrome. Somatization is a clinical situation where the patient attributes the somatic symptom to a physical problem but the condition actually is a psychiatric illness that responds to psychiatric treatment. Common dermatologic symptoms associated with somatization in chronic sensory syndrome include cutaneous pain, itching, burning, tingling and numbness.

Clinical management: A diagnosis of chronic cutaneous dysaesthesia is a clinical diagnosis of exclusion; therefore, a good history and physical examination is the key. A thorough medical, neurologic, and psychiatric work-up should be performed to exclude an organic aetiology. Patient should have basic labs and be up to date on cancer screenings. The duration and nature of the dysaesthesia should be well-documented, including exacerbating and alleviating qualifiers. Once diagnosed, physicians should first acknowledge and validate the patient's symptoms and experience. Irritating and possible contributing factors should be avoided. Inquiries into the patient's sleep hygiene are important, as sleep disruptions are known to enhance perception of chronic cutaneous dysaesthesia. It is important to identify whether or not the patient has a diagnosable psychiatric comorbidity, most commonly depression and anxiety. If present, the psychiatric comorbidity should be treated regardless, if the psychiatric comorbidity is related since psychiatric disease can also enhance the perception of chronic cutaneous dysaesthesia. Pharmacologic management targets molecules involved in sensation of pain both peripherally and centrally.[53–55] Benefit is seen within 4–6 weeks; resolution is achieved within 2–3 months. While some patients may eventually be tapered off pharmacologic therapy without recurrence of pain, other patients may require long-term pharmacologic therapy. In our clinical experience, it is possible for a patient to continue long-term pharmacologic therapy safely and without waning efficacy. Pharmacologic therapy for chronic cutaneous dysaesthesia targets molecules involved in the pathophysiology of pain. Doxepin and paroxetine are typically used when pruritus is the predominant symptom. TCAs, SSRIs, anticonvulsants, and capsaicin are typically used when pain is involved. Antipsychotics have been found to be very effective in cases refractory to treatment.[56] A therapeutic dose can be reached, followed by eventual tapering to a lower maintenance dose or to no medication at all. More studies are needed to elucidate our understanding of chronic cutaneous dysaesthesia; however, many available pharmacologic treatments have been shown to be successful in the off-label treatment of chronic cutaneous dysaesthesia.[57–59]

PSYCHOGENIC PRURITUS (PP)

A poorly defined entity in which the patient has intractable or persistant itch, not ascribed to any physical or dermatological illness. Misery et al have proposed diagnostic criteria. There are three subtypes of PP (Table 29.5). Pruritic episodes are unpredictable with abrupt onset and termination, predominantly occurring at the time of relaxation. PP can be generalized or localized. The commonest sites of predilection are legs, arms, back, and genitals. Often there is history of a major psychological stress preceding the onset of PP.[60] A significant number of patients have associated anxiety and/or depression. Detailed cutaneous and systemic examination and routine baseline investigation should be performed to rule out cutaneous and systemic causes of pruritus before diagnosing PP.

Diagnostic Criteria for Psychogenic Pruritus[61]

Three compulsory criteria are as follows:

1. Localized or generalized pruritus sine material
2. Chronic pruritus (>6 weeks)
3. The absence of a somatic cause

Three additional criteria from following seven:

1. A chronological relationship of pruritus with one or several life events that could have psychological repercussions
2. Variations of intensity associated with stress
3. Nocturnal variation
4. Predominance during rest or inaction
5. Associated psychological disorders
6. Pruritus that is improved by psychogenic drugs.
7. Pruritus that is improved by psychotherapy.

Commonest Sites

Legs, Arms, Back and Genitals

Often there is history of a major psychological stress preceding the onset and a significant number of patients have associated anxiety and/or depression. It is diagnosed when other cutaneous and systemic conditions have been ruled out after detailed evaluation and investigations.

Management

Usually psychotherapy helps. In addition, SSRIs are useful.

Dermatitis Para-artefacta Syndrome

In this condition, patient seems to have lost control over manipulation of the skin. A minimal primary lesion is often characteristically excessively traumatized, leading to pronounced, serious clinical findings. Most common underlying psychiatric condition is impulse control disorder.

TABLE 29.5: Subtypes of pychogenic pruritus[62]

Compulsive type	Impulsive type	Mixed type
Skin excoriation performed to avoid anxiety or to prevent a dreaded event elicited by obsession	Skin excoriation linked with arousal, pleasure or reduction of tension	Features of both the other types are present
Executed in full awareness	Executed at times with minimal awareness (automatically)	—
Associated with some resistance to behaviour	Resistance is lesser	

Source: Primary psychiatric disorders—cutaneous manifestations. Ravindra Munoli, Pg 46. Handbook of Psychodermatology by Abdul Latheef EN 2016.

Patterns of Dermatitis Para-artefacta Syndrome

Skin and mucosa	Skin-picking syndrome (epidermotillomania, neurotic excoriations Acne excoriee Pseudo-knucle pads Morsicatio buccarum Chelitis factitia
Integument	Onychophagia Onychotillomania Onychotemnomania Trichotillomania Trichotemnomania Trichoteiromania

Source: Primary Psychiatric disorders-cutaneous manifestations. Ravindra Munoli Handbook of Psychodermatology by Abdul Latheef EN 2016

IMPULSE CONTROL DISORDERS

Trichotillomania: The term trichotillomania (TM) means a compulsive urge to pull out one's hair. It is one of the types of traumatic alopecia. ICD-10 defines it as a disorder characterized by noticeable hair loss due to a recurrent failure to resist impulses to pull out hairs. The revised DSMIV diagnostic criteria suggested for TM are:[63] (A) Recurrent pulling out of one's own hair resulting in hair loss, (B) an increasing sense of tension immediately before pulling out the hair or when attempting to resist the behaviour, (C) pleasure, gratification, or relief when pulling out the hair, (D) the disturbance is not better accounted for by another mental disorder, and (E) the disturbance provokes clinically marked distress and/or impairment in occupational, social, or other areas of functioning. This diagnosis should not be made, if there is a pre-existing inflammation of the skin or if the hair-pulling is in response to a delusion or a hallucination.

The exact incidence in the general population is unclear although was found to be 0.6% among male and female students.[64] There is evidence of bimodal age distribution. Two distinct populations include childhood cases presenting between 5 and 15 years with a good prognosis and adult cases presenting in later life with a relatively poorer outcome.[65,66] Female predominance increases with age. Automatic hair-pulling occurs in approximately three-quarters of adult patients with trichotillomania. TM is seven times more common in children as compared to adults. Childhood cases are habitual disorders with no serious psychopathology, sometimes associated with nail biting and thumb sucking.[67,68] In adults, there is female preponderance, more diversely associated with depression, anxiety disorder, and OCD.[69,70] Hair plucking is most common from the scalp and rarely from eyebrows, eyelashes, pubic hair, and torso hair. Hair loss may be minimal to extensive. There is a typical three-phase zone presentation. Zone 1: Long hair (unremarkable, not affected, normal hair/haircut); Zone 2: Missing hair (recent alopecia due to pulling). Zone 3: Regrowth of hair, shorter and less regular than the normal hair (older, former alopecia areas with irregular hair regrowth after intermittent pulling).

Plucked hairs may be hidden/stored or sometimes swallowed (trichophagia), leading to trichobezoar.[71] Typically, hairs are short, broken, irregular in length, distorted, and feel like stubble. In adults, especially, the loss of hair has psychosocial effects and patients devise means to disguise this defect.

Diagnosis is primarily clinical, but scalp biopsy can be done in ambiguous cases.[72] There will be normally growing hairs amongst the empty anagen hair follicles in a non-inflamed dermis. Trichomalacia (distorted and curled hair bulb), bizarre fractured hair shafts, pigment casts, and perifollicular haematoma are fairly specific for TM.

Psychological basis: Typically it is an impulse control disorder, there is buildup of tension prior to pulling, then plucking hair, followed by relief/pleasure/satisfaction/relaxation. Childhood cases are mostly habitual disorders with no serious psychopathology, sometimes may be associated with nail-biting and thumb sucking. In adults, comorbid conditions are depression, anxiety disorder and OCD. Management in these cases is directed by the age of the patient. Childhood cases have good prognosis.[73,74] Identification of the stressor, parent education, behaviour modification help pre-schoolers to eventually "grow out" of this condition. In adolescents and young adults unaware of their hair pulling, information/awareness of the diagnosis helps in persuading them to seeing a psychiatrist/psychologist and engaging in non-pharmacological management such as cognitive behavioural therapy (CBT). Reassurance that normal hair regrowth is possible, if the hair is left alone is also important.

Pharmacological management: Fluoxetine and clomipramine can be used.[75,76,77]

Prognosis: Childhood/adolescent cases usually have a good prognosis but adults presenting in later life have a relatively poorer outcome.

Trichotemnomania: It is a rare entity, in which the hair is intentionally cut off (Table 29.6).

Trichoteiromania (teiro (Greek)—I scratch): There is a physical damage to the hair by rubbing and scratching the the scalp, resulting in pseudoalopecia (Table 29.6).

SKIN-PICKING SYNDROME (EPIDERMOTILLOMANIA, NEUROTIC EXCORIATIONS)

Neurotic excoriations or pathological skin-picking (Table 29.7) is characterized by an unfounded, untamable urge to scratch the skin accompanied by visible tissue damage and functional impairment.[78] There is female preponderance and average age of onset varies between 30 and 50 years.[77] The exact pathophysiology is elusive; however, psychosocial stress precedes exacerbation in around 30–90% cases.[78,79] There is a compulsive quality and the associated psychological co-morbidity commonly is depression.[80–81] The picking can target real blemishes or imaginary flaws. It can involve

TABLE 29.6: Comparison of trichotillomania, trichotemnomania and trichoteiromania

	Trichotillomania	Trichotemnomania	Trichoteiromania
Injury pattern	Pulling out the hair	Cutting of the hair	Breaking of the hair by scratching
Clinical findings	Typical 3-phase configuration with long, missing and regrowing hair	Pseudoalopecia with hair stubble that appears shaved	Pseudoalopecia with broken hair of normal thickness; hair stubble with whitish-looking ragged ends
Trichogram	Telogen rate reduced	Normal hair root pattern	Dystrophic hair root pattern; sometimes reduced telogen proportion

Source: Primary Psychiatric disorders-cutaneous manifestations. Ravindra Munoli Pg-39. Handbook of Psychodermatology by Abdul Latheef EN 2016

TABLE 29.7: Skin-picking syndrome

Morphology of lesions polymorphic	Sites (accessible areas)	Differential diagnosis
Excoriations, erosions, crusting, atrophic and hyperpigmented scars secondary to self-inflicted trauma	Arms and legs, face (acne excoriee)	Prurigo nodularis Lichen simplex chronicus Insect bite reaction

Source: Primary psychiatric disorders—cutaneous manifestations. Ravindra Munoli Pg 35. Handbook of Psychodermatology by Abdul Latheef EN 2016

picking, pulling, poking, prodding, squeezing, or tearing of the skin. It can be episodic, irregular, or constant. Patients pick at areas until they can pull the material out of the skin, also referred as "pulling a thread from the skin". Patients admit to an urge to pick and gouge (unconscious or deliberate) at their skin unlike patients with dermatitis artefacta. The lesions are polymorphic. Newer lesions are angulated excoriated crusted erosions, while older lesions have depigmented scarred centre and hyperpigmented periphery. Lesion numbers vary from few to hundred and are in all stages of development. Prurigo nodularis is an extreme variant of this entity. Distribution of the lesions reflects their self-inflicted nature with lesions concentrated over the most accessible sites. Neurotic excoriation is differentiated from dermatitis artefacta by its conscious and compulsive nature. However, patient should be evaluated for all cutaneous and systemic causes of pruritus before making this diagnosis.

Psychological basis: Invariably seen in impulse control disorders. Psychosocial stress preceeds excacerbation in around 30–90% cases. Supportive psychotherapy, CBT, and habit reversal programmes along with anti-depressants help all patients.[82]

Acne Excoriee

Acne excoriee is a variant of neurotic excoriation, a form of skin-picking syndrome where patients either have only facial or predominant facial involvement. Few patients develop lesions after picking acne lesions while majority did not have acne at any time. It is commoner in females with a mean age of 30 years. Psychiatric comorbidity includes BDD, depression, anxiety, OCD, delusional disorder, personality disorder, and social phobias. Lesions morphologically resemble chronic excoriation or neurotic excoriations and are found predominantly distributed around the hairline, forehead, preauricular cheek, and chin areas. Minimal lesions are extensively manipulated by squeezing and pressing, usually with the finger nails or sharp instruments by the person. If the patient has concomitant acne, aggressive treatment with systemic antibiotic and/or systemic retinoids must be considered. Topical non-irritating anti-acne drugs should be prescribed. Due to the face involvement, patient feels embarrassed, guilty, stigmatized. Disease coping strategies need to be addressed first.[83,84]

Morsicatio Buccarum

Here patients will have continuous, unconscious sucking and chewing on the oral mucosa. These lead to to benign, sharply demarcated, usually leukodermic lesions around the tooth base and buccal mucosa. Again, compulsive disorders may be the underlying condition. It is found more often among denture wearers without other psychiatric symptoms.

Onychophagia, Onychotillomania, Onychotemnomania

Usually these are behaviours, which are normally seen in population and not disease entities as such. These become troublesome when the behaviour leads to problems in structure or function of nail appendages.

Onychophagia (nail biting or nail chewing): Patient bites, chews and swallows nail fragments. These behaviours may lead to bacterial or fungal infections, inflammation, bleeding and malformations triggered by the repeated trauma, with shortening of the distal nail plate. Usually, it is seen in nearly 45% adolescents, so not everyone with this condition will have underlying psychological problem. In a few cases, unresolved conflicts or tensions may exist.

Onychotillomania: Here trauma of the paranychium or constant manipulation, picking and removal of the cuticle and/or nail is seen as the elicitor of self-induced nail diseases. These may range from onychodystrophy to serious paronychias.

Onychotemnomania: Cutting nails too short leads to traumatization of the nail body or nail fold.

FACTITIOUS SKIN DISEASES/ SELF-INFLICTED DERMATITIS

Factitious disorders (ICD-10: F 68.1, L98.1; DSM-IV, 300.16/300.19) are defined as self-harming behaviours that directly or indirectly cause subjective, clinically-relevant harm without being directly linked to suicidal intent. The prevalence of factitious disorders ranges from 0.05–0.4% in the general population. Except for malingering, this is seen mostly in women (5–8:1) and the onset will be during puberty or early adulthood. The current classification differentiates between four groups:

1. Dermatitis artefacta syndrome—as unconscious/dissociated self-injury
2. Dermatitis para-artefacta syndrome: Disorders of impulse control, often as manipulation of an existing specific dermatoses (often semi-conscious, admitted self-injury)
3. Malingering: Consciously simulated injuries and diseases to obtain material gain
4. Special forms, such as the Gardner-Diamond syndrome, Münchausen syndrome, and Münchausen by proxy syndrome.

Dermatitis Artefacta (DA)

It is a skin disease caused by the deliberate harm by a fully aware patient on skin, hair, nails, or the mucosa. The DSM-IV-TR criteria for factitious disorder include: (a) Intentional feigning of physical or psychological signs or symptoms, (b) the motivation is to assume the sick role, (c) external incentives for the behaviour (such as economic gain, avoiding legal responsibility, or improving physical well-being, as in malingering), are absent. The female to male ratio varies between 20:1 and 4:1, while in children, there is equal sex incidence. Although reported to be more common in health care workers and their families; recent studies do not suggest the same.[85]

The pathophysiology of DA is poorly understood, but may be multifactorial including complex interplay by genetics, psychosocial factors, and personal/family history of psychiatric illness. The underlying psychopathology is assuming a sick role. Affected children have anxiety disorder or immaturity of coping styles in response to dysfunctional parent–child relationship, bullying, sexual, and substance abuse. Adults may be neurotic, depressed, hysterical, or may have paranoid personality disorder.

The two characteristics of DA are the physical signs and the fabrication. The most common site of involvement is face, followed by dorsum of hands and forearm. The lesions are polymorphic, bizarre, clearly demarcated from the surrounding normal skin and can resemble many inflammatory reactions in the skin like ulcerations, deep necrosis, irritant reaction pinpoint scars and star shaped. They are crude, angulated, and have the tendency for linear configuration. They are produced by every known means of damaging the skin. Self-inflicted chemical burn may show a "drip sign". Punched-out necrotic areas or uniform circular blisters or erosions are typical of cigarette burns. Oedema of limbs from tied bands is described as Secretan's syndrome.[86–88] Dramatic dermal induration and necrosis occur from foreign body injection of milk, oil, or grease into breasts, thighs, abdomen, and penis. The other common presentation is chronic, non-healing infected wounds. Infectious complications are of serious nature and sometime supervene. A patient is unable to provide clear history of evolution of the lesions and typically denies any role in the production of the lesions. Lesions evolve overnight without prior signs and symptoms. Phenomenon of La belle indifference is often seen, i.e. patients will explain about their symptoms but appear emotionally uninvolved, as if it is happening to someone else.[89, 90] In dermatitis simulata, the patient uses external disguise to simulate a disease, and there is no significant damage to the skin. Make-up has been used to simulate a rash or a birthmark, and topical printing dyes has been used to produce a discoloured sweat.[91, 92] Bizarre crude presentations are easy to diagnose. At times, lesions mimic specific dermatosis, where a skin biopsy must be considered. Histopathology is usually non-specific, but can sometimes provide supportive information. The behaviour of patient usually occurs in dissociative states, i.e. patient will be unable to remember or remember partially and unanable to comprehend the event emotionally. Doctor should avoid immediate confrontation regarding the suspicion that the lesions are self-inflicted. This can be counter-productive and the patient may flee from the treatment. Clinician needs to build-up a relationship with the patient by frequent visits, symptomatic treatment, and gradually explore the complex personality and behavioural derangement that underlies this condition. Münchausen syndrome is a special form of factitious disorder in which the affected person feigns disease or illness to draw attention or sympathy. Dermatological complaints are uncommon in this syndrome.[93–95]

Prognosis

Mild cases secondary to identifiable psychosocial stressors, usually have a good outcome. However, if associated with chronic dermatologic or medical issues, prognosis is poor. Continuous or repeated episodes of self-mutilation may result in disfiguring scars on exposed areas of the body. Drugs like SSRI, tricyclic antidepressants, typical antipsychotics (pimozide) and atypical antipsychotics (risperidone, olanzapine, etc.) are used.[96–98]

Dissociative Somatization

Symptoms with no explainable underlying physical pathology are commonly encountered in clinical practice such as unexplained cutaneous sensory syndromes, body memories in post-traumatic stress syndrome that manifest as pruritus, urticaria, or angioedema, self-induced dermatoses such as dermatitis artefacta and trichotillomania associated with dissociative states, and BDD, when the patient has a somatic preoccupation involving the skin or hair. About 20% patients of acne have aspects of BDD. These patients are more responsive to active non-pharmacological treatments such as exercise and psychotherapy as compared with pharmacological treatment. Drugs with central nervous system action generally are more effective than those that affect peripheral physiologic function. It should be emphasized that psychiatric referral and consultation should be attempted whenever feasible. Yet, for a significant proportion of patients who refuse psychiatric referral, the judicious use of psychotropic medications by dermatologists may provide much needed assistance in the recovery. Frequent and regular follow-ups of these patients are required to evaluate clinical response or worsening and adverse effects.[99]

Cutaneous phobias: Irrational obsessional fear which causes anxiety. Mole phobia, venereophobia, wart phobia and steroid phobia, fear of emotional display flushing, sweating.

Dermatoses as a Result of Compulsive Disorder

Compulsive thoughts/obsessions are recurrent and persistent thoughts, impulses, or ideations that are intrusive, irrational which elicit pronounced anxiety and great malaise. Compulsive acts are repeated behaviour patterns such as washing the hands, controlling for tidiness, or imagined acts. Compulsive disorders may also be present as comorbidity with certain dermatoses.

Categorization of compulsive disorders:

1. Certain compulsive disorders
   - Washing eczema
   - Primary lichen simplex chronicus
2. Frequent compulsive disorders
   - Trichotillomania
   - Body dysmorphic disorder
   - Cutaneous hypochondrias
   - Special multifactorial dermatoses (anal eczema, seborrhoeic eczema)

Washing Eczema

Here the patient has an obsession of contamination with germ, dirt, infections. This leads to anxiety and distress, to relieve this anxiety, patient repeatedly washes hands, feet, face, etc. The washing practice may be very frequent to the extent of 50–200 times or duration of washing may be more like 5–10 minutes for hand washing, 1 hour for bathing, etc. All these lead to eczematous changes, mycotic infections, nail dystrophies.

Management includes pharmacotherapy with SSRIs, TCAs, and low dose antipsychotics clubbed with cognitive behavioural therapy focussing on exposure to dirt and preventing response of washing.

Primary Lichen Simplex Chronicus

It is a chronic pruritic lichenoid plaque with thickening of the skin areas, which is provoked and maintained by rubbing or scratching. There is primarily an emotional disorder with skin manifestations, occasionally it is associated with atopic eczema.

Sites involved: Posterior neck, extensor aspect of the extremities, axillae and genital area.

Psychiatric symptoms: Obsession of itch and compulsion of scratching are seen.

Differential diagnosis: The group of prurigo diseases (prurigo simplex acuta and prurigo simplex chronica), para-artefactas.

Managements: Pharmacotherapy with SSRIs, TCAs and low dose antipsychotic clubbed with cognitive behavioural therapy focusing on preventive scratching/rubbing.

Secondary Psychiatric Disorders

This category of disorders includes patients who have psychological symptoms secondary to the skin disorder, which is usually chronic and disfiguring, taxing on the patients coping skills and decimating their self-confidence, interpersonal relationships and quality of life. The course of such dermatoses is characterized by exacerbations and remissions and the patient's initial enthusiasm to new treatments wanes off leading to a stage where they have to learn to live with the condition and how successfully they would be able to do this depends on their psychological resources. Skin disorders are rarely life-threatening, but are associated with significant morbidity and bearing on the quality of life. Overall prevalence of psychological disorders among patients with skin disease is 30–60%.[100] These skin problems, especially chronic skin diseases, affecting exposed body parts because of the visibility and resultant disfigurement lead to embarrassment, depression, anxiety, poor self-image, low self-esteem, and suicidal ideation in the patients.[101–103] Also, patients have to commonly face social isolation and discrimination and, at times, have difficulty getting jobs.[104] Many patients are able to cope up with the disease while a few develop secondary psychiatric morbidity. When skin patients were screened for depression, the prevalence of major depressive disorder was found to be 8.4%.[3] The study by Gupta and Gupta showed the prevalence of suicidal ideation as 5.5% and 5.6% in severe psoriasis and acne patients, respectively.[105] A study by Shenoi et al in 2013 showed a prevalence of depression in 17%, adjustment disorder in 5% and anxiety disorder in 2.5 % in all patients attending the psychodermatology clinic.[106] Alcohol abuse is more common in psoriasis patients and the amount of daily intake correlates with the severity of psoriasis and its poor response to treatment.[107,108]

The prevalence of psychosomatic disorders among dermatological patients is more than that of general population and prevalence rates among patients is twice that of outpatients. The prevalence of psychiatric disorders among dermatological patients is slightly higher than that of neurological, oncology and cardiac patients combined. Patients with psoriasis, atopic dermatitis, hand eczema and leg ulcers had highest associations with anxiety and depression and adjustment disorder.

Mattoo et al[109] found 25% of vitiligo patients to have psychiatric morbidity. Majority of the cases had a diagnosis of adjustment disorder. A General Health Questionnaire (GHQ) study assessed psychiatric morbidity rates at 33.63% and 24.7% for vitiligo and psoriasis, respectively.[110] Adjustment disorder (56% vs 62%), depressive episode (22% vs 29%), and dysthymia (9% vs 4%) were the most common psychiatric disorders in vitiligo and psoriasis patients, respectively. Most of the time, patients do not discuss the psychological effects of their disease with the treating physician. If the dermatologist suspects significant secondary psychological morbidity, then interrogation, counselling, psychiatric referral, and help of dermatologic support group should be sought.

The onset of a psychiatric disorder in a patient after a dermatological condition has been diagnosed could be due to the following reasons:

1. ***As a comorbidity:*** The predisposing factors for dermatoses and psychiatric disorder are same. Cytokines and inflammatory factors, which are elevated in conditions like psoriasis, can also predispose to depression; but alopecia areata which does not have abnormal cytokine levels, is also associated with depression; brain-derived neurotrophic factor has been seen to be reduced in vitiligo and depression. Medical conditions like diabetes, hypothyroidism, SLE can cause dermatoses and organic psychiatric disorders secondary to medical cause. Delirium may result from metabolic changes secondary to the dermatological condition.
2. ***As a reaction to dermatoses:*** Skin not only has physiological function but also is an organ of importance for social interaction. The initial social assessment of a person by another is solely based on skin and facial features. Chronic skin diseases are often disfiguring and cause embarrassment and discrimination and social isolation. Person's perception of body image, self-esteem and confidence are lowered and lead to strained relationship with partner and sexual dysfunction.
3. ***Stigma*** is not just external (from the society) but also internal (from the patient). Many patients are able to cope with it, some are unable to and develop depression, anxiety disorders (including social anxiety), adjustment disorders, substance abuse and suicidal ideations. To cope up depends on their childhood experiences and personality traits. Excessive importance to physical attractiveness, sensitivity to criticism , poor self-esteem, inability to maintain relationships, high neuroticism and use of maladaptive defences are some factors that predict poor coping. Patients with psoriasis have high scores of alexithymia deficiency in understanding, processing and describing emotions. This was connected with both anxiety and depression, whereas difficulty in describing was related to anxiety. Psychological morbidity is higher in chronic, resistant and exposed site dermatoses. Associated psychiatric condition results in further worsening of the quality of llife, poor compliance to treatment and poor doctor–patient relationship. Fear of certain medications like corticosteroids, methotrexate and cyclosporine may have a neagative impact on treatment adherence. The dermatological malignancies could be associated with excessive anxiety about recurrence after treatment, body image disturbance after surgery.
4. ***Treatment emergent psychiatric conditions:*** The drugs used for treatment of dermatoses may cause psychiatric symptoms, especially in the elderly, those with pre-existing psychiatric disorder and with polypharmacy. Such adverse effects lead to emotional suffering, increase in disability, length of stay in hospital, mortality (including suicide), non-compliance, lack of recovery from the primary condition , harm

to others and self and increased utilization of health care services.

There are some of the psychological adverse effects of dermatological medications. Management includes substituting with a safer medicine, if possible. In severe cases, psychotropics may be required. Patients who are on medications that are known to cause psychological adverse effects should be screened frequently as depression and anxiety may be not easily detectable.

Management of Psychophysiologic Disorders

Treatment of psychophysiologic conditions involves a two-pronged approach. Firstly, the role of stress in the intiation and exacerbation of the condition has to be ascertained and managed. Secondly and most important is the treatment of the dermatological diseases. Ideally, these patients should be managed in a psychodermatology liaison clinic alongside clinical psychologists and psychiatrists.

Stepwise Plan for Psychophysiologic Disorders

Standard dermatological management: Psychological intervention (depending on the situation, we can use singly or in combination)—psychosomatic primary care, psychoeducation, cognitive behaviour therapy, relaxation therapy, mindful stress reduction , hypnosis, guided imageries, habit reversal, supportive therapy, disease coping skill training, group therapy, family therapy, and psychopharmacotherapy (depending on the psychiatric comorbidity).

Pharmacology management in geriatric psychodermatology: Psychotropic medications play an important and frequently essential role in the treatment of psychodermatologic conditions in the geriatric population.

In many cases, pharmacologic management ideally involves coordination of care with a psychiatrist and concurrent nonpharmacologic treatment.

Psychodermatology patients often decline psychiatric referral, however, because they may present with limited insight into the psychological component of their dermatological symptoms. Therefore, it is helpful for the practicing dermatologist to be knowledgeable about the characteristics of psychotropic medications and their use in elderly patients.

The use of pharmacologic management in geriatric patients requires individualized consideration due to the unique characteristics of this population. Geriatric patients are more likely to have complex medical histories and be prescribed multiple medications than younger patients. Physiologic changes associated with ageing, such as changes in hepatic metabolism, renal clearance, and body composition, are likely to affect the pharmacokinetics and pharmacodynamics of drugs and may increase the sensitivity of elderly patients to the side effects of psychoactive medications.

Further, the dermatologist should be aware that geriatric patients are at an increased risk of falls, particularly if prescribed sedating medications.

Most of the patients with psychocutaneous disorders can be broadly categorized under four diagnoses: (a) Anxiety, (b) depression, (c) psychosis, and (d) OCD. The choice of a psychotropic medication is based primarily on the nature of the underlying psychopathology. The initial and the most important step in successful management of these patients are to establish rapport. It is important to recognize that the patient expects the clinician to treat him or her as having a bonafide skin disease, rather than a psychiatric condition. Patients with psychophysiological disorders or SPsDs usually welcome an opportunity to discuss their psychological status, but patients with PPsDs are extremely resistant to it. It is necessary to start both somatic (i.e. dermatologic) and psychotropic treatment simultaneously in these patients. In PPsD, psychotropic therapy is the mainline of treatment and somatic modalities are supportive. For secondary psychiatric cases, the approach is treating the dermatoses by using a potent therapeutic option because of the great emotional distress suffered by the patient such as the use of isotretinoin for borderline acne with severe psychosocial or occupational impact although there is much debate over the potential psychiatric side-effects of oral isotretinoin as a recent systemic review did not find any conclusive evidence for such an association. Management includes standard psychotropic drugs, placebo effect, suggestion, cognitive-behavioral methods, biofeedback, and hypnosis. Whenever simple measures fail to produce the results desired, combination of drugs or an addition of non-pharmacological therapy may be required. Psychophysiological skin disorders respond to non-pharmacological therapies that counteract stress, supplemented by anxiolytics, or antidepressants when indicated. Treatment of PPsDs that affects the skin often results in improvement of the associated skin disorders.[112,113]

Working classification

A simple classification of psychotropic drugs based on the major actions:

Antipsychotics: Earlier called major tranquilizers. These are drugs used in major psychotic disorders like schizophrenia, bipolar disorder, etc.

Antidepressants: Drugs used for treatment of condition with depressive and anxiety symptoms.

Anxiolytics: For relief of anxiety symptoms.

Mood stabilizers: Drugs used for control of manic phase of bipolar disorders. These are also used for preventing recurrence of mood episodes in such patients.

Anti-parkinsonian agents: Usually used to prevent occurrence of extrapyramidal symptoms in patients who are receiving antipsychotic drugs.

Drugs useful in addictions: Used as anti-craving agents for preventing relapse in addiction medicine.

Drugs Used in Dementia

Adjuvants

Anxiety: Therapeutic modalities for anxiety include BDZ, non-BDZ, and CBT. Risk of dependence on BDZ is quite high; hence, they are indicated only for short-term treatment (2–4 weeks) for severe and disabling symptoms and should be avoided in milder forms. Diazepam, alprazolam, chlordiazepoxide, and clobazam are longer-acting drugs. Lorazepam and oxazepam are shorter-acting compounds with a greater risk of withdrawal symptoms and addiction.

Non-BDZ used in the treatment of anxiety are selective SSRIs (citalopram escitalopram, paroxetine), serotonin-norepinephrine re-uptake inhibitors (SNRIs) (venlafaxine XL, duloxetine), antihistamines (hydroxyzine), beta-blockers (propranolol), and the anti-epileptic pregabalin. Antidepressants and pregabalin are non-addictive, but those with a short half-life (paroxetine) may cause discontinuation symptoms when they are stopped abruptly. In the treatment of anxiety, SSRIs may have to be used in a dose higher than that used in depression. Occasionally, an increase in anxiety symptoms may be observed for 1 week when the SSRIs are initiated.[112,114]

Depression: Depression can be a PPsD or secondary to dermatological condition. Treatment depends on the severity of symptoms; in cases with mild symptoms, if a patient does not wish treatment, then watchful waiting or CBT is recommended. Moderate symptoms can be managed with SSRI and CBT. But in cases with severe symptoms and suicidal ideation admission, antidepressants with possibly electroconvulsive therapy (ECT) are recommended.[115] Currently available antidepressants are equally effective. The clinical response is gradual and usually begins 2–3 weeks after the therapeutic dosage is reached, but for complete therapeutic effectiveness minimum of 6 weeks of full-dose treatment is required. Side-effect profiles and toxicity vary substantially, thus the choice of antidepressant medication depends primarily on tolerability and safety.

Older drugs: Tricyclics—imipramine, amitriptyline, doxepin.

Newer drugs: SSRI—selective serotonin reuptake inhibitors.

Escitalopram, fluoxetine, sertraline, fluvoxamine, newer drugs SNRIs—venlafaxine, duloxetine.

Newer drugs: NASSAs—non-adrenergic and specific serotonergic antidepressants mirtazapine.

DNRI norepinephrine and dopamine reuptake inhibitor—bupropion, SPARI serotonin partial agonist and reuptake inhibitor—vilazodone.

Antipsychotics: Antipsychotics are used in the therapy of psychocutaneous disorders such as delusions of parasitosis, dermatitis artefacta, and monosymptomatic hypochondriasis. Compliance is the most challenging aspect in the management of these patients, as they lack insight. It is difficult to convince them to participate in a behavioral modification or to seek psychiatric advice. Therefore, the goal of the dermatologist is not to relieve the patients of their delusion, but to help them function better with the delusion.

Typical antipsychotics: First generation drugs: Chlorpromazine, trifluperazine, thioridazine, haloperidol, fluphenazine. Second-generation antipsychotics are considered the treatment of choice for patients with psychosis, because of a better side effect profile and compliance. Risperidone, ziprasidone, iloperidone. Other drugs like olanzapine, quietapine, clozapine, newer drugs include: Aripiprazole the main side-effects of these agents are sedation and weight gain; however, aripiprazole and ziprasidone are least likely to cause these effects. Risperidone and olanzapine are useful in patients who are rapidly deteriorating or have a severe negative effect on the quality of life.[112,114,116]

OBSESSIVE COMPULSIVE DISORDER

Disorders like BDD and impulse control disorder (acne excoriee, trichotillomania, onychotillomania, neurodermatitis) are treated on the lines of OCD. The approach to these patients is different from that of the delusional patient, and one may directly confront these patients about their activities. However, we should avoid exacerbating the existing embarrassment in patients. Initially, we should try to build a rapport with them and start by and once patients develop insight into the etiology of their problem, they are more amenable to see a psychiatrist and engage in non-pharmacological management (CBT). For patients who are unwilling or unable to initiate behavioral modification, pharmacological therapy can be helpful.[95] Currently, three SSRIs—fluoxetine, paroxetine, and sertraline—are the first-line therapy for the management of OCD. Patients here often require higher doses and more time to respond than those with depression. Initial response to SSRI may require up to 4–8 weeks, and maximal response may take as long as 20 weeks. The response should be assessed after 6 weeks and then the dose is increased for patients with partial response. If the patient does not respond to 10–12 weeks at therapeutic dosage, a psychiatric referral is required. If it is not feasible, then it is advisable to switch to another SSRI. Therapy should be continued for at least 6 months to 1 year once a therapeutic response is achieved.[90,92] Medications require slow tapering during discontinuation and restarted if symptoms reappear. Behavioral modification is the cornerstone in the management of OCD, therefore, the most effective treatment is a combination of medication and CBT. However, if patients are resistant to psychiatric referral, they should be encouraged to pursue other resources such as self-help books on habit reversal training and/or self-help groups for OCD.[117]

Non-pharmacology Treatments

The aim of psychotherapy is to recognize the emotional issues that may affect the skin problems respond to medical treatment. As there is well-established connection between skin and mind, there is no doubt that many of the dermatological conditions are result of stress. Therefore, intervention needs to target stress, anxiety and worry which may be secondary to skin condition or may lead to aggravation of illness.

There is a significant psychosomatic/behavioral component in many dermatologic conditions, hence complementary non-pharmacological psychotherapeutic interventions like biofeedback, CBT, hypnosis, placebo, and suggestion have positive impacts on many dermatologic disorders. These psychocutaneous modalities cause beneficial modification of immune, autonomic, and endocrine function leading to a decreased release of catecholamines and modification of numerous cytokines and neuropeptides. Moreover, these interventions are reported to enhance compliance with therapeutic regimens, which is a big advantage.[113]

Special Challenges of Psychotherapy with Older Adults

Although psychotherapy has proven to be successful in the treatment of older adults, it is not without some challenges. Sensory decline especially hearing deficit, vision decline, and physical limitations in mobility are the most commonly encountered challenges in practice.

The therapist may have to accommodate to the physical and sensory challenges of their older adult clients in their office setting. For instance, an office should be handicapped friendly, well lit, and should not have loose rugs or other objects crowding the hallways or walking area to avoid any risk of falls. Furthermore, efficient therapy may require a therapist to sit more closer to the patient, face them directly so they can observe the lip movements, speak clearly while emphasizing consonants, and speak in a low pitch voice. Additionally, cognitive decline related with ageing, may cause difficulties in therapy unless therapists help patients develop some techniques to remember and recall the information they are working on. They may have to mutually develop some ways to counter the cognitive problems by using techniques of memory cueing; use of mnemonics, or some other homework assignments to ensure progress.

Another challenge in treating older adults with psychotherapy may arise from complications in scheduling. Older adults may deal with physical frailty and medical issues that may surface from time to time, impacting scheduling because of unexpected cancellations. Also older patients may be dependent on others to come to appointments due to inability to drive. Psychotherapists must be aware of these challenges and be willing to accommodate patients when needed and to provide psychotherapy in an optimal way despite these challenges. On the other hand, psychotherapy can be utilized effectively to enhance compliance in older adults with major health issues including psychodermatological issues of chronic nature requiring strict and multiple regimen of biologic treatments. Psychotherapeutic alliance and support can motivate older adults to adhere to the proposed treatment plan, help them adapt to change in level of functioning, and to move them forward psychologically to accept the consequences of non-adherence with treatment. Lack of mobility remains a challenge in treating older adults with psychotherapy.[118]

Patients may be housebound or even immobilized to the extent that they are confined to their room or bed. This can be very relevant in a patient with illness like severe psoriatic arthropathy. This should not preclude them from engaging in psychotherapy and in fact may be the only outlet they have to engage in a therapeutic alliance besides the visits from nurses and related health care workers. The interactions they have with nurses are generally limited to focus on the task at hand and do not engage or stimulate the patient psychologically.

Medicare covers at-home therapy, and if such service is available psychotherapist should take advantage and strive to engage patients in such therapeutic alliance.

Transference and counter transference can be much more pronounced in working with older adults in comparision to other populations. The older adults are usually not comfortable with the idea of being considered as in need of receiving mental health treatment especially psychotherapy and they may consider it as a sign of weakness, being labeled in certain way or fear of being called—crazy creating transference issues. While on the other hand, therapist specially if they are not used to working with older adults may have difficulties with counter-transference because of unique aspects of treating older adults like concerns about their frailty and physical difficulties, social issues like transportation, insurance issues, etc. causing difficulties in engaging and keeping them in treatment. Younger therapist may have countertransference issue to identifying older patient with their parents, grandparents or teachers which they had difficulties with while growing up.[118,119]

The following psychological interventions will be discussed:

- Habit reversal
- Supportive therapy
- Relaxation procedures
- Cognitive behaviour therapy

Habit reversal is used successfully in the treatment of trichotillomania and body focused repetitive behaviour (skin picking).

It has four important components: Awareness training, competing response, habit control motivation and generalization.

Awareness training is the most important step and aims at the patient being aware of the whole behaviour chain. Patient is trained in performing movements which are in compatible with pulling hair or skin picking, etc. competing response has to be applied before the problemative behaviour occurs. Motivation and social support, regular feedback and positive reinforcement should be given.

Supportive therapy: There are some dermatological conditions in which the damage is irreversible or chronic. These patients loose self-confidence, become dysfunctional and hopeless. Supportive therapy brings about equilibrium by promoting psychological and social adaptation, by restoring and reinforcing abilities to cope with challenges of life which are caused by the illness.

Relaxation procedures: These procedures help to calm down and include muscular relaxation training, autogenic training, biofeedback, meditation, imagery and paced breathing. These techniques basically help the patients to reduce the arousal. Deep state of relaxation could reduce arousal in both central nervous system and autonomic nervous system and as a result it could resort or promote psychological and physical well-being.

Biofeedback: Biofeedback is a non-invasive conditioning technique with wide applications in the field of medicine. It gives feedback about involuntary physiological changes, e.g. electromyography (EMG, muscle tension) and blood flow (temperature) training are the most commonly used modalities. Patients are taught relaxation techniques and their effects can be directly observed by the patients in terms of changes in muscle tension, blood flow, heart rate, or other parameters paralleling desired improvements. Patients are often enthusiastic about this modality because the monitoring and feedback displays suggest that they are receiving a high-tech intervention. Besides the auditory or visual feedback endpoints, the patients also experience/observe enhanced feelings of relaxation, well-being, symptom reduction, and an increased patient's sense of bodily control. BF techniques can be applied in many medical conditions like hypertension, chronic pain, migraine headache and in psychiatric conditions. Biofeedback training encompasses a wide variety of progressive muscle-relaxing techniques, autogenic training, imagery techniques, transcendental, and other meditation techniques as well as other relaxation directed programs (i.e. breathing techniques, self-talk, and others). Relaxation training is primarily directed at minimizing sympathetic reactivity and enhancing parasympathetic function. Biofeedback is useful in skin disorders that have an autonomic nervous system component (Table 29.8), such as biofeedback of galvanic skin resistance (GSR) for hyperhidrosis and biofeedback of skin temperature for Raynaud's syndrome. Using biofeedback, individuals may learn consciously how to alter the autonomic response and with enough repetition (20–40 sessions) may establish new habit patterns. Hypnosis or autogenic training may enhance the effects obtained by biofeedback.[113] An example of autogenic imagery training in a patient of psoriasis can be imagery focused on slowing the hyperproliferating keratinocytes by using guided imagery of a calm, serene, beachside/hill station, and the warm, sun gently soothing, and slowing his racing skin cells.

COGNITIVE BEHAVIOURAL THERAPY (CBT)

The basic assumption of cognitive behaviour therapy is thinking influence our emotions and emotions influence our thinking. So, the aim of the therapy is to modify thinking so that it brings positive changes in emotions. It deals with dysfunctional thought patterns (cognitive) or actions (behavioral) that damage

TABLE 29.8: Non-pharmacological treatment modalities for psychocutaneous disorders

Biofeedback	Cognitive behavioural methods	Hypnosis
Hyperhidrosis	Atopic dermatitis	Atopic dermatitis
Raynaud's phenomenon	Acne excoriee	Acne excoriee
Psoriasis	Factitious cheilitis	Urticarial
Atopic dermatitis	Hyperhidrosis	Onychotillomania
Lichen planus	Lichen simplex	Trichotillomania
Urticaria	Prurigo nodularis	Alopecia areata
Post-herpetic neuralgia	Urticaria	Erythroderma
	Onychotillomania	Congenital ichthyosiform erythroderma of Brocq
	Trichotillomania	Pompholyx
	Body dysmorphic disorder	Hyperhidrosis
	Neurotic excoriation	Pruritus
	Needle phobia	Herpes simplex
		Warts
		Vitiligo
		Glossodynia
		Post-herpetic neuralgia
		Rosacea
		Erythromelalgia
		Recurrent furunculosis

Source: Yadav S et al. Psychodermatology: A comprehensive review. Indian J Dermatol Venereol Leprol 2013; 79:176–92.

the skin or interfere with dermatologic therapy (Table 29.7). There are well-established cognitive models for depression, anxiety, personality and psychosis, etc. In addition to hypnosis, CBT can facilitate aversive therapy and enhance desensitization. The various steps involved are as follows:

- First identify specific problems by listening to the patient's verbalization of thoughts and feelings or by observing behaviors.
- Determine the goals of CBT such as reduction in anxiety or stop a harmful action.
- Develop a hypothesis about the underlying beliefs or environmental events that precede (stimulate), maintain (reinforce), or minimize (extinguish) these thought patterns and behaviours.
- Test the hypothesis of cause and effect by altering the underlying cognitions, the behavior, the environment, or all three, and observe and document the effects on the patient's dysfunctional thoughts, feelings, and actions.
- Revise the hypothesis if the desired results are not obtained or to continue the treatment if the desired results are obtained until the goals of therapy are reached (modified from Levenson and colleagues.[120] The cognitive techniques are used to restructure NAT, beliefs, assumptions and schemes.

Hypnosis: Hypnosis is an intentional induction, deepening, maintenance, and termination of a trance state for a specific purpose. Hypnotic trance can be defined as a heightened state of focus that can be helpful in reducing unpleasant sensations (i.e. pain, pruritus, dysesthesias), while simultaneously inducing favorable physiologic changes. Hypnosis may improve or clear many skin disorders.[121] There are many myths about hypnosis; however, the main purpose of medical hypnotherapy is to reduce suffering, promote healing, or help the person alter a destructive behaviour. Although the exact mechanism is unknown, it can help to regulate blood flow and other autonomic functions that are usually not under conscious control. The relaxation response during hypnosis alters the neurohormonal systems that in turn regulate many body functions. Hypnosis may be used to help control harmful habits such as scratching. It also can be used to provide immediate and long-term analgesia, reduce pruritus, improve recovery from surgery, and facilitate the mind-body connection to promote healing. Although psychotherapeutic interventions have come of age and are being incorporated in all spheres of medicine. These non-pharmacological approaches are currently underused and underpromoted in dermatology especially in our country. Selection of patients is very important as there are subsets who are a more resistant and difficult population such as patients with personality disorders including borderline, narcissistic, and schizotypal disorders and patients with any active psychotic process. Therapeutic success in these patients is not as good as expected; however, they are often the ones in the greatest subjective distress and certainly can profit from any of the described interventions. A multipronged approach to the problem is more effective than using only one mode of treatment. While psychoactive drugs have reasonable efficacy in the areas of anxiety, depression, and psychosis, they also have significant side effects. Use of non-pharmacological therapies can often reduce the amount of conventional drugs required, thereby reducing side effects while synergistically contributing to effectiveness. All these interventions require more commitment and lifestyle changes than just swallowing a drug, but the side effects are far less and the benefits often are greater than with a drug.

Complementary psychocutaneous therapies: These include herbs and supplements, lavender oil aromatherapy, passion flower, St. John's wort, S-adenosyl-L-methionine (SAM), and melatonin (Table 29.9).[112,113,122,123] The role of these interventions is rather ill-defined and

TABLE 29.9: Pharmacological complementary psychocutaneous therapies

Therapy	Indications
Lavender oil aromatherapy/magnolia bark	Anxiety
Lemon balm/passion flower	Nervousness and insomnia
St. John's wort	Depression
S-adenosyl-L-methionine (SAM)	Depression
Melatonin/valerian	Insomnia due to nervousness

Source: Yadav S, et al. Psychodermatology: A comprehensive review. Indian J Dermatol Venereol Leprol 2013; 79:176–92.

vague. They have been used as anxiolytics, antidepressants, soporifics, and few studies have compared these with standard therapies; however, it is difficult to interpret these studies due to variable results, heterogenous designs, and end points. An analysis of 29 clinical trials with more than 5000 patients was conducted by Cochrane collaboration.[124] The review concluded that extracts of St. John's wort were superior to placebo in patients with major depression. St. John's wort had similar efficacy to standard antidepressants. The rate of side-effects was half that of newer SSRI antidepressants and onefifth that of older tricyclic antidepressants.[4] The exact mechanism by which St. John's wort functions is unclear and subject to conjecture. Its mechanism is believed to involve inhibition of serotonin (5-HT) reuptake, much like the conventional SSRIs. The major active antidepressive constituents in St. John's wort are believed to be hyperforin and hypericin. Standardized extracts are available in the form of tablets, capsules, teabags, and tinctures. Most studies of St. John's wort for treating depression used doses varying from 300–1,800 mg daily. Similarly, a meta-analysis of studies that compared SAM with controls showed significant clinical improvement with SAM similar to that of the standard SSRI treatment with fewer side effects.

Epigenetics is a new concept in the arena of psychiatry that suggests novel pathophysiology and entirely new approach to prevention and treatment of various psychosomatic disorders.[19] Epigenetics suggests that there is a regulation of gene expression via molecular mechanisms (DNA methylation, histone modification, and microRNA dysregulation) in response to environmental stimuli, drugs, and chemicals and that epigenomes reside at the interface between genome and the environment. This field is still in its infancy, but has added newer dimension to our understanding of comorbidity and multimorbidity in psychosomatic medicine. It has great potential to explain how external factors can affect our genes and possibly lead to various diseases.

References

1. Yadav S, Narang T, Kumaran M S. Psychodermatology: A comprehensive review. Indian J Dermatol Venereol Leprol. 2013; 79:176–92.
2. Picardi A, Abeni D, Melchi CF, Puddu P, Pasquini P. Psychiatric morbidity in dermatological outpatients: an issue to be recognized. Br. J. Dermatol. 2000; 143(5):983–91.
3. Picardi A, Adler DA, Abeni D, Chang H, Pasquini P, Rogers WH, et al. Screening for depressive disorders in patients with skin diseases: A comparison of three screeners. Acta Derm Venereol. 2005; 85:414–9.
4. Katon WJ. Epidemiology and treatment of depression in patients with chronic medical illness. Dialogues Clin Neurosci 2011; 13:7–23.
5. Johnson TJ, Basu S, Pisani BA, Avery EF, Mendez JC, Calvin JE Jr, et al. Depression predicts repeated heart failure hospitalizations. J Card Fail. 2012; 18:246–52.
6. O'Sullivan RL, Lipper G, Lerner EA. The neuro-immunocutaneous-endocrine network: Relation-

ship of mind and skin. Arch Dermatol. 1998; 134:1431–5.

7. Slominski A, Pisarchik A, Zbytek B, Tobin DJ, Kauser S, Wortsman J. Functional activity of serotoninergic and melatoninergic systems expressed in the skin. J Cell Physiol. 2003; 196:144–53.
8. Azmitia EC. Serotonin neurons, neuroplasticity, and homeostasis of neural tissue. Neuropsychopharmacology. 1999; 21:S33–45.
9. Arck PC, Slominski A, Theoharides TC, Peters EM, Paus R. Neuroimmunology of stress: Skin takes center stage. J Invest Dermatol. 2006; 126: 1697–704.
10. Nemiah JC, Sifneos PE. Psychosomatic illness: A problem in communication. Psychother Psychosom. 1970; 18:154–60
11. Taylor GJ, Bagby RM. New trends in alexithymia research. Psychother Psychosom. 2004; 73:68–77.
12. Sayar K, Köse O, Ebrinç S, Setin M. Hopelessness, depression and alexithymia in young Turkish soldiers suffering from alopecia areata. Dermatol Psychosom 2001; 2:12–5.
13. Richards HL, Fortune DG, Griffiths CE, Main CJ. Alexithymia in patients with psoriasis: Clinical correlates and psychometric properties of the Toronto Alexithymia Scale-20. J Psychosom Res. 2005; 58:89–96.
14. Maniaci G, Epifanio MS, Marino MA, Amoroso S. The presence of alexithymia investigated by the TAS-20 in chronic urticaria patients: A preliminary report. Allerg Immunol (Paris), 2006; 38:15–9.
15. Picardi A, Pasquini P, Cattaruzza MS, Gaetano P, Melchi CF, Baliva G, et al. Stressful life events, social support, attachment security and alexithymia in vitiligo. A case-control study. Psychother Psychosom. 2003; 72:150–8.
16. Griffiths CE, Richards HL. Psychological influence in psoriasis Clin Exp Dermatol. 2001; 26:338–342.
17. Harvima RJ, Viinamak H, Harvima IT, et al. Association of psychic stress with clinical severity and symptoms of psoriatric patients. Acta Derm Venereol. 1996; 76:467–471.
18. Gupta MA, Gupta AK.Psoriasis and sex: a study of moderately to severely affected patients. Int J Dermatol. 1997; 36:259–262.
19. Ginsburg IH, Link BG. Feelings of stigmatization in patients with psoriasis. J Am Acad Dermatol 1989; 20:53–63.
20. Gupta MA, Gupta AK, Ellis CN, et al. Some psychosomatic aspects of psoriasis. Adv Dermatol. 1990; 5:21–30.
21. Ito.T. Recent advances in the pathogenesis of autoimmune hair loss disease alopecia areata. J Immunol Res 2013, http: //dx.doi.org/10.1155/2013/348546.
22. Peters EM, Imfeld D, Graub R. Graying of the human hair follicle. J. Cosmet. Sci. 2011 Mar.-Apr.; 62(2):121–5.
23. Shi Y, Luo LF, Liu X M, Zhou Q, Xu SZ, Lei TC. Premature graying as a consequence of compromised antioxidant activity in hair bulb melanocytes and their precursors. PLoS One, 2014; 9(4):e93589.
24. Ortonne JP, Thivolet J, Guillet R. Graying of hair with age and sympathectomy. Arch. Dermatol., 1982 Nov.; 118(11):876-7.
25. Otberg N., Finner A. M., Shapiro J. Androgenetic alopecia. Endocrinol. Metab. Clin. North Am. 2007 Jun.; 36(2):379–98.
26. Wang TL, Zhou C, Shen YW, Wang XY, Ding X. L, Tian S, et al. Prevalence of androgenetic alopecia in China: a community-based study in six cities. Br. J. Dermatol. 2010 Apr.; 162(4):843-7.
27. Shin H, Jo SJ, Kim DH, Kwon O, Myung SK. Efficacy of interventions for prevention of chemotherapy-induced alopecia: A systematic review and meta-analysis. Int. J. Cancer, 2014 Aug. 1.
28. Trueb R. M. Chemotherapy-induced alopecia. Curr. Opin. Support Palliat. Care, 2010 Dec.; 4(4):281–4.
29. Can G, Demir M, Erol O, Aydiner A. A comparison of men and women's experiences of chemotherapy–induced alopecia. Eur. J. Oncol. Nurs., 2013 Jun.; 17(3):255–60.
30. Jafferany M. Psychodermatology: A Guide to Understanding Common Psychocutaneous Disorders. Prim Care Companion J Clin Psychiatry. 2007; 9(3):203–213.
31. Gil KM, Keefe FJ, Sampson HA, et al. The relation of stress and family environment to atopic dermatitis symptoms in children. J Psychosom Res. 1987; 31:673–684.

32. Schut C, Bosbach S, Gieler U, Kupfer J. Personality traits, depression and itch in patients with atopic dermatitis in an experimental setting: A regression analysis. Acta Derm Venereol. 2014; 94:20–25.
33. Kreydon OP, Heckmann M, Peschen M. Delusional hyperhidrosis as a risk for medical overtreatment: a case of botuliniphilia. Arch Dermatol. 2002; 138:538–539.
34. Davidson JR, Foa EB, Connor KM, et al. Hyperhidrosis in social anxiety disorder. Prog Neuropsychopharmacol Biol Psychiatry, 2002; 26: 1327–1331.
35. Gupta MA, Gupta AK, Schork NJ, et al. Depression modulates pruritus perception: a study of pruritus in psoriasis, atopic dermatitis, and chronic idiopathic urticaria. Psychosom Med. 1994; 56:36–40.
36. Sainz B, Loutsch JM, Marquart ME, et al. Stress associated immunomodulation and herpes simplex virus infection. Med Hypotheses. 2001; 56:348–356.
37. Manolache L, Benea V. Stress in patients with alopecia areata and vitiligo. J Eur Acad Dermatol Venereol. 2007; 21:921–8.
38. Poli F, Dreno B, Verschoore M. An epidemiological study of acne in female adults: Results of a survey conducted in France. J Eur Acad Dermatol Venereol. 2001; 15:541–5.
39. Jaworek AK, Wojas-Pelc A, Pastuszczak M. [Aggravating factors of rosacea]. Przegl Lek. 2008; 65:180–3.
40. Hebbar S, Ahuja N, Chandrasekaran R. High prevalence of delusional parasitosis in an Indian setting. Indian J Psychiatry. 1999; 41:136–9.
41. Phillips KA, Menard W, Pagano ME, Fay C, Stout RL. Delusional versus nondelusional body dysmorphic disorder: Clinical features and course of illness. J Psychiatr Res. 2006; 40:95–104.
42. Otto MW, Wilhelm S, Cohen LS, Harlow BL. Prevalence of body dysmorphic disorder in a community sample of women. Am J Psychiatry 2001; 158:2061–3.
43. Veale D. Body dysmorphic disorder. Postgrad Med J 2004;80: 67–75. 33. Phillips KA, Menard W, Fay C. Gender similarities and differences in 200 individuals with body dysmorphic disorder. Compr Psychiatry. 2006;47:77–87.
44. Crerand CE, Franklin ME, Sarwer DB. Body dysmorphic disorder and cosmetic surgery. Plastic Reconstr Surg. 2006; 118:167e–80.
45. Veale D, Boocock A, Gournay K, Dryden W, Shah F, Willson R, et al. Body dysmorphic disorder: A survey of fifty cases. Br J Psychiatry, 1996; 169: 196–201.
46. Phillips KA, Menard W. Suicidality in body dysmorphic disorder: A prospective study. Am J Psychiatry, 2006; 163:1280–2.
47. Phillips KA. Treating body dysmorphic disorder using medication. Psychiatr Ann 2004; 34:945–52.
48. Gupta, MA, and Gupta, AK. Evaluation of cutaneous body image dissatisfaction in the dermatology patient. Clinics in Dermatology, 21013; 31(1), 72–79.
49. Gupta MA. Somatization disorders in dermatology. Int Rev Psychiatry, 2006; 18:41–7.
50. Koo J, Gambla C. Cutaneous sensory disorder. Dermatologic clinics, 1996; 14:497–502.
51. Cotterill JA. Dermatological non-disease. Dermatology nursing/Dermatology Nurses' Association, 1981; 3:315–7.
52. Bergdahl M, Bergdahl J. Burning mouth syndrome: prevalence and associated factors. Journal of oral pathology and medicine: official publication of the International Association of Oral Pathologists and the American Academy of Oral Pathology, 1999; 28:350–4.
53. Grushka M. Clinical features of burning mouth syndrome. Oral surgery, oral medicine, and oral pathology, 1987; 63:30–6.
54. Hoss D, Segal S. Scalp dysesthesia. Archives of dermatology 1998; 134:327–30.
55. McKay M. Dysesthetic (essential) vulvodynia. Treatment with amitriptyline. The Journal of reproductive medicine, 1993; 38:9–13.
56. Park KK, Koo J. Use of psychotropic drugs in dermatology: unique perspectives of a dermatologist and a psychiatrist. Clinics in dermatology, 2013; 31:92–100.
57. Nagashima W, Kimura H, Ito M, Tokura T, Arao M, Aleksic B, et al. Effectiveness of duloxetine for the treatment of chronic nonorganic orofacial pain. Clinical neuropharmacology, 2012; 35:273–7.

58. Miranda Sivelo A, Nunez Rodriguez MH. Venlafaxine for depression and glossovulvodynia: a case report. Primary care companion to the Journal of clinical psychiatry 2010;12.
59. Ventolini G, Barhan S, Duke J. Vulvodynia, a stepwise therapeutic prospective cohort study. Journal of obstetrics and gynaecology: the journal of the Institute of Obstetrics and Gynaecology 2009; 29:648–50.
60. Misery L, Alexandre S, Dutray S, Chastaing M, Consoli SG, Audra H, et al. Functional itch disorder or psychogenic pruritus: Suggested diagnosis criteria from the French psychodermatology group. Acta Derm Venereol. 2007; 87:341–4.
61. Radmanesh M, Shafei S. Underlying psychopathologies of psychogenic pruritic disorders. Dermatol Psychosom. 2001; 2:130–3.
62. Gieler U, Neimeir V. Psychosomatic aspects of pruritus. Dermatol Psychosom. 2002; 3:6–13.
63. American Psychiatric Association. Diagnostic and Statistical Manual of Mental Disorders. DSM-IV, 4th ed. Text revision. Washington DC: American Psychiatric Press, Inc.; 2000.
64. Christenson GA, Pyle RL, Mitchell JE. Estimated lifetime prevalence of trichotillomania in college students. J Clin Psychiatry, 1991; 52:415–7.
65. Swedo SE, Rapoport JL. Annotation: Trichotillomania. J Child Psychol Psychiatry, 1991;32:401–9.
66. Christenson GA, Mackenzie TB, Mitchall JE. Characteries of 60 adult chronic hair pullers. Am J Psychiatry, 1991; 148:365–70.
67. Keren M, Ron-Miara A, Feldman R, Tyano S. Some reflections on infancy-onset trichotillomania. Psychoanal Study Child 2006; 61:254–72.
68. Demaret A. Nail-biting, hair-plucking, and grooming. Ann Med Psychol (Paris), 1973; 2: 235–42. 44. Hautmann G, Hercogova J, Lotti T. Trichotillomania. J Am Acad Dermatol. 2002; 46:807–26.
69. Cohen LJ, Stein DJ, Simeon D, Spadaccini E, Rosen J, Aronowitz B, et al. Clinical profile, comorbidity, and treatment history in 123 hair pullers: A survey study. J Clin Psychiatry, 1995; 56:319–26.
70. Radmanesh M, Shafiei S, Naderi AH. Isolated eyebrow and eyelash trichotillomania mimicking alopecia areata. Int J Dermatol. 2006; 45:557–60.
71. Kohler JE, Millie M, Neuger E. Trichobezoar causing pancreatitis: First reported case of Rapunzel syndrome in a boy in North America. J Pediatr Surg. 2012; 47:e17–9.
72. Muller SA. Trichotillomania: A histopathologic study in sixty-six patients. J Am Acad Dermatol. 1990; 23:56–62.
73. Dougherty DD, Loh B, Jenike MA, Keuthen NJ. Single modality versus dual modality treatment for trichotillomania: Sertraline, behavioral therapy, or both? J Clin Psychiatry, 2006; 67:1086–92.
74. Bloch MH, Landeros-Weisenberger A, Dombrowski P, Kelmendi B, Wegner R, Nudel J, et al. Systematic review: Pharmacological and behavioural treatment for trichotillomania. Biol Psychiatry, 2007; 62:839–46
75. Bruce TO, Barwick LW, Wright HH. Diagnosis and management of trichotillomania in children and adolescents. Paediatr Drugs, 2005; 7:365–76.
76. Gupta MA, Gupta AK. The use of psychotropic drugs in dermatology. Dermatol Clin. 2000; 18:711–25.
77. Franklin ME, Zagrabbe K, Benavides KL. Trichotillomania and its treatment: A review and recommendations. Expert Rev Neurother. 2011; 11:1165–74.
78. Flessner CA, Woods DW. Phenomenological characteristics, social problems, and the economic impact associated with chronic skin picking. Behav Modif. 2006; 30:944–63.
79. Fruensgaard K. Neurotic excoriations. Int J Dermatol. 1978; 17:761–7. 56. Gupta MA, Gupta AK, Haberman HF. Neurotic excoriations: A review and some new perspectives. Compr Psychiatry, 1986; 27:381–6.
80. Arnold LM, Auchenbach MB, McElroy SL. Psychogenic excoriation. Clinical features, proposed diagnostic criteria, epidemiology and approaches to treatment. CNS Drugs, 2001; 15:351–9.
81. Arnold LM. Phenomenology and therapeutic options for dermatotillomania. Expert Rev Neurother. 2002; 2:725–30.
82. Bloch MR, Elliott M, Thompson H, Koran LM. Fluoxetine in pathologic skin-picking: Open-label and double-blind results. Psychosomatics 2001; 42:314–9.

83. Wrong NM. Excoriated acne of young females. AMA Arch Derm Syphilol. 1954; 70:576–82.

84. Sneddon J, Sneddon I. Acne excoriée: A protective device. Clin Exp Dermatol. 1983; 8:65–68.

85. Millard L. Dermatitis artefacta in the 1990s. Br J Dermatol. 1996; 135:27.

86. Koblenzer CS. Dermatitis artefacta: Clinical features and approaches to treatment. Am J Clin Dermatol. 2000; 1:47–55.

87. Verraes-Derancourt S, Derancourt C, Poot F, Heenen M, Bernard P. Dermatitis artefacta: Retrospective study in 31 patients. Ann Dermatol Venereol. 2006; 133:235–8.

88. Rogers M, Fairley M, Santhaman R. Artefactual skin disease in children and adolescents. Australas J Dermatol. 2001; 42:264–70.

89. Smith RJ. Factitious lymphedema of the hand. J Bone Joint Surg Am. 1975; 57:89–94.

90. Behar TA, Anderson EE, Barwick WJ, Mohler JL. Sclerosing lipogranulomatosis. A case report of scrotal injection of automobile transmission fluid and literature review of subcutaneous injection of oils. Plast Reconstr Surg. 1993; 91:352–61.

91. Angus JE, Affleck AG, Leach IH, Millard LG. Factitious disease presenting as nonhealing wounds. J Eur Acad Dermatol Venereol 2005;19:70.

92. Murray SJ, Ross JB, Murray AH. Life-threatening dermatitis artefacta. Cutis, 1987; 39:387–8.

93. Vrij A, Mann S. Non-verbal and verbal characteristics of lying. In: Halligan P, Bass C, Oakley D, editors. Malingering and Illness Deception. Oxford: Oxford University Press; 2003: pp. 351–4.

94. King CM, Chalmers RJ. Another aspect of contrived disease: "Dermatitis simulata". Cutis, 1984; 34: 463–4.

95. MacSween RM, Millard LG. A green man. Arch Dermatol. 2000; 136:115–118.

96. McSween R, Stevens A, Millard L. Sex, lies and dermatopathology. Br J Dermatol. 1996; 135:27.

97. Gattu S, Rashid RM, Khachemoune A. Self-induced skin lesions: A review of dermatitis artefacta. Cutis, 2009; 84:247–51.

98. Koblenzer CS. Dermatitis artefacta. Clinical features and approaches to treatment. Am J Clin Dermatol. 2000; 1:47–55.

99. Henningsen P, Zipfel S, Herzog W. Management of functional somatic syndromes. Lancet, 2007; 369:946–55.

100. Picardi A, Abeni D, Melchi CF, Puddu P, Pasquini P. Psychiatric morbidity in dermatological outpatients: An issue to be recognized. Br J Dermatol. 2000; 143:983–91.

101. Saitta P, Keehan P, Yousif J, Way BV, Grekin S, Brancaccio R. An update on the presence of psychiatric comorbidities in acne patients, Part 2: Depression, anxiety, and suicide. Cutis, 2011; 88:92–7.

102. Shulman LH, DeRogatis L, Spielvogel R, Miller JL, Rose LI. Serum androgens and depression in women with facial hirsutism. J Am Acad Dermatol. 1992; 27:178–81.

103. Picardi A, Mazzotti E, Pasquini P. Prevalence and correlates of suicidal ideation among patients with skin disease. J Am Acad Dermatol. 2006; 54:420–6.

104. Adam JE, Weatherhead L. Lamellar ichthyosis in a recluse. Int J Dermatol. 1983; 22:427–9.

105. Gupta MA, Gupta AK. Depression and suicidal ideation in dermatology patients with acne, alopecia areata, atopic dermatitis and psoriasis. Br J Dermatol. 1998; 139:846–50.

106. Shenoi SD, Prabhu S, Nirmal B, Petrowala S. Our experience in a psychodermatology liaison clinic at Manipal, India. Indian Journal of Dermatology. 2013; 58(1):53.

107. Hill L, Kennedy P. The role of coping strategies in mediating subjective disability in psoriasis. Psychol Health Med. 2002; 7:261–9.

108. Gupta MA, Schnork NJ, Gupta AK, Ellis CN. Alcohol intake and treatment responsiveness of psoriasis: A prospective study. J Am Acad Dermatol. 1993; 28:730–2.

109. Mattoo SK, Handa S, Kaur I, Gupta N, Malhotra R. Psychiatric morbidity in vitiligo: Prevalence and correlates in India. J Eur Acad Dermatol Venereol. 2002; 16:573–8.

110. Mattoo SK, Handa S, Kaur I, Gupta N, Malhotra R. Psychiatric morbidity in vitiligo and psoriasis: A comparative study from India. J Dermatol. 2001; 28:424–32.

111. Picardi A, Lega I, Tarolla E. Suicide risk in skin disorders. Clinics in Dermatology, 2013; 31(1): 47–56.

112. Shenefelt PD. Therapeutic management of psychodermatological disorders. Expert Opin Pharmacother. 2008; 9:973–85.
113. Fried RG. Nonpharmacologic treatment in psychodermatology. Dermatol Clin. 2002; 20:177–85.
114. Lee CS, Koo JY. The use of psychotropic medications in dermatology. In: Koo JY, Lee CS, editors, Psychocutaneous medicine. New York: Marcel Dekker; 2003: pp. 427–51.
115. National Institute for Health and Clinical Excellence. Depression: Management of Depression in Primary and Secondary Care. Clinical Guideline 23 (Amended). Available from: http://www.nice.org.uk/nicemedia/pdf/CG23quickrefguideamended.pdf. [Last accessed on 2012 Jun 22].
116. Lee CS, Koo J. Psychopharmacologic therapies in dermatology: An Update. Dermatol Clin. 2005; 23:735–44.
117. Rasmussen SA, Eisen JL. Treatment strategies for chronic and refractory obsessive-compulsive disorder. J Clin Psychiatry, 1997; 58:9–13.
118. Morgan AC. Psychodynamic psychotherapy with older adults. Psychiatric Services. 2013; 54(12): 1592–94.
119. Dewald PA. Principles of supportive psychotherapy. Am. J. Psychotherapy, 1994; 48(4): 505–18.
120. Levenson H, Persons JB, Pope KS. Behavior therapy and cognitive therapy. In: Goldman HH, editor. Review of General Psychiatry. 5th ed. New York: McGraw-Hill; 2000: pp. 472.
121. Shenefelt PD. Hypnosis in dermatology. Arch Dermatol. 2000; 136:393–9.
122. Levin C, Maibach H. Exploration of "alternative" and "natural" drugs in dermatology. Arch Dermatol. 2002; 138:207–11.
123. Bedi MK, Shenefelt PD. Herbal therapy in dermatology. Arch Dermatol. 2002; 138: 232–42.
124. Linde K, Berner MM, Kriston L. St John's wort for major depression. Cochrane Database Syst Rev. 2008:CD000448.

CHAPTER 30

Dermoscopy of Common Dermatological Disorders in the Geriatric Age Group

• Samipa S Mukherjee • Subrata Malakar

Introduction

Dermoscopy is a non-invasive diagnostic modality first used for the diagnosis of melanoma, however, over the last decade its utility in various dermatological disorders is being explored. It is advantageous over histopathology in being non-invasive, an office based *in vivo* procedure with zero downtime. It helps not only in diagnosis but also is a great tool to convince the patient with regards to diagnosis, monitor the treatment improvement and serves as an adjunctive tools in patients where biopsy may not be feasible. In the elderly the levels of anxiety, comorbidities and multiple ongoing medications and polypharmacy may limit the usage of an invasive investigative technology thereby giving dermoscopy an edge over the conventional diagnostic modalities.

INFECTIONS AND INFESTATIONS

Molluscum Contagiosum

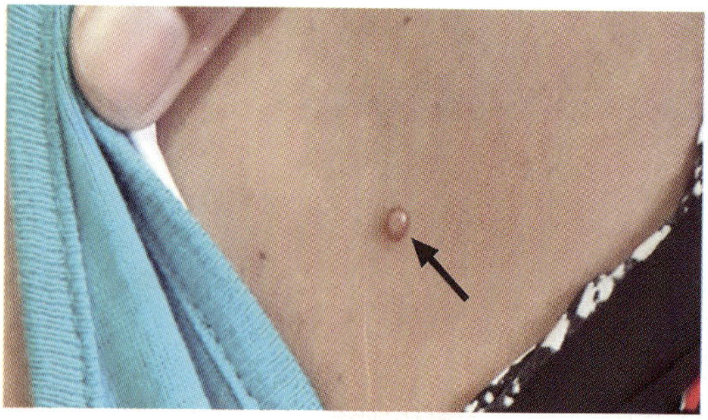

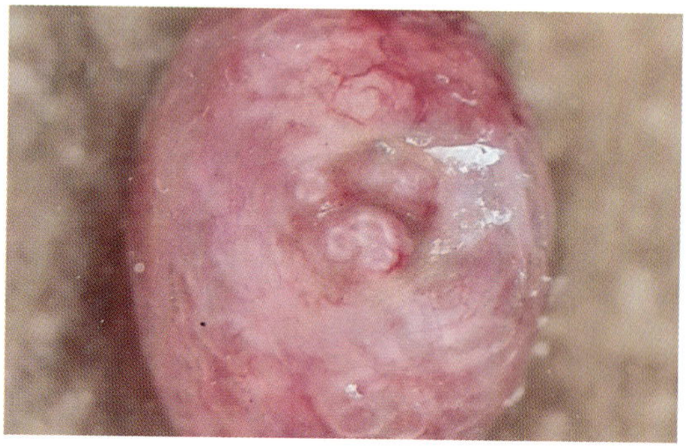

Key Observation Points

- Crown vessels
- Central white amorphous material
- Additionally rosettes were also seen.

Viral Warts

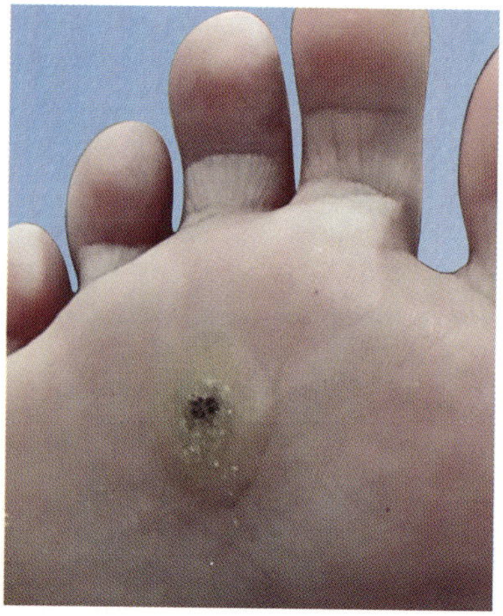

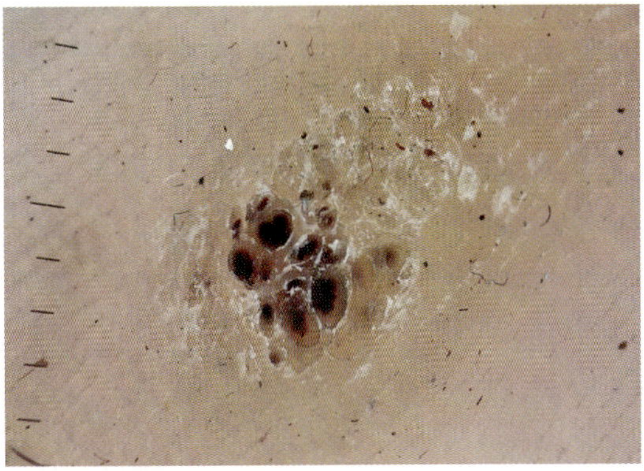

Key Observation Points

- Irregularly distributed red/brown/black dots, loops or linear streaks
- Keratotic halo
- Verrucous yellowish structureless area
- Disruption of dermatoglyphics

Filiform Warts

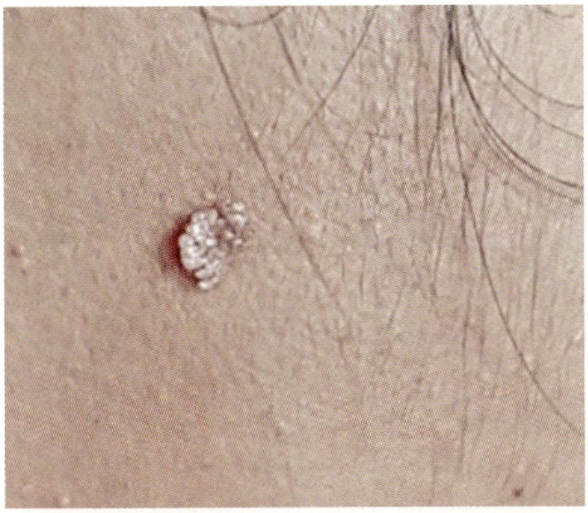

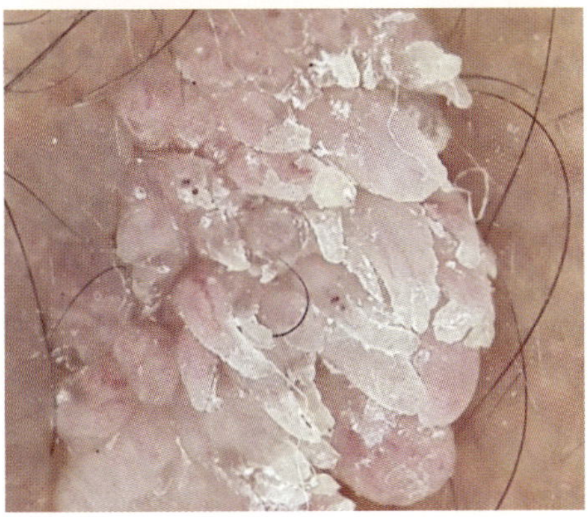

Key Observation Points

- Finger-like projections
- Knob-like projections
- Hairpin vessels

Scabies

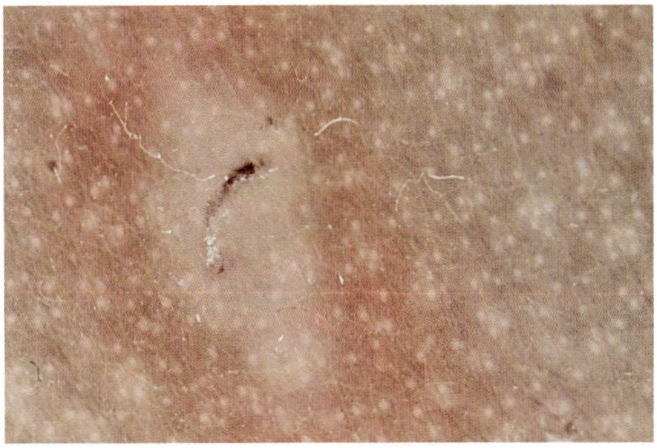

Key Observation Points

- Burrows
- A black dot at the end of the burrow represents the mite
- Delta wing jet, transluscent scabies body and scabious eggs

Pediculosis

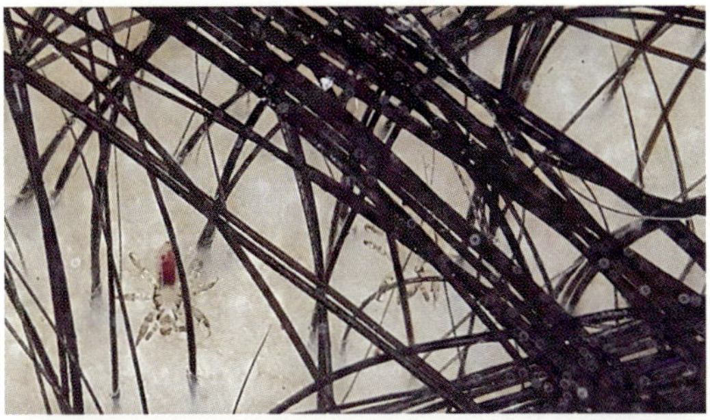

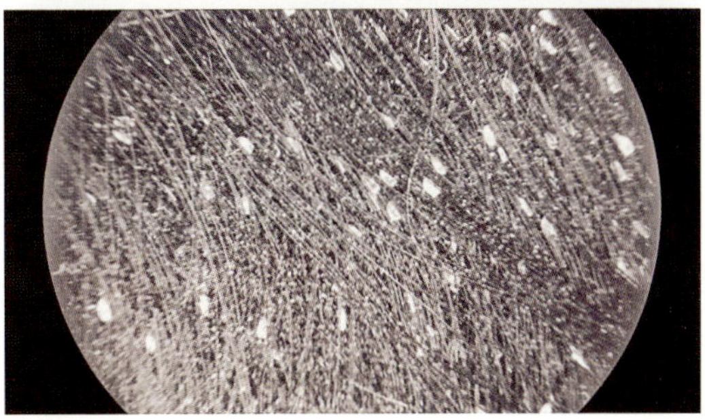

Key Observation Points

- Nit—louse egg attached to hair shaft.
- Nit cast—empty egg appearing as a translucent structure fixed to a hair shaft.
- Head louse

INFLAMMATORY CONDITIONS

Psoriasis

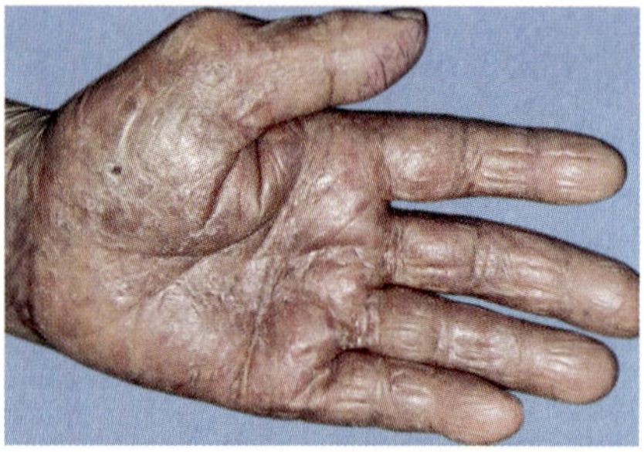

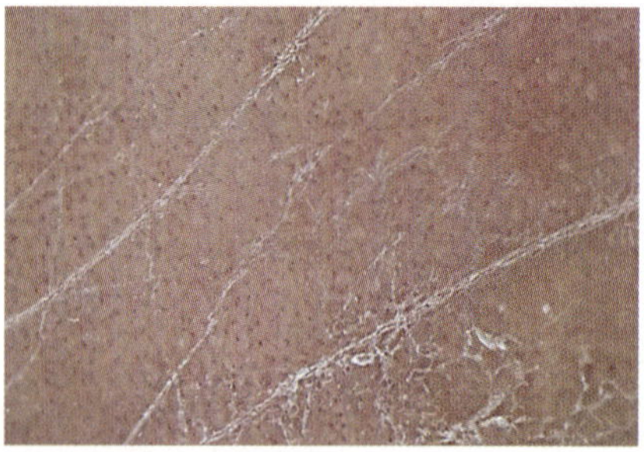

Key Observation Points

- Sheets of red dots and globules throughout the lesions
- Presence of white micaceous scales

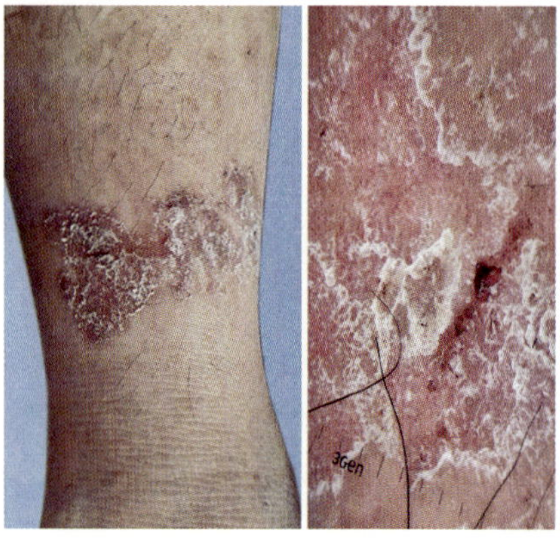

Key Observation Points

- Regularly distributed dotted vessels
- White scales
- Dermoscopic 'Auspitz sign'

Lichen Planus

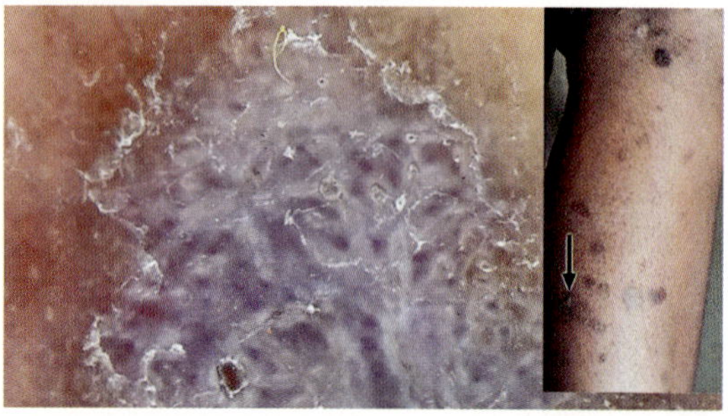

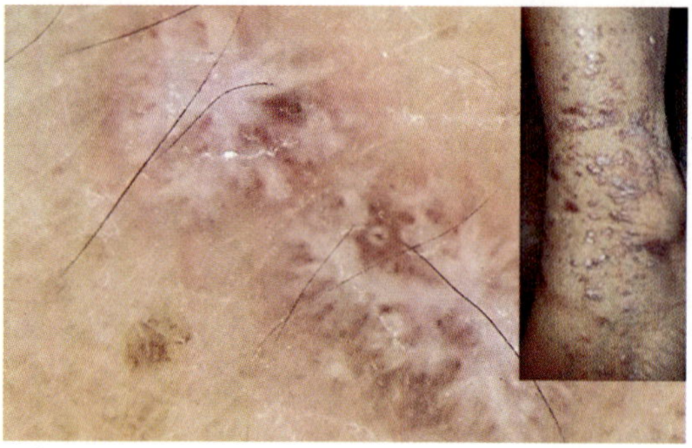

Key Observation Points

- Wickham's striae (WS)
- Dotted/linear vessels at the periphery of the lesion
- Structureless homogeneous brown-gray areas or gray dots in regressing lesions of lichen planus
- Comedo-like structures in hypertrophic lichen planus

Eczema

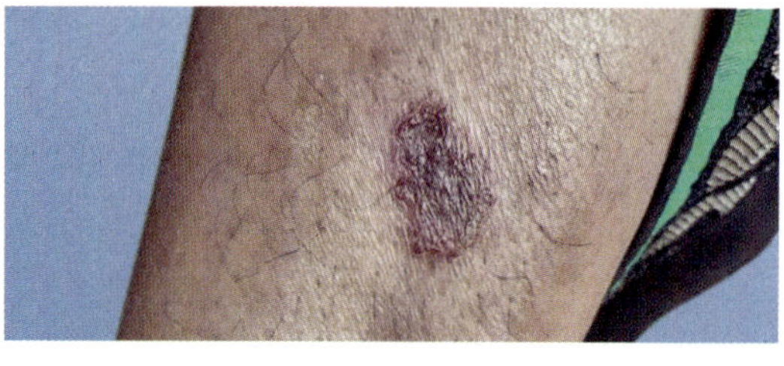

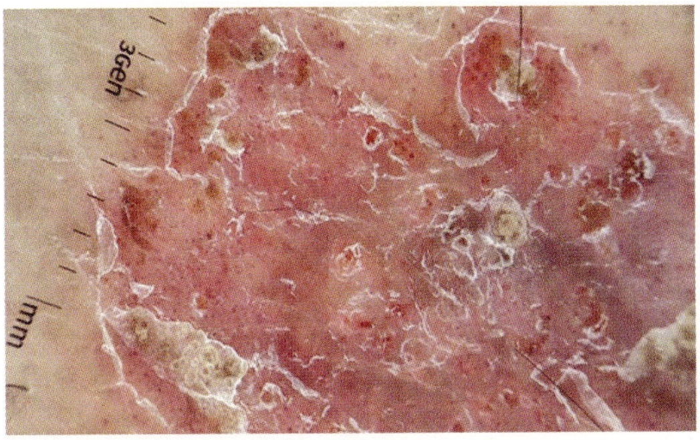

Key Observation Points

- Dotted vessels in a patchy distribution
- Yellow clods (serocrusts)

Lichen Sclerosus et Atrophicus

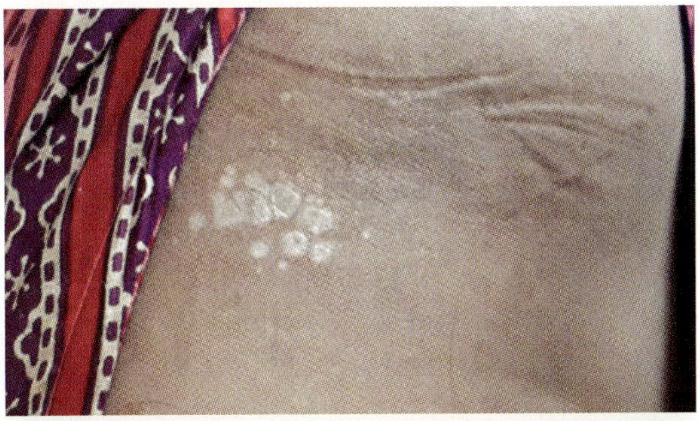

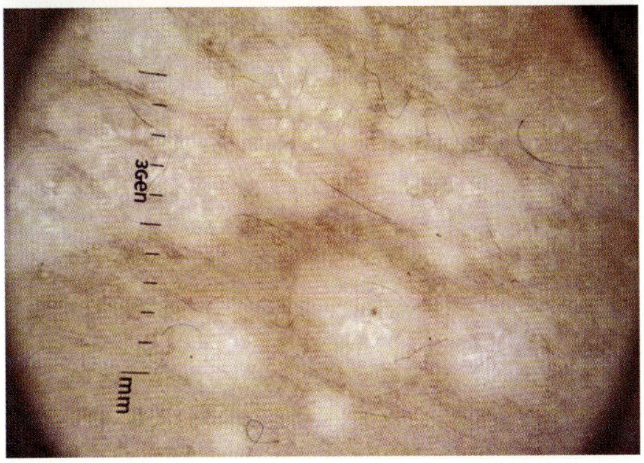

Key Observation Points

- Comedo-like openings
- White structureless areas
- Chrysalis structures
- Linear branching vessels
- Non-branching vessels such as dotted, comma-like and hairpin

Morphea

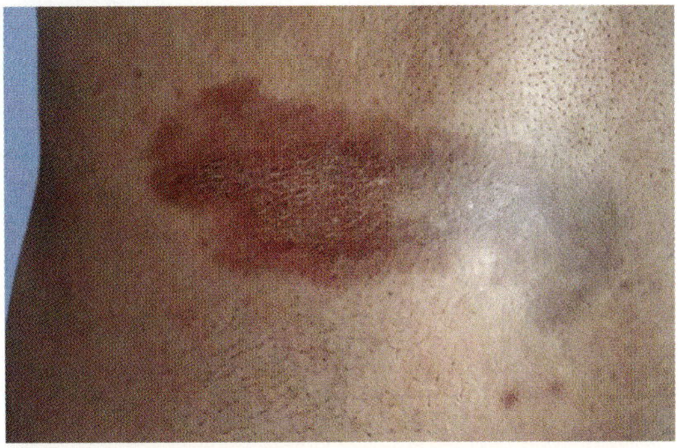

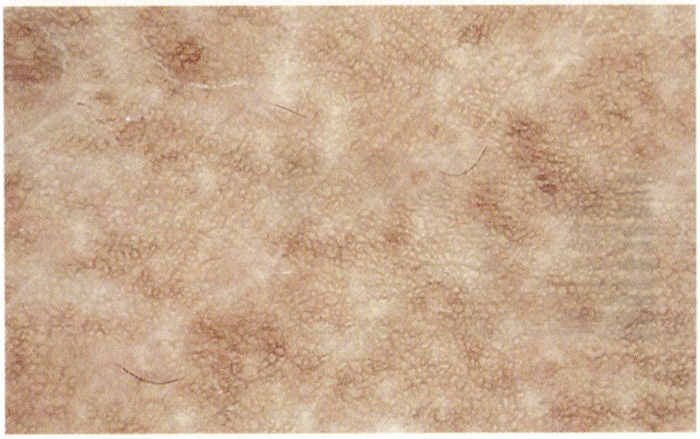

Key Observation Points

Superficial morphea

- White fibrotic beam
- Linear branching vessels
- White shiny structures (personal observation)

Vascular Lesions

Cherry Angioma

Key Observation Points

- Red to purplish lagoons of variable sizes from round to oval
- Milky-white veil was prominent in older lesions.

Pyogenic Granuloma

Key Observation Points

- Homogeneous reddish or reddish-white areas

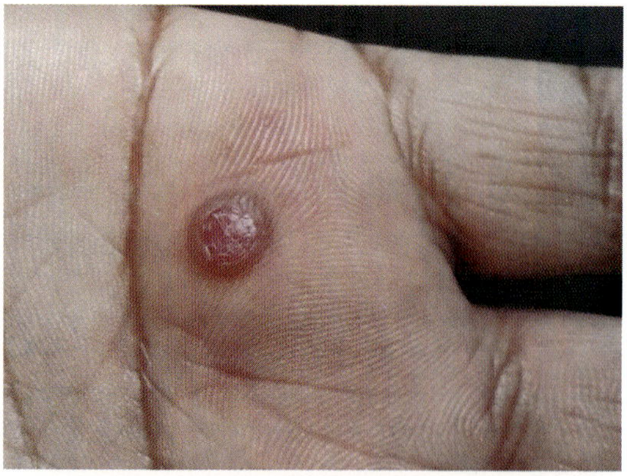

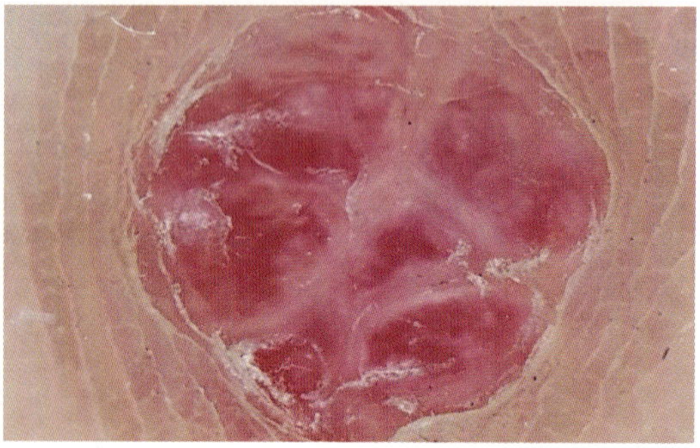

- A whitish collarette which surrounds the reddish-white area
- White rail lines
- Various vascular patterns such as hairpin, dotted, linear irregular, and polymorphous vessels
- Haemorrhagic crusts

Lymphangioma

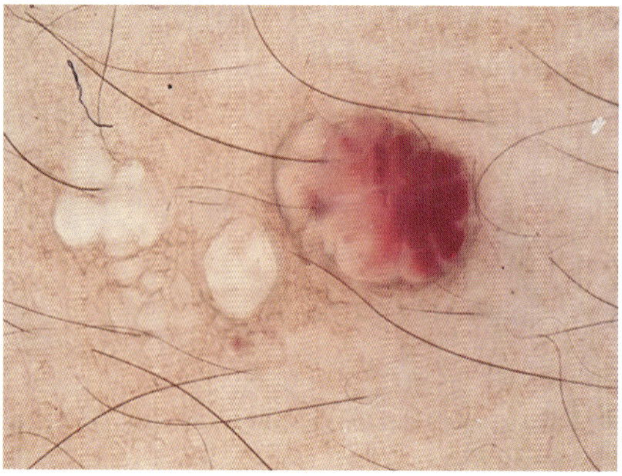

Key Observation Points

- Yellow/brown lacunae surrounded by pale septa; thin linear vessels may or may not be visible
- Reddish to bluish lacunae
- Hypopyon-like lesions

Pigmentary Disorders

Idiopathic guttate hypopigmentation

Key Dermoscopic Patterns

Amoeboid pattern

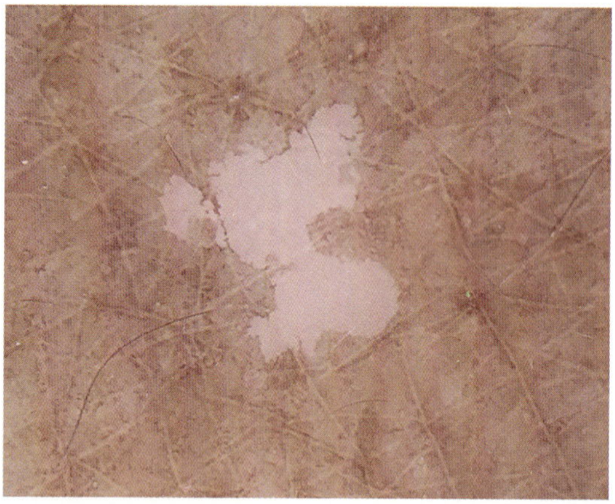

Feathery pattern

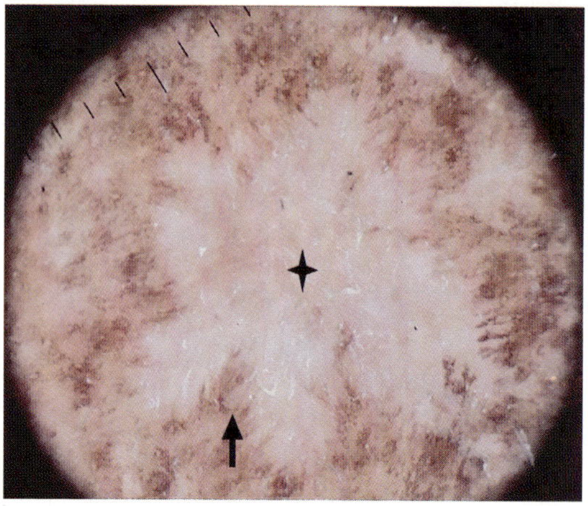

(*Courtesy:* Dr Balachandra Ankad)

Petaloid pattern

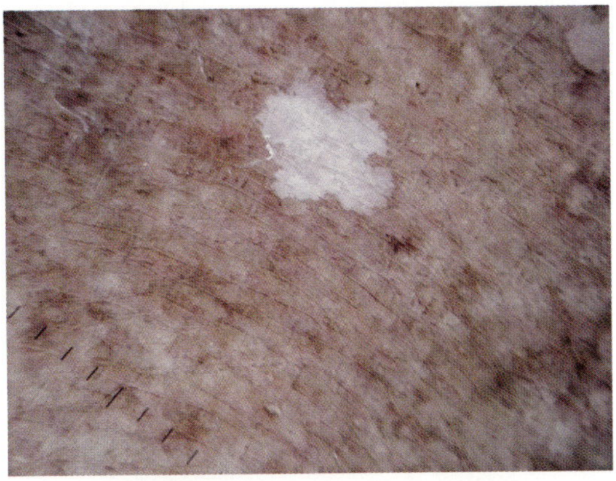

Nebuloid pattern

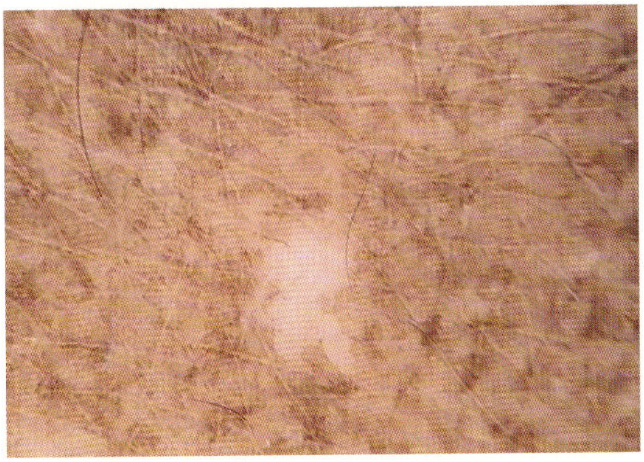

Freckles

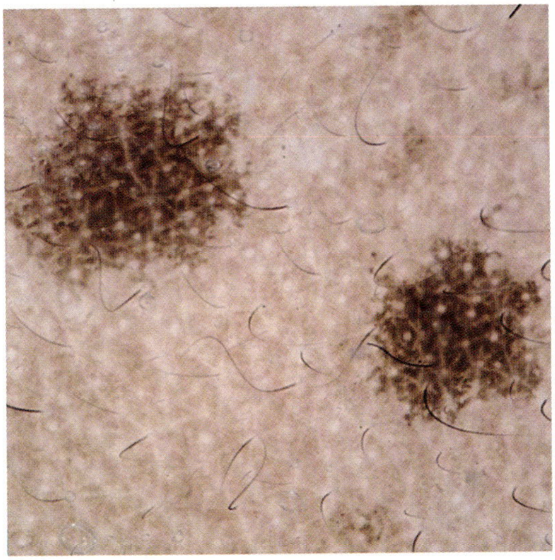

Key Observation Points

- Pigmentation in a light-brown, intertwined, tight, pigment network
- A moth-eaten edge
- Uniform areas of pigmentation may also be seen

TUMOURS

Seborrhoeic Keratoses

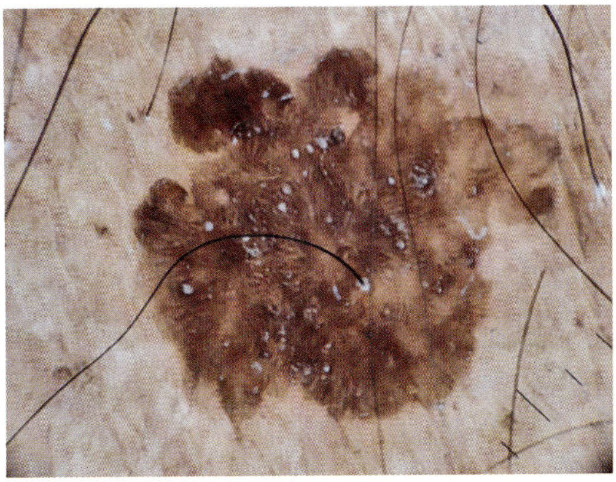

Key Observation Points

1. Milia-like cyst: These are intraepidermal keratin cysts which appear as multiple bright white-yellowish structures. They are visualized better on non-polarised dermoscopy.
2. Comedo-like openings: They are black to brown keratin plugs within dilated follicular openings.
3. Cerebriform pattern: Multiple fissures (linear and curvilinear) and ridges resulting in cerebriform pattern are seen. Fissures are keratin filled deep invaginations of the epidermis.
4. Fingerprint structures and moth-eaten border.
5. Hairpin vessels: They are U-shaped vessels twisted upon themselves, with a whitish halo. Hairpin vessels may also be seen in melanomas, where they are surrounded by a pink halo.

Dermatofibroma

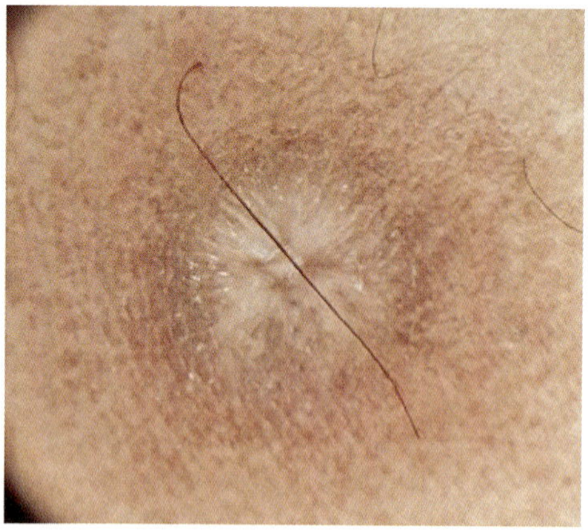

Key Observation Points

1. Delicate pigment network distributed throughout the lesion.
2. Peripheral pigment network surrounding a central white network.
3. Peripheral homogeneous pigmentation surrounding a central scar-like area.
4. Areas of multifocal scar-like patches.
5. White scar-like patch throughout the lesion.
6. Homogeneous pigmentation throughout the lesion.
7. Peripheral pigment network surrounding a central homogeneous patch.
8. White network throughout the lesion.
9. Atypical pattern comprises combination of various features, some may exhibit bluish red homogeneous areas, white linear streaks (chrysalis-like structure), various vascular patterns (dotted vessels, coma vessels, hairpin vessels, glomerular vessels, telangiectasias, linear irregular vessels, polymorphous/atypical vessels) and erythema.

MALIGNANT TUMOURS

Squamous Cell Carcinoma

Key Observation Points

- White circles (targetoid hair follicles)
- Central keratin and blood spots
- White structureless area
- Highly polymorphous vascular structures.

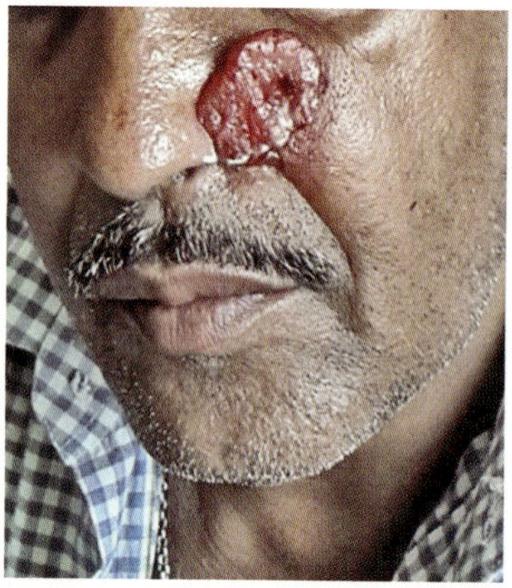

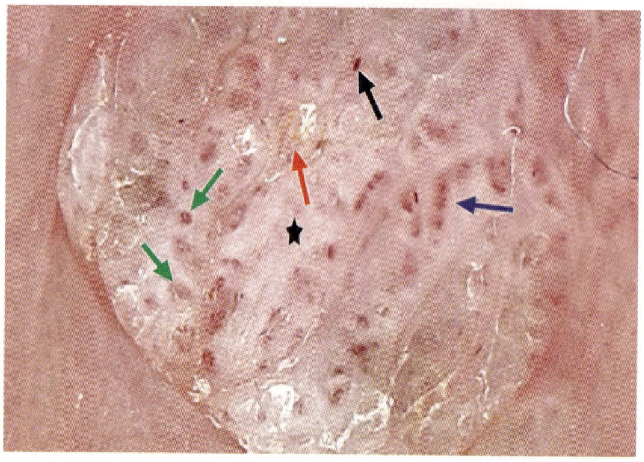

White circles (green arrow), central keratin (red arrow), blood spots (black arrow), white structureless area (star), polymorphous vascular structures (blue arrow).

Basal Cell Carcinoma

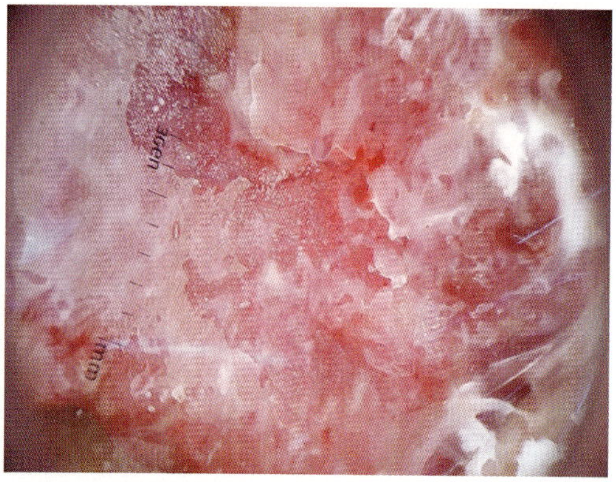

Structureless homogeneous areas with blood spots

Non-pigmented Basal Cell Carcinoma

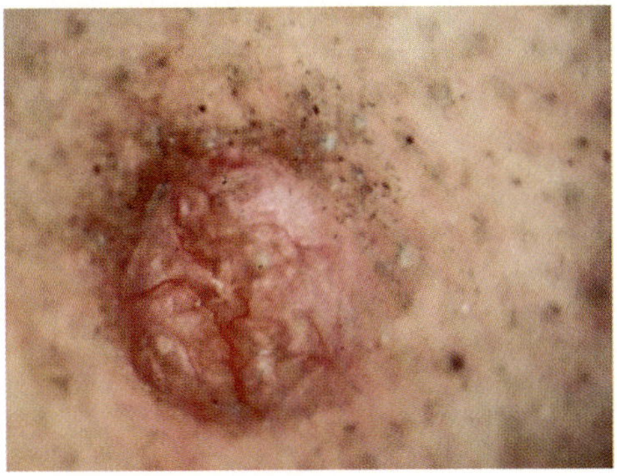

Key Observation Points

- Arborizing vessels
- Superficial fine telangiectasia
- Multiple small erosions
- Shiny white-red structureless areas
- Tiny white streaks

TRICHOSCOPY

Nonscarring Alopecia

1. Alopecia Areata

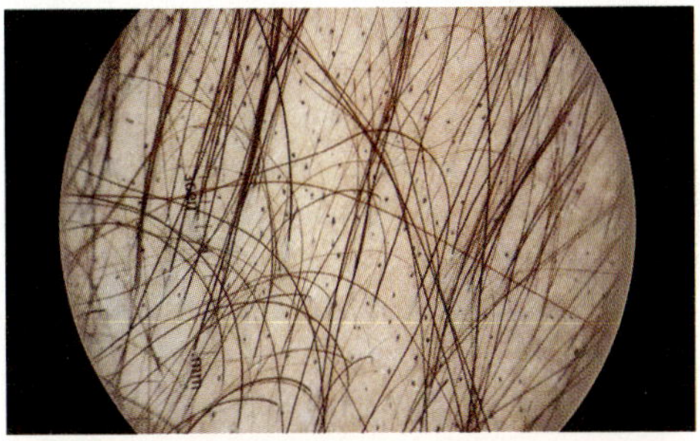

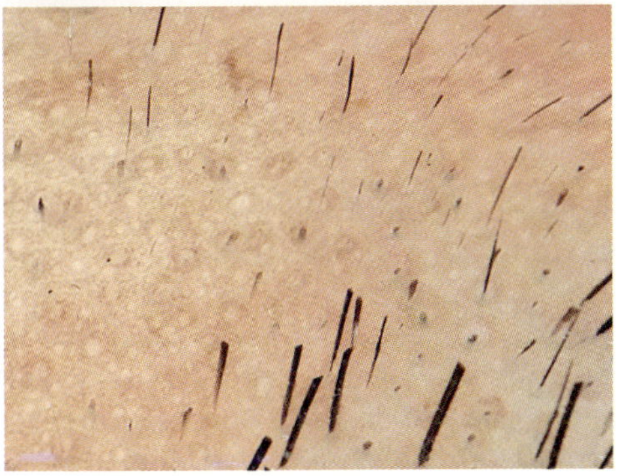

Key Observation Points

- Yellow dots
- Black dots
- Tapered hair
- Broken hair
- Vellus hair
- Pohl-Pinkus constriction

2. Trichotillomania

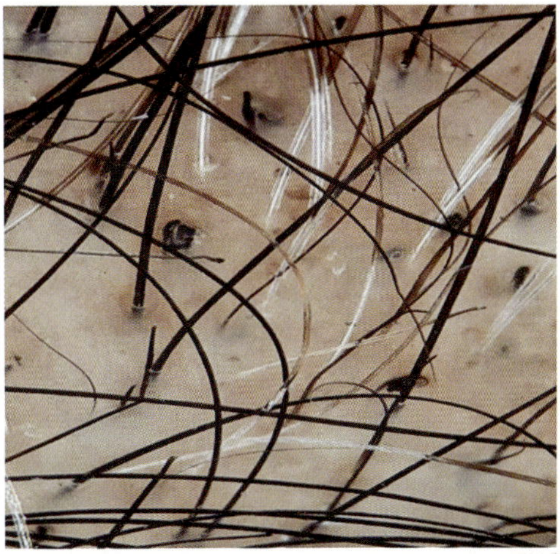

Key Observation Points

- Hair dust
- Black dots
- Broken hair of varying lengths
- Perifollicular haemorrhage
- Flame hair
- Mace sign and burnt matchstick sign resulting from manipulation of the hair

3. Androgenetic Alopecia

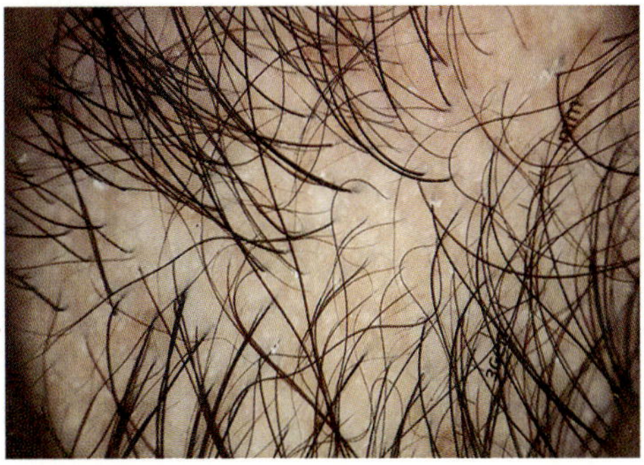

Key Observation Points

- Hair diameter diversity
- Peripilar sign
- Yellow dots
- Vellus hair
- Reduced number of hair per follicular unit
- Increased interfollicular distance

Scarring Alopecia

1. Lichen Planopilaris

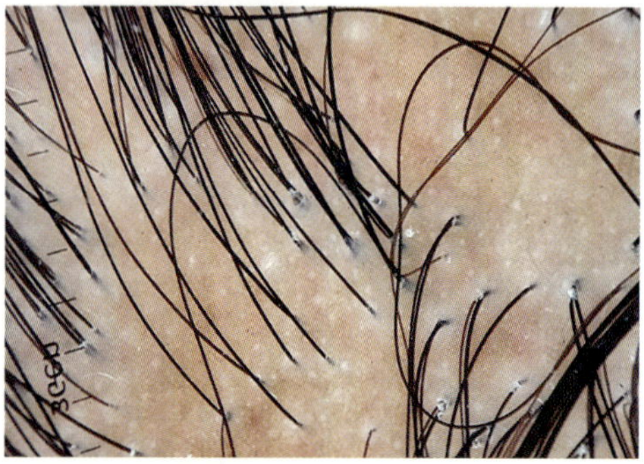

Key Observation Points

- Absence of follicular openings
- Absence of vellus hair
- Fibrotic white patches
- Blue grey dots in a target pattern around hair follicles
- Scalp erythema
- Broken hair
- Presence of a group of 2–3 hairs surrounded by peripilar casts

2. Discoid Lupus Erythematosus

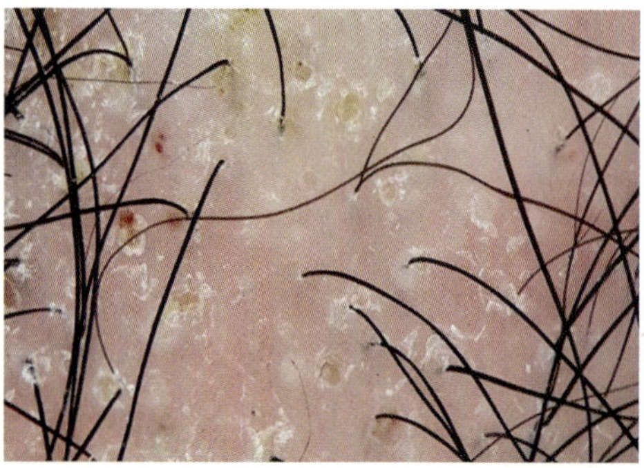

Key Observation Points

- Loss of pigmentation and disruption of honeycomb pattern
- Follicular keratotic plugs
- Red dots
- Giant irregular capillaries
- Peri and inter follicular blue grey dots
- Loss of follicular openings

CONCLUSION

Dermoscopy is rapidly gaining grounds in the routine dermatology practice owing to its non-invasive nature, ready results and conclusive identification of certain disorders without the need for invasive and extensive investigations. In the geriatric age group where patients have multiple comorbidities and may already be on polypharmacy usage of this non-invasive diagnostic technique is beneficial since it takes away the anxiety and stress of an invasive investigation. Awareness of dermoscopic features of common dermatological conditions encountered in the geriatric age group will enable the clinician to effectively screen, diagnose and monitor response to treatment in this age group.

Further Reading

1. Ankad BS, Beergouder SL. Dermoscopic evaluation of idiopathic guttate hypomelanosis: A preliminary observation. Indian Dermatol Online J. 2015; 6(3):164–7.
2. Errichetti E, Stinco G. Dermoscopy in General Dermatology: A Practical Overview. Dermatol Ther (Heidelb). 2016; 6(4):471–507.
3. Lallas A, Apalla Z, Argenziano G, Moscarella E, Longo C, Zalaudek I. Clues for differentiating discoid lupus erythematosus from actinic keratosis. J Am AcadDermatol. 2013; 69:e5-e6.
4. Malakar S. Pattern of hair shafts. In: Malakar S, Chandrashekhar BS, Mukherjee S, Mehta P, Pradhan P (editors). Trichoscopy: A Text and Atlas. New Delhi: Jaypee; 2017.
5. Vázquez-López F, Kreusch J, Marghoob AA. Dermoscopic semiology: further insights into vascular features by screening a large spectrum of nontumoral skin lesions. Br J Dermatol. 2004; 150:226–31.

Index